Massachusetts General Hospital
Psychopharmacology and Neurotherapeutics

SECOND EDITION

Massachusetts General Hospital Psychopharmacology and Neurotherapeutics

SECOND EDITION

Created with content from:
Massachusetts General Hospital Comprehensive Clinical Psychiatry (Third Edition). ISBN: 9780443118449
Massachusetts General Hospital Handbook of General Hospital Psychiatry (Eighth Edition). ISBN: 9780443118951

Editors

THEODORE A. STERN, MD
Psychiatrist and Chief Emeritus
Avery D. Weisman Psychiatry Consultation Service
Director, Thomas P. Hackett Center for Scholarship in Psychosomatic Medicine
Massachusetts General Hospital
Boston, MA, USA
Ned H. Cassem Professor of Psychiatry in the Field
Psychosomatic Medicine/Consultation
Harvard Medical School
Boston, MA, USA

JOAN A. CAMPRODON, MD, MPH, PHD
Chief, Division of Neuropsychiatry
Massachusetts General Hospital
Director, Laboratory for Circuit Neuroscience and Neuromodulation
Massachusetts General Hospital
Director, Transcranial Magnetic Stimulation Clinical Service, Psychiatry
Massachusetts General Hospital
Boston, MA, USA
Associate Professor of Psychiatry
Harvard Medical School
Boston, MA, USA

MAURIZIO FAVA, MD
Psychiatrist-in-Chief
Department of Psychiatry
Vice Chair, Executive Committee on Research
Massachusetts General Hospital
Boston, MA, USA
Executive Director, Clinical Trials Network & Institute (CTNI)
Massachusetts General Hospital
Boston, MA, USA
Associate Dean for Clinical & Translational Research & Slater Family Professor of Psychiatry
Harvard Medical School
Boston, MA, USA

ELSEVIER

Elsevier
1600 John F. Kennedy Blvd.
Ste 1800
Philadelphia, PA 19103-2899

MASSACHUSETTS GENERAL HOSPITAL PSYCHOPHARMACOLOGY AND NEUROTHERAPEUTICS, SECOND EDITION

ISBN: 978-0-443-11972-9

Previous edition copyrighted 2016.

Content Strategist: Mary Hegeler
Senior Content Development Specialist: Lisa Barnes
Publishing Services Manager: Deepthi Unni
Project Manager: Nandhini Thanga Alagu
Design Direction: Christian Bilbow

Printed in India

Last digit is the print number: 9 8 7 6 5 4 3 2 1

Working together
to grow libraries in
developing countries

www.elsevier.com • www.bookaid.org

Preface

The field of Psychiatry continues to evolve, and practitioners of all disciplines now need to know more about psychopharmacologic and somatic treatments of psychiatric and neurologic conditions. This second edition of *MGH Psychopharmacology and Neurotherapeutics* was created by a stalwart group of psychiatrists, neurologists, and psychologists, largely from the Massachusetts General Hospital (MGH). It was designed to solidify and expand the knowledge base of busy practitioners to enhance clinical care; to them we owe our deepest gratitude.

This book would not have been possible if not for the helping hands of our partners at Elsevier – Mary Hegeler and Lisa Barnes – to whom we owe our unending thanks.

On behalf of patients who suffer, we hope this updated edition facilitates the conceptualization, diagnosis, understanding, and treatment of psychiatric problems while providing solace, solutions, and much needed relief.

Contributors

Gregory Alexander Acampora, MD
Psychiatrist
Massachusetts General Hospital
Boston, MA, USA
Assistant Professor of Psychiatry
Harvard Medical School
Boston, MA, USA
Consultant Psychiatrist
Department of Anesthesiology Critical
    Care and Pain Medicine
Massachusetts General Hospital
Boston, MA, USA

Zeba N. Ahmad, PhD
Psychologist, Department of Psychiatry
Massachusetts General Hospital
Boston, MA, USA
Instructor in Psychology in the
    Department of Psychiatry
Harvard Medical School
Boston, MA, USA

Menekse Alpay, MD
Psychiatrist
Massachusetts General Hospital
Boston, MA, USA
Instructor in Psychiatry
Harvard Medical School
Boston, MA, USA

Jonathan E. Alpert, MD, PhD
Chair, Department of Psychiatry and
    Behavioral Sciences
Montefiore Medical Center and Albert
    Einstein College of Medicine
Bronx, NY, USA
Professor of Psychiatry, Neuroscience
    and Pediatrics
Albert Einstein College of Medicine
Bronx, NY, USA

Ji Hyun Baek, MD, PhD
Associate Professor of Psychiatry
Sungkyunkwan University School of
    Medicine Samsung Medical Center
Seoul, Republic of Korea
Visiting Scholar, Department of
    Psychiatry
Massachusetts General Hospital
Boston, MA, USA

Ashika Bains, MD, MSc
Psychiatrist
Massachusetts General Hospital
Boston, MA, USA
Instructor in Psychiatry
Harvard Medical School
Boston, MA, USA

Scott R. Beach, MD
Psychiatrist
Massachusetts General Hospital
Boston, MA, USA
Associate Professor of Psychiatry
Harvard Medical School
Boston, MA, USA

Joseph Biederman, MD (Deceased)
Chief, Clinical and Research Programs
    in Pediatric Psychopharmacology and
    Adult ADHD
Massachusetts General Hospital
Boston, MA, USA
Professor of Psychiatry
Harvard Medical School
Boston, MA, USA

Rebecca W. Brendel, MD, JD
Director, Center for Bioethics
Harvard Medical School
Boston, MA, USA
Associate Professor of Psychiatry, Global
    Health, and Social Medicine
Harvard Medical School
Boston, MA, USA

Eric Bui, MD, PhD
Professor of Psychiatry
University of Caen Normandy
Caen, France

Joan A. Camprodon, MD, MPH, PhD
Chief, Division of Neuropsychiatry
Massachusetts General Hospital
Director, Laboratory for Circuit
    Neuroscience and Neuromodulation
Massachusetts General Hospital
Director, Transcranial Magnetic
    Stimulation Clinical Service,
    Psychiatry
Massachusetts General Hospital
Boston, MA, USA
Associate Professor of Psychiatry
Harvard Medical School
Boston, MA, USA

Paolo Cassano, MD, PhD
Director of Photobiomodulation at
    the Division of Neuropsychiatry and
    Neuromodulation, Psychiatry
Massachusetts General Hospital
Boston, MA, USA
Associate Professor of Psychiatry
Harvard Medical School
Boston, MA, USA

Zeina Chemali, MD, MPH
Director, Neuropsychiatry Clinics and
    Education
Massachusetts General Hospital
Boston, MA, USA
Director, McCance Center for Brain
    Health
Departments of Neurology and
    Psychiatry
Massachusetts General Hospital
Boston, MA, USA
Associate Professor of Neurology and
    Psychiatry
Harvard Medical School
Boston, MA, USA

Sun Young Chung, BS
Harvard Medical School
Boston, MA, USA

Lee S. Cohen, MD
Director, Ammon-Pinizzotto Center for
    Women's Mental Health
Massachusetts General Hospital
Boston, MA, USA
Edmund and Carroll Carpenter
    Professor of Psychiatry
Harvard Medical School
Boston, MA, USA

Cristina Cusin, MD
Psychiatrist
Massachusetts General Hospital
Boston, MA, USA
Associate Professor of Psychiatry
Harvard Medical School
Boston, MA, USA

Darin D. Dougherty, MD
Director, Division of Neurotherapeutics,
Massachusetts General Hospital
Boston, MA, USA
Associate Professor of Psychiatry
Harvard Medical School
Boston, MA, USA

Judith Edersheim, JD, MD
Psychiatrist and Founding
    Co-Director
The Center for Law, Brain, and
    Behavior
Massachusetts General Hospital
Boston, MA, USA
Assistant Professor of Psychiatry
Harvard Medical School
Boston, MA, USA

Maurizio Fava, MD
Psychiatrist-in-Chief
Department of Psychiatry
Vice Chair, Executive Committee on
 Research
Massachusetts General Hospital
Boston, MA, USA
Executive Director, Clinical Trials
 Network & Institute (CTNI)
Massachusetts General Hospital
Boston, MA, USA
Associate Dean for Clinical &
 Translational Research & Slater Family
 Professor of Psychiatry
Harvard Medical School
Boston, MA, USA

Carlos G. Fernandez Robles, MD, MBA
Chief of Psychiatry
Brigham and Women's Faulkner
 Hospital
Jamaica Plain, MA, USA
Vice Chair of Faulkner Psychiatry,
 Department of Psychiatry
Brigham and Women's Hospital
Boston, MA, USA
Assistant Professor of Psychiatry
Harvard Medical School
Boston, MA, USA

Alice W. Flaherty, MD, PhD
Neurologist
Massachusetts General Hospital
Boston, MA, USA
Associate Professor of Neurology and
 Psychiatry
Harvard Medical School
Boston, MA, USA

Oliver Freudenreich, MD
Co-Director, MGH Psychosis Clinical
 and Research Program
Department of Psychiatry
Massachusetts General Hospital
Boston, MA, USA
Professor of Clinical Psychiatry
Harvard Medical School
Boston, MA, USA

Jennifer R. Gatchel, MD, PhD
Psychiatrist
Massachusetts General Hospital
Boston, MA, USA
Assistant Professor of Psychiatry
Harvard Medical School
Boston, MA, USA
Staff Psychiatrist, Mental Health Care
 Line, Psychiatry
Baylor College of Medicine/MEDVAMC
Houston, TX, USA

Sharmin Ghaznavi, MD, PhD
Psychiatrist
Massachusetts General Hospital
Boston, MA, USA
Instructor in Psychiatry
Harvard Medical School
Boston, MA, USA

Michael E. Henry, MD
Director, Somatic Therapies Service
Department of Psychiatry
Massachusetts General Hospital
Boston, MA, USA
Associate Professor of Psychiatry
Harvard Medical School
Boston, MA, USA

John B. Herman, MD
Associate Chief of Psychiatry
Massachusetts General Hospital
Boston, MA, USA
Medical Director, Employee Assistance
 Program
Partners HealthCare
Boston, MA, USA
Associate Professor of Psychiatry
Harvard Medical School
 Boston, MA, USA

Jeff C. Huffman, MD
Director, Clinical Services
Department of Psychiatry
Massachusetts General Hospital
Boston, MA, USA
Professor of Psychiatry
Harvard Medical School
Boston, MA, USA

Ana Ivkovic, MD
Psychiatrist
Massachusetts General Hospital
Boston, MA, USA
Assistant Professor of Psychiatry
Harvard Medical School
Boston, MA, USA

Masoud Kamali, MD
Psychiatrist
Massachusetts General Hospital
Boston, MA, USA
Assistant Professor of Psychiatry
Harvard Medical School
Boston, MA, USA

Rebecca Leval, MD, MPH
Psychiatrist, The Center for Women's
 Mental Health
Massachusetts General Hospital
Boston, MA, USA
Psychiatrist, Acute Psychiatry Services
Massachusetts General Hospital
Boston, MA, USA
Instructor in Psychiatry
Harvard Medical School
Boston, MA, USA

Carol Lim, MD, MPH
Medical Director, MGH Clozapine
 Clinic
Massachusetts General Hospital
Boston, MA, USA
Instructor in Psychiatry
Harvard Medical School
Boston, MA, USA

James Luccarelli, MD, DPhil
Psychiatrist
Massachusetts General Hospital
Boston, MA, USA
Instructor in Psychiatry
Harvard Medical School
Boston, MA, USA

David Mischoulon, MD, PhD
Psychiatrist and Director
Depression Clinical and Research
 Program
Department of Psychiatry
Massachusetts General Hospital
Boston, MA, USA
Joyce R. Tedlow Professor of Psychiatry
Harvard Medical School
Boston, MA, USA

Shamim H. Nejad, MD, FASAM
Medical Director, Addiction Medicine &
 Psychiatry
Consultation Services UW Medicine
 Valley Medical Center
Renton, WA, USA

Andrew Nierenberg, MD
Co-Director, Center for Clinical Research
 Education
Massachusetts General Hospital
Boston, MA, USA
Director, Dauten Family Center for
 Bipolar Treatment Innovation
Harvard Medical School
Boston, MA, USA
Thomas P. Hackett, MD, Professor of
 Psychiatry
Harvard Medical School
Boston, MA, USA

Mladen Nisavic, MD
Director, Burns and Trauma Psychiatry
Massachusetts General Hospital
Boston, MA, USA
Instructor in Psychiatry
Harvard Medical School
Boston, MA, USA

Ruta Nonacs, MD, PhD
Psychiatrist
Massachusetts General Hospital
Boston, MA, USA
Instructor in Psychiatry
Harvard Medical School
Boston, MA, USA

Henry K. Onyeaka, MD, MPH
Psychiatrist
Massachusetts General Hospital
Boston, MA, USA
Research Fellow in Psychiatry
Harvard Medical School
Boston, MA, USA

Michael J. Ostacher, MD, MPH, MMSc
Director, Bipolar and Depression
   Research Program
VA Palo Alto Health Care System
Palo Alto, CA, USA
Professor of Psychiatry and Behavioral
   Sciences
Stanford University School of Medicine
Stanford, CA, USA

George I. Papakostas, MD
Psychiatrist and Scientific Director
Clinical Trials Network
Institute Director of Treatment-Resistant
   Depression Studies
Professor of Psychiatry
Harvard Medical School
Boston, MA, USA

Shreedhar Paudel, MD, MPH
Psychiatrist
Massachusetts General Hospital
Boston, MA, USA
Assistant Professor of Psychiatry
Harvard Medical School
Boston, MA, USA

Celeste Peay, MD, JD
Assistant Professor of Psychiatry,
   Psychiatry
University of Southern California Keck
   School of Medicine
Los Angeles, CA, USA

Roy H. Perlis, MD, MSc
Associate Chief (Research), Department
   of Psychiatry
Massachusetts General Hospital
Boston, MA, USA
Director, Center for Quantitative Health
Massachusetts General Hospital
Boston, MA, USA
Professor of Psychiatry
Harvard Medical School
Boston, MA, USA
Affiliate Faculty, Center or Genomic
   Medicine/Harvard Stem Cell Institute/
   Broad Institute of MIT
Boston, MA, USA

Jefferson B. Prince, MD
Director, Child Psychiatry
Vice-Chair, Department of Psychiatry
MGB Salem Hospital
Salem, MA, USA
Psychiatrist, Child Psychiatry
Massachusetts General Hospital
Boston, MA, USA

Joshua L. Roffman, MD, MMSc
Co-Director, Mass General
   Neuroscience
Director, Mass General Early Brain
   development Institute
Massachusetts General Hospital
Boston, MA, USA
Associate Professor of Psychiatry
Harvard Medical School
Boston, MA, USA

**Ronald Schouten, MD, JD, CTM,
DLFAPA**
Director, Forensic Psychiatry Fellowship
   Program
Saint Elizabeth's Hospital
Washington, District of Columbia, USA
Associate Professor of Psychiatry
Harvard Medical School
Boston, MA, USA
Affiliate Professor, Psychiatry &
   Behavioral Sciences
Howard University College of Medicine
Washington, District of Columbia, USA

Linda Carol Shafer, MD
Psychiatrist
Massachusetts General Hospital
Boston, MA, USA
Assistant Professor of Psychiatry
Harvard Medical School
Boston, MA, USA

Felicia A. Smith, MD
Associate Chief of Psychiatry
Massachusetts General Hospital
Chief, Division of Psychiatry and
   Medicine
Massachusetts General Hospital
Boston, MA, USA
Assistant Professor of Psychiatry
Harvard Medical School
Boston, MA, USA

Theodore A. Stern, MD
Psychiatrist and Chief Emeritus
Avery D. Weisman Psychiatry
   Consultation Service
Director, Thomas P. Hackett Center
   for Scholarship in Psychosomatic
   Medicine
Massachusetts General Hospital
Boston, MA, USA
Ned H. Cassem Professor of Psychiatry
   in the Field
Psychosomatic Medicine/Consultation
Harvard Medical School
Boston, MA, USA

Mira Stone, BA
Clinical Research Coordinator
Department of Psychiatry
Massachusetts General Hospital
Boston, MA, USA

Craig B.H. Surman, MD
Psychiatrist and Scientific Coordinator
   for the Adult ADHD Research
   Program
Clinical and Research Programs in
   Pediatric Psychopharmacology and
   Adult ADHD
Massachusetts General Hospital
Boston, MA, USA
Associate Professor of Psychiatry
Harvard Medical School
Boston, MA, USA

Lara Traeger, PhD
Psychologist, Department of Psychiatry
Massachusetts General Hospital
Boston, MA, USA
Associate Professor of Psychology
University of Miami
Coral Gables, FL, USA

Nhi-Ha Trinh, MD, MPH
Psychiatrist
Massachusetts General Hospital
Boston, MA, USA
Associate Professor of Psychiatry
Harvard Medical School
Boston, MA, USA
Associate Director, Hinton Society
Harvard Medical School
Boston, MA, USA

Mai Uchida, MD
Director, MGH Child Depression
   Program
Massachusetts General Hospital
Boston, MA, USA
Associate Professor of Psychiatry
Harvard Medical School
Boston, MA, USA

Adele C. Viguera, MD, MPH
Psychiatrist, Department of Psychiatry
Cleveland Clinic
Cleveland, OH, USA
Senior Investigator, Department of
   Psychiatry
Massachusetts General Hospital
Boston, MA, USA

Betty Wang, MD
Psychiatrist
Massachusetts General Hospital
Boston, MA, USA
Instructor in Psychiatry
Harvard Medical School
Boston, MA, USA

Marc S. Weinberg, MD, PhD
Psychiatrist
Massachusetts General Hospital
Boston, MA, USA
Instructor in Psychiatry
Harvard Medical School
Boston, MA, USA

Timothy E. Wilens, MD
Psychiatrist and Chief, Division of Child
   and Adolescent Psychiatry
Co-Director, Center for Addiction
   Medicine
Massachusetts General Hospital
Boston, MA, USA
Professor of Psychiatry
Harvard Medical School
Boston, MA, USA

Contents

1 Psychiatric Neuroscience: Incorporating Pathophysiology into Clinical Case Formulation

Joan A. Camprodon and Joshua L. Roffman

KEY POINTS

- One can approach the study of the brain and its pathophysiology from various perspectives with different levels of resolution: molecular, genetic, cellular, synaptic, systems, and behavioral.
- Pathological processes and therapeutic interventions can target one or more of these levels, leading to a cascade of events that changes each of them.
- Affect, behavior, and cognition are processed in specific brain circuits, and their altered function leads to the signs, symptoms, and syndromes that clinicians can identify.
- Clinical presentation reflects an interaction of static and dynamic factors, including biological and environmental, often mediated by adaptive or maladaptive plasticity.
- Neurobiological knowledge provides mechanistic insights, explanations for abnormal behaviors, and a rationale for treatment selection (by clinicians) and discovery (by scientists), which are important to patients and providers.

OVERVIEW

People with major mental illnesses suffer as a result of abnormal and maladaptive brain function. This is the fundamental premise of psychiatric neuroscience, which seeks to identify biological mechanisms that underlie mental illness, often with the translational goal of developing novel diagnostic, prognostic, and therapeutic tools to support clinical practice. Critically, this approach does not negate the critical role of psychological, social, and environmental factors; to the contrary, it provides an integrated non-reductionistic framework for understanding how these higher levels of resolution affect and are affected by (in a bi-directional causal relationship) neural function.

Psychiatric neuroscience is one of the most interesting and challenging endeavors in all of medicine. Although much is already known, a wide gap remains between the clinical phenomena that disturb affect, behavior, and cognition and neuroscientific explanations. However, recent advances, particularly in neuroimaging and genetics, have provided important tools for tackling these problems. Indeed, we are starting to enjoy the benefits of decades of work with the development, approval, and implementation in clinical practice of biomarker-driven novel treatments, such as neuro-steroids for rapid response in post-partum depression[1] or functional magnetic resonance imaging (MRI)–guided individualized non-invasive brain stimulation for treatment-resistant depression.[2] As the neuroscience pipeline continues to introduce innovations in mental health practice, clinicians will need to incorporate this knowledge into everyday clinical decision-making and be ready to communicate neuroscience-informed clinical decisions to patients, families, and members of the general public.

One might ask if the term "psychiatric neuroscience" is still valid. Although it has traditionally related to neuroscience research with clinical relevance to disorders embedded within the limits of psychiatry, as opposed to neurology or other medical specialties interested in the brain, these boundaries are becoming more porous as knowledge progresses and clinical practice adapts. The unclear limits between psychiatry and neurology have been defined historically by amorphous criteria, such as differences in clinical attitude (diagnostic vs therapeutic) or brain function of interest (motor and sensory vs affective and behavioral, with cognition always occupying an unclear intermediate frontier). Whereas neurology once focused mainly on pathologies that resulted in major structural changes that one could observe in an autopsy or under a microscope, psychiatry focused on detailed phenomenological descriptions (including inferences about psychological dynamics) and neurochemical processes. As new generations of clinician-scientists emerge who trained in systems neuroscience rather than in psychiatric or neurological neuroscience, translational efforts are highlighting the common principles of brain structure and function to study pathophysiology, identify biomarkers, and develop treatments. From this effort, new models are emerging with a clinical focus on brain circuits, as opposed to focal lesions or clinical syndromes. For clinicians who treat patients with disorders of affect, behavior, and cognition (whether in psychiatry, neurology, or other clinical neuroscience specialties), it will be particularly important to understand the circuit level because this is where mental states, including the pathological affective, behavioral, and cognitive states that we treat, are processed.

This chapter aims to explain the different neurobiological approaches relevant to study brain biology and pathophysiology, from molecular to genetic to cellular to circuit to organ dynamics to psychological processes. Other higher levels are also relevant to the study of the healthy and diseased brain, although outside the scope of this chapter, including syndromal combinations of signs and symptoms, population dynamics, and even cultural and sociological phenomena. All levels of resolution are important, and all interact with each other casually, but it is critical to understand what approach is framing our thought process at any given time. With this background, we will offer a framework to incorporate the biological components of clinical cases into enriched diagnostic formulations and more nuanced treatment plans.

PSYCHIATRIC DIAGNOSIS: BIOMARKERS AND BIOLOGICAL VALIDITY

In the context of psychiatric neuroscience, the recent diagnostic system (*Diagnostic and Statistical Manual of Mental Disorders, Fifth Edition, Text Revision* [DSM-5-TR])[3] has both strengths and weaknesses. A major advance of the post-1980s DSM was the development of diagnostic categories of psychiatric illness with good inter-rater reliability, largely based on phenomenological observation and epidemiological data collection. This provided a firm starting point for scientific investigation, in contrast to previous diagnostic systems based on etiological theories with limited evidence and associated ill-defined terminology. However, the intentional avoidance of etiological models in generating DSM diagnoses also made their biological validity uncertain. Unlike most medical *illnesses*, most psychiatric *disorders* have so far not been tightly linked to specific biological markers: the descriptive criteria demarcating current diagnoses are likely several steps removed from homogeneous pathological processes. In part, this is because "psychiatric disorders" are not diseases but clinical syndromes (i.e., constellations of signs and symptoms that present together with some frequency). Like all clinical syndromes, these are heterogeneous and associated with different pathophysiological processes (i.e., different diseases) that can converge under a similar phenomenological clinical presentation. For example, in the same way that many diseases may lead to the clinical syndrome of left-sided heart failure (e.g., myocardial disease, valvular pathology, electrical rhythm abnormalities), many diseases and pathophysiological mechanisms may lead to the clinical syndrome of major depressive disorder or schizophrenia. Importantly, although there may be common symptomatic treatments for left-sided heart failure regardless of the specific underlying etiology, myocardial disease, valvular pathology, and electrical rhythm abnormalities require disease-specific interventions. One of the major goals of psychiatric neuroscience is to identify pathophysiological mechanisms to define specific diseases that are linked to the clinical syndromes described in the DSM, with a primary goal of supporting the rational biomarker-informed development of disease-specific treatments. In line with this strategy, the National Institute of Mental Health (NIMH) developed the Research Domain Criteria (RDoC)[4] nosological system of empirically defined dimensional domains of emotion, cognition, and behavior relevant to psychopathology, each associated with an evolving evidence-based explanatory matrix encompassing different levels of mechanistic resolution and methodological approaches, from genes to molecules, cells, circuits, physiology, behavior, and clinical constructs. The goal of this dimensional approach, which can co-exist with the more established DSM system, is to move beyond syndromes, their inherent heterogeneity and limited biological validity to facilitate multilayer biological, behavioral, and clinical explanatory models better suited to the rational bottom-up development of clinical innovations.

METHODS IN PSYCHIATRIC NEUROSCIENCE

Researchers have adopted a variety of methods for studying the neural mechanisms of mental illness and behavior (Box 1.1). Each of these methods has strengths and weaknesses.

Lesion Studies

There is a strong tradition within classical neuropsychology and behavioral neurology of understanding neuroanatomical circuitry by studying the emergent or lost behaviors in patients with focal brain lesions.[5] These studies have provided us with

---

BOX 1.1 Methods in Psychiatric Neuroscience

Animal models
Brain lesion cases
Brain stimulation and neuromodulation
Genetics and molecular biology
Neuroimaging
Neuropathology
Neurophysiology
Neuropsychology and endophenotypes
Psychopharmacology

---

a rich view of various brain regions and their relationship to behavior. Perhaps the most famous case is that of Phineas Gage, the Vermont railway worker who sustained a traumatic lesion bilaterally to the medial frontal lobes and developed personality changes.[6] Another famous patient (known by his initials) is H.M., who underwent bilateral medial temporal lobe resection for intractable epilepsy and as a result lost the ability to form new declarative memories.[7] Although striking and informative, findings from these rare cases may be difficult to extrapolate to the pathophysiology of common psychiatric illnesses, which generally do not involve focal lesions. Traditionally, biological psychiatry has relied more on biometrics and quantitative methods; these population-based approaches risk losing insights available from rare cases but are more likely to produce broadly generalizable findings. A novel take on lesion studies has recently emerged integrating larger samples of lesions associated with clinical phenotypes and combining neuroimaging data with data science approaches to define the circuits, not the regions, affected by lesions causing clinical phenomena.[8]

Neuropsychology and Dimensional Behavioral Endophenotypes

An increasingly important approach in psychiatric neuroscience is to identify and study intermediate behavioral phenotypes. These are quantitative phenotypes that are closely associated with the clinical syndrome of interest but that are more specific and easier to link to the anatomy and physiology of specific neural circuits. They can also be used to identify biologically relevant subtypes within a syndromal diagnostic category (i.e., biotypes), reducing heterogeneity that may limit the power of scientific investigations. Endophenotypes are intermediate phenotypes that can be present both in affected individuals and in their unaffected relatives, reflecting dimensional (not categorical) behavioral variation and genetic risk independent of actual disease. Neuropsychological and behavioral assessments are commonly used to identify endophenotypes. For example, impairment of working memory, which is closely related to the function of the dorsolateral prefrontal cortex (DLPFC), is found within a subgroup of patients with schizophrenia.[9] Endophenotypes thus help bridge the gap between brain circuits, which are amenable to study at the molecular and cellular level, and clinical syndromes, which are less tractable biologically. This approach, core to the NIMH RDoC framework,[4] becomes especially powerful when combined with other methods, such as neuroimaging or genetics.

Neuroimaging

Neuroimaging has provided one of the best modern tools for examining the pathophysiology of mental illness in the living brain. Because this topic is covered in greater depth in another chapter, we will only briefly summarize it here. Neuroimaging can provide many different quantitative measures, including morphometry, functional activity, blood flow, metabolism, neurotransmitter receptor dynamics, chemical composition, and distribution of toxic deposits. Neuroimaging research using groups of subjects can determine whether mental illness is associated with changes in the size or shape of specific brain regions; the functional activity within these regions; or their concentrations of particular neurotransmitters, receptors, or key metabolites.[10] Although neuroimaging methods can be used to measure cellular and molecular phenomena, the currently achievable spatial resolution still represents an important limitation in examining the microscopic pathological changes implicated in psychiatric illness. That said, recent innovations in high-field MRI and the development of novel positron emission tomography ligands are overcoming such limitations and assessing processes such as the physiology of neuronal cortical columns and inflammatory glial activation, respectively.

Neurophysiology

There is a strong tradition within psychiatric neuroscience of studying the electrical activity of the brain and its relation to function. These methods include use of the electroencephalogram (including event-related potentials, neuronal oscillations, functional connectivity, and source localization), magnetoencephalography, and transcranial magnetic stimulation (TMS). These modalities provide information about the living brain with excellent temporal and good spatial resolution, and they are invaluable in studying the coordinated function of widely distributed neural circuits. Abnormalities in the timing of oscillations in neural circuit activity have been associated with psychiatric illnesses, and this is an area of intense research activity. For example, the reduction of gamma frequency (30–80 Hz) oscillations in schizophrenia has been ascribed to impaired N-methyl-D-aspartate (NMDA) receptor activity on gamma aminobutyric acid (GABA)-ergic interneurons.[11] At present, non-invasive electrophysiological techniques cannot provide cellular or synaptic resolution, and they are limited to the study of populations of neurons. That said, invasive neurophysiological methods with either intraoperative temporary assessments or surgically implanted devices are pushing the traditional limits of resolution in human neurophysiology studies, improving pathophysiological models and supporting the development of closed-loop surgical neuromodulation devices, such as deep brain stimulation (DBS).[12]

Brain Stimulation and Neuromodulation

Brain stimulation and neuromodulation techniques encompass a variety of device-based methodologies that can generate focal electrical currents in pre-selected brain regions. These currents can increase or decrease the excitability of the target neurons and modulate the networks they belong to by acting as neural pacemakers.[13]

Brain stimulation can be divided among invasive, convulsive, and non-invasive approaches. Invasive techniques require the surgical implantation of stimulating electrodes in the brain and are therefore exclusively used in therapeutic settings where the risk-to-benefit analysis is favorable. They include DBS and vagus nerve stimulation. Convulsive techniques do not require surgical intervention but do involve the use of general anesthesia and pharmacological paralysis to avoid iatrogenic consequences from an artificially induced therapeutic seizure. Electroconvulsive therapy (ECT) is the best know example in this category. Non-invasive methods do not require surgery or anesthesia; are very safe; and alter brain function, via inducing long-term plasticity and symptomatic

change. The better-known and most commonly used methods are TMS and transcranial direct current stimulation (tDCS). Chapter 18 describes these methods and their therapeutic applications in detail. That said, neuromodulation techniques, primarily non-invasive examples, can be used as neurophysiological and brain mapping tools to study brain biology and pathophysiology and develop biomarkers of clinical diagnostic utility.[14] TMS has been used since the mid-1980s, initially as a tool to study human motor neurophysiology in vivo and later expanded to non-motor questions in cognitive neuroscience and systems neurophysiology. Event-related paradigms using single pulses that are time-locked to a given stimulus or task have been used to determine the chronometry of the computations in a given brain region with great temporal resolution (in the order of milliseconds). Repetitive TMS can increase or decrease the excitability of a given area beyond the time of stimulation, creating a "virtual lesion" that lasts 15 to 60 minutes after the stimulation. This virtual lesion approach has been used, following the tradition of classical lesion studies, to understand the functional role of discrete brain regions. Although neuroimaging and electrophysiological techniques are defined by their spatial and temporal resolution, what sets brain stimulation methods apart is their *causal resolution*.[15] Neuroimaging and electrophysiological methods are observational; they measure patterns of brain activity (the dependent variable) in the context of a given task or disease state (independent variable). Such a design can establish correlations among these measures, but it can never determine that a given pattern of brain activity is *causing* a mental state (or vice versa). On the other hand, brain stimulation techniques are interventional: they modify the system by changing brain activity (now the independent variable) and measure the behavioral, cognitive, or affective changes that follow. This design offers causal explanatory power, which makes it a useful tool to answer several questions.[16]

Neuropathology

Many researchers have examined post-mortem neural tissue from people with psychiatric illnesses. Post-mortem analysis reaches a level of molecular and cellular resolution currently unachievable in vivo; however, it is commonly limited by confounds (such as age, effects of chronic medication, and non-specific effects of chronic psychiatric illness).

Neuropathology was the primary, if not only, method used to study brain disorders in the late 1800s and early 1900s, when Alzheimer first described plaques in the brain of his patient with dementia[17] and identified frontal cortex abnormalities in those with schizophrenia.[18] Although some skeptics described schizophrenia as the "graveyard of neuropathologists," recent studies have provided reproducible descriptions of deficits (such as those in parvalbumin-expressing GABA-ergic interneurons in deep layers 3 and 4, akin to Alzheimer's findings) in the cortex. These neuropathological findings have provided one of the strongest etiological hypotheses for schizophrenia.

Psychopharmacology

More than any other methodology in psychiatric neuroscience, pharmacology has been used to understand the neurochemical basis of behavior and to develop hypotheses regarding psychopathological mechanisms. Famous examples include the dopamine and glutamate hypotheses of schizophrenia, the catecholamine depletion hypothesis of depression, and the dopaminergic models of attention-deficit hyperactivity disorder (ADHD) and substance abuse. In relating pharmacological effects to potential disease mechanisms, it is important to note that the effects of drugs on clinical symptoms may reflect mechanisms that are downstream of the core pathophysiology or even unrelated to core disease mechanisms. By analogy, diuretics can improve the symptoms of congestive heart failure while providing less direct insight into its core pathophysiology. Nonetheless, by clearly connecting cellular and synaptic mechanisms with clinical symptoms, pharmacology provides mechanistic tools and information with enormous clinical and scientific utility.[19]

Human Genetics and Molecular Biology

Adoption, twin, and familial segregation studies have proven that many psychiatric conditions are highly heritable (i.e., caused in large part by the additive effect of genes). Following up on seminal work in the early 2000s such as the Human Genome Project and HapMap project, large-scale genome-wide association studies are providing new insights into the cellular and molecular basis of psychopathology. These studies, which involve tens and (increasingly) hundreds of thousands of patients and healthy control participants, have identified two broad categories of genes that contribute to risk for psychopathology: common variants, which are present in at least 1% of the population and contribute tiny amounts of risk; and rare variants, which occur far less frequently but account for substantially greater increases in risk. For most patients, the presence of a single genetic variant does not determine disease risk; rather, it is the combination of hundreds or thousands of variants that underlie genetic risk. Large-scale studies of polygenic risk scores, which reflect the summed effects of thousands of risk variants for a given individual, show promise as markers for disease risk, although they do not yet provide sufficient sensitivity or specificity for routine clinical use.[20]

This lack of resolution represents one of several other important challenges that will need to be overcome before routine clinical use of genetic markers in psychiatry. For example, there exists significant overlap in the genetic underpinnings of psychiatric disorders, meaning that the same set of genes may confer risk for multiple disorders.[21] Genomic studies also fail to capture important environmental determinants of risk, and their use in populations with non-European ancestry currently is limited at present by insufficient sample size in research studies. However, as in other areas of medicine, it is likely that genetic markers will take on increasing importance in the realms of risk stratification, diagnosis, and prognosis in psychiatry soon.

Methodologies in molecular genetics and molecular neuroscience also promise improved understanding of gene function in the brain. These methods include the following: comparison of gene sequences in human with non-human primate and other animals, a deeper understanding of how non-coding elements within the genome may regulate important brain genes and thereby play a role in psychiatry, the study of gene expression using microarrays, the study of gene function in mice in which specific genes have been modified by recombinant methods (e.g., "knock-out" or "knock-in" studies), and studies examining how experience and the environment alter gene expression. In summary, genomics and molecular genetics hold great promise for identifying genes and thus biological mechanisms at the core of psychiatric pathophysiology.[22]

Animal Experiments

Complex psychiatric symptoms (such as delusions) cannot be modeled well in animals, and anthropomorphic interpretations of animal behavior should be taken with due skepticism. Despite these caveats, animal behaviors with known neuroanatomical correlates have been critical in elucidating the neurocircuitry and neurochemistry that underlie psychiatric phenomena.[23] For example, anxiety- and fear-related behaviors have been very productively modeled in animals, leading to a detailed understanding of the role of the amygdala and its subnuclei in these behaviors.[24] Of course, animal studies also permit a wider range of experimental perturbations than possible with human investigations. Independent of their value as behavioral models, animal models offer the opportunity to explore cellular and molecular pathophysiology in ways that are ethically or technically impossible in human participants. For example, the fragile X knock-out mouse is an excellent model for fragile X syndrome, the most common form of inherited cognitive impairment. Studying these mice has led to a deep understanding of relevant defects in dendrite formation and neurophysiology.[25]

BIOLOGICAL CASE FORMULATION: NEUROSCIENTIFIC CONTENT AND PROCESS

Clinical case formulation in psychiatry is structured around the bio-psycho-social model. In this chapter, we offer a framework for formulating the biological aspects of this model. Specifically, neuroscientific explanations may be organized in two broad conceptual areas: process and content. *Process* refers to dynamic brain mechanisms that lead to illness, and *content* refers to the brain properties (including neural circuits, brain regions, synapses, cells, and molecules) that form the substrate for these changes.

Process

A key concept in basic neuroscience and its clinical specialties is neuroplasticity. Although it is defined in different ways and can be studied at various levels of resolution (e.g., circuits, synapses), this term generally refers to the capacity of the neural system to change in response to external or internal stimuli following predetermined rules. Neuroplasticity provides a great deal of flexibility and adaptive capacity to the brain, permitting variable computational strategies and patterns of connectivity in a changing environment.[26] Despite the significant potential for reactive (and adaptive) change, this happens around an exquisitely regulated homeostatic equilibrium point. Nevertheless, when the plastic changes are restricted, excessive, or occur around an altered equilibrium state, pathology develops. Luckily, the brain remains plastic, and any intervention (e.g., medications, psychotherapy, or brain stimulation) that is effective in changing pathological cognition, behavior, or affect induces adaptive plasticity. That is, a pathological mental state is sustained by a given pattern of brain activity, and changing this mental state will require changing its associated neural computational algorithm. Therefore, neuroplasticity is a key dynamic property of the brain that allows adaptive change (including learning and memory), but it is also an important source of pathology and a necessary mechanism of action of effective neuropsychiatric treatments.

Although the pathophysiological mechanisms that lead to neuropsychiatric disease are many, we will consider different biological processes associated with neurodevelopment. Under neurodevelopment, we include related processes that continue into adulthood. Previously underestimated, adult neurogenesis is now known to continue in select regions of the human brain, most notably the dentate gyrus of the hippocampus.[27] Although the role of adult neurogenesis in humans remains a topic of inquiry, evidence has connected maladaptive hippocampal neurogenesis to the pathophysiology of mood disorders and stress-related conditions and has also linked effective antidepressant therapy (using medications or ECT) with adaptive engagement of this very same process.[28] Beyond neurogenesis, neurodevelopmental processes shaping

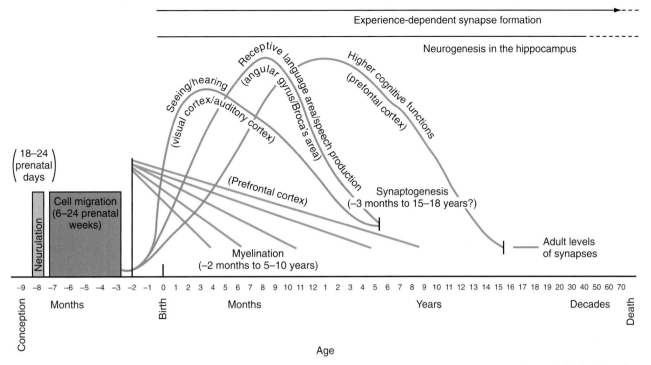

Figure 1.1 A depiction of the processes of brain development, including intrauterine neuronal patterning, neurogenesis, cortical migration, gliogenesis, myelination, and experience-dependent synapse modification. (From Thompson RA, Nelson CA. Developmental science and the media. Early brain development, *Am Psychol.* 2001;56(1):5–15.)

brain circuits have lifelong effects on patterns of affect, behavior, and cognition with direct relevance to mental health. The effects of childhood experience have always been central to psychiatric understanding; psychiatric neuroscience has also attempted to provide a biological grounding for this understanding. In the first years and decade of life, the brain undergoes a process of synapse formation and pruning. Figure 1.1 shows the processes of brain development, including intrauterine neuronal patterning, neurogenesis, cortical migration, gliogenesis, myelination, and experience-dependent synapse modification.[29,30] Figure 1.2 shows age-related changes in synaptic density and frontal gray matter.

GENES, ENVIRONMENT, AND EPIGENETICS

At the beginning of this chapter, we stated that major mental illnesses reflect abnormal brain function. However, although neuropsychiatric conditions are frequently highly heritable, the emergence of psychopathology likely requires a complex interaction of a genetic susceptibility and exposure to environmental risk factors.[31,32] Note that the "environment" must be understood broadly and includes the prenatal environment as well as peri-natal and post-natal events into childhood, adolescence, and adulthood. It is likely that environmental exposures affect the structure of the genome in ways that affect gene expression, a process known as epigenetics. These epigenetic changes can also be heritable and contribute to risk (or resiliency) in subsequent generations.[33] An animal model demonstrating cross-generational effects of child abuse provides proof of concept for analogous epigenetic effects in humans.[34] Although it has been widely noted in psychiatry that child abuse or mistreatment can have long-term effects on cognition and behavior, a model system of rodent maternal care has also demonstrated that rodent pups mistreated during development will have long-standing dysfunctional programming of their hypothalamic–pituitary–adrenal axis and thereby their response to stress. Investigators have further demonstrated that these occur because of specific

changes in chromatin structure and subsequent gene expression, and they have also shown that these changes and downstream effects may be heritable. These effects may be treatable or even reversible with novel medicines that affect chromatic structure, and, indeed, some of our older medicines, most notably valproic acid,[35] may act in part through such mechanisms. This is an important example of how a detailed mechanistic understanding of gene–environment interactions may truly make vast contributions to the understanding and treatment of major mental illness.

Content

The "content" of a psychiatric illness comprises the different structural and functional levels of biological resolution that form the nervous system: ions, proteins, genes, cells, synapses, circuits, behavior, and mental states. These can all be the target of pathological changes, leading to clinical syndromes. This is the subject of the remaining sections of this chapter. Characterizing neuropsychiatric conditions in terms of both biological processes and substrates (content) can provide a framework to facilitate an understanding of etiology, loci of intervention, and potential treatments.

OVERVIEW OF THE STRUCTURE OF THE CENTRAL NERVOUS SYSTEM

The structural organization of the central nervous system (CNS) is shown in Figure 1.3A–D. The human brain is organized into the cerebrum (including the cerebral cortex and subcortical structures), the brainstem, and the cerebellum. These anatomical structures are made of inter-connected elements that create distributed and highly inter-connected circuits. It is in these circuits where cognition, behavior, and affect are processed. This section provides an overview of neuroanatomy with a structural focus.

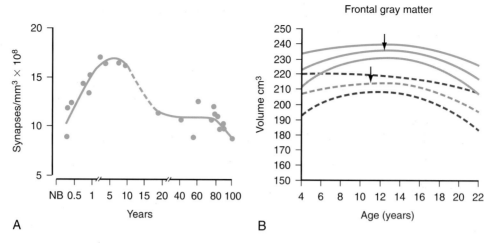

Figure 1.2 A, Depiction of the number of synapse counts in layer 3 of the middle frontal gyrus as a function of age. **B,** Graph of the volume, in cubic centimeters, of frontal gray matter with respect to age in years. Males represented by *solid lines* and females by *dashed lines* with 95% confidence intervals, respectively. *Arrows* indicate peak volume. *NB,* Newborn. (A, Data from Huttenlocher PR. Synaptic density in human frontal cortex: developmental changes and effects of aging. *Brain Res.* 1979;163(2):195–205. B, Data from Lenroot RK, Giedd JN. Brain development in children and adolescents: insights from anatomical magnetic resonance imaging. *Neurosci Biobehav Rev* 2006;30(6):718–729.)

The cerebral cortex is the outermost layer of the cerebrum and consists of a foliated structure, encompassing gyri and sulci. Within the most highly evolved cortical regions (isocortex), a structure composed of six cellular layers orchestrates complex brain functions. Cortical anatomy can be subdivided in different ways, including macroscopic anatomical regions (such as the occipital, parietal, temporal, insular, limbic, and frontal lobes) (see Figure 1.3). The limbic "lobe" is a ring (limbus) of phylogenetically older cortex surrounding the upper brainstem and includes the hippocampus, amygdala, hypothalamus, parahippocampal gyrus, and cingulate cortex (see Figure 1.3). Structures within the medial temporal lobe are especially important in psychiatry; the hippocampus plays a critical role in memory, and the amygdala is an important element of fear circuitry and for assigning emotional valence to stimuli.[36]

Functionally, the cortex may be divided into primary sensory or motor, unimodal association (where complex information from a single modality is processed, e.g., integrating shape and color into a visual percept), and multi-modal association regions that receive inputs from multiple systems. Multi-modal association cortex may be subdivided into three areas: frontal executive (involved in a wide variety of higher functions, such as planning, attention, abstract thought, problem-solving, judgment, initiative, and inhibition of impulses), limbic (involved in emotion and memory), and posterior sensory and spatial (at the interface of the parietal, occipital, and temporal lobes, involved in integrating sensory information and both perceiving and organizing behavior in space).[36]

In addition to the cerebral cortex, many other brain regions are of critical importance to psychiatry. The cerebellum (see Figure 1.3A and B), traditionally known for its role in motor coordination and learning, has more recently been implicated in cognitive and affective processes as well.[37] The thalamus is a major relay station for incoming sensory information and other critical circuitry, including connections between association cortices (via the mediodorsal nucleus) and outputs regulating motor activity.[38] Interestingly, the mediodorsal nucleus, a critical relay station between association cortices, is a region of the thalamus found to be smaller in some neuropathological studies of patients with schizophrenia. Figure 1.3C shows the parts of the basal ganglia, which comprise the striatum (i.e., caudate, putamen, and nucleus accumbens) and globus pallidus rostrally and the subthalamic nucleus and substantia

nigra caudally. The basal ganglia orchestrate multiple functions;[39] the dorsal striatum plays an important role in motor control, and the ventral striatum (especially the nucleus accumbens) plays key roles in emotion and learning via connections with the hippocampus, amygdala, and prefrontal cortex. The hypothalamus plays a critical role in neuroendocrine regulation of the internal milieu.[40] Via its effects on pituitary hormone release and connections to other regions of the brain, the hypothalamus exerts homeostatic effects on numerous psychiatrically relevant factors, including mood, motivation, sexual drive, hunger, temperature, and sleep. Finally, several discrete nuclei in the brainstem synthesize key modulatory neurotransmitters, exerting major effects on brain function via their widespread projections to striatal and corticolimbic regions of the brain. These neuromodulatory nuclei include the dopaminergic ventral tegmental area (VTA) in the midbrain, serotonergic raphe nuclei in the brainstem, noradrenergic locus coeruleus neurons in the pons, and cholinergic neurons of the basal forebrain and brainstem.

CELLULAR DIVERSITY IN THE BRAIN: NEURONS AND GLIA

The cellular diversity of the primate nervous system is truly fantastic. There are two broad classes of cells in the brain: neurons and glia. The Spanish neuroanatomist Santiago Ramon y Cajal prolifically and painstakingly documented the cellular diversity of the nervous system (Figure 1.4).[41] Images made with modern fluorescent staining techniques also convey the exquisite beauty of the cells of the CNS (Figure 1.5). Based on his observations, Ramon y Cajal proposed that neurons act as physically discrete functional units within the brain, communicating with each other through specialized junctions. This theory became known as the "neuron doctrine," and Ramon y Cajal's enormous contributions were recognized with a Nobel Prize in 1906.[42]

Neurons

There are approximately 100 billion neurons in the human brain, and each neuron makes up to 10,000 synaptic connections. At the peak of synapse formation in the third year of

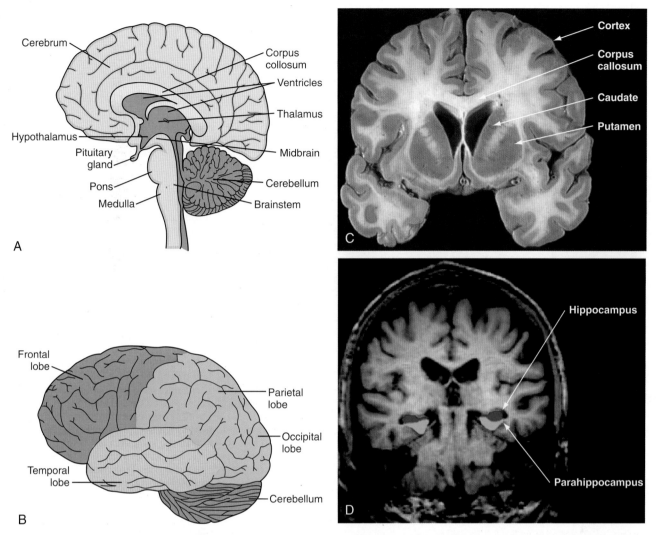

Figure 1.3 A, Schematic of the human brain organized into the cerebral cortex, brainstem, subcortical structures (e.g., basal ganglia, brainstem, thalamus, hypothalamus, and pituitary), and cerebellum. **B**, Depiction of the cortical anatomy divided into anatomical regions (such as the occipital, parietal, temporal, insular, limbic, and frontal lobes). **C**, Brain cut demonstrating the limbic "lobe" as a ring (limbus) of phylogenetically older cortex surrounding the upper brainstem. **D**, Brain cut highlighting the hippocampus, amygdala, hypothalamus, parahippocampal gyrus, and cingulate cortex. (C, From http://library.med.utah.edu/WebPath/HISTHTML/NEURANAT/CNS213A.html. D, From Dickerson BC, Salat DH, Bates JF, et al. Medial temporal lobe function and structure in mild cognitive impairment. *Ann Neurol*. 2004;56(1):27–35.)

life, the total number of brain synapses is estimated at 10,000 trillion, thereafter declining and stabilizing in adulthood to between 1000 trillion and 5000 trillion synapses.

Consistent with their functional diversity, neurons come in a wide variety of shapes and sizes. Nonetheless, all neurons share several characteristic features (Figure 1.6), including the cell soma (housing the nucleus with its genomic DNA), the axon, the pre-synaptic axon terminal, and the dendritic field (the receptive component of the neuron containing post-synaptic dendritic structures). Axon length is highly variable; short axons are found on inhibitory inter-neurons, which make only local connections, and axons many inches long are found on cortical projection neurons, which must reach to the contralateral hemisphere or down to the spinal cord. Motor and sensory neurons have axons that may be several feet long.

There are many ways to classify neurons: by their connectivity arrangement (i.e., projection neuron or local inter-neuron), morphology (i.e., bipolar, multi-polar, or unipolar), function (i.e., excitatory, inhibitory, or modulatory), electrophysiological pattern (i.e., tonic, phasic, or fast-spiking), or neurotransmitter type.

Glia

Although neurons have captured the lion's share of attention since the time of Ramon y Cajal, there are up to 10-fold more glial cells in the brain than neurons. The word "glia" means "glue," aptly summarizing the structural and supportive role traditionally attributed to them. Indeed, glia support neuronal function in many ways by supplying nutrition, maintaining homeostasis, stabilizing synapses, and myelinating axons. They also play important roles in synaptic transmission. In the CNS, there are two large categories of glia: microglia and macroglia. Microglia are small, phagocytic cells related to peripheral macrophages. Macroglia can be further classified into two types: astrocytes that maintain the synaptic milieu and oligodendrocytes that myelinate axons. Astrocytes play an active and critical role in glutamatergic neurotransmission, releasing co-agonists required for glutamate receptor function and transporting glutamate to terminate its synaptic action. New functions of glia continue to be discovered, and a belated appreciation of their importance to psychiatric neuroscience continues to grow. Mood disorders are associated with a reduction in the number

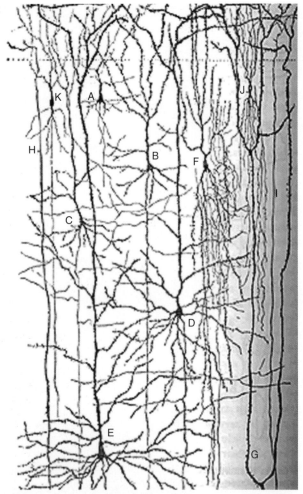

Figure 1.4 Ramon y Cajal's drawing from his classic *Histologie du Système Nerveux de l'Homme et des Vertébrés* showing the cellular diversity of the nervous system. (From Ramon y Cajal S. *Histologie du Système Nerveux de l'Homme et des Vertébrés*. A Maloine; 1909.)

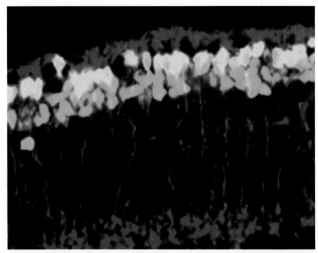

Figure 1.5 Images made with modern fluorescent staining techniques also convey the exquisite beauty of the cells of the central nervous system. (*Courtesy of Dr. Eric Morrow*)

of glia in select brain regions.[43] The mechanisms of action of ECT have been association with effective glial activation. In adult-onset metachromatic leukodystrophy, a genetic enzyme deficiency produces diffuse myelin destruction; the illness may manifest in mid-adolescence with neuropsychiatric symptoms resembling schizophrenia. Furthermore, studies looking for genes whose expression is altered in schizophrenia have identified prominent changes in myelin-related genes.

THE STRUCTURE OF THE SYNAPSE

The previous section described how inter-cellular communication serves as an organizing feature of neuroanatomy. Neurons and glia are elegantly situated within the brain to facilitate signaling between adjacent cells and between cells in distinct brain regions. Depending on the specific neurotransmitters released pre-synaptically and the specific receptors located post-synaptically, the transmitted signal may have excitatory, inhibitory, or other modulatory effects on the post-synaptic neuron. Detailed knowledge of the neurochemical anatomy of the brain is therefore a prerequisite to the optimal use of psychotropic medicines in psychiatry. Important aspects of neurochemical anatomy include how neurotransmitters are distributed within brain circuits, how these neurotransmitter systems function, and how these systems are altered either by disease or by our treatments.

Neurotransmitters

Neurotransmitters are defined by four essential characteristics (Figure 1.7 and Box 1.2): they are synthesized within the pre-synaptic neuron, they are released with depolarization from the pre-synaptic neuron to exert a discrete action on the post-synaptic neuron, their action on the post-synaptic neuron can be replicated by administering the transmitter exogenously (as a drug), and their action in the synaptic cleft is terminated by a specific mechanism. However, they otherwise differ considerably in structure, distribution, and function. Their chemical make-up varies substantially, including small molecules such

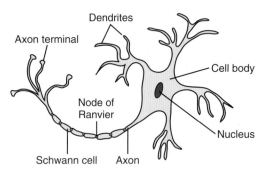

Figure 1.6 Depiction of a neuron with its components.

BOX 1.2 Schema of Neurochemical Systems
Neurotransmitter biosynthesis
Neurotransmitter storage and synaptic vesicle release
Neurotransmitter receptors
• Post-synaptic
• Pre-synaptic autoreceptors
Post-synaptic ion channels
Post-synaptic second messenger systems
Activity-dependent gene regulation
Neurotransmitter degradation
Neurotransmitter reuptake
Functional neurochemical anatomy

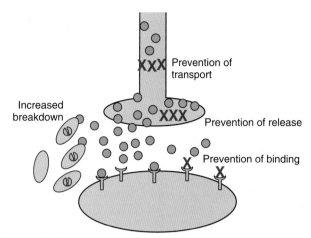

Figure 1.8 Psychopharmacology and a synapse.

BOX 1.3 Major Neurotransmitter Systems in the Brain

AMINO ACIDS
Glutamate
GABA

MONOAMINES
Dopamine
Norepinephrine (noradrenaline)
Epinephrine (adrenaline)
Serotonin
Histamine

SMALL MOLECULE NEUROTRANSMITTER
Acetylcholine

PEPTIDES
Opioids (enkephalins, endorphin, dynorphin)
Hypothalamic factors (CRH, orexins and hypocretins, and others)
Pituitary hormones (ACTH, TSH, oxytocin, vasopressin, and others)
Neuroactive CNS peptides also expressed in the GI system (substance P, VIP, and others)
Others (leptin and others)

ACTH, Adrenocorticotropic hormone; *CNS,* central nervous system; *CRH,* corticotropin-releasing hormone; *GABA,* gamma aminobutyric acid; *GI,* gastrointestinal; *TSH,* thyroid-stimulating hormone; *VIP,* vasoactive intestinal polypeptide.

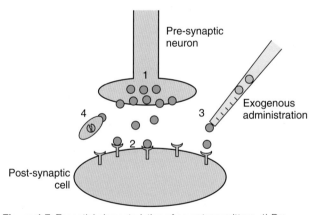

Figure 1.7 Essential characteristics of neurotransmitters. 1) Presynaptic neuron. 2) Post-synaptic cell. 3) Exogenous administration. 4) Catalytic enzyme.

as amino acids, biogenic amines, and nitrous oxide, as well as larger peptides, such as opioids and substance P. Certain neurotransmitters are found ubiquitously throughout the cortex, whereas others act in more select locations. Moreover, whereas certain neurotransmitters are always excitatory (e.g., glutamate) or inhibitory (e.g., GABA) in the adult brain, others can exert variable downstream neuromodulatory effects based on where they are located (functional neuroanatomy) and to which receptors they bind (synaptic physiology).

More than 100 neurotransmitters have been identified within the mammalian brain. However, we will focus on several well-characterized neurotransmitter systems with major relevance to neuropsychiatric phenomena (Box 1.3). Each of these neurotransmitters plays an important role in normal brain function; thus, abnormal activity in any of these neurotransmitter systems may contribute to neuropsychiatric dysfunction. We will consider the normal "life cycle" for each neurotransmitter system, including synthesis, synaptic release,

receptor binding, neurotransmitter degradation, post-synaptic signaling through ion channels or second messengers, and activity-dependent changes in gene expression and subsequent neuronal activity (see Box 1.2). We will focus particularly on the various points in this cycle that are amenable to pharmacological intervention.

For example, consider the hypothetical synapse in Figure 1.8. Suppose a specific psychiatric symptom was related to abnormally high synaptic concentrations of a specific neurotransmitter. The diversity of biochemical steps involved in the neurotransmitter cycle provides many targets for pharmacological intervention:[44] one could inhibit neurotransmitter synthesis; interfere with neurotransmitter transport, vesicle formation, or release; block post-synaptic receptor effects; or increase the clearance rate from the synapse by degradation or transport. We will re-visit this model as we consider each of the neurotransmitter systems and their relation to normal and abnormal brain function below.[44]

Synaptic Transmission, Second Messenger Systems, and Activity-Dependent Gene Expression

Neurotransmitter signals alter post-synaptic neuron function via a complex collection of receptors and second messenger systems. These signals ultimately result in changes in neuronal activity, often associated with changes in gene expression. Although neurotransmitter receptors are the classic targets of pharmacological intervention, it has become apparent that second messenger systems may also provide important targets for existing and novel therapies.

In general, neurotransmitter receptors trigger either rapid or slow effector systems. Rapid-effect neurotransmitter receptors are either themselves ion channels (e.g., NMDA glutamate receptors) or are coupled to ion channels. Ion flux through these transmitter-activated channels rapidly alters electrical membrane potential and neuronal activity. Other neurotransmitter receptors, including the large family of G-protein–coupled receptors (GPCRs), work via slower second messenger systems. Such second messenger systems usually involve sequential multi-enzyme cascades. Post-translational modifications, such as protein phosphorylation (introduced by kinase proteins and removed by phosphatase proteins), can act as on–off switches to propagate or terminate the signal at specific branch points. Second messenger systems convert receptor signals into a coordinated set of cellular effects by altering the function of multiple target proteins. These targets may include ion channels that control neuronal firing, synaptic proteins that regulate synaptic efficacy, and cytoskeletal elements that determine cellular morphology. Although there are more than 500 different kinases in the human genome, several that have been heavily studied in psychiatry are worthy of special mention, such as the cyclic adenosine monophosphate (cAMP)–dependent kinase (also known as protein kinase A [PKA]) and calcium/calmodulin-dependent protein kinase, which both play critical roles in memory formation. Another second messenger pathway, involving glycogen synthase kinase, has been proposed to mediate at least some of the therapeutic efficacy of lithium salts in bipolar disorder.[45]

Transcription factors are also critical downstream targets of neurotransmitter signals and second messenger systems. By modifying gene expression in the nucleus, transcription factors can produce persistent plastic changes in neural function. The most widely studied neuronal transcription factors include immediate early genes *c-Jun*, *c-Fos*, and cAMP response element binding protein (CREB), whose activity is quickly regulated by neurotransmitter signals.[46] CREB has been shown to be up-regulated and phosphorylated in neurons in response to antipsychotic medication as well as drugs of abuse and in response to neurotrophic factors, such as brain-derived neurotrophic factor (BDNF). BDNF and related neurotrophic factors are of particular interest to psychiatric neuroscience because they exert effects both as growth factors during embryonic neurodevelopment and synaptic signaling in adults. BDNF signaling modulates CREB activity and gene expression; both factors play important roles in neural plasticity and have been heavily studied in genetic association studies in psychiatric disorders.[47]

A REVIEW OF CLINICALLY RELEVANT NEUROTRANSMITTER SYSTEMS

This section reviews the major neurotransmitter systems, all of which have clinical importance in psychiatry. In each subsection, emphasis is placed on the "content" of neuropsychiatric explanation.

Glutamate

As the major excitatory neurotransmitter in the CNS, glutamate is found ubiquitously throughout the brain. A non-essential amino acid, glutamate does not cross the blood–brain barrier; thus, synthesis of the glutamate neurotransmitter pool relies entirely on conversion from its precursors (glutamine or aspartate) within nerve terminals (Figure 1.9). Aspartate is converted to glutamine via transamination, and glutamine is converted to glutamate within mitochondria via glutaminase. Glutamate is packaged within synaptic vesicles and, when released into the synapse, binds post-synaptic glutamate receptors. Unable to diffuse across cell membranes, glutamate is cleared from the synapse primarily by sodium (Na^+)–dependent uptake into astrocytic processes that unsheathe the glutamatergic synapse ("tripartite synapse"), where it is converted back to glutamine (which is then transported back to the presynaptic glutamatergic terminal).

Glutamate receptors are varied in structure and function, capable of imparting either rapid (ionotropic) or gradual (metabotropic) change in the function of the post-synaptic neuron. The ionotropic family of glutamate receptors, which includes NMDA, α-amino-3-hydroxy-5-methyl-4-isoxazolepropionic acid (AMPA), and kainate receptors, act rapidly by opening channels for Na^+ and (to a variable degree) calcium (Ca^{2+}) influx. This influx causes post-synaptic depolarization, which, if present in sufficient force, causes the neuron to fire. The metabotropic glutamate receptors (mGluRs) effect gradual change in neuronal function. These seven membrane-spanning GPCRs are linked to cytoplasmic enzymes via G proteins embedded within the cell membrane. After being activated, these enzymes can induce second messenger cascades that can influence intra-cellular processes, including gene transcription.

The *N*-Methyl-D-Aspartate Receptor and the Role of Glutamate in Neuropsychiatric Illness

The NMDA receptor deserves special attention because of its role in normal and abnormal cognitive processes. When activated, the NMDA receptor serves as a channel for the influx of Ca^{2+} into the neuron (Figure 1.10). This process relies on both the binding of ligands (such as glutamate and a co-agonist, glycine) to the receptor and on recent depolarization of the post-synaptic cell membrane, which displaces a magnesium (Mg^{2+}) ion that normally blocks the channel. NMDA

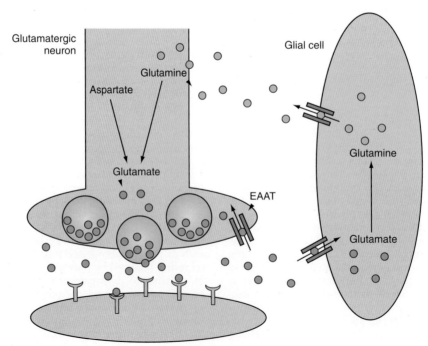

Figure 1.9 The glutamate life cycle. *EAAT*, Excitatory amino acid transporters.

receptor signaling thus requires near-simultaneous activity of the pre-synaptic and post-synaptic neurons; this provides a molecular mechanism for associating two temporally linked inputs, a key ingredient in basic forms of learning. Indeed, NMDA receptors, along with AMPA receptors, mediate long-term potentiation in the hippocampus, a process critical for neuroplasticity and hippocampal-dependent memory formation.

When NMDA receptors are activated in sufficient numbers, however, the resulting large calcium influx can result in cell death, a process known as excitotoxicity (see Figure 1.10). Excitotoxicity is thought to contribute to neurodegenerative disorders (such as AD, Huntington disease, and amyotrophic lateral sclerosis).[48] Memantine, an NMDA antagonist, is used for the treatment of AD and is hypothesized to slow disease progression by dampening excitotoxic injury. Although over-active NMDA receptors may contribute to neurodegeneration and memory loss in dementia, blockade of these receptors can also cause profound cognitive disruption. NMDA antagonists (such as ketamine and phencyclidine [PCP]) produce psychotic symptoms (e.g., disorganization, dissociation, hallucinations, delusions) in healthy people and exacerbate psychosis in patients with schizophrenia. This pattern, in concert with observed alterations in glutamate-related proteins, has spurred the "glutamate hypothesis" of schizophrenia. The glutamate system thus represents a promising target for the development of new antipsychotic medications. The NMDA receptor, in addition to its binding site for glutamate, also has a co-regulatory site for the amino acids, glycine or D-serine, which must be occupied for glutamate to open the channel. Based on the hypothesis of a hypoactive glutamatergic system in schizophrenia, these amino acids and the related D-cyclo-serine have been studied as potential augmentation strategies for antipsychotic treatment.

Last, the role of glutamate in mood disorders has been the focus of attention since the discovery of the rapid antidepressant effects of ketamine, an NMDA antagonist. Although the mechanisms of action of ketamine in depression are not fully understood, the role of NMDA modulation may be part but not a critical causal component. Modulation of other receptors and downstream effects beyond the NMDA receptor are also being investigated. Still, the repurpose of ketamine as an old drug with such a novel therapeutic indication, an antidepressant that works in hours not weeks, has generated a growing interest in NMDA modulators as potential novel treatments for mood and cognitive disorders.[49]

GABA

Another amino acid, GABA, serves as the major inhibitory transmitter in the CNS. When bound to membrane receptors, GABA causes hyperpolarization either directly, by causing chloride channels to open, or indirectly, through second messenger systems. Although found throughout the CNS, GABA is concentrated specifically in both cortical and spinal interneurons and plays a major role in dampening excitatory signals. As such, GABA receptors have been of considerable interest to researchers concerned about the normal and abnormal function of neural networks.

GABA is synthesized primarily from glucose, which is converted via the Krebs cycle into α-ketoglutarate and then to glutamate (Figure 1.11). Conversion from glutamate to GABA occurs through the action of glutamic acid decarboxylase (GAD). Because GAD is found only in GABA-producing neurons, antibodies to the enzyme have been used to identify GABA-ergic neurons with high specificity. After depolarization of the pre-synaptic neuron, vesicles containing GABA discharge it into the synapse, where binding to post-synaptic receptors occurs. GABA is then cleared from the synapse and transported into pre-synaptic terminals and surrounding glia. It is then broken down by GABA α-oxoglutarate transaminase (GABA-T), and downstream products are returned to the Krebs cycle. GABA synthesis and metabolism are thus referred to as the *GABA shunt reaction.*

GABA Receptors

There are two major classes of GABA receptors: $GABA_A$ and $GABA_B$ receptors. Binding of GABA to the $GABA_A$ receptor causes a chloride channel to open, which, under most circumstances, renders the post-synaptic membrane potential more negative (Figure 1.12). Of note, several other agents bind allosterically to the $GABA_A$ receptor, including alcohol, barbiturates, and benzodiazepines, and render it more sensitive to GABA. The anticonvulsant activity of benzodiazepines and barbiturates is thought to reflect neural inhibition mediated through the $GABA_A$ receptor.

$GABA_B$ receptors, akin to the metabotropic glutamate receptors, are GPRCs rather than ion channels. Activation of $GABA_B$ causes downstream changes in potassium (K^+) and Ca^{2+} channels, largely via G-protein–mediated inhibition of cAMP. Specific interactions between $GABA_B$ receptors and Ca^{2+} channel activity may be linked to absence seizures.

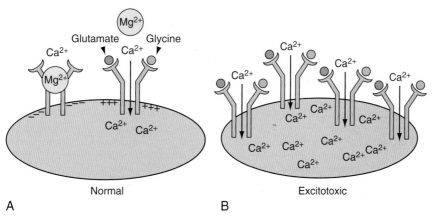

Figure 1.10 *N*-methyl-D-aspartate receptors and excitotoxicity. **A**, Normal. **B**, Excitotoxic.

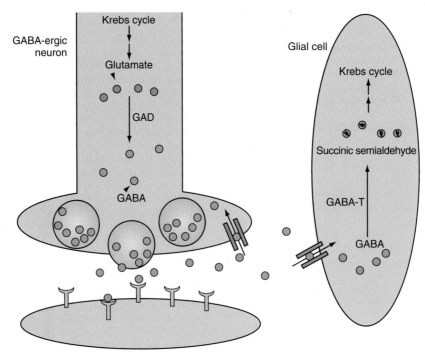

Figure 1.11 The gamma aminobutyric acid (GABA) life cycle. *GAD*, Glutamic acid decarboxylase.

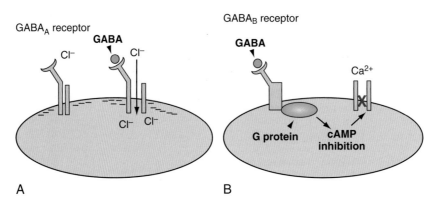

Figure 1.12 Gamma aminobutyric acid (GABA) receptors. **A**, GABA$_A$ receptor. **B**, GABA$_B$ receptor. *cAMP*, Cyclic adenosine monophosphate.

GABA in Neuropsychiatric Illness

Altered GABA activity may contribute significantly to psychiatric disorders. In schizophrenia, reduced GABA synthesis in a select population of inter-neurons within the DLPFC is thought to affect inhibition of pyramidal neurons in this region. Reduced inter-neuron input may thus disrupt synchronized neuronal activity, which in turn may underlie working memory deficits in schizophrenia. Furthermore, although the exact mechanism remains uncertain, the chronic action of alcohol, benzodiazepines, and barbiturates on specific GABA$_A$ receptor subunits is hypothesized to underlie such clinical phenomena as tolerance and withdrawal. GABA-ergic dysfunction has also been posited to contribute to panic disorder. The recent discovery of neuro-steroids such as brexanolone as rapid antidepressants for post-partum depression has invigorated the investigation on the role of GABA in mood disorders because this drug acts by modulating GABA$_A$ receptors.[1]

Dopamine

Although glutamate and GABA are found throughout the brain, other neurotransmitter systems are localized to specific neural pathways. The monoamines (e.g., norepinephrine, serotonin, dopamine) and acetylcholine are synthesized in several discrete brainstem nuclei, yet they project widely, affecting most brain systems. Dopamine, a catecholamine neurotransmitter, affects many brain regions that are consistently implicated in psychiatric disorders. It is hardly surprising, then, that a host of psychopharmacological interventions target the dopamine system.

Dopamine Pathways and Relevance to Neuropsychiatry

There are four major dopamine projections (Figure 1.13), each with great relevance to neuropsychiatric phenomena. The name of each projection indicates the location of the dopaminergic cell bodies, as well as the region targeted by their axons; for example, the nigrostriatal system consists of dopamine cell bodies in the substantia nigra, with axons projecting to the striatum. Degeneration of the nigrostriatal pathway leads to extrapyramidal motor symptoms (such as tremor, bradykinesia, and rigidity), as seen in Parkinson's disease. An analogous mechanism underlies extrapyramidal symptoms (EPSs) associated with antipsychotic medications, which block dopamine receptors in the striatum.

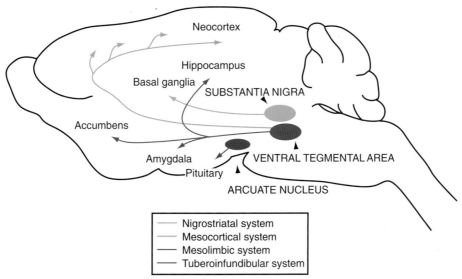

Figure 1.13 Dopaminergic projections. (Adapted from NIAAA. http://www.niaaa.nih.gov/Resources/GraphicsGallery/EndocrineReproductiveSystem/LengthwiseView.htm.)

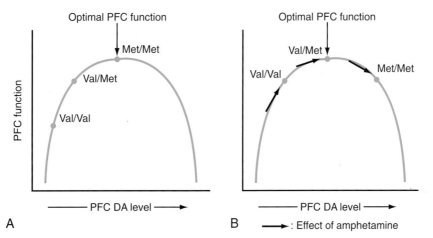

Figure 1.14 A, and **B**, Dopamine (DA) and prefrontal cortex *(PFC)* function. *Met*, Methionine; *Val*, valine. (Adapted from Mattay VS, Goldberg TE, Fera F, et al. Catechol O-methyltransferase val158-met genotype and individual variation in the brain response to amphetamine. *Proc Natl Acad Sci U S A.* 2003;100:6186–6191.)

Dopamine neurons in the mesolimbic pathway project from the VTA, also in the mid-brain, to limbic and paralimbic structures, including the nucleus accumbens, amygdala, hippocampus, and septum. Given the importance of these downstream structures to emotion, sensory perception, and memory, it has been speculated that altered activity in the mesolimbic pathway may underlie the perceptual disturbances common to positive symptoms of schizophrenia, hallucinogen use, and even temporal lobe seizures. The mesolimbic pathway is also implicated in the addictive actions of drugs of abuse, which share the common feature of enhancing dopamine release in the nucleus accumbens. In addition, loss of mid-brain nigrostriatal dopaminergic neurons in Parkinson's disease may spread to VTA neurons, and this may underlie the depressive symptoms commonly seen in Parkinson's disease.

Mesocortical dopamine neurons also have their cell bodies in the VTA but project to the neocortex, primarily the prefrontal cortex (e.g., anterior cingulate and orbitofrontal cortex). Release of dopamine in the prefrontal cortex is believed to affect the efficiency of information processing, attention, and wakefulness. The relationship between prefrontal dopamine and frontal lobe function does not appear to be linear but rather reflects an "inverted-U" shape (Figure 1.14).[50] For example, brain activation during working memory tasks, largely mediated by prefrontal activation, is inefficient under conditions of either low or high prefrontal dopamine release. Altered availability of prefrontal dopamine may underlie cognitive impairment in schizophrenia, ADHD, Parkinson's disease, and other neuropsychiatric conditions.

The tuberoinfundibular dopamine system projects from the arcuate nucleus of the hypothalamus to the stalk of the pituitary gland. When released in the pituitary, dopamine inhibits the secretion of prolactin. Individuals who take dopamine-blocking medications (including some antipsychotics) are therefore at risk for hyperprolactinemia, which can in turn cause menstrual cycle abnormalities, galactorrhea, gynecomastia, and sexual dysfunction.

Dopamine Synthesis, Binding, and Inactivation and More Clinical Correlates

The catecholamines (dopamine, norepinephrine, and epinephrine) are synthesized sequentially in the same biosynthetic

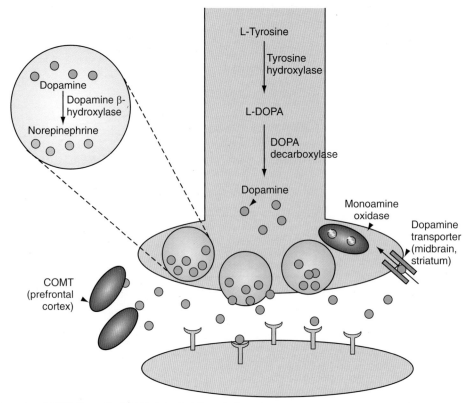

Figure 1.15 The dopamine *(DOPA)* life cycle. *COMT*, Catechol-*O*-methyltransferase.

pathway. First, dopamine is synthesized from tyrosine through the actions of tyrosine hydroxylase (the rate-limiting enzyme for catecholamine synthesis) and 3,4-dihydroxy-L-phenylalanine (DOPA) decarboxylase (Figure 1.15). The dopamine precursor, L-DOPA, crosses the blood–brain barrier and is given systemically to ameliorate symptoms of Parkinson's disease. Dopamine is packaged and stored in synaptic vesicles by the vesicular monoamine transporter (VMAT) and when released binds to post-synaptic dopamine receptors.

Although numerous classes of dopamine receptors have been described, they each affect intra-cellular signaling through second messenger systems. Dopamine receptors fall into one of two families: D_1-like or D_2-like receptors. D_1-like receptors (which include D_1 and D_5) activate adenylyl cyclase, and D_2-like receptors (including D_2, D_3, and D_4) inhibit cAMP production. D_1 and D_2 receptors significantly outnumber other dopamine receptor types. Most typical antipsychotics were developed as D_2 antagonists, but atypical antipsychotics usually have less activity at D_2 receptors (clozapine, for example, has a high affinity for the D_4 receptor).

There are several mechanisms for inactivating dopamine. Within the neuron, extra-vesicular dopamine may be catabolized by the mitochondrial enzymes, monoamine oxidase-A or -B (MAO-A or MAO-B). MAO-A metabolizes norepinephrine, serotonin, and dopamine; inhibitors of this enzyme, such as clorgyline and tranylcypromine, are used to treat depression and anxiety. MAO is also present in the liver and gastrointestinal tract, where it degrades dietary amines (such as tyramine and phenylethylamine), thereby preventing their access to the general circulation. Phenylethylamine can cause hypertension when systemically absorbed; thus, patients receiving MAO inhibitors are at risk of hypertensive crisis if they ingest food products containing these amines. MAO-B targets dopamine most specifically, and therefore agents that inhibit this enzyme are used in Parkinson's disease.

Two other molecules, catechol-*O*-methyltransferase (COMT) and the dopamine transporter (DAT), can clear dopamine from the synaptic cleft. In the mid-brain and striatum, DAT plays a more substantial role than COMT, but in the prefrontal cortex, COMT predominates. A common, functional polymorphism in the *COMT* gene, Val 108/158 Met, has been identified; individuals with one or more copies of the Met allele have significantly reduced COMT activity. Thus, these individuals presumably have greater concentrations of prefrontal dopamine (see Figure 1.14). In humans, in the setting of a challenging working memory task, healthy individuals homozygous for the Met allele (Met/Met) may exhibit more efficient brain activation than Val/Val or Val/Met participants. However, if given amphetamine, which blocks dopamine reuptake and increases synaptic dopamine, Val/Val individuals are shifted to a more optimal position in the curve, but those with Met/Met are shifted to the less efficient downward slope of the curve.[51] Among individuals with altered prefrontal dopamine levels, such as patients with schizophrenia and Parkinson's disease, variation in the *COMT* genotype may play a significant role in determining prefrontal efficiency and hence performance on tasks involving planning, sequencing, and working memory. Similarly, patients with velo-cardio-facial syndrome (VCFS) often have psychotic symptoms that may relate to altered COMT function. VCFS is caused by a 3-Mb (million base pairs) deletion of the genome on chromosome 22q11.2, which results in the complete loss of one parental copy of approximately 30 genes, one of which is *COMT*. These patients, who exhibit a somewhat variable phenotype (which may also include abnormalities of the heart, thymus, parathyroid, and palate), also have an increased risk for psychotic disorders. Almost 30% of patients with VCFS have a psychiatric condition akin to bipolar disorder or schizophrenia.

Norepinephrine

Like dopamine, norepinephrine (noradrenaline [NE]) is a catecholamine neurotransmitter that is present in discrete neural projections. NE cell bodies are concentrated in the locus

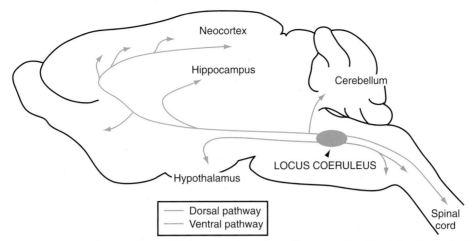

Figure 1.16 Noradrenergic projections. (Adapted from NIAAA at www.niaaa.nih.gov/Resources/GraphicsGallery/EndocrineReproductiveSystem/ LengthwiseView.htm; and from Siegel GJ, Agranoff BW, Albers RW, et al. *Basic neurochemistry*. 7th ed. Philadelphia: Lippincott-Raven; 1999: 252.)

coeruleus, which is in the pons near the fourth ventricle (Figure 1.16). Whereas this dorsal collection of noradrenergic neurons innervates the cerebral cortex, hippocampus, cerebellum, and spinal cord, a ventral collection projects to the hypothalamus and other CNS sites.

Noradrenaline overlaps substantially with dopamine regarding synthesis and degradation pathways; in fact, dopamine is the immediate precursor to NE, which is produced within synaptic vesicles by dopamine β-hydroxylase (see Figure 1.15). Like dopamine, NE is also degraded by COMT and MAO.

There are three families of noradrenergic receptors: α_1, α_2, and β. Like the dopamine receptors, NE receptors are all coupled to G proteins and thus modify intra-cellular signaling pathways. The α_1 receptors augment protein kinase C activity through the release of inositol 1,4,5-triphosphate and diacylglycerol. Although activated α_2 receptors decrease cAMP through inhibition of adenylyl cyclase, β receptors do the opposite, stimulating cAMP production. In this sense, α_2 receptors are somewhat akin to D_2, and β receptors to D_1. In the CNS, α_2 receptors frequently act as "autoreceptors" present pre-synaptically on noradrenergic neurons themselves, providing negative-feedback regulation of noradrenergic output.

Norepinephrine in Opiate Withdrawal

Clonidine, a drug commonly used to treat hypertension, activates CNS α_2 autoreceptors and thereby dampens noradrenergic tone. Use of clonidine in the treatment of opiate withdrawal provides a wonderful example of a case in which psychiatric neuroscience has successfully characterized the links between a clinical disorder; therapeutic drug effects; and mechanisms at the molecular, cellular, and neural circuit levels. Acutely, opiates act through GPCRs to inhibit the cAMP system and reduce the activity of locus coeruleus neurons; this partly mediates their calming and sedating effects. With chronic opiate administration, tolerance develops, in part because of homeostatic up-regulation in the activity of cAMP pathway elements (such as PKA and CREB). In opiate withdrawal, this adaptive up-regulation is no longer balanced by the opiate inhibition. Rebound hyperactivity of the locus coeruleus then occurs, with a great increase in NE release from its widespread projections. This in turn leads to the autonomic and psychological hyperarousal seen during withdrawal; these symptoms are greatly dampened by clonidine.[52]

Serotonin

The serotonin system is involved in many processes in psychiatry, including most prominently mood, sleep, and psychosis.[53,54] Serotonin (5-hydroxytryptamine [5-HT]), a monoamine and indolamine, is synthesized from the amino acid tryptophan by tryptophan hydroxylase (Figure 1.17). Serotonin is synthesized in mid-line neurons of the brainstem, known as the raphe nuclei.[55] Serotonergic neurons project diffusely to numerous targets (including cerebral cortex, thalamus, basal ganglia, mid-brain dopaminergic nuclei, hippocampus, and amygdala) (Figure 1.18).

Like the catecholamines, serotonin is transported into vesicles by VMAT. Serotonin is subsequently released into the synaptic cleft, and after receptor binding, is inactivated either by pre-synaptic reuptake via the serotonin transporter or degradation via MAO. The serotonin transporter is a critical molecule in neuropsychopharmacology. Drugs that block the serotonin transporter (SERT) prolong serotonin's action; these agents include the selective serotonin reuptake inhibitors commonly used in treating patients with depression and anxiety disorders. Like the norepinephrine transporter (NET) and DAT, SERT is also a common target of drugs of abuse. For example, both cocaine and amphetamine prolong the action of serotonin by inhibiting SERT. Similarly, MDMA (3,4-methylenedioxymethamphetamine), a drug also known as ecstasy or molly, prohibited since the 1980s because of its recreational uses and recently rediscovered for its potential therapeutic applications in conditions such as post-traumatic stress disorder (PTSD), is a fast-acting SERT inhibitor.

Seven classes of serotonin receptors exhibit distinct patterns of expression in CNS and peripheral tissues and activate distinct second messenger systems. For example, 5-HT$_{1A}$ receptors are GPCRs that are inhibitory and thereby decrease cAMP; agonists at this receptor (e.g., buspirone) have anxiolytic properties. 5-HT$_2$ receptors (which have three subtypes, A–C) act through a different G protein to activate inositol triphosphate and diacylglycerol second messenger systems. 5-HT$_2$ signaling is particularly relevant to psychosis: whereas the hallucinogen lysergic acid diethylamide (LSD) activates 5-HT$_2$ receptors, many atypical antipsychotics inhibit them.[54]

Acetylcholine

The first neurotransmitter to be discovered, acetylcholine (ACh), was initially characterized by Otto Loewi as *Vagusstoff*,

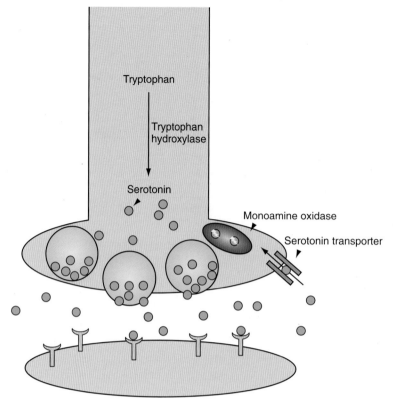

Figure 1.17 The serotonin life cycle.

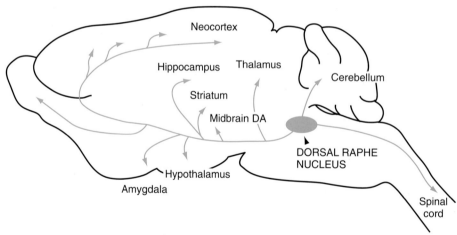

Figure 1.18 Serotonergic projections. (Adapted from NIAAA at www.niaaa.nih.gov/Resources/GraphicsGallery/EndocrineReproductiveSystem/LengthwiseView.htm.)

the mediator of vagal parasympathetic outflow to the heart. As we now know, ACh plays important roles in central as well as peripheral neurophysiology, including the modulation of a host of cognitive functions. In the periphery, ACh is the neurotransmitter for the neuromuscular junction, for pre-ganglionic neurons in the autonomic nervous system and for parasympathetic post-ganglionic neurons. In the CNS, cholinergic neurons are concentrated in the nucleus basalis of Meynert in the basal forebrain and project diffusely to the neocortex (Figure 1.19). There are also cholinergic projections from the septum and diagonal band of Broca to the hippocampus. Cholinergic inter-neurons are found in the basal ganglia.

Acetylcholine is formed in nerve terminals through the action of choline acetyltransferase (Figure 1.20). Its precursor, choline, is supplied through both breakdown of dietary phosphatidylcholine and recycling of synaptic ACh (which

is catabolized by acetylcholinesterase to choline and actively transported back into the pre-synaptic terminal).

There are two classes of ACh receptors: muscarinic and nicotinic. Although muscarinic receptors are G-protein–coupled, nicotinic receptors are ion channels, which allows for rapid influx of Na^+ and Ca^{2+} into the post-synaptic neuron. Both receptor types are abundant in brain tissue.

The cholinergic system is an important target in the psychopharmacology of dementia (pro-cholinergics) and movement disorders (anti-cholinergics).

Acetylcholine and Cognition

Anticholinergic medications affect the balance of dopamine and ACh in the basal ganglia, which can improve EPSs in patients with movement disorders (either primary or secondary

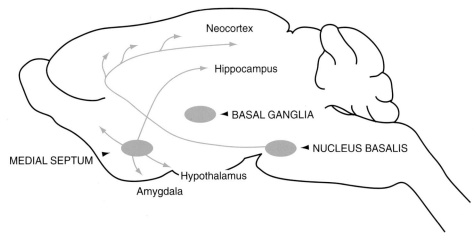

Figure 1.19 Cholinergic projections. (Adapted from NIAAA at www.niaaa.nih.gov/Resources/GraphicsGallery/EndocrineReproductiveSystem/LengthwiseView.htm.)

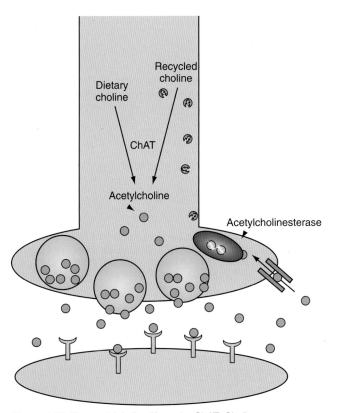

Figure 1.20 The acetylcholine life cycle. *ChAT*, Choline acetyltransferase.

to antipsychotic use). However, alterations in cholinergic transmission caused by medications or to underlying disease can profoundly affect cognition. Anticholinergic medications, such as diphenhydramine, are common sources of delirium in older adults or medically ill patients. Many antipsychotic and tricyclic antidepressant drugs have some anticholinergic activity, which can affect cognition (and produce significant peripheral side effects, including dry mouth, urinary retention, constipation, and tachycardia). The degeneration of cholinergic neurons in AD contributes strongly to cognitive decline; acetylcholinesterase inhibitors may slow this effect somewhat but do not reverse the degeneration process.[56] Nicotine, acting through nicotinic ACh receptors, may produce significant cognitive effects (as well as addictive rewarding effects).

Histamine

Like ACh and NE, histamine serves important functions both in the CNS and peripherally. Histamine is best known for its roles outside the brain in activating immune and inflammatory responses and in stimulating gastric acid secretion. Within the brain, it acts both as a classical neurotransmitter and as a neuromodulator, potentiating the excitability of other neurotransmitter systems.

Histaminergic neurons are concentrated within the hypothalamus in the tuberomammillary nucleus. They project diffusely to cortical and subcortical targets, as well as to the brainstem and spinal cord. Histamine is derived from its precursor, L-histidine, through the action of L-histidine decarboxylase. Histamine can be broken down either through oxidation (via diamine oxidase) or methylation (via histamine N-methyltransferase and subsequently MAO).

Three classes of histamine receptors—H_1, H_2, and H_3—have been found both within brain tissue and in the periphery. Each affects second messenger systems through coupling to G proteins. H_3 may also function as an inhibitory autoreceptor. More recently, a fourth class of histamine receptor (H_4) has also been described but apparently is not expressed in human brain.

Histamine stimulates wakefulness, suppresses appetite, and may enhance cognition through its excitatory effects on brainstem, hypothalamic, and cortical neurons. Drugs with antihistaminic properties can cause significant disruptions of these processes, producing the therapeutic effects of sleep medications, as well as side effects (sedation and weight gain) of some atypical antipsychotics and, in particular, the antidepressant mirtazapine.[57] Animal research shows that whereas histamine depletion adversely affects short-term memory, H_3 autoreceptor antagonists may have the opposite effect; these findings have fueled the development of H_3 antagonists as a potential treatment for memory disorders.

Other Neurotransmitters and Interactions Among Neurotransmitters

Many additional neurotransmitters mediate important effects in the brain; some with relevance to psychiatry include neuropeptides (e.g., endogenous opioids), neurohormones (e.g., corticotropin-releasing hormone), steroids, cannabinoids, and short-acting gases (such as nitric oxide). And although we have focused on one neurotransmitter at a time, numerous and complex interactions occur among neurotransmitter systems. Although discussion of these other neurotransmitters and neurotransmitter interactions is beyond the scope of this chapter, they are of great importance to psychiatric neuroscience and the subject of intensive research.

CONCLUSION

We are fortunate in psychiatry to have multiple treatment choices for most conditions. However, existing treatments are frequently only partially effective. Side effects may interfere with compliance and produce their own morbidity, and even after successful treatment, relapse is common. Despite decades of progress in neuropsychiatric treatment development, we still need better treatments for individuals with mental illness. Greater understanding of the biological mechanisms underlying brain function and dysfunction will be essential in the development of new and better behavioral, pharmacological, or device-based therapies. Important insights will also come from clarifying the specific therapeutic mechanisms of existing treatments.

Over the past century, psychiatric neuroscience has made great strides in linking neural mechanisms to conditions of abnormal affect, behavior, and cognition. However, because of challenges inherent to the study of psychiatric phenomena and brain function, the gap between mechanistic understanding and clinical practice remains wide for most conditions. Genetics and neuroimaging have dramatically enhanced our ability to bridge these gaps, and the accelerating development of these fields provides great hope.

Although our biological knowledge is incomplete, there is already a great deal of information that may be incorporated into our clinical problem-solving. This will be facilitated by applying a systematic framework when evaluating the neuroscientific aspects of clinical cases. Biological formulations should involve consideration of two broad domains: process (the dynamic mechanisms of neurodevelopment, neurotransmission, and neurodegeneration) and content (key regional, cellular, and molecular neural substrates). These biological components of major mental illnesses, identified through decades of research, are extremely valuable in our explanations to patients and families.

REFERENCES

1. Meltzer-Brody S, Colquhoun H, Riesenberg R, et al. Brexanolone injection in post-partum depression: two multicentre, double-blind, randomised, placebo-controlled, phase 3 trials. *Lancet.* 2018; 392(10152):1058–1070.
2. Cole EJ, Phillips AL, Bentzley BS, et al. Stanford Neuromodulation Therapy (SNT): a double-blind randomized controlled trial. *Am J Psychiatry.* 2022;179(2):132–141.
3. American Psychiatric Association.Text Revision. *Diagnostic and Statistical Manual of Mental Disorders.* 5th ed. American Psychiatric Association; 2022.
4. Insel T, Cuthbert B, Garvey M, et al. Research Domain Criteria (RDoC): toward a new classification framework for research on mental disorders. *Am J Psychiatry.* 2010;167(7):748–751.
5. Geschwind N. Mechanisms of change after brain lesions. *Ann N Y Acad Sci.* 1985;457:1–11.
6. Phineas FJ. Gage: A Gruesome But True Story About Brain Science. Houghton Mifflin; 2002.
7. Corkin S. What's new with the amnesic patient H.M. *Nat Rev.* 2002; 3(2):153–160.
8. Fox MD. Mapping symptoms to brain networks with the human connectome. *N Engl J Med.* 2018;379(23):2237–2245.
9. Gur RE, Calkins ME, Gur RC, et al. The consortium on the genetics of schizophrenia: neurocognitive endophenotypes. *Schizophrenia Bull.* 2007;33(1):49–68.
10. Camprodon JA, Stern TA. Selecting neuroimaging techniques: a review for the clinician. *Prim Care Companion CNS Disord.* 2013;15(4).
11. Cunningham MO, Hunt J, Middleton S, et al. Region-specific reduction in entorhinal gamma oscillations and parvalbumin-immunoreactive neurons in animal models of psychiatric illness. *J Neurosci.* 2006;26(10):2767–2776.
12. Widge AS, Ellard KK, Paulk AC, et al. Treating refractory mental illness with closed-loop brain stimulation: progress towards a patient-specific transdiagnostic approach. *Focus (Am Psychiatr Publ).* 2022;20(1):137–151.
13. Camprodon JA, Rauch SL, Greenberg BD, Dougherty DD, eds. *Psychiatric Neurotherapeutics: Contemporary Surgical & Device-Based Treatments in Psychiatry.* Humana Press (Springer); 2016.
14. Camprodon JA, Pascual-Leone A. Beyond therapeutics: multimodal TMS applications for circuit-based psychiatry. *JAMA Psychiatry.* 2016;73(4):407–408.
15. Paus T. Inferring causality in brain images: a perturbation approach. *Philos Trans R Soc Lond B Biol Sci.* 2005;360(1457):1109–1114.
16. Camprodon JA. Transcranial magnetic stimulation. In: Camprodon JA, Rauch SL, Greenberg BD, Dougherty DD, eds. *Psychiatric Neurotherapeutics: Contemporary Surgical & Device-Based Treatments in Psychiatry.* Humana Press; 2016:165–186.
17. Alzheimer A, Stelzmann RA, Schnitzlein HN, et al. An English translation of Alzheimer's 1907 paper, "Uber eine eigenartige Erkankung der Hirnrinde". *Clin Anat.* 1995;8(6):429–431.
18. Alzheimer A. Beitrage zur pathologischen Anatomie der Dementia praecox. *Monatsschr Psychiatr Neurol.* 1897;2:82–120.
19. Stern TA, Camprodon JA, Fava M, eds. *Massachusetts General Hospital Psychopharmacology and Neurotherapeutics.* 2nd ed. Elsevier; 2023.
20. Hyman SE. The daunting polygenicity of mental illness: making a new map. *Philos Trans R Soc Lond B Biol Sci.* 2018;373(1742): 20170031.
21. Smoller JW, Andreassen OA, Edenberg HJ, et al. Psychiatric genetics and the structure of psychopathology. *Mol Psychiatry.* 2019;24(3):409–420. Erratum in: *Mol Psychiatry.* 2018 Mar 14; PMID: 29317742; PMCID: PMC6684352.
22. Report of the National Advisory Mental Health Council Workgroup on Genomics: opportunities and challenges of psychiatric genetics 2017. https://www.nimh.nih.gov/about/advisory-boards-andgroups/namhc/reports/report-of-the-national-advisory-mental-health-council-workgroup-ongenomics.shtml.
23. Milton AL, Holmes EA Of mice and mental health: facilitating dialogue and seeing further. *Philos Trans R Soc Lond B Biol Sci.* 2018;373(1742):20170022. https://doi.org/10.1098/rstb.2017.0022.
24. LeDoux J. The amygdala. *Curr Biol.* 2007;17(20):R868–874.
25. Bear MF, Huber KM, Warren ST. The mGluR theory of fragile X mental retardation. *Trends Neurosci.* 2004;27(7):370–377.
26. Pascual-Leone A, Amedi A, Fregni F, et al. The plastic human brain cortex. *Ann Rev Neurosci.* 2005;28:377–401.
27. Bergmann O, Spalding KL, Frisén J. Adult neurogenesis in humans. *Cold Spring Harb Perspect Biol.* 2015;7(7):a018994.
28. Kang E, Wen Z, Song H, et al. Adult neurogenesis and psychiatric disorders. *Cold Spring Harb Perspect Biol.* 2016;8(9):a019026.
29. Tau GZ, Peterson BS. Normal development of brain circuits. *Neuropsychopharmacology.* 2010;35(1):147–168.
30. Thompson RA, Nelson CA. Developmental science and the media. Early brain development. *Am Psychol.* 2001;56(1):5–15.
31. Caspi A, Moffitt TE. Gene-environment interactions in psychiatry: joining forces with neuroscience. *Nat Rev.* 2006;7(7): 583–590.
32. Caspi A, Sugden K, Moffitt TE, et al. Influence of life stress on depression: moderation by a polymorphism in the 5-HTT gene. *Science.* 2003;301(5631):386–389.
33. Petronis A, Gottesman II, Crow TJ, et al. Psychiatric epigenetics: a new focus for the new century. *Mol Psychiatry.* 2000;5(4):342–346.
34. Meaney MJ, Szyf M. Maternal care as a model for experience-dependent chromatin plasticity? *Trends Neurosci.* 2005;28(9):456–463.
35. Gottlicher M. Valproic acid: an old drug newly discovered as inhibitor of histone deacetylases. *Ann Hematol.* 2004;83(suppl 1): S91–S92.
36. Mesulam MM. *Principles of Behavioral and Cognitive Neurology.* 2nd ed. Oxford University Press; 2000,
37. Schmahmann JD. The cerebellum and cognition. *Neurosci Lett.* 2019;688:62–75.
38. Schmahmann JD. Vascular syndromes of the thalamus. *Stroke.* 2003;34(9):2264–2278.
39. Graybiel AM. The basal ganglia: learning new tricks and loving it. *Curr Opin Neurobiol.* 2005;15(6):638–644.

40. Saper CB, Cano G, Scammell TE. Homeostatic, circadian, and emotional regulation of sleep. *J Comp Neurol.* 2005;493(1):92–98.

41. Ramon y Cajal S. *Histology of the Nervous System of Man and Vertebrates.* Oxford University Press; 1995.

42. Lopez-Munoz F, Boya J, Alamo C. Neuron theory, the cornerstone of neuroscience, on the centenary of the Nobel Prize award to Santiago Ramon y Cajal. *Brain Res Bull.* 2006;70(4–6):391–405.

43. Ongur D, Drevets WC, Price JL. Glial reduction in the subgenual prefrontal cortex in mood disorders. *Proc Natl Acad Sci U S A.* 1998; 95(22):13290–13295.

44. Nestler EJ, Kenny PJ, Russo SJ, Schaefer A, eds. *Nestler, Hyman & Malenka's Molecular Neuropharmacology: A Foundation for Clinical Neuroscience.* 4th ed. McGraw-Hill; 2020.

45. Gould TD, Manji HK. Glycogen synthase kinase-3: a putative molecular target for lithium mimetic drugs. *Neuropsychopharmacology.* 2005;30(7):1223–1237.

46. Herdegen T, Leah JD. Inducible and constitutive transcription factors in the mammalian nervous system: control of gene expression by Jun, Fos and Krox, and CREB/ATF proteins. *Brain Res Brain Res Rev.* 1998;28(3):370–490.

47. Schumacher J, Jamra RA, Becker T, et al. Evidence for a relationship between genetic variants at the brain-derived neurotrophic factor (BDNF) locus and major depression. *Biol Psychiatry.* 2005; 58(4):307–314.

48. Bossy-Wetzel E, Schwarzenbacher R, Lipton SA. Molecular pathways to neurodegeneration. *Nat Med.* 2004;10(suppl):S2–S9.

49. Sanacora G, Katz R. Ketamine: a review for clinicians. *Focus (Am Psychiatr Publ).* 2018;16(3):243–250.

50. Goldman-Rakic PS. The cortical dopamine system: role in memory and cognition. *Adv Pharmacol.* 1998;42:707–771.

51. Mattay VS, Goldberg TE, Fera F, et al. Catechol *O*-methyltransferase Val158Met genotype and individual variation in the brain response to amphetamine. *Proc Natl Acad Sci U S A.* 2003;100(10):6186–6191.

52. Nestler EJ, Alreja M, Aghajanian GK. Molecular control of locus coeruleus neurotransmission. *Biol Psychiatry.* 1999;46(9):1131–1139.

53. Arango V, Underwood MD, Mann JJ. Serotonin brain circuits involved in major depression and suicide. *Prog Brain Res.* 2002;136: 443–453.

54. Meltzer HY. The role of serotonin in antipsychotic drug action. *Neuropsychopharmacology.* 1999;21(2 suppl):106S–115S.

55. Hornung JP. The human raphe nuclei and the serotonergic system. *J Chem Neuroanat.* 2003;26(4):331–343.

56. Cummings JL. Alzheimer's disease. *N Engl J Med.* 2004;351(1): 56–67.

57. Witkin JM, Nelson DL. Selective histamine H3 receptor antagonists for treatment of cognitive deficiencies and other disorders of the central nervous system. *Pharmacol Ther.* 2004;103(1):1–20.

2 Treatment Adherence

Lara Traeger, Zeba N. Ahmad, John B. Herman, and Theodore A. Stern

KEY POINTS

Background

- Among patients with a psychiatric illness, adherence to psychiatric treatments is associated with better treatment outcomes, a lower risk of relapse and hospitalization, and better adherence to treatments for co-morbid medical illnesses. However, barriers to adherence are common, and rates of suboptimal adherence to psychiatric treatments remain critically high.

History

- Over the past several decades, approaches have evolved to help patients continue treatment for chronic health problems.
- The term "adherence," promoted by the World Health Organization, reflects that optimal health outcomes require multi-level efforts to reduce treatment barriers encountered by patients.

Clinical and Research Challenges

- Patient adherence is a necessary component of treatment response and remission of illness.
- Standardized definitions and measures of adherence are needed to support comparisons of risk factors and intervention outcomes across studies and translation to clinical work.
- Adherence curricula should be included in mental health professional training and continuing education programs.

Practical Pointers

- Practitioners are encouraged to collaborate actively with patients to select and monitor psychiatric treatment regimens.
- Optimal patient adherence requires a complex series of behaviors.
- Routine assessment of both modifiable and non-modifiable barriers to adherence throughout the course of treatment enables practitioners to tailor treatment approaches and adherence interventions for individual patients.
- Patient education, including cognitive and behavioral strategies, can enhance adherence to care plans.

OVERVIEW

Poor adherence to psychiatric treatments is a widespread clinical problem that negatively impacts rates of treatment response and remission.[1] Although empirically supported medications and psychotherapies are available for many psychiatric disorders, these treatments are not universally effective. Patients commonly face difficulties in taking prescribed psychotropic medications or attending psychotherapy sessions as recommended and therefore may not achieve optimal outcomes. Moreover, some patients who adhere to treatment recommendations may not experience a clinically significant response, resulting in the need to remain in care and to tolerate treatment plan modifications.[2]

The World Health Organization (WHO) has defined *adherence* as the extent to which patients' health behaviors are consistent with recommendations that they have agreed to with their practitioners.[3] This definition emphasizes that practitioners must collaborate with their patients in making decisions throughout treatment. However, researchers frequently evaluate patient adherence to psychiatric regimens in ways that do not capture the dynamics among patients, practitioners, and health care systems.[4,5] A consensus study across experts in psychiatry ranked treatment adherence to be the most important factor in predicting treatment outcomes, but the least likely to be measured accurately.[6] Common measures include the extent to which patients take their medications at the prescribed dose and timing, attend scheduled clinic appointments, and remain in care. These broad measures are discussed in this chapter (summarizing findings on the prevalence of, and the barriers to, psychiatric treatment adherence). This chapter also highlights the fact that optimal adherence is a moving target that involves complex patient behaviors and multi-factorial challenges and may be enhanced by targeted strategies for patients, practitioners, and systems.

EPIDEMIOLOGY OF ADHERENCE

The estimated prevalence of patient adherence to the use of psychotropic medications has varied widely because of differences in study populations, diagnoses, medication classes, and the definition of adherence. However, evidence strongly supports the notion that poor adherence is common across groups. A meta-analysis of medication non-adherence in individuals with psychiatric disorders indicated that among 120,134 individuals pooled from 35 studies, 49% reported medication non-adherence. For individuals with schizophrenia, major depressive disorder, and bipolar disorder, rates of non-adherence were 56%, 50%, and 44%, respectively.[1]

Reports of adherence to psychotropic medications further reflect problems with premature treatment discontinuation. Moreover, many patients do not inform their physicians about having stopped their medications. Across studies of treatment trials for anxiety disorders (generally lasting 10–12 weeks), 18% to 30% of patients discontinued their treatment prematurely.[7] Among patients with depression, nearly half may discontinue antidepressant treatment within 6 months.[8] Some studies have shown that adults with depression prefer psychotherapy over antidepressants.[9] However, 20% to 70% of those who enter psychotherapy stop attending sessions before the therapy has been completed, with variability based on the clinical population under study.[10]

CLINICAL AND ECONOMIC IMPACT OF NON-ADHERENCE

Lower adherence to psychiatric treatments leads to worse clinical outcomes and to excess health care utilization; these factors contribute in turn to the economic burden of mental illness.[1] Among patients with depression, non-adherence to antidepressants is associated with higher medical costs, hospitalization, and emergency department (ED) visits.[11] Medication non-adherence is also the most powerful predictor of relapse after a first episode of schizophrenia, independent of gender, age of onset, pre-morbid function, patient insight, or other key factors.[12,13] Although little-studied, patient non-adherence also may increase the risk of burnout and fatigue among psychiatric practitioners. Findings emphasize that intervening at multiple levels to enhance adherence has the potential to improve population health and well-being and to reduce excess health care utilization beyond individual improvements in specific treatments.[3]

RISK FACTORS FOR NON-ADHERENCE

Risk factors for non-adherence are complex and varied. In clinical settings, practitioners must consider and address multifactorial challenges to optimal patient adherence (Table 2.1). Key risk factors are summarized next.

Clinical Factors

Mood

Mood symptoms can increase patients' perceptions of barriers to psychiatric care and can adversely affect treatment adherence.[14] Dysphoria and hopelessness may reduce intrinsic motivation for treatment. Patients who experience psychomotor slowing, decreased energy, and poor concentration also may have difficulty engaging in self-care, attending appointments, completing cognitive-behavioral therapy (CBT) assignments, or taking their medications appropriately. In comparison, when patients enter a manic episode, they may experience elevated mood and energy as positive and may not want to take their medications that slow them down. Moreover, when insight and judgment are impaired, patients may not believe that they have an illness that requires treatment.

Anxiety

Anxiety disorders are associated with hyper-vigilance to internal or external stimuli (or both), which may affect a patient's adherence to treatment recommendations in several ways. Some patients become too anxious to leave their homes and to attend scheduled clinic appointments. Anxiety also may interfere with the optimal upward titration or tapering of

TABLE 2.1 Multi-Factorial Influences on Treatment Adherence

Factor	Examples
Clinical	Psychiatric symptoms that may interfere with adherence
	Substance misuse
	Cognitive impairment
Treatment related	Treatment efficacy
	Side effects
	Dose timing and frequency
	Psychotherapy modality
Patient level	Knowledge about psychiatric symptoms and their treatments
	Attitudes, beliefs, and concerns about psychiatric symptoms or treatments
	Attitudes, beliefs, and concerns about health care systems
Practitioner level	Knowledge, attitudes, and beliefs about psychiatric symptoms or treatments
	Knowledge, attitudes, and beliefs about barriers to patient adherence
	Use of adherence assessments and interventions throughout treatment
	Facilitation of therapeutic alliance
	Collaboration with the patient in treatment decision-making
Systems level	Mental health care coverage
	Fragmentation of patient care
	Distance from the patient's home to the clinic and availability of care
	Financial barriers (transportation, co-payments, childcare)
	Barriers to mental health care among racial or ethnic minorities
Sociocultural	Attitudes and beliefs about psychiatric symptoms or treatments within the patient's identified communities (e.g., family, cultural, and religious)
	Mental health stigma within communities
Interactions among factors	The practitioner–patient therapeutic alliance
	The match between the patient's preferences or values and treatments
	The match between the patient's resources or needs and prescribed treatments
	The level of a patient's trust in the practitioner and the health care system
	The patient's access to or use of support for navigating barriers to adherence

medications because patients may attribute transient physical symptoms to changes in medication doses. Among patients with obsessive-compulsive disorder, counting rituals and fears of contamination may preclude adherence to both medication and psychotherapy regimens.

Psychosis

Most studies of adherence to psychiatric treatment regimens have focused on psychotic disorders, including schizophrenia. Problems related to both the disorders and their treatments present significant barriers to adherence. Factors such as younger age, severe positive symptoms, reduced insight into illness, substance use, and treatment side effects (e.g., akathisia) have predicted poor adherence.[15,16] A consensus survey of experts in schizophrenia and bipolar disorder indicated that non-adherence was associated with inadequate treatment efficacy, fear of side effects, and an inability to tolerate the medications.[17]

Substance Misuse

Misuse of substances is an important risk factor for non-adherence in patients with a variety of psychiatric disorders.[1,14] Patients who believe that mixing alcohol or illicit drugs with prescribed medications can be dangerous may eschew use of their medication in favor of alcohol or drugs. Drug intoxication and withdrawal also affect a patient's attention, memory, and mood state, which in turn can interfere with adherence. The financial burden of substances may also negatively affect a patient's ability to make co-payments for medications and clinic appointments.

Patient Factors: Knowledge, Attitudes, and Beliefs

Across psychiatric diagnoses, patients' perceptions of their disorder and its treatment consistently predict adherence or the lack thereof. Higher self-efficacy and an increased locus of control are associated with better adherence.[18] Patients with severe mental illness are more likely to adhere to their medication regimens if they believe that their need for the medications is high and that risk of adverse effects related to the medications is low.[16,17] On the other hand, mental health stigma, denial of one's diagnosis, a poor therapeutic alliance, and lack of insight all increase the risk for treatment non-adherence.[14,19,20] With regard to psychotherapy, trials of CBT for anxiety have shown that patients with a low motivation for treatment, little readiness for change, or low confidence in CBT, in comparison with other treatments, have an elevated risk for early treatment discontinuation.

Economic and Racial or Ethnic Disparities

Structural and financial barriers to taking medications and attending appointments (e.g., a lack of resources for stable housing, transportation, or co-payments) are important risk factors for non-adherence.[21] US health insurance providers historically have restricted mental health services more than other medical services. Some patients may be more likely to forego psychiatric medications if they are balancing medication costs for multiple health conditions.

Racial or ethnic disparities in access to quality psychiatric care are well-documented.[22] However, among patients who do initiate medication or psychotherapy, evidence for differences in treatment adequacy or retention in care is more equivocal. Some studies of severe mental illness suggest that racially or ethnically minoritized patients have poorer adherence to psychiatric medications relative to white patients.[23] A combination of factors, such as access to psychiatric care; differences in medication metabolism, response, and side effects; clinicians' implicit bias; and patients' beliefs and concerns about treatment, may underlie these disparities.[24,25] Practitioners should consider these factors during treatment selection, titration, and management.

Clinical Encounters

Poor practitioner–patient therapeutic alliances and a lack of follow-up increase the risk for treatment non-response and attrition.[19,26] Adherence and medication effects need to be monitored on an ongoing basis. Practitioners can help patients manage expectations by discussing with patients that certain treatments may cause side effects or require adjustments before they confer benefits on psychiatric symptoms and quality of life. The following sections summarize suggestions for assessing adherence and integrating adherence into all phases of treatment.

ASSESSING ADHERENCE

Currently, there is no "gold standard" measure of treatment adherence or a consensus on the adequate or optimal level of adherence among patients. Available tools for assessing

patient adherence to psychotropics include self-report measures, daily diaries, electronic pill containers, ingestible event monitoring systems, prescription refill records, pill counts, laboratory assays, directly observed therapy, and collateral information.[5,27] Practitioners should consider the strengths and limitations of each method, such as cost-effectiveness and reliability, in the context of available resources and the intended purpose of assessment. Self-report measures may be subject to the impact of social desirability or forgetting.[28] Electronic pill containers yield detailed adherence data, but may be impractical when tracking multiple medications. Having free samples and leftover pills from other prescriptions reduces the accuracy of pill counts. Laboratory assays may identify the presence of medication classes or individual agents but cannot confirm daily administration. When appropriate, multiple measures can be used to support a more complete view of adherence.

INTEGRATING ADHERENCE INTO THE TREATMENT COURSE

Initial Consultation

Practitioners commonly underestimate patient barriers to treatment adherence.[29] Adherence must be an explicit, core element of treatment, starting with the initial consultation (Table 2.2). Moreover, practitioners can facilitate a therapeutic alliance early on by transmitting a warm, non-judgmental stance and by demonstrating support and commitment to the patient's well-being. Key tasks include exploring the patient's values and perspectives about symptoms and which treatments

TABLE 2.2 Incorporation of Adherence-Related Inquiries Into Initial Consultation

Component	Areas of Inquiry
History of present illness	What are the patient's beliefs about symptoms and acceptable treatments?
	To what extent are barriers to adherence related to the present symptoms?
	How may the current symptoms affect adherence behaviors?
Past psychiatric history	To what extent were barriers to adherence related to prior psychiatric risk?
	What were the patient's attitudes about medication and psychotherapy?
Substance abuse	Is the patient actively using alcohol or illicit drugs?
Medical history	What are the patient's beliefs about their medical conditions and treatments?
Medications	What are the patient's attitudes, beliefs, and concerns about their current medications?
	How does the patient cope with current medication side effects?
	What types of barriers to adherence does the patient experience?
Family history	What are familial attitudes, beliefs, and coping regarding psychiatric symptoms?
Social history	What are attitudes and beliefs about psychiatric symptoms and treatments within the patient's identified cultural and religious communities?
	How may non-modifiable financial concerns or living situations influence the ability to obtain, store, and take certain medications or to attend the clinic?
	What role should the family play in treatment decision-making and monitoring?
Mental status examination	To what extent may insight, judgment, or cognitive impairments influence treatment adherence?

will be acceptable to them.[30] By evaluating modifiable barriers (e.g., misinformation about medications), practitioners may identify opportunities for intervention. In addition, they should also assess non-modifiable barriers to adherence (e.g., problems created when the patient lives far from the clinic) to recommend feasible treatment options.

Treatment Planning

Active collaboration helps practitioners and patients develop an appropriate, acceptable, and feasible treatment plan. Practitioners may present the pros and cons of available treatment options to arrive at treatment recommendations. Following treatment selection, practitioners may express belief in the treatment and thereby promote optimism that the treatment will result in positive change. As mentioned earlier, however, practitioners also should manage patients' expectations by stating that medications may require adjustments before they confer benefits. Patients are told that treatments can be discontinued if they are ineffective, cause intolerable side effects, or create other issues that are personally important. Notably, the best way for some patients to commit to a specific plan is to enhance their sense of agency to otherwise say "no."

Introduction to Adherence

As early as possible, practitioners should explicate the role of adherence in facilitating treatment goals. This includes normalizing adherence challenges, preparing the patient for regular adherence assessments, and adopting a non-judgmental attitude toward the risk of adherence lapses. Depending on a patient's barriers to adherence, practitioners may integrate specific strategies into the treatment plan, such as increasing the frequency of clinic visits, using a long-acting injectable antipsychotic, reducing the complexity of a medical regimen, and selecting medications based on tolerable side effects.[31]

Ongoing Assessment

Adherence can vary over the course of care and be based on symptom trajectories, although additional data on long-term patterns are needed.[32] The patient's initial evaluation, evolving symptom profile, and barriers to adherence should guide the nature and extent of follow-up adherence assessments (Table 2.3). Engaging in regular discussions helps practitioners foster a treatment relationship in which the patient feels comfortable discussing adherence challenges.

Practitioners should also ask about adherence in an empathic, non-judgmental manner using a tone of genuine curiosity (*How is it going with taking your medications?*). After introducing the topic, they may ask their patient which medications they are taking and how they are taking them. Open-ended questions will identify when the patient is taking medications incorrectly (deliberately or unknowingly). Disarming inquiries are less likely to seem shaming or punitive (*Many people find it difficult to take medication—have you ever forgotten to take yours?*).

PROBLEM-SOLVING BARRIERS TO ADHERENCE

Most patients face barriers to optimal adherence during their treatment course. Practitioners should invest time during clinic appointments exploring non-adherence and tailoring adherence strategies accordingly. A foundational approach focuses on developing and maintaining a strong therapeutic alliance with the patient. The following sections and Table 2.4 provide examples of more targeted strategies.

TABLE 2.3 Patterns of Poor Medication Adherence and Corresponding Concerns to Explore

Adherence Pattern	Potential Concerns to Explore
Takes higher dose than recommended	Are treatment recommendations understood and acceptable? Are symptoms inadequately managed at the lower dose? Is the patient abusing the medication?
Takes lower dose than recommended	Are treatment recommendations understood and acceptable? Are side effects too bothersome? Has the desired effect been achieved at the lower dose? Is the patient concerned about medication tolerance or dependence? Is the patient misusing the remaining medication?
Misses one dose per week	Are treatment recommendations understood and acceptable? Is the patient facing barriers to treatment on days when the dose is missed? Is the patient skipping the dose or doubling the next dose?
Takes pills every other day	Are treatment recommendations understood and acceptable? Is the patient facing barriers on days when the dose is missed? Is the patient having difficulty with medication expenses?
Takes medications sporadically	Are treatment recommendations understood and acceptable? Does the patient have a sufficient understanding or acceptance of the illness being treated or the treatment's mechanism of action?

Education

Patients benefit from building knowledge and from insight gained about their condition and its treatment. Education should be provided in multiple formats (e.g., oral, written, graphic) to illustrate the rationale for the treatment's dose and timing and the reason for the expected treatment duration. However, patients commonly face complex challenges in managing their medication regimens. Interventions that combine patient education with cognitive and behavioral strategies are more effective than the use of educational strategies alone. Across diverse health conditions, multi-component approaches have led to moderate improvements in both adherence and clinical outcomes.[33] When available, some patients also benefit from CBT or other problem-focused therapies for more intensive adherence intervention.

Motivation

Based on the transtheoretical model, readiness to change may fluctuate across five stages, from *pre-contemplation* (not yet committed to the need for psychiatric treatment) to *maintenance* (already adhering to treatment).[34] Practitioners should explore their patient's motivations for treatment on an ongoing basis. Motivational interviewing techniques can be used, as needed, to elicit intrinsic motivation and resolve ambivalence toward treatment.[35] Patients who are mandated or urged by others to start treatment are at higher risk for non-adherence, relative to patients who are ready to change.[7]

Skills

Even with knowledge about and motivation for treatment, many patients need to enhance their problem-solving skills to

TABLE 2.4 Components of Patient-Focused Interventions to Enhance Adherence

Component	Sample Strategies
Education	Education about target symptoms, their treatments, and treatment side effects
	Information in multiple formats (oral, written, visual)
Motivation	Development of a strong practitioner–patient therapeutic alliance
	Identification of intrinsic motivation for adherence (e.g., life goals)
	Identification of other rewards and reinforcements for adherence
	Initiation of peer mentoring
Skills	PROBLEM-SOLVING
	Identification of steps involved in optimal adherence and potential barriers
	Generation and testing of potential solutions to barriers
	Use of incremental goals to reach desired level of adherence
	ADAPTIVE THINKING
	Socratic questioning to guide the patient in the discovery of problematic patterns about adherence (e.g., depressive hopelessness)
	Cognitive re-structuring to generate more realistic and helpful thoughts
	USE OF CUES
	Daily alarms (mobile phone or wristwatch)
	A pill box or electronic pill container
	A mobile phone app for adherence
	Written reminders or stickers in key areas of a patient's home
	Reminders from an informal caregiver
	Tailoring of the medication schedule to the patient's daily life schedule and activities
	Telephone- or computer-based reminders for pill taking, appointments, and refills
	SUPPORT
	Patient counseling or education on support-seeking skills
	Family or group-based interventions
Logistics	Case management or financial counseling to increase access to care
	Simplified dose schedule
	Adherence monitoring via diary or electronic pill cap

BOX 2.1 Adherence-Related Tasks for Patients Taking Psychiatric Medications

- Describe psychiatric symptoms (frequency, severity, characteristics).
- Comprehend information about recommended medications.
- Collaborate with the practitioner to make treatment decisions.
- Obtain prescribed medications.
- Safely store medications.
- Follow the regimen's dose and timing (or make decisions about taking as-needed medications).
- Identify, manage, and cope with side effects.
- Obtain informal caregiver support as needed.
- Attend regular follow-up clinic appointments.
- Identify and raise concerns about medications.
- Continue collaborating to titrate and modify the regimen as needed.

schedules and revising medication times to match specific activities that the patient never forgets (e.g., brushing one's teeth or filling a coffee pot in the morning). Finally, patients may benefit from learning adaptive thinking strategies, such as cognitive re-structuring, to reduce severe interfering thoughts (e.g., *My need for medication is a sign that I am a weak person*). Practitioners can review the success of their patient's strategies at each visit, revising them as needed and setting incremental goals for achieving optimal adherence.

Patients also may benefit from developing communication skills to increase social support for adherence within their families or communities. Occasionally, a patient's loved ones may have concerns about the treatment or may have high expressed emotion at home, which in turn may impede adherence. Practitioners and their patients may plan to initiate an open discussion of these issues directly with loved ones to engage them in the collaborative relationship and invite them to "walk the treatment path" with the patient. Family interventions may be needed to address problems with high expressed emotion.[7]

Logistics

As mentioned earlier, many non-modifiable barriers, such as limitations in mental health insurance coverage and limited resources or mobility to attend clinic appointments, reduce a patient's access to care. Moreover, problems (such as depression) exacerbate hopelessness in navigating these types of barriers.[38] Patients with limited resources need specific, practical support to problem-solve ideas and gain access to available services. Practitioners may consider lower-cost alternatives, explore how patients pay for other medications, and refer patients to resource specialists when available.

FUTURE DIRECTIONS
Research

Standardized terminology and measures of treatment adherence are needed to compare study outcomes and translate this information into clinical practice. The *perceptions and practicality approach* describes how patient perceptions (e.g., beliefs about medication) coincide with practical aspects of care (e.g., resources) to predict adherence.[29] A taxonomy of adherence identifies *initiation*, *discontinuation*, and *implementation* of a medication regimen as key points for defining and reporting on adherence across populations.[39] Prospective studies of non-adherence (including *a priori* measures of potential risk factors, multiple adherence measures and longer follow-up periods)

improve adherence to their prescribed regimens.[35] Adherence comprises a complex series of tasks. Practitioners may use Box 2.1 as a starting point to help their patients organize adherence into practical steps and to identify potential barriers at each step, such as obtaining medication (e.g., difficulty with co-payments), storing medication (e.g., unstable housing or desire to conceal one's psychiatric diagnosis from a housemate), taking medications on time (e.g., problems with forgetting or a co-morbid attention deficit disorder), or raising concerns with the practitioner (e.g., desire to avoid being a "bad" patient). Socratic questioning may help patients further uncover problematic thought or behavior patterns that interfere with their adherence to treatment.

After barriers are identified, practitioners can work with the patient to generate and test solutions for reducing obstacles to care. Forgetting is one of the most common reasons that patients cite for missing or delaying use of psychiatric medications.[36] Based on an adherence intervention for patients with co-morbid depression and medical conditions,[37] patients are encouraged to identify both a plan (e.g., set up a daily alarm) and a back-up plan (e.g., stick a written reminder on one's bathroom mirror) to address each specific barrier. Moreover, practitioners can help by reviewing their patients' daily will increase our understanding of adherence and our ability to identify patients at risk for non-adherence or treatment attrition over time. These findings, in turn, will help researchers and clinicians target modifiable risk factors in patients who need more intensive adherence interventions.

More research is also needed to establish effective, cost-efficient ways to improve adherence, particularly among patients who are medically complex or lower functioning. In stepped or collaborative care models, care managers provide patients with support in consultation with a supervising psychiatrist and each patient's primary medical provider.[32] Telephone or text messaging might support patient engagement in care or treatment response monitoring, although more research is needed to establish its efficacy.[40] Quantitative economic studies will provide leverage with privatized managed care and government agencies by allowing researchers to demonstrate that interventions to improve adherence result in cost benefits such as decreasing ED visits and hospitalizations.

Education

Critical gaps remain in the training of psychiatric practitioners on the assessment and management of treatment adherence. Residency training programs can, and should, provide opportunities to teach about the integration of adherence into routine clinical care. Several curricular components have been recommended along these lines (e.g., defining adherence, identifying the relationship between adherence and treatment efficacy, assessing adherence, intervening to enhance adherence, maintaining the therapeutic alliance).[41,42] National conferences and continuing medical education (CME) programs provide further opportunities to disseminate state-of-the-art interventions and outcomes research.

CONCLUSION

The importance of treatment adherence among patients with psychiatric disorders cannot be overstated. Adherence increases the likelihood that patients will attain treatment response and remission, thereby reducing the burden of mental illness for patients and health care systems. Improving adherence requires strategies that target multi-factorial barriers. In the clinic setting, practitioners should use a collaborative approach with patients and integrate adherence assessment and interventions into all phases of treatment. Brief motivational and cognitive-behavioral strategies can be tailored to help patients increase their knowledge about treatment, as well as their motivation, skills, and support for treatment adherence. CME and training programs can increase the attention to adherence as an integral part of clinical care and as an opportunity to improve patient quality of life and optimize health care utilization.[43]

REFERENCES

1. Semahegn A, Torpey K, Manu A, et al. Psychotropic medication non-adherence and its associated factors among patients with major psychiatric disorders: a systematic review and meta-analysis. *Syst Rev.* 2020;9:17.
2. Gaynes BN, Warden D, Trivedi MH, et al. What did STAR★D teach us? Results from a large-scale, practical, clinical trial for patients with depression. *FOCUS J Lifelong Learn Psychiatry.* 2012;10:510–517.
3. Sabaté E, Sabaté E, eds. *Adherence to long-term therapies: evidence for action.* World Health Organization; 2003. Accessed May 8, 2023. https://apps.who.int/iris/handle/10665/42682.
4. Sajatovic M, Velligan DI, Weiden PJ, et al. Measurement of psychiatric treatment adherence. *J Psychosom Res.* 2010;69:591–599.
5. Lam WY, Fresco P. Medication adherence measures: an overview. *Biomed Res Int.* 2015;2015:217047.
6. Hatch A, Docherty JP, Carpenter D, et al. Expert consensus survey on medication adherence in psychiatric patients and use of a digital medicine system. *J Clin Psychiatry.* 2017;78:e803–e812.
7. Taylor S, Abramowitz JS, McKay D. Non-adherence and non-response in the treatment of anxiety disorders. *J Anxiety Disord.* 2012;26:583–589.
8. Hung Ching-I. Factors predicting adherence to antidepressant treatment. *Curr Opin Psychiatry.* 2014;27:344–349.
9. Givens JL, Houston TK, Van Voorhees BW, et al. Ethnicity and preferences for depression treatment. *Gen Hosp Psychiatry.*. 2007;29:182–191.
10. Gearing RE, Townsend L, Elkins J, et al. Strategies to predict, measure, and improve psychosocial treatment adherence. *Harv Rev Psychiatry.* 2014;22:31–45.
11. Ho SC, Chong HY, Chaiyakunapruk N, et al. Clinical and economic impact of non-adherence to antidepressants in major depressive disorder: a systematic review. *J Affect Disord.* 2016;193:1–10.
12. Dufort A, Zipursky RB. Understanding and managing treatment adherence in schizophrenia. *Clin Schizophr Relat Psychoses.* 2019 online ahead of print.
13. Alvarez-Jimenez M, Priede A, Hetrick SE, et al. Risk factors for relapse following treatment for first episode psychosis: a systematic review and meta-analysis of longitudinal studies. *Schizophr Res.* 2012;139:116–128.
14. Mert DG, Turgut NH, Kelleci M, et al. Perspectives on reasons of medication nonadherence in psychiatric patients. *Patient Prefer Adherence.* 2015;9:87–93.
15. El Abdellati K, De Picker L, Morrens M. Antipsychotic treatment failure: a systematic review on risk factors and interventions for treatment adherence in psychosis. *Front Neurosci.* 2020;14:531763.
16. García S, Martínez-Cengotitabengoa M, López-Zurbano S, et al. Adherence to antipsychotic medication in bipolar disorder and schizophrenic patients: a systematic review. *J Clin Psychopharmacol.* 2016;36(4):355–371.
17. Velligan DI, Weiden PJ, Sajatovic M, et al. The expert consensus guideline series: adherence problems in patients with serious and persistent mental illness. *J Clin Psychiatry.* 2009;70(S4):1–46. quiz 47-8.
18. Marrero RJ, Fumero A, de Miguel A, et al. Psychological factors involved in psychopharmacological medication adherence in mental health patients: a systematic review. *Patient Educ Couns.* 2020;103:2116–2131.
19. Jawad I, Watson S, Haddad PM, et al. Medication nonadherence in bipolar disorder: a narrative review. *Ther Adv Psychopharmacol.* 2018;8:349–363.
20. Deng M, Zhai S, Ouyang X, et al. Factors influencing medication adherence among patients with severe mental disorders from the perspective of mental health professionals. *BMC Psychiatry.* 2022;22:22.
21. Aznar-Lou I, Iglesias-González M, Gil-Girbau M, et al. Impact of initial medication non-adherence to SSRIs on medical visits and sick leaves. *J Affect Disord.* 2018;226:282–286.
22. Puyat JH, Daw JR, Cunningham CM, et al. Racial and ethnic disparities in the use of antipsychotic medication: a systematic review and meta-analysis. *Soc Psychiatry Psychiatr Epidemiol.* 2013;48:1861–1872.
23. Maura J, Weisman de Mamani A. Mental health disparities, treatment engagement, and attrition among racial/ethnic minorities with severe mental illness: a review. *J Clin Psychol Med Settings.* 2017;24:187–210.
24. Londono Tobon A, Flores JM, Taylor JH, et al. Racial implicit associations in psychiatric diagnosis, treatment, and compliance expectations. *Acad Psychiatry.* 2021;45:23–33.
25. Cook BL, Trinh NH, Li Z, et al. Trends in racial-ethnic disparities in access to mental health care, 2004–2012. *Psychiatr Serv.* 2017;68:9–16.
26. Farooq S, Farooq N. Tackling nonadherence in psychiatric disorders: current opinion. *Neuropsychiatr Dis Treat.* 2014;10:1069–1077.
27. Liberman JN, Davis T, Velligan D, et al. Mental health care provider's perspectives toward adopting a novel technology to improve medication adherence. *Psychiatr Res Clin Pract.* 2022;4:61–70.
28. Stirratt MJ, Dunbar-Jacob J, Crane HM, et al. Self-report measures of medication adherence behavior: recommendations on optimal use. *Translat Behav Med.* 2015;5:470–482.

29. Chapman SC, Horne R. Medication nonadherence and psychiatry. *Curr Opin Psychiatry*. 2013;26:446–452.

30. Julius RJ, Novitsky MA, Dubin WR. Medication adherence: a review of the literature and implications for clinical practice. *J Psychiatr Pract*. 2009;15:34–44.

31. Costa E, Giardini A, Savin M, et al. Interventional tools to improve medication adherence: review of literature. *Patient Prefer Adherence*. 2015;9:1303–1314.

32. El-Mallakh P, Findlay J. Strategies to improve medication adherence in patients with schizophrenia: the role of support services. *Neuropsychiatr Dis Treat*. 2015;11:1077–1090.

33. Conn VS, Ruppar TM, Enriquez M, et al. Medication adherence interventions that target subjects with adherence problems: systematic review and meta-analysis. *Res Social Admin Pharm*. 2016;12:218–246.

34. Kini V, Ho PM. Interventions to improve medication adherence: a review. *JAMA*. 2018;320:2461–2473.

35. Spoelstra SL, Schueller M, Hilton M, et al. Interventions combining motivational interviewing and cognitive behaviour to promote medication adherence: a literature review. *J Clin Nurs*. 2015;24:1163–1173.

36. Velligan DI, Sajatovic M, Hatch A, et al. Why do psychiatric patients stop antipsychotic medication? A systematic review of reasons for nonadherence to medication in patients with serious mental illness. *Patient Prefer Adherence*. 2017;11:449–468.

37. Safren S, Gonzalez J, Soroudi N. *Coping with Chronic Illness: A Cognitive-Behavioral Approach for Adherence and Depression Therapist Guide*. 1st ed. Oxford University Press; 2007.

38. Gast A, Mathes T. Medication adherence influencing factors—an (updated) overview of systematic reviews. *Syst Rev*. 2019;8:112.

39. Vrijens B, De Geest S, Hughes DA, et al. A new taxonomy for describing and defining adherence to medications. *Br J Clin Pharmacol*. 2012;73:691–705.

40. Mistry N, Keepanasseril N, Wilczynski NL, et al. Technology-mediated interventions for enhancing medication adherence. *J Am Med Inform Assoc*. 2015;22:e177–e193.

41. Weiden PJ, Rao N. Teaching medication compliance to psychiatric residents: placing an orphan topic into a training curriculum. *Acad Psychiatry*. 2005;29:203–210.

42. Witry MJ, LaFever M, Gu X. A narrative review of medication adherence educational interventions for health professions students. *Am J Pharm Educ*. 2017;81:95.

43. Rosenbaum L, Shrank W. Taking our medicine—improving adherence in the accountability era. *N Engl J Med*. 2013;22:694–695.

3 Pharmacological Approaches to Depression and Treatment-Resistant Depression

Maurizio Fava, Ji Hyun Baek, Andrew Nierenberg, David Mischoulon, Cristina Cusin, Paolo Cassano, and George I. Papakostas

KEY POINTS

- The immediate mechanism of action of modern antidepressants ("immediate effects") involves influencing the function of one or more monoamine neurotransmitter systems (serotonin, norepinephrine [noradrenaline], or dopamine).

- Influencing monoaminergic function has been shown to result in changes in second-messenger systems and gene expression and regulation ("downstream effects"), which may explain the delayed onset of antidepressant response seen with all contemporary agents (with most patients improving after at least 3 weeks of treatment).

- For the most part, all contemporary antidepressants are equally effective when treating patients with major depressive disorder, but relative tolerability and safety vary among agents.

- Despite the recent advances in the treatment of depression, only 30% to 40% of patients achieve remission after initial treatment. An inadequate response to at least one antidepressant given in sufficient doses and for an appropriate duration is called treatment-resistant depression (TRD).

- Various strategies (including switching antidepressants, combining two different antidepressants, augmenting antidepressants, and using non-pharmacological approaches) can be applied to TRD. However, the standard approach for TRD has not been established largely because of a lack of comprehensive investigations.

- Biomarkers to identify the predicting factors of TRD can help clinicians determine an appropriate treatment plan.

- Many patients with TRD are either inadequately treated or misdiagnosed. Clinicians need to systematically re-evaluate the primary diagnosis of depression as well as search for medical and psychiatric co-morbidities.

OVERVIEW

Numerous compounds have been developed to treat depression. Traditionally, these compounds have been called "antidepressants" even though most of these drugs are also effective in the treatment of a variety of anxiety disorders (such as panic disorder and obsessive-compulsive disorder [OCD]) as well as other conditions (Box 3.1).

The antidepressant drugs are a heterogeneous group of compounds that have been traditionally subdivided into major groups according to their chemical structure or, more commonly, according to their effects on monoamine neurotransmitter systems: selective serotonin reuptake inhibitors (SSRIs), tricyclic antidepressants (TCAs) and the related cyclic antidepressants (i.e., amoxapine and maprotiline), monoamine oxidase inhibitors (MAOIs), serotonin norepinephrine reuptake inhibitors (SNRIs), norepinephrine reuptake inhibitors (NRIs), norepinephrine/dopamine reuptake inhibitors (NDRIs), serotonin receptor antagonists/agonists, and alpha$_2$-adrenergic receptor antagonists. Because they overlap, the mechanisms of action and the indications for use for the antidepressants are discussed together, and separate sections are provided for methods of administration and side effects of the more commonly used and newer agents.

MECHANISMS OF ACTION

The precise mechanisms by which antidepressant drugs exert their therapeutic effects remain unknown, although much is known about their immediate actions within the nervous system. All currently marketed antidepressants interact with the monoamine neurotransmitter systems in the brain, particularly the norepinephrine and serotonin systems and to a lesser extent the dopamine system. All these antidepressants essentially target components of monoamine synapses, including the reuptake transporters (that terminate the action of neurotransmitters in synapses), monoamine receptors, or enzymes that serve to metabolize monoamines. What remains unknown is how these initial interactions produce a therapeutic response.[1] The search for the molecular events that convert altered monoamine neurotransmitter function into the lifting of depressive symptoms remains a matter of active research.

Inhibition of monoamine reuptake or inhibition of MAO by antidepressants represents an initiating event that occurs rapidly. However, the actual therapeutic actions of antidepressants take several weeks and result from slower adaptive responses within neurons to these initial biochemical perturbations ("downstream events"). Receptor studies have been useful in understanding and predicting some side effects of contemporary antidepressants. For example, the binding affinity of antidepressants at muscarinic cholinergic receptors generally parallels the prevalence of certain side effects that develop during treatment (e.g., dry mouth, constipation, urinary hesitancy, poor concentration). Similarly, treatment with agents that have high affinities for histamine H$_1$ receptors (e.g., doxepin, amitriptyline) appears to be more likely to result in sedation and increased appetite. Such information is very useful to clinicians and patients when making treatment decisions and to researchers when attempting to develop new antidepressants.

BOX 3.1 Possible Indications for Antidepressants

- Major depressive disorder and other unipolar depressive disorders
- Bipolar depression
- Panic disorder
- Social anxiety disorder
- Generalized anxiety disorder
- Post-traumatic stress disorder
- Obsessive-compulsive disorder (e.g., clomipramine and SSRIs)
- Depression with psychotic features (in combination with an antipsychotic drug)
- Bulimia nervosa
- Neuropathic pain (tricyclic drugs and SNRIs)
- Insomnia (e.g., trazodone, amitriptyline)
- Enuresis (imipramine best studied)
- Atypical depression (e.g., monoamine oxidase inhibitors)
- ADHD (e.g., desipramine, bupropion)

ADHD, Attention-deficit hyperactivity disorder; *SNRI*, serotonin norepinephrine reuptake inhibitor; *SSRI*, selective serotonin reuptake inhibitor.

CLINICAL USES OF ANTIDEPRESSANTS

Since the introduction of fluoxetine, the SSRIs and the SNRIs have become the most frequently prescribed initial pharmacological treatment for patients with major depressive disorder (MDD). The success of these newer agents in displacing TCAs as first-choice agents is not based on established differences in efficacy, but rather on a generally more favorable side effect profile (such as a lack of anticholinergic and cardiac side effects, and a high therapeutic index, i.e., the ratio of lethal dose to therapeutic dose), combined with ease of administration. Furthermore, with certain co-morbidities of depression (such as OCD), SSRIs offer advantages in efficacy over the TCAs. Nonetheless, the TCAs remain useful alternatives for the treatment of some patients with depression. In contrast, because of their inferior safety profile, MAOIs are a class of drugs reserved for patients in whom other treatments have failed. Clearly, the newer antidepressants (SSRIs, SNRIs, NRIs, NDRIs, and serotonin receptor antagonists) all have major safety or tolerability advantages over the TCAs and MAOIs. The newer serotonin receptor antagonist vortioxetine may have the additional advantage of distinctive pro-cognitive effects.

Continuation and Maintenance of Antidepressant Treatment

Originally, based on studies with TCAs, patients with unipolar depressive disorders were observed to be at high risk for relapse when treatment was discontinued within the first 16 weeks of therapy. Therefore, in treatment responders, most experts favor a continuation of antidepressant therapy for a minimum of 6 months after the achievement of remission. The value of continuation of therapy for several months to prevent relapse into the original episode has also been established for virtually all the newer agents. Risk of recurrence after this 6- to 8-month continuation period (i.e., the development of a new episode after recovery from the index episode) is particularly elevated in patients with a chronic course before recovery, residual symptoms, and multiple prior episodes (three or more).[2] For these individuals, the optimal duration of maintenance treatment is unknown, but it is assumed to be much longer (measured in years). In fact, based on research, the prophylactic efficacy of antidepressants has been observed for as long as 5 years with clear benefit. In contrast to the

initial expectation that maintenance therapy would be effective at dosages lower than those required for acute treatment, the current consensus is that full-dose therapy is required for effective prophylaxis.[3] About 20% to 30% of patients treated with each class of antidepressant will experience a return of depressive symptoms despite continued treatment. In such patients, a dose increase of the antidepressant is typically the first-line approach, and this is discussed further later in this chapter (see the Treatment-Resistant Depression section).[4]

Suicide Risk

Unlike the SSRIs and other newer agents, the MAOIs, TCAs, and related cyclic antidepressants (maprotiline and amoxapine) are potentially lethal in overdose. Thus, a careful evaluation of impulsiveness and suicide risk influences not only the decision to hospitalize a person with depression but also the choice of an antidepressant. For potentially suicidal or highly impulsive patients, SSRIs and the other newer agents are a better initial choice than are cyclic compounds or MAOIs. Patients at elevated suicide risk who cannot tolerate these safer compounds or who do not respond to them should not receive large quantities or refillable prescriptions for TCAs or MAOIs. In general, patients who are new to treatment, who are at more than minimal risk for suicide, or who are in an unstable therapeutic relationship should receive a limited supply of all medication. Evaluation for suicide risk must continue even after the initiation of treatment. Although suicidal thoughts are often among the first symptoms to improve with antidepressant treatment, they may also be slow to respond to treatment, and patients may become demoralized before therapeutic efficacy is evident. Side effects (such as agitation and restlessness) and, most important, inter-current life events may exacerbate thoughts of suicide before achieving a full therapeutic response. Thus, rarely, for a variety of reasons, patients may temporarily become more suicidal after the initiation of treatment. If such worsening occurs, appropriate interventions include management of side effects, more frequent monitoring, discontinuation of the initial treatment, or hospitalization. In 2004, the U.S. Food and Drug Administration (FDA) asked manufacturers of almost all the newer antidepressants to include in their labeling a warning statement that recommended close observation of adult and pediatric patients treated with these drugs for worsening depression or the emergence of suicidality. This warning was based on the analyses of clinical trials data that compared the relative risk of emergence of suicidal ideation on these drugs with placebo after initiation of treatment. The difference was small but statistically significant. This finding underscores the need for good clinical practice, which includes education of patients (and families if the patient is a child) about drug side effects (including the possible emergence of suicidal thoughts and behaviors), close monitoring (especially early in treatment), and the availability of a clinician in the event that suicidality emerges or worsens. However, the consensus is that the risks associated with withholding antidepressant treatment from patients, including pediatric patients with serious depression, vastly outweigh the risks associated with the drugs by many orders of magnitude.

CHOICE OF AN ANTIDEPRESSANT

Antidepressants are widely available (Table 3.1), including SSRIs, SNRIs, NRIs, NDRIs, serotonin receptor antagonists/agonists, alpha$_2$-adrenergic receptor antagonists, TCAs and related compounds, and MAOIs. All are roughly equivalent in efficacy. The available formulations and their typical dosages are listed in Table 3.1, and aspects of their successful use are listed in Box 3.2. Selected agents are discussed next.

BOX 3.2 Requirements for Successful Use of Antidepressants

1. Good patient selection as determined by a thorough and comprehensive diagnostic evaluation. Attention should be paid to co-morbid psychiatric and medical disorders.
2. Choice of a drug with an acceptable side effect profile for the given patient.
3. Adequate dosage. In the absence of side effects and response, dose escalations within the recommended range should be pursued aggressively.
4. Use of the antidepressant for at least 6–12 weeks to determine whether it is helping or not.
5. Consideration of drug side effects. Although there are some differences in efficacy across the class of antidepressants for subtypes of depression, the major clinically significant differences among the antidepressants are in their side effects.
6. Use of a drug that was clearly effective in the past if it was well tolerated by the patient.
7. Selection of an appropriate agent for patients with initial insomnia, for example, a sedating secondary amine TCA (e.g., nortriptyline) given at bedtime (a strategy used by some clinicians), avoidance of agents with anticholinergic and cardiovascular side effects (therefore, the sleep-enhancing, alpha$_2$-adrenergic receptor antagonist mirtazapine would be preferred, with the expectation that daytime sedation will abate over time with these medications). An alternative to prescribing a sedating antidepressant is the temporary use of a short-acting benzodiazepine or other hypnotic combined with an SSRI or another non-sedating newer antidepressant, with the expectation of tapering and discontinuing the hypnotic when the depression has improved. Trazodone at lower doses (50–300 mg at bedtime) has been used in place of benzodiazepines or other hypnotics to treat insomnia, particularly middle to late insomnia, in patients treated for depression with an SSRI.
8. Consideration of effects on sexual function. Decreased libido, delayed orgasm or anorgasmia, arousal difficulties, and erectile dysfunction have been reported with almost all of the classes of antidepressants.
9. Awareness of co-morbid conditions. The co-morbid disorder should influence initial treatment selection in choosing an agent thought to be efficacious for the co-morbid condition, as well as the depression, as with SSRIs and OCD or the NDRI bupropion and attention-deficit disorder.
10. Consideration of metabolic effects on drug levels and elimination half-life. Older adults may have alterations in hepatic metabolic pathways, especially so-called phase I reactions, which include demethylation and hydroxylation, which are involved in the metabolism of both SSRIs and cyclic antidepressants. In addition, renal function may be decreased, and there may be increased end-organ sensitivity to the effects of antidepressant compounds. Because the elimination half-life of antidepressants can be expected to be significantly greater than what it is in younger patients, accumulation of active drug will be greater and occur more slowly. Clinically this means that older adults should be started on lower doses, that dosage increases should be slower, and that the ultimate therapeutic dose may be lower than in younger patients.

NDRI, Norepinephrine/dopamine reuptake inhibitor; *OCD,* obsessive-compulsive disorder; *SSRI,* selective serotonin reuptake inhibitor.

Selective Serotonin Reuptake Inhibitors

Because of their favorable side effect profile, SSRIs are used as first-line treatment in most cases of MDD. However, depressed patients with certain characteristics (including those with co-morbid anxiety disorders[5] and more somatic symptoms [such as pain, headaches, and fatigue]) may respond less well to SSRIs than those without such characteristics.

Dosage

Because of their relatively low side-effect burden, the starting dose of SSRIs is often the minimally effective daily dose (Table 3.1A-J). Starting at lower doses and increasing the dose shortly thereafter (i.e., after 1–2 weeks) may further improve tolerability. Maximum therapeutic doses for SSRIs are typically one-fold to four-fold greater than the starting dose. The dosages and formulations of SSRIs marketed in the United States are listed in Table 3.1. Although all SSRIs are effective antidepressants, fluvoxamine is approved in the United States only for the treatment of OCD.

Side Effect Profile

The most common side effects of SSRIs are nausea, tremor, excessive sweating, flushing, headache, insomnia, activation or sedation, jitteriness, dizziness, rash, and dry mouth. The use of SSRIs is also associated with the emergence of sexual dysfunction (including decreased libido, delayed ejaculation, impotence, and anorgasmia) or the worsening of pre-existing sexual dysfunction in depression.[6] Some patients treated with SSRIs may also experience cognitive impairment (such as mental slowing and diminished attention), psychological symptoms (such as apathy and emotional blunting),[7] and motor symptoms (such as bruxism and akathisia). Other less common adverse events associated with SSRI treatment include diarrhea, tremor, bruxism, rash, hyponatremia, hair loss, and the syndrome of inappropriate antidiuretic hormone secretion. There are also case reports of SSRIs worsening motor symptoms in those with Parkinson disease, as well as creating increased requirements for levodopa in Parkinson patients after initiation of an SSRI for depression. SSRIs have been associated with abnormal bleeding (e.g., bruising and epistaxis) in children and adults who have unremarkable routine hematological laboratory results, except for an abnormal bleeding time or platelet count. Although many patients may also experience reduced appetite and weight loss during the acute treatment with SSRIs, this effect does not seem to persist during the continuation and maintenance phases of treatment; one study revealed a greater risk for significant weight gain during long-term treatment with paroxetine.[8] For depressed patients who are unable to tolerate one SSRI, switching to another SSRI has been effective and well tolerated in most cases.[9,10] For patients complaining of gastrointestinal (GI) side effects with paroxetine, the continued-release formulation (Paxil CR) has led to lower incidence of nausea, and it may be used in place of the standard formulation. As with other antidepressants, the potential adverse neuroendocrine and skeletal effects of SSRIs have yet to be systematically explored. SSRIs also appear to possess extremely low toxicity in overdose.

Selective Serotonin Reuptake Inhibitors Discontinuation Syndrome

Several reports also describe discontinuation-emergent adverse events (including dizziness, insomnia, nervousness, irritability, nausea, and agitation) after abrupt cessation of

TABLE 3.1 A Available Preparations of Antidepressants: Selective Serotonin Reuptake Inhibitors

Drug	Therapeutic Dosage Forms	Usual Daily Dose (mg/day)	Extreme Dosage (mg/day)	Plasma Levels (ng/mL)
Fluoxetine (Prozac and generics)	C: 10, 20, 40 mg LC: 20 mg/5 mL Weekly: 90 mg	20–40	5–80	
Fluvoxamine (Luvox and generics)[a]	T: 50, 100 mg	50–150	50–300	
Paroxetine (Paxil and generics)	T: 10, 20, 30, 40 mg LC: 10 mg/5 mL	20–40	10–50	
	CR: 12.5, 25, 37.5 mg	25–50	12.5–50	
Sertraline (Zoloft and generics)	T: 25, 50, 100 mg LC: 20 mg/mL	50–150	25–300	
Citalopram (Celexa and generics)	T: 10, 20, 40 mg LC: 10 mg/5 mL	20–40	10–60	
Escitalopram (Lexapro and generics)	T: 10, 20 mg	10–20	10–30	

[a]Not marketed for depression in the United States.
C, Capsules; CR, controlled release; LC, liquid concentrate or solution; T, tablets.

TABLE 3.1B Available Preparations of Antidepressants: Serotonin Norepinephrine Reuptake Inhibitors

Drug	Therapeutic Dosage Forms	Usual Daily Dose (mg/day)	Extreme Dosage (mg/day)	Plasma Levels (ng/mL)
Venlafaxine (Effexor and generics)	T: 25, 37.5, 50, 75, 100 mg XR: 37.5, 75, 150 mg	75–300	75–450	
Duloxetine (Cymbalta and generics)	C: 20, 30, 60 mg	60–120	30–180	
Desvenlafaxine (Pristiq)	T: 50, 100 mg	50–100	25–200	
Levomilnacipran ER (Fetzima)	C: 20, 40, 80, 120 mg	40–120	20–240	

C, Capsules; T, tablets; XR, extended release.

TABLE 3.1C Available Preparations of Antidepressants: Norepinephrine Reuptake Inhibitors

Drug	Therapeutic Dosage Forms	Usual Daily Dose (mg/day)	Extreme Dosage (mg/day)	Plasma Levels (ng/mL)
Reboxetine[a]	T: 4 mg	4–10	4–12	
Atomoxetine (Strattera)	T: 10, 18, 25, 40, 60 mg	40–80	40–120	

[a]Not marketed for depression in the United States.
T, Tablets.

TABLE 3.1D Available Preparations of Antidepressants: Serotonin Receptor Antagonists/Agonists

Drug	Therapeutic Dosage Forms	Usual Daily Dose (mg/day)	Extreme Dosage (mg/day)	Plasma Levels (ng/mL)
Trazodone (Desyrel and generics)	T: 50, 100, 150, 300 mg	200–400	100–600	
Trazodone Extended Release (Oleptro)	T: 150, 300 mg	150–300	75–600	
Nefazodone (Serzone and generics)	T: 50, 100, 150, 200, 250 mg	200–400	100–600	
Vilazodone (Viibryd)	T: 10, 20, 40 mg	40–80	20–160	
Vortioxetine (Brintellix)	T: 5, 10, 20 mg	10–20	5–40	

T, Tablets.

TABLE 3.1E Available Preparations of Antidepressants: Norepinephrine Dopamine Reuptake Inhibitors

Drug	Therapeutic Dosage Forms	Usual Daily Dose (mg/day)	Extreme Dosage (mg/day)	Plasma Levels (ng/mL)
Bupropion (Wellbutrin and generics)	T: 75, 100 mg XR: 100, 150, 200 mg XL: 150, 300 mg Soltabs: 15, 30, 45 mg	200–300	100–450	

Soltabs, Orally disintegrating tablet; T, tablets; XL, extended release; XR, extended release.

TABLE 3.1F Available Preparations of Antidepressants: Alpha₂-Receptor Antagonists

Drug	Therapeutic Dosage Forms	Usual Daily Dose (mg/day)	Extreme Dosage (mg/day)	Plasma Levels (ng/mL)
Mirtazapine (Remeron and generics)	T: 15, 30, 45 mg Soltabs: 15, 30, 45 mg	15–45	7.5–90	

Soltabs, Orally disintegrating tablet; *T*, tablets.

TABLE 3.1G Available Preparations of Antidepressants: Tricyclic Antidepressants and Other Cyclic Compounds

Drug	Therapeutic Dosage Forms	Usual Daily Dose (mg/day)	Extreme Dosage (mg/day)	Plasma Levels (ng/mL)
Imipramine (Tofranil and generics)	T: 10, 25, 50 mg C: 75, 100, 125, 150 mg INJ: 25 mg/2 mL	150–200	50–300	>225[a]
Desipramine (Norpramin and generics)	T: 10, 25, 50, 75, 100, 150 mg C: 25, 50 mg	150–200	50–300	>125
Amitriptyline (Elavil and generics)	T: 10, 25, 50, 75, 100, 150 mg INJ: 10 mg/mL	150–200	50–300	>120[b]
Nortriptyline (Pamelor and generics)	C: 10, 25, 50, 75 mg LC: 10 mg/5 mL	75–100	25–150	50–150
Doxepin (Adapin, Sinequan, and generics)	C: 10, 25, 50, 75, 100, 150 mg LC: 10 mg/mL	150–200	25–300	100–250
Trimipramine (Surmontil and generics)	C: 25, 50, 100 mg	150–200	50–300	
Protriptyline (Vivactil and generics)	T: 5, 10 mg	10–40	10–60	
Maprotiline (Ludiomil and generics)	T: 25, 50, 75 mg	100–150	50–200	
Amoxapine (Asendin and generics)	T: 25, 50, 100, 150 mg	150–200	50–300	
Clomipramine (Anafranil and generics)	C: 25, 50, 75 mg	150–200	50–250	

[a]Sum of imipramine plus desipramine.
[b]Sum of amitriptyline plus nortriptyline.
C, Capsules; *INJ*, injectable form; *LC*, liquid concentrate or solution; *T*, tablets.

TABLE 3.1H Available Preparations of Antidepressants: Monoamine Oxidase Inhibitors

Drug	Therapeutic Dosage Forms	Usual Daily Dose (mg/day)	Extreme Dosage (mg/day)	Plasma Levels (ng/mL)
Phenelzine (Nardil and generics)	T: 15 mg	45–60	15–90	
Tranylcypromine (Parnate and generics)	T: 10 mg	30–50	10–90	
Isocarboxazid (Marplan and generics)	T: 10 mg	30–50	30–90	
Selegiline Transdermal System (patch) (Emsam)	P: 6, 9, 12/day	6–12	6–18	

P, Patch; *T*, tablets.

TABLE 3.1I Available Preparations of Antidepressants: Gamma-Aminobutyric Acid Type A Modulators

Drug	Therapeutic Dosage Forms	Usual Daily Dose (mg/day)	Extreme Dosage (mg/day)	Plasma Levels (ng/mL)
Brexanolone (Zulresso)	IV: Infusion over 2.5 days	Hours 0–4: 30 mcg/kg/hr Hours 4–24: 60 mg/kg/hr Hours 24–52: 90 mg/kg/hr Hours 52–56: 60 mg/kg/hr Hours 56–60: 30 mg/kg/hr		

IV, Intravenous infusion.

TABLE 3.1J Available Preparations of Antidepressants: *N*-Methyl-D-Aspartate Receptor Antagonists

Drug	Therapeutic Dosage Forms	Usual Daily Dose (mg/day)	Extreme Dosage (mg/day)	Plasma Levels (ng/mL)
Ketamine	IV	0.5 mg/kg once/week or twice/week	1 mg/kg	
Esketamine	IN	56 mg or 84 mg twice/week	112 mg twice/week	
Dextromethorphan-bupropion (Auvelity)	T: 45 mg dextromethorphan hydrobromide + 105 mg bupropion hydrochloride	Initial dose: 1 tablet daily in the morning for 3 days; may increase to 1 tablet orally twice a day		

IV, Intravenous infusion; *IN*, intranasal administration; *T*, tablets.

SSRIs.[11] The risk of such adverse events occurring appears to be inversely related to the half-life of the SSRI, with fluoxetine reported as having a significantly lower risk than paroxetine in two studies. For more severe discontinuation-related adverse events, re-institution of the SSRI and a slow taper may be necessary to alleviate these symptoms.

Drug Interactions

With the possible exception of citalopram and its stereoisomer escitalopram, SSRIs may inhibit cytochrome P (CYP) 450 isoenzymes to varying degrees, potentially causing substrate levels to rise or reducing conversion of a substrate into its active form. Concern about drug interactions, however, is pertinent to patients who take medications with a narrow therapeutic margin and that are metabolized by isoenzymes inhibited by an SSRI, especially when the prescriber is unfamiliar with or unable to determine the appropriate dose adjustment. Reports of clinically significant interactions with the SSRIs are remarkably rare. For all SSRIs, some vigilance is necessary concerning the possibility of an increased therapeutic or a toxic effect of other co-administered drugs metabolized by P450 2D6. If a TCA is combined with an SSRI, the TCA should be initiated at a low dose, and plasma levels should be monitored. The augmentation and combination of SSRIs with other serotonergic agents, tryptophan, 5-HT, or MAOIs may also result in the serotonin syndrome, which has been associated with fatalities.

Use of Selective Serotonin Reuptake Inhibitors in Pregnancy and the Post-partum Period

There is accumulating information about the use of SSRIs in pregnancy, although the bulk of the available data are on fluoxetine. One prospective study of 128 pregnant women who took fluoxetine,[12] 10 to 80 mg/day (mean, 25.8 mg), during their first trimester did not find elevated rates of major malformations compared with matched groups of women taking TCAs or drugs thought not to be teratogenic. There was a higher, albeit not statistically significant, rate of miscarriages in the fluoxetine (13.5%) and TCA (12.2%) groups compared with the women exposed to known non-teratogenic drugs (6.8%). Whether this increased rate of miscarriages is biologically significant and, if so, whether it relates to the drugs or to the depressive disorder could not be determined. Decisions on continuing antidepressant drugs during pregnancy must be individualized, but it must be remembered that the effects of severe untreated depression on maternal and fetal health may be far worse than the unknown risks of fluoxetine or tricyclic drugs. Information from a large registry of fluoxetine exposure during pregnancy is consistent with generally reassuring data from the TCA era that antidepressant agents are not clearly teratogens.

On the other hand, infants exposed to SSRIs during late pregnancy may be at increased risk for serotonergic central nervous system (CNS) adverse effects, although the incidence of these events has not been well established. The FDA has issued a warning for all SSRIs, reporting an increased risk for neonatal toxicity and recommending cessation of treatment before delivery. However, in clinical practice, the risk of postpartum depression often warrants continued treatment and close monitoring of newborns.

Whenever possible, unnecessary exposure to any drug should be minimized, and thoughtful pre-pregnancy treatment planning and consideration of alternative interventions, such as psychotherapies (e.g., cognitive-behavioral therapy [CBT]), are to be recommended.

The SSRIs are secreted in breast milk. Because their effects on normal growth and development are unknown, breast-feeding should be discouraged for mothers who are taking SSRIs.

Serotonin Norepinephrine Reuptake Inhibitors

Venlafaxine, duloxetine, desvenlafaxine, and levomilnacipran share the property of being relatively potent reuptake inhibitors of serotonin and norepinephrine and are therefore considered SNRIs. All of them are approved for the treatment of depression in the United States.

Venlafaxine and Desvenlafaxine

Venlafaxine (Effexor) was the first SNRI to gain FDA approval for the treatment of depression. At daily doses greater than 150 mg, venlafaxine inhibits the reuptake of both serotonin and norepinephrine while mostly inhibiting the reuptake of serotonin at lower doses. The augmentation and combination of venlafaxine with other serotonergic agents, tryptophan, 5-HT, or MAOIs may also result in serotonin syndrome. Venlafaxine is metabolized by CYP 450 2D6, of which it is also a very weak inhibitor. The half-lives of venlafaxine and its active metabolite O-desmethylvenlafaxine are about 5 and 11 hours, respectively. The drug and this metabolite reach steady state in the plasma within 3 days in healthy adults. Venlafaxine is generally effective at daily doses at or above 150 mg, and it is often started at 75 mg or even 37.5 mg, typically in its extended-release (XR) formulation.

Venlafaxine, along with the SSRIs and bupropion, is also commonly selected as a first-line treatment for depression. It is reported as the most popular switch strategy for refractory depression in one large survey of clinicians.

Common side effects of venlafaxine include nausea, insomnia, sedation, sexual dysfunction, headache, tremor, palpitations, and dizziness, as well as excessive sweating, tachycardia, and palpitations; there are also reports of bruxism. Between 2% and 6% of patients experience an increase in diastolic blood pressure, which appears to be dose-related.[13] The abrupt discontinuation of venlafaxine, given its short half-life, also carries a risk of discontinuation-related adverse events similar to those described for the SSRIs.[14] Finally, in one uncontrolled study, 4 of 13 patients treated with venlafaxine during electroconvulsive therapy (ECT) experienced asystole.[15] Although this is a small sample, the use of venlafaxine in patients requiring ECT and perhaps even general anesthesia should be avoided.

Desvenlafaxine (Pristiq) is a major active metabolite of venlafaxine and an SNRI with little affinity for muscarinic, histaminic, or adrenergic receptors. Desvenlafaxine is metabolized by CYP 450 3A4 and it is a very weak inhibitor of 2D6. The half-life of desvenlafaxine is about 10 hours. The augmentation and combination of desvenlafaxine with other serotonergic agents, tryptophan, 5-HT, or MAOIs may also result in the serotonin syndrome. Side effects of desvenlafaxine have included nausea, dry mouth, sweating, somnolence, anorexia, constipation, asthenia, vomiting, tremor, nervousness, abnormal vision, and sexual dysfunction. There have also been reports of increased diastolic blood pressure, and the abrupt discontinuation of desvenlafaxine carries a risk of discontinuation-related adverse events like those described for the SSRIs. In addition, liver enzymes may increase in patients treated with desvenlafaxine. Desvenlafaxine is commonly administered at doses between 50 and 100 mg daily in a single administration.

Duloxetine

Duloxetine (Cymbalta) also inhibits the reuptake of both serotonin and norepinephrine. Duloxetine appears to be as effective as the SSRIs in the treatment of MDD, although in more severe depression, it may have some advantages.

Duloxetine lacks significant cholinergic, antihistaminergic, and alpha$_1$-adrenergic–blocking effects. Duloxetine is extensively metabolized to a variety of metabolites that are primarily excreted into the urine in a conjugated form. The major metabolites in plasma are glucuronide conjugates of 4-hydroxy duloxetine (M6), 6-hydroxy-5-methoxy duloxetine (M10), 4,6-dihydroxy duloxetine (M9), and a sulfate conjugate of 5-hydroxy-6-methoxy duloxetine (M7). Duloxetine is metabolized by CYP 450 2D6, of which it is also a moderate inhibitor, intermediate between paroxetine and sertraline. The half-life of duloxetine is about 12.5 hours. Abrupt discontinuation of duloxetine is associated with a discontinuation-emergent adverse event profile like that seen with SSRIs and SNRIs. Therefore, duloxetine's discontinuation should be accomplished with a gradual taper (over at least 2 weeks) to reduce the risk of discontinuation-emergent adverse events. Duloxetine is commonly used at daily doses of 60 to 120 mg, often started at 30 mg. Duloxetine also appears to be effective for the somatic symptoms of depression, such as pain. Common side effects associated with duloxetine include dry mouth, headache, nausea, somnolence, sweating, insomnia, and fatigue. Duloxetine does not appear to cause hypertension.

Levomilnacipran and Milnacipran

Levomilnacipran (Fetzima) is an SNRI and the 1S-2R enantiomer of milnacipran, an SNRI approved for depression in Europe (brand names: Dalcipran, Ixel). Levomilnacipran is metabolized by CYP 450 3A4, and it is not an inhibitor of CYP 450 systems. Its half-life is about 12 hours. The augmentation and combination of milnacipran or levomilnacipran with other serotonergic agents, tryptophan, 5-HT, or MAOIs may also result in serotonin syndrome. Because of its potent norepinephrine reuptake inhibition, levomilnacipran appears to be particularly effective in treating depression-associated fatigue. Common side effects of milnacipran include headaches, dry mouth, dysuria, tremor, tachycardia, weight gain, and sedation. Levomilnacipran's frequently reported adverse events (≥5% in levomilnacipran ER and twice the rate of placebo) are nausea, dizziness, constipation, tachycardia, urinary hesitation, hyperhidrosis, insomnia, vomiting, and elevated blood pressure. Daily doses of milnacipran range from 50 to 200 mg, often divided in twice-daily dosing, whereas the usual dosage of levomilnacipran ER is 40 to 120 mg once daily.

Norepinephrine/Dopamine Reuptake Inhibitors

Bupropion

Bupropion is a phenethylamine compound that is structurally related to amphetamine and the sympathomimetic diethylpropion; it primarily blocks the reuptake of dopamine and norepinephrine, with minimal or no affinity for postsynaptic receptors.[16] Although some researchers have argued that bupropion's effect on norepinephrine is primarily through an increase in presynaptic release, there is convincing evidence for binding of both norepinephrine and dopamine transporters. Bupropion is rapidly absorbed after oral administration, and it demonstrates biphasic elimination, with an elimination half-life of 11 to 14 hours. Bupropion lacks anticholinergic properties, and it does not cause postural hypotension or alter cardiac conduction in a clinically significant manner. It is a substrate of CYP 450 2B6 and appears to have the potential for CYP 450 2D6 inhibition, which suggests that when it is combined with fluoxetine or paroxetine, both 2D6 substrates, levels of SSRIs may increase. One advantage with bupropion treatment compared with use of SSRIs is the lower risk of sexual dysfunction. Treatment with bupropion is also associated with a lower incidence of GI side effects (e.g., nausea and diarrhea) and sedation than with SSRIs.[17,18] Long-term (44 weeks) bupropion treatment appears to result in weight changes that

are no different than those of placebo in MDD. Thus, long-term treatment with bupropion may convey a lower risk of weight gain than long-term treatment with an SSRI.

The dose range for the sustained-release (SR) formulation of bupropion (Wellbutrin SR) is 150 to 450 mg administered in twice a day or three times a day dosing, with 100 or 150 mg being a common starting dose. A once-daily dose formulation (Wellbutrin XL), available in 150-, 300-, and 450-mg doses, has been subsequently introduced. Common side effects include agitation, insomnia, weight loss, dry mouth, headache, constipation, and tremor. The major medically important adverse event associated with bupropion use is seizure. With the immediate-release formulation the rate is 0.4% (4 per 1000) at doses up to 450 mg/day, whereas with bupropion SR the rate is 0.1% (1 per 1000) at doses up to the target antidepressant dose of 300 mg/day (Wellbutrin SR Prescribing Information). SSRI antidepressants are also associated with seizures at a rate of approximately 0.1% (Wellbutrin SR Prescribing Information). Patients should only be prescribed bupropion with extreme caution if there is a predisposition to having seizures. For this reason, the maximum daily dose for bupropion SR and bupropion XL is 450 mg, with no single dose being greater than 200 mg for the SR formulation. In addition, bupropion may be more likely to induce seizures in those with bulimia nervosa and a history of head trauma; therefore, it should not be used in patients with these disorders. Because the risk of seizure appears to be dose-related and related to peak plasma concentrations, the SR and XL formulations are thought to be associated with a somewhat lower seizure risk, estimated at 0.1% when daily doses lower than 450 mg are used.

Serotonin Receptor Antagonists/Agonists

Trazodone

Although the serotonin receptor antagonists trazodone (Desyrel) and nefazodone (Serzone) have been as effective as SSRIs in the treatment of depression,[19] they are used infrequently as monotherapy for depression. Trazodone is rapidly absorbed after oral administration, achieving peak levels in 1 to 2 hours. It has a relatively short elimination half-life (3–9 hours), and it is excreted predominantly in the urine (75%); its metabolite mCPP has a similar pharmacokinetic profile. Despite its short half-life, once-daily dosing at bedtime is the usual route of administration because of its sedating properties. When used as monotherapy for the treatment of depression, the starting dose is usually 100 to 150 mg daily, given either in divided doses or as a single bedtime dose and gradually increased to 200 to 300 mg/day. An extended-release formulation of trazodone (Oleptro) is available. The dose range for the extended-release form is between 150 and 300 mg every night at bedtime. For optimal benefit, doses in the range of 400 to 600 mg may be needed for either formulation. Low-dose trazodone (25–150 mg at bedtime) is commonly used in the treatment of insomnia from myriad causes, a strategy that may result in improvement of depressive symptoms. The most common side effects of trazodone are sedation, orthostatic hypotension, and headaches. Trazodone lacks the quinidine-like properties of the cyclic antidepressants, but it has been associated, rarely, with cardiac arrhythmias, which may be related to trazodone's ability to inhibit potassium channels. Thus, trazodone should be used with caution in those with known cardiac disease. A rare but serious side effect of trazodone is priapism (of the penis or clitoris), a condition that requires immediate medical attention. Rare cases of hepatotoxicity have been associated with the use of trazodone, and fatal cases of trazodone overdose have also been reported. The minimal effective dose of trazodone for depression is usually 300 mg daily.

Nefazodone

Nefazodone has less affinity for the alpha$_1$-adrenergic receptor; therefore, it is less sedating. The half-life of nefazodone is approximately 5 hours. The usual starting dosage is 50 mg/day, given at bedtime or twice a day and titrated up in the absence of daytime sedation as rapidly as tolerated to achieve a usually effective antidepressant dosage in the range of 450 to 600 mg/day administered in divided doses. A slower dose titration is recommended for older adults. Nefazodone inhibits CYP 3A4 and can result in serotonin syndrome when combined with SSRIs. Common side effects include somnolence, dizziness, dry mouth, nausea, constipation, headache, amblyopia, and blurred vision. An unusual but occasional adverse effect is irritability (possibly related to its mCPP metabolite, which may occur in higher levels in the presence of a CYP 450 2D6 inhibitor). Treatment with nefazodone is associated with a lower risk of long-term weight gain, perhaps because of the appetite-reducing effects of mCPP. Nefazodone also has the advantage of a lower risk of sexual side effects than the SSRIs. A rare but serious side effect of nefazodone is priapism (of the penis or clitoris), which requires immediate medical attention. In addition, an increasing number of reports suggest that treatment with nefazodone is associated with an increased risk of hepatotoxicity (occurring in ~29 cases over 100,000 patient-years), often severe (in >80% of cases) and often appearing during the first 6 months of treatment. Therefore, this agent should be avoided in those with present or past liver abnormalities; liver enzymes should be checked periodically in patients taking nefazodone. The minimal effective dosages for nefazodone are usually 300 mg daily, with 600 mg daily being the optimal dosage.

Vilazodone

Vilazodone (Viibryd) is a serotonin 5-HT$_{1A}$ receptor partial agonist and a selective serotonin reuptake inhibitor. The augmentation and combination of vilazodone with other serotonergic agents, tryptophan, 5-HT, or MAOIs may also result in the serotonin syndrome. Vilazodone lacks significant cholinergic, antihistaminergic, and alpha$_1$-adrenergic–blocking effects. Vilazodone is metabolized primarily by CYP 450 3A4, and it is a moderate inhibitor of 2C19 and 2D6. The terminal half-life of vilazodone is about 25 hours. Vilazodone therapy is typically initiated at a dosage of 10 mg once daily and then incrementally adjusted over 14 days to the recommended target daily dose of 40 mg; for optimal bioavailability and effectiveness, it should be taken after a light or high-fat meal. The adverse effects most commonly reported in clinical trials of vilazodone have been diarrhea, nausea, vomiting, dizziness, insomnia, and dry mouth. Treatment-related sexual side effects may be less likely than with SSRIs. Vilazodone was not associated with clinically relevant weight change in short-term trials. In an open-label 1-year study of vilazodone, mean weight increased by 1.7 kg.[20]

Vortioxetine

Vortioxetine (Trintellix) is an antidepressant with multimodal activity that functions as a serotonin 5-HT$_3$, 5-HT$_7$ and 5-HT$_{1D}$ receptor antagonist, serotonin 5-HT$_{1B}$ receptor partial agonist, serotonin 5-HT$_{1A}$ receptor agonist, and inhibitor of the serotonin transporter in vitro. Vortioxetine increases extracellular serotonin, dopamine, and norepinephrine levels in the medial prefrontal cortex and ventral hippocampus. The augmentation and combination of vortioxetine with other serotonergic agents, tryptophan, 5-HT, or MAOIs may result in serotonin syndrome. Vortioxetine lacks significant cholinergic, anti-histaminergic, and alpha$_1$-adrenergic–blocking effects. Vortioxetine is metabolized primarily by CYP 450 2D6. The terminal half-life of vortioxetine is about 66 hours. Vortioxetine therapy is typically initiated at a dosage of 10 mg once daily and incrementally adjusted by 20 mg once daily; if tolerability is limited, the dose can be lowered to 5 mg daily. Nausea, dry mouth, diarrhea, nasopharyngitis, headache, dizziness, somnolence, vomiting, dyspepsia, constipation, and fatigue were reported in 5% or more of patients receiving vortioxetine. Treatment-emergent sexual dysfunction and weight gain are minimal. Recently presented data suggest that vortioxetine may have the additional advantage of distinctive procognitive effects.

Buspirone

Buspirone (BuSpar) acts as a full agonist at serotonin 5-HT$_{1A}$ autoreceptors and as a partial agonist at postsynaptic serotonin 5-HT$_{1A}$ receptors. Buspirone is FDA approved as a treatment for anxiety and not for depression; however, it has been reported to be effective for MDD. One possible advantage of buspirone is that its use does not appear to be related to a greater incidence of weight gain or sexual side effects than placebo, at least during the acute phase of treatment of depression. Effective antidepressant dosages of buspirone for depression range between 30 and 90 mg/day. Side effects include headache, dizziness, light-headedness, nausea, and insomnia.

Alpha$_2$-Adrenergic Receptor Antagonists

Mirtazapine

Mirtazapine shows linear pharmacokinetics over a dose range of 15 to 80 mg, and its elimination half-life ranges from 20 to 40 hours, consistent with its time to reach steady state (4–6 days). Biotransformation is mainly mediated by the CYP 2D6 and CYP 3A4 isoenzymes. Inhibitors of these isoenzymes, such as paroxetine and fluoxetine, cause modestly increase mirtazapine plasma concentrations, while mirtazapine has little inhibitory effects on CYP isoenzymes; therefore, the pharmacokinetics of co-administered drugs are hardly affected by mirtazapine. Mirtazapine is associated with more sedation and weight gain than the SSRIs.[21] The widespread use of mirtazapine as a first-line agent in depression has been primarily limited by its sedative effects and propensity to induce weight gain.[22] In addition to sedation and weight gain, common side effects associated with mirtazapine include dizziness, dry mouth, constipation, and orthostatic hypotension. Because of blockade of 5-HT$_2$ and 5-HT$_3$ receptors, mirtazapine is associated with a lower risk of headache and nausea than the SSRIs. Treatment with mirtazapine is also associated with a lower incidence of sexual dysfunction than the SSRIs. In addition, switching to mirtazapine may alleviate SSRI-induced sexual dysfunction in SSRI remitters. Severe neutropenia has been reported rarely (i.e., 1 in 1000) with an uncertain relationship to the drug, but as with other psychotropics, the onset of infection and fever should prompt the patient to contact his or her physician. The drug is most efficacious at doses of 30 to 45 mg (although 60 mg/day has been used in refractory cases) usually administered as a single bedtime dose. Available in 15-, 30-, and 45-mg scored tablets and in an orally soluble tablet formulation at 15, 30, and 45 mg, lower doses may be sub-optimal, and compared with 15 mg, the 30-mg dose also may be less or at least not more sedating, possibly as a consequence of the noradrenergic effects that are recruited at that dose. The starting daily dose can be as low as 7.5 mg in older adults.

Tricyclic and Related Cyclic Antidepressants

Although TCAs' overall efficacy in treating depression is equivalent to that of the SSRIs, they tend to have considerably more side effects when taken in very large (supra-therapeutic) quantities. As a result, TCAs are rarely chosen as first-line agents in the treatment of depression, and they are much less frequently used in general psychiatric practices. Furthermore, several studies also suggest that TCAs may be more effective than the SSRIs in the treatment of melancholic depression or in the treatment of depressed patients with certain co-morbid medical conditions. In addition, perhaps because of their ability to inhibit the reuptake of both serotonin and norepinephrine, as well as their ability to block sodium channels, TCAs appear effective in treating neuropathic pain and other somatic complaints. The TCAs may be sub-divided into tertiary amines and secondary amines (their demethylated secondary amine derivatives). In addition, maprotiline (Ludiomil), which is classified as a tetracyclic antidepressant, is commonly grouped with the TCAs because of similarities in dosing, mechanism of action, and side effects. Tertiary amine TCAs include amitriptyline (Elavil, Adepril), imipramine (Tofranil, Antidepril), trimipramine (Surmontil, Herphonal), clomipramine (Anafranil, Clopress), and doxepin (Sinequan, Deptran). Secondary amine TCAs are nortriptyline (Pamelor, Aventyl), desipramine (Norpramin, Metylyl), protriptyline (Vivactil, Concordin), and amoxapine (Ascendin, Defanyl).

Side Effect Profile

In general, the side effects of the TCAs and related cyclic antidepressants are more difficult for patients to tolerate than are the side effects of the newer drugs (Table 3.2), and they probably account for higher discontinuation rates. Thus, treatment is typically initiated at lower doses (e.g., 10 mg/day for imipramine) to minimize the risk of adverse events and premature treatment discontinuation. The side effect profile of the TCAs can be sub-categorized in terms of their relative affinity for several monoamine receptors and transporters. Overall, secondary amine TCAs tend to cause fewer anticholinergic, antihistaminergic, and anti-alpha$_1$–related side effects than tertiary amine TCAs. Amoxapine is the only TCA with documented, significant dopamine D$_2$ receptor antagonism, and it should be avoided in patients with co-morbid depression and Parkinson disease.

Anticholinergic-related side effects result from the affinity of TCAs for muscarinic cholinergic receptors and typically include dry mouth, blurred vision, constipation, urinary hesitancy, tachycardia, memory difficulties, and ejaculatory difficulties. Finally, because of their anticholinergic effects, TCAs should be avoided in patients with narrow-angle glaucoma and prostatic hypertrophy because symptoms related to these conditions may worsen because of such anticholinergic effects.

Antihistaminergic-related side effects result from histaminergic H$_1$-receptor blockade and typically include increased appetite, weight gain, sedation, and fatigue. Weight gain with TCAs can be substantial, averaging 1 to 3 lb per month of treatment.[23] As a result, TCAs may complicate the management of diabetes and worsen glycemic control and should be avoided whenever possible in those with diabetes. TCAs may also have hyperlipidemic effects, thus complicating their long-term use in patients with hyperlipidemia. Xerostomia secondary to anticholinergic and antihistaminergic effects may also increase the risk of oral pathology, particularly dental caries.

Orthostatic hypotension and reflex tachycardia may result from alpha$_1$-adrenergic receptor antagonism. Nortriptyline is generally thought to be less likely to cause orthostatic hypotension than tertiary amine TCAs, such as imipramine; however, nortriptyline's affinity for the alpha$_1$-adrenergic receptor, although less than the affinity of most TCAs, is much greater (e.g., by a factor of 2) than the affinity of desipramine and protriptyline. In addition, homozygosity for 3435T alleles of *ABCB1*, the multi-drug resistance gene that encodes a P-glycoprotein regulating the passage of many substances across the blood–brain barrier, appears to be a risk factor for occurrence of nortriptyline-induced postural hypotension. TCAs may also cause sexual dysfunction and excessive sweating.

The ability of TCAs to inhibit the sodium channel may also result in electrocardiographic changes in susceptible individuals (e.g., in post–myocardial infarction patients, as well as in patients with bifascicular heart block, left bundle branch block, or a prolonged QT interval), even at therapeutic doses, and given that contemporary psychopharmacologists have access to a multitude of alternative treatment options, TCAs should be avoided in these patients. Because of the inhibition of sodium channels and cholinergic receptors, the TCAs also carry a risk of seizures. Maprotiline and clomipramine are considered the TCAs with the greatest risk of seizures. This combined risk of seizure and arrhythmia renders the TCAs as the least safe during overdose.

Prescribing Tricyclic and Related Cyclic Antidepressants

Aside from electrocardiography, no other tests are generally indicated in healthy adults before starting a TCA. TCAs are started at a low dose followed by gradual increases until the therapeutic range is achieved. Finding the right TCA dose for a patient often involves a process of trial and error. The most common error leading to treatment failure is inadequate dosage. In healthy adults, the typical starting dose is 25 to 50 mg of imipramine or its TCA equivalent. Nortriptyline is about twice as potent; thus, its starting dose is 10 to 25 mg. In some clinical situations, especially in older adults and in patients with panic disorder, it may be necessary to start with lower doses (as low as 10 mg of imipramine or the equivalent) because of intolerance to side effects. Generally, TCAs are administered once a day at bedtime to help with compliance and, when the sedating compounds are used, to help with sleep. Divided doses are used if patients have side effects because of high peak levels. The dosage can be increased by 50 mg every 3 to 4 days, as side effects allow, up to a dose of 150 to 200 mg of imipramine or its equivalent at bedtime (see Table 3.1). If there is no therapeutic response in 3 to 4 weeks, the dosage should be slowly increased, again as side effects allow. The maximum dosage of most TCAs is the equivalent of 300 mg/day of imipramine, although uncommonly, patients who metabolize the drug rapidly may do well on higher dosages. Of the currently available cyclic antidepressants, only four drugs (imipramine, desipramine, amitriptyline, and nortriptyline) have been studied well enough to generalize about the value of their blood levels in treatment of depression. Serum levels of the other cyclic antidepressants have not been investigated well enough to be clinically meaningful, although they can confirm presence of the drug or document extremely high serum levels. There is a wide range of effective doses for TCAs. Typical antidepressant doses are 100 to 300 mg/day for imipramine. There is evidence to suggest a relationship between serum levels of TCAs and clinical response. The relationship between clinical response and blood levels for desipramine is linear, and other TCAs have a curvilinear (inverse "U"–shaped curve) relationship between blood level and clinical response.

When used, TCA blood levels should be drawn when the drug has achieved steady-state levels (at least 5 days after a dosage change in healthy adults; longer in older adults) and 10 to 14 hours after the last oral dose. Abrupt discontinuation

symptoms may emerge with TCAs and in part represent cholinergic rebound, and they include GI distress, malaise, chills,
coryza, and muscle aches.

Use of Tricyclic and Related Cyclic Antidepressants During Pregnancy and the Post-partum Period

There are limited data on the use of TCAs during pregnancy.
There have been reports of congenital malformations in association with TCA use, but there is no convincing causal association. Overall, the TCAs may be safe, but given their lack of
proven safety, the drugs should be avoided during pregnancy
unless the indications are compelling. Pregnant women who
are at risk for serious depression might be maintained on
TCA therapy. This decision should always be made very carefully and with extensive discussion of the risks and benefits.
Because of decades of clinical use, older agents, such as imipramine, may be preferred to newer drugs during pregnancy.
TCAs appear to be secreted in breast milk. Because their
effects on normal growth and development are unknown,
breast-feeding should be discouraged for mothers who are on
tricyclics.

Overdoses with Tricyclic and Related Cyclic Antidepressants

Acute doses of more than 1 g of TCAs are often toxic and may
be fatal. Death may result from cardiac arrhythmias, hypotension, or uncontrollable seizures. Serum levels should be
obtained when an overdose is suspected, both because of distorted information that may be given by patients or families
and because oral bioavailability with very large doses of these
compounds is poorly understood. In acute overdose, almost
all symptoms develop within 12 hours.

Anti-muscarinic effects are prominent, including dry
mucous membranes, warm dry skin, mydriasis, blurred vision,
decreased bowel motility, and often urinary retention. Either
CNS depression (ranging from drowsiness to coma) or an agitated delirium may occur. The CNS depressant effects of cyclic
antidepressants are potentiated by concomitantly ingested alcohol, benzodiazepines, and other sedative–hypnotics. Seizures
may occur, and in severe overdoses, respiratory arrest may occur.
Cardiovascular toxicity presents a particular danger (Box 3.3).
Hypotension often occurs, even with the patient supine.

A variety of arrhythmias may develop, including supraven-
tricular tachycardia, ventricular tachycardia, or fibrillation, and
varying degrees of heart block, including complete heart block.

Drug Interactions

The cyclic antidepressants have a variety of important pharmacodynamic and pharmacokinetic drug–drug interactions that
may worsen the toxicity of other drugs (see Box 3.3).

Monoamine Oxidase Inhibitors

Although the overall efficacy of MAOIs does not differ from
that of other commonly used antidepressants in the treatment of MDD, their use is considerably limited by the risk of
potentially lethal adverse events, such as hypertensive crises
and serotonin syndrome, and by the strict dietary restrictions
required to minimize such risks. As a result, they are rarely
chosen as first-line agents in the treatment of depression; their
use is mainly limited to the treatment of treatment-resistant
depression, either as a "next-step" strategy in TCA-resistant
depression[24,25] or even depression resistant to several antidepressants. In addition, perhaps because of their ability to
inhibit the reuptake of dopamine in addition to serotonin

BOX 3.3 Drug Interactions with Cyclic Antidepressants

WORSEN SEDATION

Alcohol
Antihistamines
Antipsychotics
Barbiturates, chloral hydrate, and other sedatives

WORSEN HYPOTENSION

α-Methyldopa (Aldomet)
β-Adrenergic blockers (e.g., propranolol)
Clonidine
Diuretics
Low-potency antipsychotics

ADDITIVE CARDIOTOXICITY

Quinidine and other type 1 antiarrhythmics
Thioridazine, pimozide, ziprasidone

ADDITIVE ANTICHOLINERGIC TOXICITY

Antihistamines (diphenhydramine and others)
Anti-parkinsonians (benztropine and others)
Low-potency antipsychotics, especially thioridazine
OTC sleeping medications
GI antispasmodics and antidiarrheals (Lomotil and others)

OTHER

Tricyclics may increase the effects of warfarin
Tricyclics may block the effects of guanethidine

GI, Gastrointestinal; *OTC*, over-the-counter.

From Rosenbaum JF, Arana GW, Hyman SE, et al., eds. *Handbook of Psychiatric Drug Therapy*. 5th ed. Lippincott Williams & Wilkins; 2005.

---

and norepinephrine, MAOIs appear to be more effective than
TCAs[26] in the treatment of atypical depression (characterized
by mood reactivity as well as by hypersomnia, hyperphagia,
extreme fatigue, and rejection sensitivity). Although to date,
there have been no double-blind studies that compare the
relative efficacy of MAOIs versus the SSRIs or TCAs in the treatment of fatigue in depression, these studies suggest a potential
advantage for MAOIs over SSRIs in atypical depression.

In the GI tract and the liver, MAO catabolizes several
dietary pressor amines (such as dopamine, tyramine, trypt-
amine, and phenylethylamine). For this reason, consumption of foods containing high levels of dietary amines while a
patient is taking an MAOI may precipitate a hypertensive crisis characterized by hypertension, hyperpyrexia, tachycardia,
tremulousness, and cardiac arrhythmias. The same reaction
may also occur during co-administration of dopaminergic
agents and MAOIs, whereas the co-administration of MAOIs
with other antidepressants that potentiate serotonin could
result in a serotonin syndrome because of toxic CNS serotonin
levels. The serotonin syndrome is characterized by alterations
in cognition (disorientation, confusion), behavior (agitation, restlessness), autonomic nervous system function (fever,
shivering, diaphoresis, diarrhea), and neuromuscular activity
(ataxia, hyperreflexia, and myoclonus). Because MAO enzymatic activity requires approximately 14 days to be restored,
such food or medications should be avoided for 2 weeks after
the discontinuation of an irreversible MAOI ("MAOI washout period"). Serotonergic and dopaminergic antidepressants
are typically discontinued 2 weeks before the initiation of an
MAOI, except for fluoxetine, which needs to be discontinued
5 weeks in advance because of its longer half-life. In addition

to its oral formulation, selegiline is also available in a transdermal form (patch), designed to minimize the inhibition of the MAO enzymes found in the lining of the GI tract. Treating MDD with transdermal selegiline appears to be both effective and safe, even in the absence of a tyramine-restricted diet when used at lower doses. Although rare, serotonin syndrome may occur when oral selegiline is combined with serotonergic agents, particularly the SSRIs. The risk of such drug interactions with the transdermal formulation of selegiline has not been studied.

Side Effect Profile

The most common side effects of MAOIs include postural hypotension, insomnia, agitation, sedation, and sexual dysfunction. Other side effects include weight changes, dry mouth, constipation, and urinary hesitancy. A list of side effects with MAOIs is presented in Table 3.2. Older adults may develop constipation or urinary retention while taking an MAOI. Alternatively, nausea and diarrhea have been reported by some patients. Sweating, flushing, or chills may occur. Rarely, hepatotoxicity (which may be serious) may occur with phenelzine. Peripheral edema, likely reflecting effects of the drug on small vessels, may prove difficult to manage. Finally, some patients complain of muscle twitching or electric shock–like sensations.

Dietary Restrictions and Drug Interactions

As discussed previously, treatment with MAOIs carries a risk of hypertensive crisis. To minimize this risk, patients on MAOIs need to adhere to a strict dietary regimen that excludes foods and beverages that have a high content of dietary amines, including all aged cheeses; sour cream; yogurt; fermented or dried meats (sausages, pastrami, pepperoni, chorizo); fava and broad bean pods (lima, lentils, snow peas); marmite yeast extract; sauerkraut; soy sauce and other soy products; overripe bananas and avocado; eggplant; spinach; pickled, dried, or salted fish; caviar; fish roe; and foods containing monosodium glutamate. Patients should also avoid consumption of caffeinated drinks and most alcoholic beverages, especially tap beer and red wine, but also certain white wines, including those that are resinated, aged (sherry), and others (Riesling, vermouth). Sympathomimetics, both prescribed and over the counter (pseudoephedrine, ephedrine, oxymetazoline, dextroamphetamine, and methylphenidate), potent noradrenergic and dopaminergic antidepressants, dextromethorphan, and meperidine (Demerol) may also precipitate a hypertensive crisis. In addition, as mentioned previously, combining MAOIs with potent serotonergic agents (such as the TCAs and SSRIs) carries a risk of serotonergic syndrome. MAOIs must be used with caution in patients with diabetes (because of possible potentiation of oral hypoglycemics and worsened hypoglycemia).

Dosage

The optimal dosages for MAOIs vary from agent to agent. Initially, MAOIs are administered at low doses, with gradual increases as side effects allow. Some tolerance may develop to side effects, including postural hypotension. Phenelzine is usually started at 15 mg twice daily (7.5–15 mg/day in older adults), isocarboxazid at 10 mg twice daily, and tranylcypromine at 10 mg twice daily (5–10 mg/day in older adults). Dosages can be increased by 15 mg weekly for phenelzine and 10 mg weekly for isocarboxazid and tranylcypromine (as side effects allow) to 45 to 60 mg/day for phenelzine (30–60 mg/day in older adults) and 30 to 40 mg/day for the others. Dosages as high as 90 mg/day of these drugs may be required, although these doses exceed the manufacturers' recommendations. When depressive symptoms remit, full therapeutic doses are protective against relapse, although when managing patients taking MAOIs, dose adjustments over time to manage side effects or clinical response are common. For transdermal selegiline, the minimal effective dosage reported is 6 mg/day. It is prudent to taper MAOIs over 2 weeks or more when discontinuing them because discontinuation reactions have been reported with abrupt discontinuation. There is little experience with the use of MAOIs in pregnancy. For this reason, their use should be avoided.

Patients have reported weight gain from all MAOIs and occasionally weight loss (more commonly on tranylcypromine). Anticholinergic-like side effects occur, although they are not caused by muscarinic antagonism. These side effects are less severe than are those seen with TCAs, although patients taking phenelzine may experience dry mouth. Older adults may develop constipation or urinary retention from use of MAOIs. Nausea and diarrhea have been reported by some

TABLE 3.2 Tricyclic Antidepressants and Monoamine Oxidase Inhibitors Side Effect Profile

Category and Drug	Sedative Potency	Anticholinergic Potency	Orthostatic Hypotensive Potency	Usual Adult Daily Dose (mg/day)	Dosage (mg/day)
TRICYCLIC AND RELATED CYCLIC COMPOUNDS[a]					
Amitriptyline	High	Very high	High	150–200	75–300
Amoxapine	Low	Moderate	Moderate	150–200	75–300
Clomipramine	High	High	High	150–200	75–250
Desipramine	Low	Moderate (lowest of the tricyclics)	Moderate	150–200	75–300
Doxepin	High	High	Moderate	150–200	75–300
Imipramine	Moderate	High	High	150–200	75–300
Maprotiline	Moderate	Low	Moderate	150–200	75–225
Nortriptyline	Moderate	Moderate	Lowest of the tricyclics	75–100	40–150
Protriptyline	Low	High	Low	30	10–60
Trimipramine	High	Moderate	Moderate	150–200	75–300
MONOAMINE OXIDASE INHIBITORS					
Isocarboxazid	—	Very low	High	30	20–60
Phenelzine	Low	Very low	High	60–75	30–90
Tranylcypromine	—	Very low	High	30	20–90

[a]Each of the tricyclic and related cyclic compounds have well-established cardiac arrhythmogenic potential.
From Rosenbaum JF, Arana GW, Hyman SE, et al., eds. *Handbook of Psychiatric Drug Therapy*. 5th ed. Lippincott Williams & Wilkins; 2005.

patients. Sweating, flushing, or chills also may occur. Rarely, hepatotoxicity, which may be serious, may occur with phenelzine. Peripheral edema, likely reflecting effects of the drug on small vessels, may prove difficult to manage. Finally, some patients complain of muscle twitching or electric shock–like sensations. The latter may respond to clonazepam, although the emergence of neurological or neuropathic symptoms may reflect interference with absorption of vitamin B_6 that should improve with dietary supplementation of pyridoxine (vitamin B_6) 50 to 100 mg/day.

Overdose

The MAOIs are extremely dangerous in overdose. Because they circulate at very low concentrations in serum and are difficult to assay, good data on therapeutic or toxic serum levels are lacking. Manifestations of toxicity may appear slowly, often taking up to 12 hours to appear and 24 hours to reach their peak; thus, even if patients appear clinically well in the emergency department, they should be admitted for observation after any significant overdose. After an asymptomatic period, a serotonin syndrome may occur, including hyperpyrexia and autonomic excitation. Neuromuscular excitability may be severe enough to produce rhabdomyolysis, which may cause renal failure. This phase of excitation may be followed by CNS depression and cardiovascular collapse. Death may occur early because of seizures or arrhythmias or later because of asystole, arrhythmias, hypotension, or renal failure. Hemolysis and a coagulopathy also may occur and contribute to morbidity and mortality risk.

Drug Interactions

Important drug interactions with MAOIs are listed in Table 3.3.

TABLE 3.3 Interactions of Monoamine Oxidase Inhibitors with Other Drugs[a]

Drug	Effect
Sympathomimetics (e.g., amphetamines, dopamine, ephedrine, epinephrine [adrenaline], isoproterenol [Isuprel], metaraminol, methylphenidate, oxymetazoline [Afrin], norepinephrine, phenylephrine [Neo-Synephrine], phenylpropanolamine, pseudoephedrine [Sudafed])	Hypertensive crisis
Meperidine (Demerol and others)	Fever, delirium, hypertension, hypotension, neuromuscular excitability, death
Oral hypoglycemics	Further lowering of serum glucose
L-dopa	Hypertensive crisis
TCAs, duloxetine, venlafaxine, SSRIs, clomipramine, tryptophan[b]	Fever, seizures, delirium Nausea, confusion, anxiety, shivering, hyperthermia, rigidity, diaphoresis, hyperreflexia, tachycardia, hypotension, coma, death
Bupropion	Hypertensive crisis

[a]This may include selegiline even at low doses.
[b]Tricyclic antidepressants (TCAs) and monoamine oxidase inhibitors are occasionally used together.
From Rosenbaum JF, Arana GW, Hyman SE, et al., eds. *Handbook of Psychiatric Drug Therapy.* 5th ed. Lippincott Williams & Wilkins; 2005.
SSRI, Selective serotonin reuptake inhibitor; *TCA,* tricyclic antidepressants.

TREATMENT-RESISTANT DEPRESSION

Treatment-resistant depression (TRD) refers to an inadequate response to adequate antidepressant treatment. TRD is common in clinical settings. In the Sequenced Treatment Alternatives to Relieve Depression (STAR*D), only 36.8% of patients with MDD who were initially treated with citalopram achieved remission.[27] A recent meta-analytic study reviewed 91 antidepressant monotherapy randomized controlled trials (RCTs) and showed an average remission rate of 44%.[28]

Treatment-resistant depression leads to worse psychosocial functioning[29] and raises the risk of suicide,[30] which increases the disease burden of MDD. Cases of TRD tend to be highly recurrent, with up to 80% of patients requiring multiple treatments. The clinical outcomes of patients who fail to remit are usually worse than those of first-episode patients.

DEFINITION OF TREATMENT-RESISTANT DEPRESSION

Although it appears simple, defining "inadequate response" and "adequate antidepressant treatment" remains controversial.

Inadequate response typically means failure to achieve remission; patients who improve but who fail to remit with initial treatment are more likely to have a recurrence. In clinical trials, remission is usually defined by scores on depression symptom severity scales (e.g., a Hamilton Depression Rating Scale-17 score ≤7). Treatment response and degree of treatment resistance is typically assessed with the Massachusetts General Hospital (MGH) Antidepressant Treatment Response Questionnaire (ATRQ). which has been validated and utilized widely in clinical trials of TRD.

At least one trial with an antidepressant with established efficacy in MDD (with sufficient duration and doses) is considered to be "adequate antidepressant treatment." However, defining "sufficient duration" and "dose" is difficult. Sufficient dose is either the minimum dosage that will produce the expected effect or the maximum dose that the patient can tolerate until the expected effect is achieved. In clinical trials, 4 to 6 weeks has been used as the threshold for sufficient duration, but some researchers suggest using a longer period, up to 8 to 12 weeks.[31] In STAR*D, many patients who initially failed to achieve remission or response, eventually achieved remission or a response by 14 weeks.[32]

STAGING MODELS OF TREATMENT-RESISTANT DEPRESSION

Another important characteristic of TRD is the number of failed trials. As previously mentioned, most clinical studies use a definition of TRD as failure to remit to at least one antidepressant. In other words, those with TRD can fail several antidepressant trials. Although there is no clear method of defining the severity of TRD, it is generally thought that as the number of failed trials increases, the chance of remission will diminish. In STAR*D, 30.6% of patients achieved remission at level 2, and about 13% achieved remission at level 3.[27]

Several staging models have been suggested involving the number of non-responses to adequate treatment strategies and the types of antidepressants used.[33] The MGH Staging Method has been recently revised and is included in Appendix 1, using a very empirical, non-hierarchical approach. In many other staging models, non-response to two agents of different classes has been thought to be more difficult to treat than non-response to two agents of the same class. In addition, there is an implicit hierarchy of antidepressant treatments, with MAOIs being considered as superior to TCAs and SSRIs and TCAs being considered as more effective than SSRIs in some populations. These two concepts have never been fully investigated.[34]

CLINICAL FEATURES ASSOCIATED WITH TREATMENT-RESISTANT DEPRESSION

Several clinical conditions (e.g., substance abuse and co-morbid anxiety disorder) have been associated with TRD.[32] Co-morbid personality disorders, subtypes of depression (including atypical depression, melancholic depression, and chronic depression), and medical co-morbidity have also been associated with a poorer response to antidepressants, though not all studies agree.

CLINICAL APPROACH TO TREATMENT-RESISTANT DEPRESSION

When patients with MDD show an inadequate response (i.e., not achieving remission) with adequate antidepressant treatment, clinicians should consider the possibility of pseudo-resistance (i.e., non-response associated with inadequate treatment).

Misdiagnosis of mood disorders is a relatively common problem in clinical practice. This may involve recall bias associated with retrospective evaluations. When remission does not occur, we recommend that clinicians reassess the patient using a structured clinical interview.

It is also important to assess whether the patient receives "adequate antidepressant treatment." Clinicians need to evaluate whether an antidepressant was used in an adequate dose for a sufficient time and whether the patient took medication as prescribed. Medical co-morbidities (including hypothyroidism, fibromyalgia, and neurological conditions) can also confound treatment response. Conducting routine blood work and a physical examination can provide additional clues. Also, co-administered medication can affect antidepressant metabolism (via inducing CYP P450 enzymes). In some cases, a patient might be a rapid metabolizer of a drug, which results in a lower blood level.

COMMON TREATMENT STRATEGIES FOR TREATMENT-RESISTANT DEPRESSION

Once TRD is confirmed, more rigorous treatment is necessary. Various strategies have been investigated, although the best sequence of treatment has not been established. In general, switching antidepressants, combining two antidepressants, and using augmenting strategies are the most reasonable for TRD. However, the optimal method has not been determined. A retrospective analysis from STAR*D showed no significant differences (in terms of remission rate, response rate, time to remission, and time-to-response) between switching and augmentation strategies.[35]

Switching an Antidepressant

One of the most common strategies is switching antidepressants; however, the superiority of switching to a different class (e.g., from an SSRI to an SNRI) or switching within the same class has not been proven. In STAR*D, switching treatments in Level 2 (i.e., those who had an unsatisfactory result or intolerance of citalopram) involved use of sertraline, venlafaxine XR, or bupropion sustained-release (SR). No significant difference was observed in terms of remission rates (24.8% for

venlafaxine XR, 21.3% for bupropion SR, and 18.1% for sertraline).[27] In addition, the ARGOS study did not find significant differences (in terms of remission rates) between venlafaxine XR and other second-generation-antidepressants (mostly SSRIs) (59.3% for venlafaxine XR, 51.5% for another antidepressant).[36] On the contrary, two of four RCTs demonstrated that switching from an SSRI to venlafaxine was superior to the switching to a second SSRI.[37] One RCT compared the efficacy of mirtazapine, venlafaxine, and paroxetine after failure of two antidepressant trials did not find statistically significant differences in remission rates.[38] A meta-analysis of four clinical trials found only modest, but statistically significant increases after switching to a non-SSRI in patients with SSRI-resistant depression.[39]

COMBINING TWO ANTIDEPRESSANTS WITH DIFFERENT MECHANISMS OF ACTION

Combining two antidepressants with different mechanisms of action is an attractive approach for managing TRD. Combination of an SSRI or an SNRI with a norepinephrine-dopamine reuptake inhibitor (bupropion) or a serotonin-norepinephrine antagonist (mirtazapine or mianserin) is a commonly used combination, with expected synergistic effects of their pharmacodynamic properties.

When using combination treatments, clinicians should be mindful of pharmacokinetic and pharmacodynamic interactions. Serotonin syndrome or the effects associated with increased drug levels (due to CYP P450 enzyme inhibition, e.g., CYP 2D6 inhibition by fluoxetine or paroxetine) might develop.

Augmentation

Lithium

Lithium is one of the most common augmenting agents in TRD. A minimum daily dose of 900 mg is generally recommended. The efficacy of lithium augmentation (with either a TCA or an SSRI) has been supported by randomized, placebo-controlled, double-blind studies. Although in the STAR*D study, lithium augmentation performed poorly (see below under Triiodothyronine). In a meta-analysis, lithium augmentation was found to be significantly more effective than placebo (odds ratio [OR], 3.1; 95% confidence interval [CI], 1.8–5.4).[40]

Triiodothyronine

A meta-analysis of triiodothyronine (T_3) augmentation of TCAs (eight clinical trials; $n = 292$)[41] showed that T_3 augmentation almost doubled the response rate. Limited data on the effect of T_3 augmentation of SSRIs are available. In the STAR*D study, T_3 and lithium augmentations were used in patients who failed to achieve remission after two trials. Although no statistically significant difference was observed (the remission rate of T_3 was 24.7% and that of lithium was 15.9%), there was a clear trend toward greater efficacy of T_3 and the use of T_3 had superior tolerability and adherence. Although T_3 augmentation appears safe, there is limited evidence to guide its long-term adjunctive use. More controlled trials are needed to determine the efficacy of T_3 as an adjunctive medication.

Atypical Antipsychotics

Recently, use of atypical antipsychotics as adjunctive agents has been increasing. A meta-analysis by Nelson and Papakostas[42] of the adjunctive use of olanzapine, quetiapine, aripiprazole, and risperidone (16 trials; $n = 3480$) demonstrated that use of adjunctive atypical antipsychotics was significantly more effective than use of placebo (remission: OR, 2; 95% CI, 2.68–5.72). Aripiprazole, brexpiprazole, quetiapine, cariprazine, and olanzapine–fluoxetine combinations are approved by the FDA for use in patients with either TRD or inadequate response to antidepressants in the United States.

Atypical antipsychotics are apt to induce adverse effects, including extrapyramidal symptoms, tardive dyskinesia, and metabolic syndrome. Discontinuation rates because of such adverse effects are also high. Use of newer atypical antipsychotics with fewer metabolic concerns might be reasonable, although limited evidence is available.

Buspirone

Buspirone is a serotonin$_{1A}$ receptor partial agonist. In the STAR*D study, adjunctive use of buspirone showed a similar remission rate to that of adjunctive bupropion SR in citalopram non-responders (30.1% vs 29.7%). Although there have been positive data from open-label studies, two randomized placebo-controlled trials have failed to find a significant benefit from buspirone.[43]

L-Methylfolate

Folate is an essential co-factor involved in methylation reactions, which are crucial for monoamine synthesis and homocysteine regulation. Abnormal folate metabolism has long been associated with mood disorders. L-methylfolate is a biologically active form of dietary folate. Papakostas and colleagues[44] examined use of L-methylfolate as an augmentation strategy for poor responders to SSRIs. The response rate was 32.3% compared with 14.6% for placebo over the course of two trials. Because L-methylfolate is a medical food, it is safe and has few (minor) side effects. Considering its safety and tolerability, it may be a promising candidate as an augmentation agent for TRD.

S-Adenosyl-L-Methionine

S-adenosyl-L-methionine (SAMe) is the major donor for methyl group in synthesis of neurotransmitters. Along with folic acid, SAMe also has received attention as a promising complementary alternative medicine for the treatment of depression. In a 6-week, double-blind, randomized trial of adjunctive SAMe with SSRI non-responders, remission rates were significantly higher for patients treated with SAMe than with placebo (25.8% vs 11.7%).[45] It is also safe and has few adverse effects.

Novel Therapeutic Agents

New drugs with mechanisms that fall outside of those associated with the classical monoamine receptor hypothesis of depression offer great promise for the treatment of TRD.[37]

Ketamine and Esketamine. Ketamine, an N-methyl-D-aspartate (NMDA) receptor antagonist, has shown rapid antidepressant effects. Recently, several open-label studies[46,47] and double-blind studies with repeated intravenous (IV) ketamine infusions have shown its efficacy in TRD populations. Similarly, a number of trials of intranasal esketamine have demonstrated its efficacy and this drug has been approved by the FDA as a TRD treatment. Both ketamine and esketamine are associated with a risk of blood pressure elevation and dissociative symptoms. Other side effects include dizziness, vertigo (feeling of dizziness and spinning), nausea, loss of feeling

in part of the body, and sedation. These compounds may have anti-inflammatory effects and inflammation is thought to be associated with poorer treatment response in depression.

Brexanolone. Brexanolone (Zulresso) was approved by the FDA for the treatment of post-partum depression in 2019.[48,49] It is a unique antidepressant, derived from allopregnanolone, and is thought to be fast-acting. It is the first antidepressant shown to be effective for post-partum depression. Its mechanism of action includes modulation of gamma-aminobutyric acid type A (GABA$_A$) receptors in the brain, and this may be a contributor to its antidepressant effect. Brexanolone is administered in a continuous IV infusion over 60 hours (2.5 days). Brexanolone is well-tolerated. The most common side effects include dizziness, sedation, dry mouth, fainting and hot flushes. Brexanolone should be avoided in patients with end-stage renal disease who have an estimated glomerular filtration rate of less than $15 \, \text{mL/min}/1.73 \, \text{m}^2$ to prevent accumulation of the solubilizing agent, betadex sulfobutyl ether sodium.

Dextromethorphan–Bupropion. Dextromethorphan-bupropion (Auvelity) was approved by the FDA in 2022 for the treatment of depression, although it is typically used as a monotherapy or augmentation in TRD. It is thought to work within a week of administration, as demonstrated by two double-blind RCTs,[50,51] including one comparing it to bupropion monotherapy. Dextromethorphan functions as an NMDA receptor antagonist, a mechanism similar to the one proposed for ketamine and esketamine; this may explain its rapid onset of antidepressant action. The combination with bupropion offers wide coverage. Doses can be tapered rapidly over 3 days to the maintenance dose of 90 mg dextromethorphan/210 mg bupropion. Common side effects include dizziness, GI upset, headache, fatigue, dry mouth, sexual dysfunction, sweating, anxiety, anorexia, sleep disturbance, joint pain, paresthesias, and blurry vision.

Non-pharmacological Interventions

Adjunctive psychotherapy can be helpful for patients with TRD. In the STAR*D study, cognitive therapy was included in level 2. No significant difference was observed in remission rates between the CBT group and the medication-only group. A randomized trial investigating the effects of CBT in women with TRD ($n = 469$), adding CBT to usual care, significantly increased treatment response compared with usual care at 6 months (46% vs 22%). However, the efficacy of other types of psychotherapy has not been investigated in TRD.

Brain stimulation focuses on the direct or indirect alteration of brain function by electrical or magnetic methods. ECT, the oldest brain stimulation method, has long been viewed as an effective treatment for those with severe depression and TRD.[52] A recent, large trial has shown similar efficacy of ECT compared to IV ketamine. Cognitive impairment is the most common side effect of ECT. Repetitive transcranial magnetic stimulation (rTMS) has emerged as an evidence-based treatment for MDD that does not respond to standard first-line therapies. The majority of data support the use of high-frequency (10 Hz) treatment delivered to the left dorsolateral prefrontal cortex. Intermittent theta burst stimulation is a new emerging treatment that reduces the time required to deliver treatment and can increase capacity and access to this treatment. rTMS is relatively very well tolerated. Vagus nerve stimulation (VNS) therapy stimulates the left vagus nerve repetitively using a small electrical pulse from a neurostimulator implanted on the patient's neck. In an open study with patients with chronic MDD who had failed to respond to more than four adequate antidepressant treatments, the response rate to VNS was approximately 30%. It has been approved as an adjunctive treatment for TRD in the United States. Side effects (such as voice alteration, dyspnea, and neck pain) from VNS are generally mild. However, it requires an invasive procedure, and most of the studies have had relatively small sample sizes. Deep brain stimulation (DBS) was initially developed for the treatment of patients with Parkinson disease. DBS therapy stimulates targeted brain region via electrodes that are permanently implanted. Subcallosal cingulate white matter, the ventral caudate, the ventral striatum, and the subcallosal cingulate white matter are commonly targeted. Several small open studies have shown promise.[53]

More recently, there has been growing evidence for the use of transcranial photobiomodulation (t-PBM) for the treatment of depression, including TRD. t-PBM refers to the application of light on the head aiming to enhance neural function, human cognition, and mood. In this method, near-infrared (NIR) light crosses several tissue layers, including the scalp, periosteum, skull bone, meninges, and dura mater, thus reaching the cortical brain surface. A fraction of the NIR directly increases neuronal metabolism through a photochemical energy transfer.[54] A study included 39 patients with chronic traumatic brain injury) and co-morbid TRD who were treated with multiple sessions of t-PBM (NIR laser devices [810 and 980 nm]). After t-PBM treatment, the depression severity (mean Hamilton Depression Rating Scale or HAM-D score) decreased from 21 to 6 points on average, thus demonstrating full remission.[55] Although there are few and still uncontrolled studies on t-PBM for TRD, this remains a promising off-label intervention.

In severe TRD, psychosurgery also has been tried. Subcaudate tractotomy, anterior cingulotomy, limbic leucotomy, and anterior capsulotomy are the most common methods. Its efficacy has been suggested, but its use is still extremely limited.

RESEARCH CHALLENGES

As previously mentioned, a precise definition of TRD is necessary. Staging models to identify the degree of TRD also need to be conducted, although the MGH Staging Method, included in Appendix 1, seems promising.

Several antidepressant combination strategies have not been confirmed through placebo-controlled RCTs. Newer *antidepressants* with novel mechanisms of action may be promising. Innovative treatment strategies need to be evaluated through more collaborative, multi-center, controlled trials.

Predictive factors to identify which patients are likely to respond well to treatment remain elusive. Biomarkers can help to predict responses to certain treatments. Several studies have suggested that brain-derived neurotrophic factor, inflammatory markers, and abnormalities in the default mode network may be potential biomarkers for antidepressant response, but definitive answers are lacking.

CONCLUSIONS

Depression and TRD are common and challenging to treat, but there are many options available. Because some cases of TRD could reflect pseudo-resistance or non-response because of suboptimal treatment, clinicians should re-evaluate the diagnosis and check the patient's drug compliance when remission is not obtained. Optimal treatment strategies for patients with TRD are not well established. To develop efficacious treatment guidelines for TRD, more rigorous studies with collaborative, multi-center, controlled trials need to be completed with a variety of promising agents. Faster-acting agents, such as ketamine and esketamine, are very promising for those with very severe depression. Identifying mechanisms and predicting factors of poor response to antidepressants will be important. Further studies on biomarkers for TRD are warranted.

APPENDIX 1

Massachusetts General Hospital Staging Model (MGH-S) definition of TRD – Revised
Depression Characteristics

Mild   1
Moderate   2
Marked   3
Severe without Psychotic Features   4
Severe with Psychotic Features   5
Presence of Suicidal Ideations   3
Presence of Anxious Distress   2

(Max score = 10)

Treatment History

No response to each adequate (at least 6 weeks of an adequate dosage of an antidepressant) trial of a marketed antidepressant (based on the Massachusetts General Hospital or Antidepressant Treatment Response Questionnaire) generates an overall score of resistance
1-2 medication trials   2
3-4 medication trials   3
5 or more medication trials   5

Augmentation

1-2 medication trials   2
3-4 medication trials   3
5 or more medication trials   5
Ketamine/Esketamine   3
Transcranial Magnetic Stimulation (TMS)   3
Electroconvulsive Therapy (ECT)   4
Vagus Nerve Stimulation (VNS)   5

(Max score = 25)

Copyright: Massachusetts General Hospital (Amita Chopra, MBBS and Maurizio Fava, MD)

REFERENCES

1. Fava M, Kendler KS. Major depressive disorder. *Neuron.* 2000;28:335–341.
2. Thase ME. Preventing relapse and recurrence of depression: a brief review of therapeutic options. *CNS Spectr.* 2006;11(12 suppl 15):12–21.
3. Papakostas GI, Perlis RH, Seifert C, et al. Antidepressant dose-reduction and the risk of relapse in major depressive disorder. *Psychother Psychosom.* 2007;76:266–270.
4. Fava M, Detke MJ, Balestrieri M. Management of depression relapse: re-initiation of duloxetine treatment or dose increase. *J Psychiatr Res.* 2006;40:328–336.
5. Fava M, Uebelacker LA, Alpert JE, et al. Major depressive subtypes and treatment response. *Biol Psychiatry.* 1997;42:568–576.
6. Fava M, Rankin M. Sexual functioning and SSRIs. *J Clin Psychiatry.* 2002;63(suppl 5):13–16. Discussion 23-25.
7. Fava M, Graves LM, Benazzi F, et al. A cross-sectional study of the prevalence of cognitive and physical symptoms during long-term antidepressant treatment. *J Clin Psychiatry.* 2006;67:1754–1759.
8. Fava M, Judge R, Hoog SL, et al. Fluoxetine versus sertraline and paroxetine in major depressive disorder: changes in weight with long-term treatment. *J Clin Psychiatry.* 2000;61:863–867.
9. Thase ME, Ferguson JM, Lydiard RB, et al. Citalopram treatment of paroxetine-intolerant depressed patients. *Depress Anxiety.* 2002;16:128–133.
10. Thase ME, Blomgren SL, Birkett MA, et al. Fluoxetine treatment of patients with major depressive disorder who failed initial treatment with sertraline. *J Clin Psychiatry.* 1997;58(1):16–21.

11. Fava M. Prospective studies of adverse events related to antidepressant discontinuation. *J Clin Psychiatry.* 2006;67(suppl 4):14–21.

12. Pastuszak A, Schick-Boschetto B, Zuber C, et al. Pregnancy outcome following first-trimester exposure to fluoxetine (Prozac). *JAMA.* 1993;269:2246–2248.

13. Thase ME. Effects of venlafaxine on blood pressure: a meta-analysis of original data from 3744 depressed patients. *J Clin Psychiatry.* 1998;59:502–508.

14. Fava M, Mulroy R, Alpert J, et al. Emergence of adverse events following discontinuation of treatment with extended-release venlafaxine. *Am J Psychiatry.* 1997;154:1760–1762.

15. Gonzalez-Pinto A, Gutierrez M, Gonzalez N, et al. Efficacy and safety of venlafaxine-ECT combination in treatment-resistant depression. *J Neuropsychiatry Clin Neurosci.* 2002;14:206–209.

16. Papakostas GI. Dopaminergic-based pharmacotherapies for depression. *Eur Neuropsychopharmacol.* 2006;16:391–402.

17. Trivedi MH, Rush AJ, Carmody TJ, et al. Do bupropion SR and sertraline differ in their effects on anxiety in depressed patients? *J Clin Psychiatry.* 2001;62:776–781.

18. Papakostas GI, Nutt DJ, Hallett LA, et al. Resolution of sleepiness and fatigue in major depressive disorder: a comparison of bupropion and the selective serotonin reuptake inhibitors. *Biol Psychiatry.* 2006;60:1350–1355.

19. Papakostas GI, Fava M. A meta-analysis of clinical trials comparing the serotonin (5HT)-2 receptor antagonists trazodone and nefazodone with a selective serotonin reuptake inhibitor for the treatment of major depressive disorder. *Eur Psychiatry.* 2007;22:444–447.

20. Citrome L. Vilazodone for major depressive disorder: a systematic review of the efficacy and safety profile for this newly approved antidepressant—what is the number needed to treat, number needed to harm and likelihood to be helped or harmed? *Int J Clin Pract.* 2012;66:356–368.

21. Papakostas GI, Homberger CH, Fava M. A meta-analysis of clinical trials comparing mirtazapine with a selective serotonin reuptake inhibitor for the treatment of major depressive disorder. *J Psychopharmacol.* 2008;22:843–848.

22. Schatzberg AF, Kremer C, Rodrigues HE, et al. Mirtazapine vs. Paroxetine Study Group: double-blind, randomized comparison of mirtazapine and paroxetine in elderly depressed patients. *Am J Geriatr Psychiatry.* 2002;10:541–550.

23. Fava M. Weight gain and antidepressants. *J Clin Psychiatry.* 2000;61(suppl 11):37–41.

24. McGrath PJ, Stewart JW, Nunes EV, et al. A double-blind crossover trial of imipramine and phenelzine for outpatients with treatment-refractory depression. *Am J Psychiatry.* 1993;150:118–123.

25. McGrath PJ, Stewart JW, Harrison W, et al. Treatment of tricyclic refractory depression with a monoamine oxidase inhibitor antidepressant. *Psychopharmacol Bull.* 1987;23:169–172.

26. Thase ME, Trivedi MH, Rush AJ. MAOIs in the contemporary treatment of depression. *Neuropsychopharmacology.* 1995;12:185–219.

27. Rush AJ, Trivedi MH, Wisniewski SR, et al. Acute and longer-term outcomes in depressed outpatients requiring one or several treatment steps: a STAR*D report. *Am J Psychiatry.* 2006;163:1905–1917.

28. Sinyor M, Schaffer A, Smart KA, et al. Sponsorship, antidepressant dose, and outcome in major depressive disorder: meta-analysis of randomized controlled trials. *J Clin Psychiatry.* 2012;73:e277–e287.

29. Fekadu A, Wooderson SC, Markopoulo K, et al. What happens to patients with treatment-resistant depression? A systematic review of medium to long term outcome studies. *J Affect Disord.* 2009;116:4–11.

30. Kiloh LG, Andrews G, Neilson M. The long-term outcome of depressive illness. *Br J Psychiatry.* 1988;153:752–757.

31. Donovan SJ, Quitkin FM, Stewart JW, et al. Duration of antidepressant trials: clinical and research implications. *J Clin Psychopharmacol.* 1994;14:64–66.

32. Trivedi MH, Rush AJ, Wisniewski SR, et al. Evaluation of outcomes with citalopram for depression using measurement-based care in STAR*D: implications for clinical practice. *Am J Psychiatry.* 2006;163:28–40.

33. Thase ME, Rush AJ. When at first you don't succeed: sequential strategies for antidepressant non-responders. *J Clin Psychiatry.* 1997;58(suppl 13):23–29.

34. Fava M. Diagnosis and definition of treatment-resistant depression. *Biol Psychiatry.* 2003;53:649–659.

35. Gaynes BN, Dusetzina SB, Ellis AR, et al. Treating depression after initial treatment failure: directly comparing switch and augmenting strategies in STAR*D. *J Clin Psychopharmacol.* 2012;32:114–119.

36. Baldomero EB, Ubago JG, Cercos CL, et al. Venlafaxine extended release versus conventional antidepressants in the remission of depressive disorders after previous antidepressant failure: ARGOS study. *Depress Anxiety.* 2005;22:68–76.

37. Carvalho AF, Berk M, Hyphantis TN, et al. The integrative management of treatment-resistant depression: a comprehensive review and perspectives. *Psychother Psychosom.* 2014;83:70–88.

38. Fang Y, Yuan C, Xu Y, et al. Comparisons of the efficacy and tolerability of extended-release venlafaxine, mirtazapine, and paroxetine in treatment-resistant depression: a double-blind, randomized pilot study in a Chinese population. *J Clin Psychopharmacol.* 2012;30:357–364.

39. Papakostas GI, Fava M, Thase ME. Treatment of SSRI-resistant depression: a meta-analysis comparing within- versus across-class switches. *Biol Psychiatry.* 2008;63:699–704.

40. Crossley NA, Bauer M. Acceleration and augmentation of antidepressants with lithium for depressive disorders: two meta-analyses of randomized, placebo-controlled trials. *J Clin Psychiatry.* 2007;68:935–940.

41. Aronson R, Offman HJ, Joffe RT, et al. Triiodothyronine augmentation in the treatment of refractory depression. A meta-analysis. *Arch Gen Psychiatry.* 1996;53:842–848.

42. Nelson JC, Papakostas GI. Atypical antipsychotic augmentation in major depressive disorder: a meta-analysis of placebo-controlled randomized trials. *Am J Psychiatry.* 2009;166:980–991.

43. Connolly KR, Thase ME. If at first you don't succeed: a review of the evidence for antidepressant augmentation, combination and switching strategies. *Drugs.* 2011;71:43–64.

44. Papakostas GI, Shelton RC, Zajecka JM, et al. L-methylfolate as adjunctive therapy for SSRI-resistant major depression: results of two randomized, double-blind, parallel-sequential trials. *Am J Psychiatry.* 2012;169:1267–1274.

45. Papakostas GI, Mischoulon D, Shyu I, et al. S-adenosyl methionine (SAMe) augmentation of serotonin reuptake inhibitors for antidepressant non-responders with major depressive disorder: a double-blind, randomized clinical trial. *Am J Psychiatry.* 2012;167:942–948.

46. Haile CN, Murrough JW, Iosifescu DV, et al. Plasma brain derived neurotrophic factor (BDNF) and response to ketamine in treatment-resistant depression. *Int J Neuropsychopharmacol.* 2014;17:331–336.

47. Shiroma PR, Johns B, Kuskowski M, et al. Augmentation of response and remission to serial intravenous subanesthetic ketamine in treatment resistant depression. *J Affect Disord.* 2014;155:123–129.

48. Kanes S, Colquhoun H, Gunduz-Bruce H, et al. Brexanolone (SAGE-547 injection) in post-partum depression: a randomised controlled trial. *Lancet.* 2017;390:480–489.

49. Meltzer-Brody S, Colquhoun H, Riesenberg R, et al. Brexanolone injection in post-partum depression: two multicentre, double-blind, randomised, placebo-controlled, phase 3 trials. *Lancet.* 2018;392:1058–1070.

50. Iosifescu DV, Jones A, O'Gorman C, et al. Efficacy and safety of AXS-05 (dextromethorphan-bupropion) in patients with major depressive disorder: a phase 3 randomized clinical trial (GEMINI). *J Clin Psychiatry.* 2022;83:21m14345.

51. Tabuteau H, Jones A, Anderson A, et al. Effect of AXS-05 (dextromethorphan-bupropion) in major depressive disorder: a randomized double-blind controlled trial. *Am J Psychiatry.* 2022;179:490–499.

52. Kellner CH, Greenberg RM, Murrough JW, et al. ECT in treatment-resistant depression. *Am J Psychiatry.* 2012;169:1238–1244.

53. Gaynes BN, Lux LJ, Lloyd SW, et al. *Nonpharmacologic Interventions for Treatment-Resistant Depression in Adults.* Rockville (MD): Agency for Healthcare Research and Quality (US); 2011 Sep.Report No.: 11-EHC056-EF.

54. Caldieraro MA, Cassano P. Transcranial and systemic photobiomodulation for major depressive disorder: a systematic review of efficacy, tolerability and biological mechanisms. *J Affect Disord.* 2019;243:262–273.

55. Henderson TA, Morries LD. Multi-watt near-infrared phototherapy for the treatment of comorbid depression: an open-label single-arm study. *Front Psychiatry.* 2017;8:187.

4 Lithium and Its Role in Psychiatry

Masoud Kamali, Michael J. Ostacher, and Roy H. Perlis

KEY POINTS

- Lithium remains a first-line treatment for all phases of bipolar disorder, including mania, depression, and the prevention of recurrence.
- A large body of evidence supports a role for lithium in decreasing the risk of suicide.
- Lithium has a narrow therapeutic window, necessitating careful titration and close monitoring of its plasma levels.
- Lithium toxicity may cause confusion and ataxia.
- Drugs that affect lithium levels include non-steroidal anti-inflammatory drugs and diuretics.

HISTORICAL CONTEXT

The first specific description of the application of lithium to treat mania occurred in 1949 by an Australian named John Cade, who observed that lithium had calming effects on animals; subsequently, he treated a series of 10 agitated manic patients with lithium. However, descriptions of lithium treatment date back to at least the American Civil War. An 1883 textbook by Union Army Surgeon General William Hammond recommended the use of lithium bromide to treat manic or agitated patients. In the early 1900s, a Danish physician, Lange, published a case series on the treatment of manic patients with lithium carbonate. Unfortunately, there is little evidence that lithium was studied further until Garrod proposed that lithium urate could be used to treat gout, which opened the door to its broader therapeutic applications. However, despite early studies by Mogen Schou and others, lithium's wider adoption in the United States was hindered by concerns about lithium toxicity. Lithium chloride had been used as a sodium substitute in the 1940s, until several deaths from lithium toxicity were reported among patients with hyponatremia. Thus, lithium was initially perceived as too dangerous for clinical application, and it was only in 1970 that lithium was approved by the US Food and Drug Administration (FDA) for the treatment of mania.[1]

Lithium's Mechanism of Action

The mechanisms by which lithium exerts its therapeutic effects are not known. Animal models and clinical studies have pointed to effects on neurotransmission, neuroprotection, and intracellular molecular pathways; however, the relationship among these findings and clinical changes in patients remains incompletely understood. Several major intracellular second-messenger pathways are influenced by lithium. For example, re-cycling of inositol is inhibited by lithium, leading to inositol depletion, which influences inositol 1,4,5-trisphosphate ($InsP_3$)–dependent intracellular second-messenger signaling.[2,3] $InsP_3$ signaling acts in part by regulating intracellular calcium release and protein kinase activation, which has broad effects.

Lithium inhibits protein kinase C, which leads to reduced excitatory neurotransmission and glycogen synthesis kinase 3 (GSK3), an important enzyme involved in regulation of glycogen synthesis, gene transcription, synaptic plasticity, and cell structure and a negative regulator of the Wnt signaling cascade.[3-7] Of course, both $InsP_3$ and GSK3 pathways have convergent effects—for example, both influence serine/threonine kinase Akt-1, which is a neuroprotective pathway.[8,9] Further evidence for the neuroprotective and neurotrophic effects of lithium come from observations that lithium-treated individuals have a greater global gray matter volume compared with patients never treated with lithium.[10] At a neuronal level, lithium acts both pre- and post-synaptically to decrease excitatory neurotransmission (of glutamate and dopamine) and increase inhibitory neurotransmission (of gamma aminobutyric acid).[5] Cellular models have also been used to try to understand lithium's mechanism of action,[11] with a range of results that have not been replicated.[12,13] However, none of these observations has been convincingly linked to efficacy in bipolar disorder.

PHARMACOKINETICS AND PHARMACODYNAMICS

Lithium is absorbed through the gut and distributes rapidly throughout body water, achieving peak plasma concentrations 1 to 2 hours after a single dose. (Slower-release forms may require 4–5 hours to reach peak concentration because of transit time through the gut.) As a monovalent cation like sodium, lithium's clearance relies entirely on renal function. It is neither metabolized by the liver, nor significantly protein bound while circulating in the bloodstream. Concomitant ingestion of food tends to increase absorption. In general, the half-life for renal excretion is approximately 18 to 36 hours, so steady-state serum levels are typically reached after 4 to 5 days. For this reason, lithium levels are typically checked approximately 5 days after its initiation or a dose change. Because lithium distributes throughout the body, it is influenced by lean body mass—for example, among older adults, lithium levels for a given dose tend to be greater than among younger individuals with a leaner body (including muscle) mass. Magnetic resonance spectroscopy studies suggest that brain lithium levels are correlated with plasma levels (typically being half of serum levels), although less so in patients at the extremes of age—that is, it is possible to have supra-therapeutic levels in the central nervous system (CNS) while maintaining a normal plasma lithium level.[14]

Drugs that affect renal function, particularly re-absorption, can have profound effects on lithium clearance. Perhaps most notable from a clinical perspective, non-steroidal anti-inflammatory drugs (NSAIDs) and other cyclooxygenase-2 inhibitors may decrease renal blood flow and thereby increase lithium levels by up to 15% to 30%. Diuretics likewise affect lithium levels, although the nature of their effect depends on their site of action. In the kidneys, lithium is primarily re-absorbed in the proximal tubules, with some subsequent absorption in the loop of Henle. Importantly, in contrast to sodium, no significant absorption occurs in the distal tubules. Therefore, thiazide diuretics, which act distally, tend to increase lithium levels by up to 50%, but those that act more proximally typically have less of an effect on lithium levels.

More broadly, hydration status can affect lithium levels: individuals who become salt avid (e.g., because of hypovolemia or hyponatremia, perhaps in the context of vomiting, diarrhea, or self-induced injury, such as long-distance-running) cause their lithium levels to rise.

EVIDENCE FOR LITHIUM'S EFFICACY

Lithium in Acute Mania

Beginning with Schou's study of lithium versus placebo for acute mania, lithium has repeatedly shown its efficacy for the treatment of mania, with the first large randomized study of lithium treatment for acute mania finding that lithium's efficacy was comparable to the antipsychotic chlorpromazine.[15]

However, few of the early studies of lithium for acute mania were undertaken with the methodological rigor that is required today for regulatory approval of a drug's use. By coincidence, the first rigorously designed study to demonstrate lithium's efficacy for acute mania was Bowden's seminal study of divalproex sodium for the treatment of acute mania in 1994, which was designed to study divalproex for FDA approval; by including lithium as an active comparator, the study also demonstrated lithium's efficacy.[16] This study was adequately powered (i.e., it included a large enough patient sample to have a high probability of finding a statistically significant difference between treatments with a low probability of error), compared a drug to an agent known to be effective (lithium), and included a placebo arm. Additionally, it was not biased by inclusion based on prior response to lithium. A recent systematic review of 36 studies of lithium in acute mania (with 4220 participants) included 7 other placebo-controlled trials.[17] Aside from Bowden and co-workers' study, the others were published after 2005 and included one study in children and adolescents (aged 7–17 years).[16] Six of the studies had a third comparator (valproate, quetiapine, lamotrigine, aripiprazole, or topiramate), and one study added lithium versus placebo to quetiapine. The meta-analysis found strong evidence in favor of lithium versus placebo with lithium being twice as effective as placebo in achieving a response (odds ratio [OR], 2.13; 95% confidence interval [CI], 1.73–2.63; 1707 participants). The same review also compared studies of lithium versus active comparators (valproate, quetiapine, clonazepam, lamotrigine, carbamazepine, chlorpromazine, haloperidol, olanzapine, risperidone, aripiprazole, topiramate, zuclopenthixol, and electroconvulsive therapy). They did not find any difference in efficacy between lithium and these agents other than lithium's being more effective than topiramate (OR of remission, 2.24; 95% CI, 1.58–3.15; 660 participants). Lithium may be less likely to improve manic symptoms compared to olanzapine (OR, 0.44; 95% CI, 0.20–0.94; 80 participants), but this was low-certainty evidence from only two studies. Comparing the acceptability of lithium with all other antimanic agents whose studies provided data, there was no significant difference between groups in term of withdrawals for any reason (OR, 1.11; 95% CI, 0.84–1.47; 832 participants; 23 studies). Overall, lithium has comparable effectiveness and acceptability when used in the treatment of patients with mania compared with other antimanic agents.

Monotherapy in any phase of bipolar disorder (BPD), however, is increasingly rare and is especially so in the treatment of acute mania.[18] It appears that mania outcomes, in terms of time to response and proportion of patients who remit, may be improved with the addition of antipsychotics to lithium.[19] The adjunctive use of typical antipsychotics (including haloperidol) and atypical antipsychotics (e.g., aripiprazole, asenapine, olanzapine, quetiapine, and risperidone) with lithium carbonate has led to improved outcomes compared with the use of lithium alone. The atypical antipsychotic ziprasidone, however, did not improve outcomes significantly compared with placebo when added to lithium.

Lithium in Acute Bipolar Depression

The options for the pharmacological treatment of major depressive episodes (MDEs) in BPD, unlike those for mania, remain few. Despite being recommended as a first-line treatment in some BPD treatment guidelines, few data support the use of lithium as an acute antidepressant in BPD. Older studies (from the 1970s) that reported on the effectiveness of lithium monotherapy for bipolar depression did not follow modern standards, and the results were difficult to interpret.[20] A more recently conducted large double-blinded randomized control trial (RCT) comparing lithium (n = 136) and placebo (n = 133) was designed to evaluate the effects of quetiapine (300 and 600 mg) and included lithium as a comparator (Efficacy of Monotherapy Seroquel in Bipolar Depression [EMBOLDEN] I).[21] Lithium dosages ranged between 600 and 1800 mg/day; by the study's endpoint (8 weeks), Montgomery-Asberg Depression Rating Scale (MADRS) total score changes for lithium (–13.6) and placebo (–11.8) were not statistically different ($P = .123$), although both doses of quetiapine were significantly more effective than placebo. A recent meta-analysis did not find lithium monotherapy to be more effective than placebo in bipolar depression.[22] They identified only three studies that met eligibility criteria (double blind, RCT): the study by Young and associates[21] had the largest sample size, and the other two studies only added 46 patients. Lithium has also seemed less effective than antidepressants in several recent studies. However, these studies were conducted in those with bipolar II disorder.

Lithium, used as monotherapy, appears to be as effective for the treatment of bipolar depression as the combination of lithium and an antidepressant. In a study comparing imipramine, paroxetine, and placebo added to lithium carbonate for the treatment of a MDE in BPD, neither antidepressant added benefit beyond lithium alone.[23] Response rates (defined as a Hamilton Depression Rating Scale [HAM-D] score of ≤ 7) were 35% for lithium alone compared with 39% for imipramine, and 46% for paroxetine. In a secondary analysis, participants with lower lithium levels (<0.8 mEq/L) had a lower response rate than those in the adjunctive antidepressant group, suggesting perhaps that higher lithium levels are as effective as lithium plus an antidepressant in the treatment of bipolar depression. In the Clinical Health Outcomes Initiative in Comparative Effectiveness (Bipolar CHOICE) study, 482 patients with bipolar I or II disorder were randomized to lithium or quetiapine, along with adjunctive personalized treatment. There was no difference in outcomes among the two groups during the 6-month trial.[24] Also in a pragmatic comparative efficacy study of moderate-dose lithium augmentation as part of optimized personalized treatment (lithium treatment moderate dose use study [LiTMUS]), the addition of lithium had no effect on outcomes, but the lithium group had less exposure to antipsychotics.[25] Overall, unlike its effects in mania, the evidence supporting lithium as a first-line treatment for bipolar depression is limited.

Lithium for Maintenance Treatment and Relapse Prevention of Bipolar Disorder

Lithium is the archetypal maintenance treatment for BPD. From Prien et al.'s[26] first maintenance study using lithium (comparing it with placebo) to more recent studies using lithium as a comparator for maintenance using other drugs, lithium demonstrates a clear benefit for maintaining both a response and preventing relapse in BPD. Lithium's clearest benefit associated with long-term use is in the prevention of relapse to mania, although relapse to depression is more common in patients with BPD. As is the case with lithium in acute mania, lithium's efficacy compared with placebo was only confirmed in later studies that were designed to establish regulatory approval for newer drugs. Earlier studies were beset by methodological problems, including on–off rather than parallel group designs, a lack of diagnostic clarity (e.g., the inclusion of unipolar depressed patients), and rapid or abrupt lithium discontinuation in those who were stable. Concerns about the sudden discontinuation of lithium are genuine because there is a high rate of manic relapse in these individuals; inclusion of patients from these studies might artificially inflate the difference between lithium and placebo in maintenance treatment.[27]

Geddes and colleagues[28] completed the definitive systematic review of lithium for maintenance treatment in BPD. After reviewing 300 studies, they included only 5 studies in their meta-analysis, limiting inclusion to randomized, double-blind, placebo-controlled trials. They found that lithium was more effective than placebo in the prevention of relapses to any mood episode (random effects relative risk [RR], 0.65; 95% CI, 0.50–0.84) and to mania (RR, 0.62; 95% CI, 0.40–0.95), with a non-significant effect on relapse to depression (RR, 0.72; 95% CI, 0.49–1.07).[28] The average risk of relapse of any kind during 1 to 2 years of follow-up was 60% for placebo versus 40% for lithium; this can be understood as lithium preventing one relapse for every five patients treated compared with placebo. Relapse rates to mania were 14% for lithium compared with 24% for placebo, and relapse rates to depression were 25% for lithium compared with 32% for placebo. However, this study had some limitations and criticisms: the outcomes were not defined uniformly across the included studies, one study included in the analysis had exclusively participants with bipolar II, and the follow-up period of 1 to 2 years was too short to adequately evaluate the benefit of lithium (because some have argued that the maintenance benefit of lithium is only apparent after 2 years of treatment).[27]

Lithium has shown similar efficacy to quetiapine and olanzapine for maintenance. In patients with BPD who were first stabilized on quetiapine and then randomized to remain on quetiapine, or switch to lithium or placebo ($n = 404$ for quetiapine; $n = 364$ for lithium; and $n = 404$ for placebo), both quetiapine and lithium prolonged the time to relapse of manic (lithium's hazard ratio [HR], 0.37; 95% CI, 0.27–0.53; $P < .0001$) and depressive events (lithium's HR, 0.59; 95% CI, 0.42–0.84; $P < .004$) compared with placebo.[29] Lithium was compared with olanzapine for the prevention of relapse of bipolar I disorder in a randomized, controlled, double-blind trial.[30] Bipolar I patients were stabilized on a combination of lithium and olanzapine, randomized to one or the other drug, and followed for 12 months. There was no difference between drugs on the primary outcome measure or time to symptomatic relapse (YMRS or HAM-D scores of ≥15), although there were fewer relapses to mania or mixed (but not depressive) episodes in the olanzapine-treated group.

Several studies have examined outcomes for participants stabilized on an antipsychotic added to lithium or valproate and then randomized to remain on lithium or valproate and the antipsychotic or lithium or valproate plus placebo. Notably, these studies included aripiprazole, quetiapine, and ziprasidone; their enriched designs were primarily intended to study the impact of the antipsychotic, but they do suggest that patients who were stabilized on lithium or valproate plus one of those antipsychotics remain on both drugs.

A study was completed specifically to examine whether the combination of lithium and valproate was more effective than use of either of these two drugs as monotherapy to prevent recurrence in bipolar I disorder. Bipolar Affective disorder: Lithium/ANticonvulsant Evaluation (BALANCE) was a randomized, open-label trial of lithium, divalproex sodium, or the combination for maintenance treatment in BPD. Participants were stabilized on both drugs during a 4- to 8-week open-label run-in phase (to screen for tolerability), then randomized to continue on lithium (titrated to 0.4–1.0 mmol/L), divalproex sodium (750 mg, 1250 mg, or valproic acid serum concentration >50 µg/mL), or the combination, with the primary outcome measure being time to intervention for a mood episode. Although combination treatment was superior to divalproex sodium (HR, 0.59; 95% CI, 0.42–0.83) and lithium was also superior to divalproex (HR, 0.71; 95% CI, 0.71–1.00), combination therapy was not superior to lithium (HR, 0.82; 95% CI, 0.58–1.17). This suggests that the role for valproate monotherapy (i.e., not in combination with lithium) is limited and that lithium alone or in combination with valproate is the preferred treatment.

Some controversy remains regarding what the adequate maintenance levels of lithium should be. To minimize adverse effects and to increase patient acceptance of lithium treatment, use of the lowest effective doses should be the goal. A randomized, double-blind study by Gelenberg and co-workers[31] stabilized patients on a standard serum level of lithium (0.8–1 mmol/L) and then assigned them to either remain at that level or to be maintained with a lower serum lithium level (0.4–0.6 mmol/L). Patients in the higher lithium level group had fewer relapses than those randomly assigned to lower lithium levels.[31] A re-analysis of the data, however, controlling for the rate at which the lithium dose was lowered, found no difference between groups, suggesting that lower maintenance lithium levels may be adequate for some patients.[32]

Lithium in Rapid-Cycling Bipolar Disorder

Rapid cycling is no longer included as a course specifier in the *Diagnostic and Statistical Manual of Mental Disorders*, Fifth Edition (DSM-5), but it continues to be used conceptually by clinicians. Rapid cycling was defined in the *Diagnostic and Statistical Manual of Mental Disorders*, Fourth Edition, Text Revision (DSM-IV-TR) as four or more distinct mood episodes (either of opposite poles or of the same pole after at least 8 weeks of partial or full recovery) within a 12-month period; patients with this course are notoriously difficult to treat and to stabilize. Some have concluded that lithium is less effective than other drugs (e.g., divalproex sodium) for this specific course of BPD, but an ambitious clinical trial and a large body of naturalistic data suggest that lithium is no less ineffective than other compounds for rapid cycling.[33,34] Calabrese and colleagues[33] compared lithium with divalproex sodium in rapid-cycling patients stabilized on both drugs and found no difference between the drugs on time to episode-recurrence. As testament to the difficulty of treating those with rapid-cycling disorders, only 60 of the original 254 participants who were randomized to the two study conditions were stabilized. In a cohort of 360 patients with BPD treated in Sardinia, time to recurrence was no different for those with or without a rapid-cycling course.[34]

Lithium in Suicide Prevention

Lithium may have anti-suicide effects in individuals with mood disorders. Several meta-analyses, smaller independent studies, and a study from two large health insurance databases generally support lithium's value as a prophylactic agent against suicidal behavior in those with mood disorders.

In an update to their 2005 meta-analysis of all randomized studies of lithium (either vs. placebo or another drug) in those with mood disorders (including BPD and major depressive disorder [MDD]) Cipriani and co-workers[35] included 16 new trials for a total of 48 RCTs with 6674 participants. In addition to placebo, 14 other comparators were included (amitriptyline, carbamazepine, valproate, fluoxetine, fluvoxamine, imipramine, lamotrigine, mianserin, maprotiline, nortriptyline, olanzapine, phenelzine, quetiapine, and thyroid hormone). The average duration of follow-up was 19 months.[35]

As in their previous report, they found that lithium-treated patients took their own lives or died from any cause significantly less often. Mainly, lithium was more effective than placebo in reducing the number of suicides (OR, 0.13; 95% CI, 0.03–0.66) and deaths from any cause (OR, 0.38; 95% CI, 0.15–0.95). However, when lithium was compared with other active treatments, although lithium was generally more favorable, no statistical difference was found in the number of suicides identified.

Another meta-analysis of 33 studies that investigated long-term lithium treatment between the years 1970 and 2000 yielded a result that favored lithium as a potential means of suicide prevention.[36] Of the 19 studies that compared groups with and without lithium treatment, 18 found a lower suicide rate in the treatment group, and 1 did not have a single suicide in either group. Overall, the meta-analysis demonstrated a 13-fold reduction in suicidality for patients with an affective illness, leading to a greatly reduced suicide risk.[36]

A recent RCT of adjunctive lithium compared to placebo in veterans with depression (in both MDD and BPD) at high risk for suicide found no benefit for lithium on the primary outcome measure, repeated episodes of suicide-related events (repeated suicide attempts, interrupted attempts, hospitalizations to prevent suicide, and deaths from suicide). While the sample was quite large and included 519 participants, it was stopped for futility prior to reaching its prespecified sample size of 1860 participants. Lithium levels obtained were only modest, and one death from all causes occurred in the lithium group while three occurred in the placebo group. Data from this study would not change the outcomes of the meta-analyses, however, even as in this trial suicide-related behaviors were unchanged.[37]

In an analysis of databases from two large health maintenance organizations in the United States, Goodwin and co-workers[38] found a strong effect that favored lithium compared with divalproex sodium or other anticonvulsants. The incidence of emergency department admissions for suicide attempts (31.3 vs. 10.8 per 1000 person-years; $P < .001$), suicide attempts resulting in hospitalization (10.5 vs. 4.2 per 1000 person-years; $P < .001$), and death by suicide (1.7 vs. 0.7 per 1000 person-years; $P = .04$) was lower in the group receiving at least one lithium prescription.[38] A United Kingdom population-based electronic health record study also found increased self-harm (HR, 1.51; 95% CI, 1.21–1.88) and unintentional injury rates (HR, 1.19; 95% CI, 1.01–1.41) in patients with BPD taking valproate, olanzapine, or quetiapine compared with lithium.[39] The non-randomized nature of the samples, however, leaves concerns that the groups were clinically different, and the results were confounded by indication. For instance, it is not known how many patients in the divalproex group had previously failed to respond to lithium and thus comprised a treatment-resistant group and whether there were

co-morbidities (such as anxiety disorders, personality disorders, or substance use disorders) that were present to a greater degree in the non–lithium-treated participants. In any case, the results strongly favored lithium and were consistent with other examinations of the effect of lithium on suicide.

Lithium discontinuation itself may increase one's suicide risk. In a sample of 165 patients who decided to discontinue lithium (whether electively or for some medical reason), there was a 14-fold increase in all suicidal acts after discontinuation of lithium.[40] It is unclear whether the rate of suicide after lithium discontinuation exceeds that found in those with untreated affective illness. Lithium discontinuation may increase suicidal behavior because of higher relapse rates, higher than would be expected even if participants had been treated with placebo or had been on no medication at all.[27] It has not been established if the lower rates of suicide and self-harm in those prescribed lithium was primarily because of improved mood stabilization compared with the other treatments, reducing impulsivity and aggression, or because of a specific anti-suicidal property of lithium. In 167 patients who were on long-term treatment with lithium (approximately 3 years), the number of suicide attempts per year was significantly reduced compared with the years immediately preceding the use of lithium in those who had responded well to lithium (0.26 suicide attempts per year vs. 0.02). However, similar statistically significant reductions were seen in those with a poor (0.33 vs. 0.10) or moderate response (0.27 vs. 0.06) to lithium. The study defined response narrowly (based on hospitalizations for depression rather than measuring mood symptom intensity).[41] It is possible that some of those deemed non-responsive have some changes in their mood symptoms, without an impact on hospital admissions. Ultimately, although the effects of lithium are promising in the realm of suicide prevention, they have not yet been definitively determined. This is reflected in the ethical and logistic complications of conducting randomized trials of treatment of suicide risk. An RCT that compared the effects of lithium and valproate on reducing suicidal behavior in 98 patients with BPD and a history of suicide attempts, with a 2.5 year follow-up did not show any significant difference among groups in the time to suicide attempt. The study had challenges with recruitment and ultimately only had the power to detect a five-fold difference between lithium and valproate. Smaller and potentially clinically meaningful differences could not be ruled out.[42]

Lithium in Children and Adolescents

Pediatric Bipolar Disorder

Findling and colleagues conducted the only double-blind placebo-controlled trial of lithium in pediatric bipolar disorder (ages 7–17 years).[43] All participants ($n = 81$) were treated as outpatients and followed for 8 weeks. Lithium led to a statistically significant reduction in YMRS scores compared with placebo (5.5; 95% CI, 0.51–10.50; $P = .03$) and was generally well tolerated, and there was no statistically significant change in weight, but those in the lithium arm had an increase in their thyrotropin concentration. Two other RCTs that compared lithium with atypical antipsychotics found that atypical antipsychotics were more effective in reducing manic symptoms than lithium. In the Treatment of Early-Age Mania (TEAM) study, higher response rates were found in the risperidone group ($n = 89$) compared with the lithium group ($n = 90$) (68.5% vs. 35.6%; χ^2_1, 16.9. $P < .001$), and the discontinuation rate was higher for those with lithium treatment ($\chi^2 1$, 6.4; $P = .011$),[44] and in a 6-week double-blind randomized trial of quetiapine ($n = 58$; target dose, 400–600 mg/day) versus lithium ($n = 51$; target serum level for lithium, 1.0–1.2 mEq/L), the response rates were 72% in the quetiapine group and 49% in the lithium group ($P = .012$).[45] There have been no RCTs of lithium in pediatric bipolar depression, but the efficacy of lithium in maintenance has been demonstrated in a double-blind placebo-controlled discontinuation study.[46] Thirty-one adolescents who had been stabilized on lithium for 24 weeks were then randomized to continue on lithium ($n = 17$) or placebo ($n = 14$) and followed for 28 more weeks. The participants who received lithium had a lower HR compared with participants who received placebo (HR, 0.28; 95% CI, 0.10–0.78; $P = .015$). Discontinuation because of mood symptoms occurred in 5 of 17 participants (29%) treated with lithium compared with 10 of 14 (71%) treated with placebo. Overall, there was evidence for efficacy of lithium in pediatric bipolar mania and for its use in maintenance therapy.

Conduct Disorder

Lithium has also been used to treat aggression associated with conduct disorder (CD) in children. In a review of four studies (lasting 2–6 weeks and including a total of 184 children) that compared lithium and placebo for the treatment of aggression in hospitalized youth with CD, three of the four studies provided data that could be incorporated into a meta-analysis using the dichotomous outcomes of responder or remission. Although lithium was associated with higher odds of response or remission than placebo (OR, 4.56; 95% CI, 1.97–10.56; $P <$ .001), the evidence for lithium was inconsistent among the studies. The quality of the studies (and possibly publication bias) made confidence in the amount of benefit achieved low.[47]

Other Uses of Lithium

Although well validated for the treatment of patients with BPD, lithium has also been studied with greater or lesser success through randomized trials in other psychiatric illnesses, including unipolar MDD, schizophrenia, and alcohol dependence.

Augmentation of Antidepressants in Treatment-Refractory Major Depressive Disorder

The use of lithium as an agent to prevent relapse in MDD has been somewhat controversial, although the evidence suggests that it may be effective in some patients. In a meta-analysis of studies of lithium augmentation of antidepressants, Nelson and colleagues[48] reported a higher odds for response to lithium versus placebo (OR, 2.89; 95% CI, 1.65–5.05; $P = .0002$). The meta-analysis included nine trials with 237 patients; seven of the antidepressants were tricyclic antidepressants, and three were selective serotonin reuptake inhibitors or other second-generation agents. Eight of the nine trials had fewer than 30 participants per arm, and the most common dosages were 800 or 900 mg/day. The duration of the augmentation with lithium was quite variable, ranging from 2 days to 6 weeks. A significant limitation of the evidence was the lack of large studies. As part of the Sequential Treatment Alternatives to Relieve Depression (STAR*D) study, lithium carbonate was compared with triio-dothyronine (T_3) as an augmentation strategy in a 14-week randomized, open-label trial for 142 patients who had failed to improve on citalopram followed by a second treatment (either a switch to another antidepressant or augmentation with another agent) and found low response rates for lithium.[49] Remission rates were 15.9% with lithium augmentation (mean dosage, 859.8 mg/day, standard deviation [SD], = 373.1) and 24.7% with T_3 augmentation (mean dose, 45.2 μg; SD, 11.4) after a mean of 9.6 weeks of treatment, although the difference between treatments was not statistically significant. Lithium, however, was more frequently associated with side effects than was T_3 ($P = .045$), and more participants in the lithium group left treatment because of side effects (23.2% vs. 9.6%; $P = .027$).

Relapse Prevention in Major Depressive Disorder

Several efforts have been made to examine the potential benefit of lithium for the prevention of relapse in MDD. A meta-analysis of 21 RCTs of long-term lithium treatment for the prevention of recurrences in unipolar MDD, either as monotherapy versus placebo ($n = 7$) or an antidepressant ($n = 5$) or as an adjunct to antidepressant treatment ($n = 9$), yielded an overall pooled OR of 2.80 (95% CI, 1.59–4.92; $P < .0001$) favoring lithium over placebo or other comparators.[50] The studies included 846 patients randomized to lithium ($n = 432$) (alone or as an add-on) or a comparator ($n = 414$) and followed up for a mean of 22.2 (95% CI, 17.4–27.0) months. Lithium was more effective than placebo (OR, 4.51; 95% CI, 1.41–14.5; $P = .011$) and effective as an adjunct to antidepressants in nine trials (OR, 2.38; 95% CI, 1.05–5.40; $P = .038$). Additional meta-analyses indicated a non-significant difference between lithium and antidepressant monotherapy in five trials (OR, 2.21; 95% CI, 0.69–7.10; $P = .18$). These results suggest a role for lithium in the prevention of MDEs.

Lithium in Psychotic Disorders

Lithium is ineffective in the treatment of psychosis, but it has been studied as an adjunct to antipsychotics in the treatment of patients with schizophrenia and schizoaffective disorders. A Cochrane review of lithium for the treatment of schizophrenia identified 22 studies with a total of 763 people that met criteria for review.[51] Although most had schizophrenia, a minority ($n = 196$) had schizoaffective disorder. Three of the studies compared lithium alone versus placebo, 8 compared lithium alone versus antipsychotics, and 13 compared lithium added to an antipsychotic drug versus placebo added to the antipsychotic regimen. Most studies lasted between 3 and 8 weeks. More participants who received lithium augmentation had a clinically significant response (10 RCTs; $n = 396$; RR, 1.81; 95% CI, 1.10–2.97; low-quality evidence). However, this effect became non-significant when participants with schizoaffective disorders were excluded (8 RCTs; $n = 272$; RR, 1.64; 95% CI, 0.95–2.81), when the analysis was limited to double-blind studies (7 RCTs; $n = 224$; RR, 1.82; 95% CI, 0.84–3.96), or when studies with high attrition were excluded (9 RCTs; $n = 355$; RR, 1.67; CI, 0.93–3.00). Overall, the evidence for the use of lithium in schizophrenia is of low methodological quality.

Lithium in Alcohol Dependence

A Veterans Administration study of lithium in those with alcohol use disorder (AUD) (depressed or non-depressed) failed to find a benefit for the drug.[52] In a year-long study of 286 individuals with AUD without depression and 171 with depression, no significant differences were found between those who took lithium and those who took placebo on any study measure (including the number of individuals with AUD who became abstinent, the number of days of drinking, the number of alcohol-related hospitalizations, the changes in the rating of severity of AUD, and the change in depression severity). No significant differences were found when the data from medication-compliant participants were reviewed.

PRINCIPLES OF LITHIUM TREATMENT
Predictors of Lithium Response

Few, if any, reliable predictors of lithium response have been identified. Indeed, on closer inspection, many of the purported predictors have proven to be untrue. Thus, the bulk of evidence suggests that patients with rapid-cycling BPD respond well to lithium. Likewise, there is little convincing evidence that discontinuation of lithium decreases the likelihood of subsequent response to lithium. There is no evidence that males or females respond differentially to lithium.

Individuals with a positive family history of BPD (rather than schizophrenia) do appear to respond better to lithium. This is often interpreted incorrectly to mean that lithium response itself is familial, which has not been established.

Laboratory Monitoring

The standard evaluation (i.e., with evaluation of renal function, thyroid function, and an electrocardiogram [ECG]) for a patient beginning lithium flows from its major potential toxicities. Specifically, standard guidelines advise checking electrolytes, blood urea nitrogen (BUN) and creatinine, thyroid-stimulating hormone (TSH), and an ECG in individuals 40 years of age and older.

Lithium levels should be checked at least 5 days after each dose change or any time a patient reports the new symptoms potentially suggestive of lithium toxicity.

Guidelines also recommend following electrolytes, BUN, and creatinine up to every 2 months for the first 6 months, with a lithium level, BUN, creatinine, and thyroid function tests every 6 months to 1 year thereafter.

Lithium Dosing

Lithium carbonate is available in 150-, 300-, and 600-mg capsules or tablets, as well as 300- and 450-mg slow-release forms. A liquid, lithium citrate, is also available, in 300-mg/5-mL form. For most patients, the immediate-release lithium carbonate is initiated first, with a switch to another form only to maximize tolerability, if necessary.

The narrow therapeutic window for lithium treatment (see Pharmacokinetics and Pharmacodynamics, earlier in this chapter) complicates lithium dosing. Indeed, in its early application lithium levels of 0.8 to 1.2 mEq/L were advised, but more recently levels of 0.6 to 0.8 mEq/L—and perhaps even lower in some cases—have been advocated. The optimal dose is driven not merely by considerations of efficacy but by tolerability as well; that is, the "best" dose for prevention of recurrence may be too high for some patients to tolerate. Drug–drug interactions must be considered, and a list of selected interactions is provided in Table 4.1.

TABLE 4.1 Medications That Commonly Interact with Lithium

Medication	Effect
COMMON	
Diuretics: thiazide, loop (e.g., furosemide)	↑
ACE inhibitors	↑
NSAIDs	↑
Metronidazole	↑
Tetracycline	↑
Diuretics: osmotic, potassium-sparing, acetazolamide	↓
Theophylline	↓
Aminophylline	↓
Drugs that alkalinize urine	↓
Caffeine	↓
RARE BUT NOTABLE	
Antipsychotics	Risk of neurotoxicity
Bupropion	Increased seizure risk
SSRIs	Serotonin syndrome
Iodide salts	Hypothyroidism

ACE, Angiotensin-converting enzyme; *NSAID*, non-steroidal anti-inflammatory drug; *SSRI*, selective serotonin reuptake inhibitor.

Typically, the clinician will begin with 600 mg once daily at bedtime and then increase it to 900 mg at bedtime. After 5 days, a lithium level is checked, and the dose is increased or decreased as required to attain a level between 0.6 to 0.8 mEq/L. However, some patients may not tolerate these initial doses because of side effects, which may lead to patient refusal of lithium and the loss of a potentially effective treatment option. Depending on the setting (inpatient, outpatient), the acuity and severity of symptoms, and clinical factors (such as age, medical co-morbidity, and concomitant medication regimen), prescription of lithium can start at even lower doses with a gradual increase based on the patient's tolerance. Although nomograms exist for predicting the necessary lithium dose based on an initial test dose, because of concerns about lithium toxicity, the authors generally prefer to observe the level that results from 900 mg before titrating further.

Some data suggest that lithium may be better tolerated by patients and possibly less likely to cause renal complications when dosed once daily. If tolerability of a single dose becomes a problem—for example, in terms of sedation or gastrointestinal (GI) distress—divided dosing may be used. This need not be morning and night; some patients prefer dinnertime and bedtime.

Adverse Effects and Their Management

Hypothyroidism has been reported as being common in lithium-treated patients, with some studies describing a prevalence of up to 35%. However, more recent studies suggest that it is substantially less common and that it is seen more often among women than men. When hypothyroidism occurs, it is typically managed with the addition of thyroxine (T_4) treatment.

Lithium has several renal effects, which range from bothersome to potentially life-threatening. Perhaps the most common, polyuria (including nocturia) and consequent polydipsia, arise when lithium prevents distal tubule re-absorption of free water, antagonizing the actions of anti-diuretic hormone. When necessary, they may be addressed with careful addition of a diuretic. Amiloride is often used first because it has little effect on lithium levels. Thiazide diuretics may also be used if required, though they will increase lithium levels and often require a dose decrease of 50% and close monitoring of lithium levels. When edema (particularly common in the lower extremities) is seen in a patient with normal renal function, the diuretic spironolactone may be used, although lithium levels and renal function require close monitoring.

Of greater concern, long-term treatment with lithium is associated with reductions in creatinine clearance in about 10% of patients, indicating a decrease in glomerular filtration rate (GFR). Small studies suggest that glomerulosclerosis and interstitial fibrosis are seen among some patients receiving long-term lithium treatment. Beyond a certain point, this deterioration may accelerate and dramatically increase the risk of lithium toxicity because small perturbations in GFR can have large effects on lithium levels. When creatinine rises above baseline by 25% or more, consultation with a nephrologist may be helpful to rule out other contributors to reduction in GFR (e.g., renal complications of diabetes), and discontinuation of lithium often becomes necessary once GFR decreases beyond a certain point.

Although rare, lithium can cause a depression of firing at the sino-atrial node, contributing to sinus arrhythmias. Lithium may also cause benign ECG abnormalities, most typically an appearance resembling hypokalemia, including widening of the QRS complex and an increased PR interval.

Weight gain is common among lithium-treated patients, and although the mechanism is not known, it is not merely a result of lithium-induced edema. Some studies suggest that up to half of lithium-treated patients will experience a 5% to 10%

increase in weight. As with any medication-induced weight gain, early and aggressive intervention is warranted, focusing on both diet and exercise. A specific concern among lithium-treated patients with polydipsia is the consumption of sodas or juices high in sugar.

Cognitive complaints are common among lithium-treated patients, sometimes characterized as feeling "foggy" or "cloudy." Adjunctive thyroid hormone is sometimes used to ameliorate these symptoms; however, there is no well-established means of treating such complaints other than decreasing the lithium dose. In a study that looked at predictors of lithium monotherapy in patients with BPD,[53] examination of neurocognitive functioning found no significant difference in any of the baseline neuropsychological tests among those on lithium ($n = 169$) or not ($n = 93$). Eighty-eight of the patients with BPD achieved mood stabilization with lithium monotherapy and had repeat neuropsychological testing. There was a significant improvement in global cognitive index scores (F, 31.69; $P < .001$) and in three of the seven individual neuropsychological tests. None of the measures worsened. Cognition is affected by multiple factors in BPD, including mood state and medications. These findings are reassuring in that lithium does not significantly impair cognition when used therapeutically.

Other Bothersome Adverse Effects

Adverse GI effects are common among lithium-treated patients and may include upper (nausea, vomiting, and dyspepsia) and lower (diarrhea and cramping) GI symptoms. Because slow-release formulations are absorbed lower in the gut, they are more often associated with the latter symptoms, and immediate-release formulations are more often associated with the former symptoms. In many cases, dividing dosages or dosing with food can minimize or eliminate these symptoms. If this is not the case, a switch to lithium citrate (in liquid form) may be helpful, though some patients object to the taste of this preparation.

Tremor is common with lithium treatment, even at therapeutic levels and particularly after each dose when peak levels are achieved. This tremor, which resembles a benign physiological tremor, may be exacerbated by caffeine and by anxiety. It is typically managed by changing the timing of the lithium dose (to ensure that peak levels occur during sleep) and when necessary by adding a beta-adrenergic blocker. This may be used on either an as-needed or a standing basis, depending on patient preference. Propranolol is often initiated first to establish an effective dose and then changed to atenolol for the convenience of once-daily dosing.

Both psoriasis and acne exacerbations have been associated with lithium treatment. Typically, these conditions do not require treatment discontinuation because they can be controlled with dermatological treatments.

Presentation of lithium toxicity develops as lithium levels rise above 1 mEq/L, and particularly beyond 1.2 mEq/L; initial symptoms may include slurring of speech, ataxia or unsteady gait, confusion, and agitation. Box 4.1 shows signs and symptoms of lithium toxicity, and Box 4.2 shows management of acute toxicity.

Lithium in Pregnancy and Breast-feeding

Lithium use during the first trimester of pregnancy has been associated with a potentially life-threatening cardiac abnormality, known as Ebstein anomaly, a spectrum of changes that typically includes insufficiency of the tricuspid valve and hypoplasia of the right ventricle. The risk appears to be about 10-fold greater among children of lithium-treated pregnant women compared with those in the general population, although the absolute risk is still quite low (on the order of 1

BOX 4.1 Signs of Lithium Toxicity

LEVELS >1.5 mEq/L[a]

Lethargy or fatigue
Coarse tremor
Nausea or vomiting
Diarrhea
Visual changes (blurring)
Vertigo
Hyperreflexia
Dysarthria
Ataxia
Confusion

LEVELS >2.5–3 mEq/L

Seizure
Coma
Arrhythmia

[a] Absence of significant symptoms does not rule out toxicity; likewise, some symptoms may be apparent at levels as low as 1 mEq/L.

BOX 4.2 Management of Lithium Toxicity

If the patient is comatose or obtunded, protect the airway.
In cases of suspected overdose, consider gastric lavage. For lithium levels >4 mEq/L[a] or >3 mEq/L and severely symptomatic or in other cases when volume load will not be tolerated, initiate dialysis.

  Hold further lithium doses.

Begin intravenous normal saline, 150–200 mL/h (as long as the patient can tolerate a volume load).
Address other electrolyte abnormalities.
Follow lithium levels approximately every 2–3 h. Initiate work-up to determine cause of toxicity.

[a] Recommendations vary about when to initiate dialysis, though most sources agree that levels >4 mEq/L merit immediate dialysis.

---

in 2000). This risk must be balanced against the substantial dangers to the fetus of a mother with uncontrolled BPD during pregnancy.

The changes in maternal fluid status during pregnancy typically cause a larger volume of distribution for lithium, which can lead to a decrease in lithium levels, entailing closer monitoring of lithium during pregnancy and in some cases a dose increase. At the time of delivery, fluid shifts may likewise lead to an increase in lithium levels. However, discontinuing lithium in the peri-partum period is no longer routinely advised because it has become clear that the risk of bipolar recurrence is extremely high in this period.

Levels of lithium in breast milk are substantial, approaching 50% of maternal plasma levels. For this reason, lithium-treated mothers should not breast-feed because the effects of lithium on newborn development are not well studied, and the risk for toxicity is high.

CURRENT CONTROVERSIES AND FUTURE DIRECTIONS

Several recent reviews have raised concern that lithium is being underused relative to other, potentially less effective treatments. This has been attributed to lithium's receiving less attention in medical education and more generally because of the marketing efforts for newer, on-patent alternatives for the treatment of patients with BPD.

If lithium's mechanism of action can be better understood, it might facilitate the identification of targets for drug therapy in BPD—that is, proteins that might be targeted by drugs that could exert similar effects to lithium, without its toxicity. Alternatively, it may be possible to explain why some patients fail to respond to lithium and "sensitize" them by combining lithium with other agents. Further mechanistic and pharmacogenetic studies of lithium will be crucial in this regard.

REFERENCES

1. Bauer M, Grof P, Muller-Oerlinghausen B. *Lithium in Neuropsychiatry: The Comprehensive Guide*. Informa Health Care; 2013.
2. Williams RS, Eames M, Ryves WJ, et al. Loss of a prolyl oligopeptidase confers resistance to lithium by elevation of inositol (1,4,5) trisphosphate. *EMBO J*. 1999;18(10):2734–2745.
3. Chalecka-Franaszek E, Chuang DM. Lithium activates the serine/threonine kinase Akt-1 and suppresses glutamate-induced inhibition of Akt-1 activity in neurons. *Proc Natl Acad Sci U S A*. 1999;96(15):8745–8750.
4. Phiel CJ, Klein PS. Molecular targets of lithium action. *Annu Rev Pharmacol Toxicol*. 2001;41:789–813.
5. Malhi GS, Tanious M, Das P, et al. Potential mechanisms of action of lithium in bipolar disorder. Current understanding. *CNS Drugs*. 2013;27(2):135–153.
6. Lucas FR, Salinas PC. WNT-7a induces axonal remodeling and increases synapsin I levels in cerebellar neurons. *Dev Biol*. 1997;192(1):31–44.
7. Snitow ME, Bhansali RS, Klein PS. Lithium and therapeutic targeting of GSK-3. *Cells*. 2021;10(2):255.
8. Hashimoto R, Hough C, Nakazawa T, et al. Lithium protection against glutamate excitotoxicity in rat cerebral cortical neurons: involvement of NMDA receptor inhibition possibly by decreasing NR2B tyrosine phosphorylation. *J Neurochem*. 2002;80(4):589–597.
9. Machado-Vieira R, Manji HK, Zarate Jr CA. The role of lithium in the treatment of bipolar disorder: convergent evidence for neurotrophic effects as a unifying hypothesis. *Bipolar Disord*. 2009;11(suppl 2):92–109.
10. Sun YR, Herrmann N, Scott CJM, et al. Global grey matter volume in adult bipolar patients with and without lithium treatment: a meta-analysis. *J Affect Disord*. 2018;225:599–606.
11. Haggarty SJ, Karmacharya R, Perlis RH. Advances toward precision medicine for bipolar disorder: mechanisms & molecules. *Mol Psychiatry*. 2021;26(1):168–185.
12. Mertens J, Wang Q-W, Kim Y, et al. Differential responses to lithium in hyperexcitable neurons from patients with bipolar disorder. *Nature*. 2015;527(7576):95–99.
13. Wang JL, Shamah SM, Sun AX, et al. Label-free, live optical imaging of reprogrammed bipolar disorder patient-derived cells reveals a functional correlate of lithium responsiveness. *Transl Psychiatry*. 2014;4(8):e428.
14. Grandjean EM, Aubry JM. Lithium: updated human knowledge using an evidence-based approach. Part II: clinical pharmacology and therapeutic monitoring. *CNS Drugs*. 2009;23(4):331–349.
15. Prien RF, Caffey Jr EM, Klett CJ. Comparison of lithium carbonate and chlorpromazine in the treatment of mania. Report of the Veterans Administration and National Institute of Mental Health Collaborative Study Group. *Arch Gen Psychiatry*. 1972;26(2):146–153.
16. Bowden CL, Brugger AM, Swann AC, et al. Efficacy of divalproex vs lithium and placebo in the treatment of mania. The Depakote Mania Study Group. *JAMA*. 1994;271(12):918–924.
17. McKnight RF, de La Motte de Broöns de Vauvert S, Chesney E, et al. Lithium for acute mania. *Cochrane Database Syst Rev*. 2019;6(6):Cd004048.
18. Frye MA, Ketter TA, Leverich GS, et al. The increasing use of polypharmacotherapy for refractory mood disorders: 22 years of study. *J Clin Psychiatry*. 2000;61(1):9–15.
19. Perlis RH, Welge JA, Vornik LA, et al. Atypical antipsychotics in the treatment of mania: a meta-analysis of randomized, placebo-controlled trials. *J Clin Psychiatry*. 2006;67(4):509–516.
20. Fountoulakis KN, Tohen M, Zarate Jr CA. Lithium treatment of bipolar disorder in adults: a systematic review of randomized trials and meta-analyses. *Eur Neuropsychopharmacol*. 2022;54:100–115.
21. Young AH, McElroy SL, Bauer M, et al. A double-blind, placebo-controlled study of quetiapine and lithium monotherapy in adults in the acute phase of bipolar depression (EMBOLDEN I). *J Clin Psychiatry*. 2010;71(2):150–162.
22. Rakofsky JJ, Lucido MJ, Dunlop BW. Lithium in the treatment of acute bipolar depression: a systematic review and meta-analysis. *J Affect Disord*. 2022;308:268–280.
23. Nemeroff CB, Evans DL, Gyulai L, et al. Double-blind, placebo-controlled comparison of imipramine and paroxetine in the treatment of bipolar depression. *Am J Psychiatry*. 2001;158(6):906–912.
24. Nierenberg AA, McElroy SL, Friedman ES, et al. Bipolar CHOICE (clinical health outcomes initiative in comparative effectiveness): a pragmatic 6-month trial of lithium versus quetiapine for bipolar disorder. *J Clin Psychiatry*. 2016;77(1):90–99.
25. Nierenberg AA, Friedman ES, Bowden CL, et al. Lithium treatment moderate-dose use study (LiTMUS) for bipolar disorder: a randomized comparative effectiveness trial of optimized personalized treatment with and without lithium. *Am J Psychiatry*. 2013;170(1):102–110.
26. Prien RF, Caffey Jr EM, Klett CJ. Prophylactic efficacy of lithium carbonate in manic-depressive illness. Report of the Veterans Administration and National Institute of Mental Health collaborative study group. *Arch Gen Psychiatry*. 1973;28(3):337–341.
27. Goodwin GM. Recurrence of mania after lithium withdrawal. Implications for the use of lithium in the treatment of bipolar affective disorder. *Br J Psychiatry*. 1994;164(2):149–152.
28. Geddes JR, Burgess S, Hawton K, et al. Long-term lithium therapy for bipolar disorder: systematic review and meta-analysis of randomized controlled trials. *Am J Psychiatry*. 2004;161(2):217–222.
29. Weisler RH, Nolen WA, Neijber A, et al. Continuation of quetiapine versus switching to placebo or lithium for maintenance treatment of bipolar I disorder (Trial 144: a randomized controlled study). *J Clin Psychiatry*. 2011;72(11):1452–1464.
30. Tohen M, Greil W, Calabrese JR, et al. Olanzapine versus lithium in the maintenance treatment of bipolar disorder: a 12-month, randomized, double-blind, controlled clinical trial. *Am J Psychiatry*. 2005;162(7):1281–1290.
31. Gelenberg AJ, Kane JM, Keller MB, et al. Comparison of standard and low serum levels of lithium for maintenance treatment of bipolar disorder. *N Engl J Med*. 1989;321(22):1489–1493.
32. Perlis RH, Sachs GS, Lafer B, et al. Effect of abrupt change from standard to low serum levels of lithium: a reanalysis of double-blind lithium maintenance data. *Am J Psychiatry*. 2002;159(7):1155–1159.
33. Calabrese JR, Bowden CL, Sachs G, et al. A placebo-controlled 18-month trial of lamotrigine and lithium maintenance treatment in recently depressed patients with bipolar I disorder. *J Clin Psychiatry*. Sep 2003;64(9):1013–1024.
34. Baldessarini RJ, Tondo L, Davis P, et al. Decreased risk of suicides and attempts during long-term lithium treatment: a meta-analytic review. *Bipolar Disord*. 2006;8(5 pt 2):625–639.
35. Cipriani A, Hawton K, Stockton S, et al. Lithium in the prevention of suicide in mood disorders: updated systematic review and meta-analysis. *BMJ*. 2013;346:f3646.
36. Baldessarini RJ, Tondo L, Hennen J. Treating the suicidal patient with bipolar disorder. Reducing suicide risk with lithium. *Ann N Y Acad Sci*. 2001;932:24–38. Discussion 39-43.
37. Katz IR, Rogers MP, Lew R, et al. Lithium treatment in the prevention of repeat suicide-related outcomes in veterans with major depression or bipolar disorder: a randomized clinical trial. *JAMA Psychiatry*. 2022;79(1):24–32.
38. Goodwin FK, Fireman B, Simon GE, et al. Suicide risk in bipolar disorder during treatment with lithium and divalproex. *JAMA*. 2003;290(11):1467–1473.
39. Hayes JF, Pitman A, Marston L, et al. Self-harm, unintentional injury, and suicide in bipolar disorder during maintenance mood stabilizer treatment: a UK population-based electronic health records study. *JAMA Psychiatry*. 2016;73(6):630–637.
40. Tondo L, Baldessarini RJ. Reduced suicide risk during lithium maintenance treatment. *J Clin Psychiatry*. 2000;61(suppl 9):97–104.

41. Ahrens B, Müller-Oerlinghausen B. Does lithium exert an independent antisuicidal effect? *Pharmacopsychiatry*. 2001;34(4):132–136.

42. Oquendo MA, Galfalvy HC, Currier D, et al. Treatment of suicide attempters with bipolar disorder: a randomized clinical trial comparing lithium and valproate in the prevention of suicidal behavior. *Am J Psychiatry*. 2011;168(10):1050–1056.

43. Findling RL, Robb A, McNamara NK, et al. Lithium in the acute treatment of bipolar I disorder: a double-blind, placebo-controlled study. *Pediatrics*. 2015;136(5):885–894.

44. Geller B, Luby JL, Joshi P, et al. A randomized controlled trial of risperidone, lithium, or divalproex sodium for initial treatment of bipolar I disorder, manic or mixed phase, in children and adolescents. *Arch Gen Psychiatry*. 2012;69(5):515–528.

45. Patino LR, Klein CC, Strawn JR, et al. A randomized, double-blind, controlled trial of lithium versus quetiapine for the treatment of acute mania in youth with early course bipolar disorder. *J Child Adolesc Psychopharmacol*. 2021;31(7):485–493.

46. Findling RL, McNamara NK, Pavuluri M, et al. Lithium for the maintenance treatment of bipolar I disorder: a double-blind, placebo-controlled discontinuation study. *J Am Acad Child Adolesc Psychiatry*. 2019;58(2):287–296. e4.

47. Pringsheim T, Hirsch L, Gardner D, et al. The pharmacological management of oppositional behaviour, conduct problems, and aggression in children and adolescents with attention-deficit hyperactivity disorder, oppositional defiant disorder, and conduct disorder: a systematic review and meta-analysis. Part 2: antipsychotics and traditional mood stabilizers. *Can J Psychiatry*. 2015;60(2):52–61.

48. Nelson JC, Baumann P, Delucchi K, et al. A systematic review and meta-analysis of lithium augmentation of tricyclic and second generation antidepressants in major depression. *J Affect Disord*. 2014;168:269–275.

49. Nierenberg AA, Fava M, Trivedi MH, et al. A comparison of lithium and T(3) augmentation following two failed medication treatments for depression: a STAR*D report. *Am J Psychiatry*. 2006;163(9):1519–1530. Quiz 1665.

50. Undurraga J, Sim K, Tondo L, et al. Lithium treatment for unipolar major depressive disorder: systematic review. *J Psychopharmacol*. 2019;33(2):167–176.

51. Leucht S, Helfer B, Dold M, et al. Lithium for schizophrenia. *Cochrane Database Syst Rev*. 2015;2015(10): Cd003834.

52. Dorus W, Ostrow DG, Anton R, et al. Lithium treatment of depressed and nondepressed alcoholics. *JAMA*. 1989;262(12):1646–1652. 22–29.

53. Burdick KE, Millett CE, Russo M, et al. The association between lithium use and neurocognitive performance in patients with bipolar disorder. *Neuropsychopharmacology*. 2020;45(10):1743–1749.

5 The Use of Antiepileptic Drugs in Psychiatry

Ashika Bains and Sharmin Ghaznavi

KEY POINTS

- A "kindling hypothesis" of mood instability led to the search for anticonvulsant medications that might improve the course of illness in bipolar disorder (BPD).
- Divalproex sodium (valproate) and carbamazepine (in an extended-release form) are effective in the treatment of acute mania.
- Lamotrigine is effective in the prevention of relapse in BPD, especially to major depression.
- The risk of the development of polycystic ovarian syndrome is elevated in women of childbearing age when BPD is treated with divalproex sodium.
- Other anticonvulsants (such as gabapentin, topiramate, zonisamide, pregabalin, tiagabine, and oxcarbazepine) have been ineffective in the treatment of BPD, worsen the course of illness, or lack data from randomized trials to support their use; none can be recommended for the treatment of any phase of BPD.

OVERVIEW: HISTORICAL CONTEXT

There has been great hope for the utility of anticonvulsants in the treatment of bipolar disorder (BPD) but in this hope lies a cautionary tale. In the 1980s, work on BPD (especially that of Robert Post, MD, at the National Institutes of Mental Health [NIMH]) suggested that the mood instability that characterized the illness bore a resemblance to characteristics of epilepsy, and hypotheses about the pathophysiologic origins of BPD evolved.[1,2] Post and others have suggested that a stress model of kindling may be responsible for the onset of mood episodes and that worsening of the course of illness over time may be caused by either kindling or sensitization phenomena.[1,2] These hypotheses led directly to the use of carbamazepine (effective as a treatment for partial seizures) for the treatment of mania and later to the use of valproate in BPD. Many anticonvulsants (with different mechanisms for seizure reduction in epilepsy) have been used in BPD, but only three—valproate, lamotrigine, and carbamazepine—have proved effective in any phase of the illness.

Although anticonvulsant therapy in BPD remains attractive, its historical use has often exceeded the limit of its evidence base. The use of gabapentin as a treatment for BPD became popular in the late 1990s, propelled in part by the drug's favorable qualities: no need for blood monitoring, few interactions with other drugs, simple metabolism, and the perception of good tolerability. Even as studies demonstrated

its ineffectiveness for mania (gabapentin was significantly worse than placebo as an adjunctive treatment for mania), its use persisted. Ultimately, Pfizer Incorporated (which had acquired Warner-Lambert, gabapentin's original marketing company) settled a $430 million civil and criminal lawsuit with the United States Justice Department for the inappropriate marketing of the drug.[3] Although the kindling hypothesis has not been abandoned with regard to an understanding of the pathophysiology of BPD, there remains limited evidence in support of the phenomenon.[4] In the NIMH Collaborative Study of Depression, no evidence was found for cycle length shortening in a cohort of patients (followed prospectively) with BPD.[5]

It is likely that the efficacy of anticonvulsant drugs in BPD is independent of their efficacy in epilepsy, in that the mechanisms of mood improvement and relapse prevention may not be the same as those that underlie seizure prevention. Sodium channel inhibition is unlikely to be the primary mechanism underlying efficacy of these compounds in BPD, for example, because newer-generation carbamazepine family drugs and many other anticonvulsants have failed to demonstrate efficacy in BPD.[6] Of the three anticonvulsants currently in use for BPD, possible common mechanisms of action include inhibition of phosphatidylinositol recycling, inhibition of glycogen synthase kinase 3-beta signaling, or inhibition of histone deacetylases, culminating in the modulation of synaptic plasticity or neuronal survival mechanisms.[7] At this point, however, these hypotheses are speculative, and the biological mechanisms of anticonvulsant therapy in patients with BPD remain unclear.

Valproic Acid

Valproic acid is approved by the US Food and Drug Administration (FDA) for use in acute mania and mixed episodes. The acute anti-manic efficacy of valproic acid has been established by several controlled studies because these randomized and placebo-controlled studies have found divalproex sodium to be an effective and safe treatment for manic episodes, even in patients in whom lithium treatment previously failed.[8,9] In comparison with lithium, a randomized, open-label trial of 300 patients with acute mania showed no difference between the two medications in mania remission or tolerability at 12 weeks.[10] A meta-analysis of multiple different anti-manic treatments showed that valproate was slightly (but not significantly) less efficacious than lithium and slightly better tolerated (although as a class, antipsychotics were overall more effective than anticonvulsants and lithium in treating acute mania).[11] There also appears to be a linear relationship between the valproate serum concentration and symptom response, and the target dosage with optimal response in acute mania is above 94 µg/mL.[12]

Valproate is not approved by the FDA for the maintenance treatment of BPD; in fact, there is growing evidence in disfavor of such a role. The largest trial of valproate for BPD maintenance to date ($n = 372$) failed to find a difference between valproate, lithium, and placebo for the primary outcome measure (time to any mood episode) for up to 1 year.[13] A large randomized, open-label trial (the Bipolar Affective Disorder: Lithium/Anti-Convulsant Evaluation [BALANCE] study; $n = 330$) compared valproate and lithium monotherapies in BPD maintenance with the combination of lithium and valproate for up to 2 years.[14] This innovative study examined physician interventions for a mood episode as the primary outcome and used an initial run-in period when patients were stabilized on both medications before randomization to different maintenance arms, which ensured patient tolerance to either medication. The study found that patients taking a combination of lithium and valproate were significantly less likely to relapse than patients taking valproate alone and were as equally likely to relapse as patients taking lithium alone. The study was not designed to compare valproate and lithium monotherapies directly, although it appeared that lithium monotherapy was more effective than valproate alone. For patients on valproate alone, the study indicated there was a potential benefit of adding lithium for maintenance, although the question remains whether patients should simply be on lithium alone in the first place. Interestingly, a meta-analysis of six studies, including the BALANCE study, found that valproic acid was more effective than placebo for preventing any mood episode. The authors also found that there was no strong evidence that valproate was inferior or superior for preventing episodes of a mood disorder.[15] In contrast, more recently, in a study examining lithium, valproate, olanzapine, and quetiapine monotherapy for BPD using UK health records, the time-to-treatment failure (defined as stopping medication or requiring an add-on) was significantly shorter for valproate (0.98 years) than for lithium (2.05 years).[16]

It is intriguing that the same investigators who demonstrated a role for divalproex sodium in acute mania treatment conducted a second randomized double-blind study of the same drug in the same setting but subsequently found no difference between divalproex sodium and placebo in acute mania.[17] The investigators attributed this discrepancy to methodological differences in the study design (lower drug dose, allowance of early study termination, more liberal use of adjunctive medications, and two-to-one randomization in favor of the study drug); however, in the context of other well-established options for acute mania treatment and BPD maintenance therapy, one wonders whether the overall use of valproate for any phase of BPD should be limited.

Anticonvulsants, including valproate, are often viewed as more effective for rapid cycling than lithium. However, it appears that this may not be the case. In a rigorous and ambitious double-blind study, rapid-cycling patients were stabilized on open-label lithium and divalproex sodium and then randomized in a double-blind fashion to either lithium or divalproex and followed prospectively.[18] There were no significant differences between the lithium-treated or the valproate-treated groups in time to drop-out or time to additional psychopharmacology.

Last, there are inadequate data to support a role for valproate in acute bipolar depression. Two independent meta-analyses of four randomized placebo-controlled trials suggested possible efficacy in acute depressive symptoms of BPD; however, the study sizes were very small ($n = 9-28$).[19,20] These findings need to be replicated before valproate can be recommended for this indication.

Lamotrigine

Lamotrigine represents a significant advance in the long-term management of bipolar depression, especially given the prominent burden of depression and depressive relapses in BPD.[21-25] Lamotrigine is approved for the maintenance treatment of BPD and is efficacious when compared with placebo in maintenance studies.[26] Long-term studies found an overall reduction in bipolar depressive relapse compared with placebo. In a key study in which patients who were most recently depressed were first stabilized on lamotrigine and randomly assigned to maintenance treatment with lamotrigine, lithium, or placebo, the overall sustained response rate was 57% with lamotrigine compared with 46% for lithium and 45% for placebo; this indicates that lamotrigine is effective in the prevention of relapse to depression compared with placebo.[23] A recent meta-analysis of double-blind randomized clinical trials of lamotrigine in the treatment of all phases of BPD found that lamotrigine is effective for reducing the risk of any mood episode or depressive episode in patients with type I BPD. There was equivocal or no evidence for the utility of lamotrigine in patients with rapid cycling disorder or for acute depression or mania.

No single trial of lamotrigine for acute bipolar depression found the drug better than placebo on the primary outcome measure of the study.[27] One widely referenced study found that although lamotrigine was not statistically different from placebo as measured by total Hamilton Depression Rating Scale (HDRS) scores, it was superior on several other measures, including the Montgomery-Asberg Depression Rating Scale (MADRS) and the Clinical Global Impression Improvement (CGI-I) scale.[21] This effect has never been replicated in individual trials, but a meta-analysis and meta-regression of pooled individual data from all five lamotrigine trials in acute bipolar depression (both bipolar I and II disorders) found that response (defined as a $\geq 50\%$ decrease in scores) on both the HDRS and the MADRS was significantly greater than for placebo.[28] The effect size was small, however, and the number needed to treat was about 11, a finding the authors note is at the "margins" of clinical utility. Remission was greater than for placebo on the MADRS but not the HDRS. The antidepressant effect of lamotrigine was greatest in the most severely depressed participants in a subgroup analysis. These data suggest that any potential benefit of lamotrigine in acute depression is likely to be small, except perhaps in severely depressed patients. It is notable that the study of lamotrigine in maintenance of bipolar depression was designed to follow patients after they were first stabilized on lamotrigine for an acute depressive episode[23]; taken together, these studies suggest that lamotrigine should be continued for maintenance therapy in patients who responded to lamotrigine during acute bipolar depression and that the patients most likely to respond are those who are most severely depressed.

A small randomized, double-blind study was performed comparing lamotrigine and placebo as add-on medications to lithium in acutely depressed bipolar patients; it showed that lamotrigine plus lithium significantly improved MADRS scores at the end of week 8 compared with lithium alone.[29] To be eligible for the study, however, patients had to be depressed despite taking a therapeutic dose of lithium for at least 2 weeks (most had been taking lithium for at least 3 months), suggesting that this study population was likely enriched for non-responders to lithium monotherapy. The study also consisted of only 124 patients; therefore, it needs to be replicated. Follow-up of these patients showed that lamotrigine plus lithium was essentially as effective as lithium alone for the prevention of mood relapse or recurrence up to 68 weeks; however, the small sample size and the study design precluded formal statistical analyses.[30] At this point, evidence for any additional benefit of combination lamotrigine–lithium therapy in treating BPD versus use of either of these medications alone remains limited.

Lamotrigine has not demonstrated efficacy for the acute treatment of mania. Multiple meta-analyses of treatment with anti-manic drugs also indicated that lamotrigine is not more effective than placebo in the treatment of acute mania.[11] No single trial found lamotrigine to be of benefit for the prevention of manic episodes; however, pooled analysis revealed a small but significant effect size for the prevention of mania.[23,26,31] Although lamotrigine is more effective than lithium in the prevention of depressive episodes, lithium appears to be more effective than lamotrigine in the prevention of manic episodes.

No validated treatments for treatment-refractory bipolar depression exist, but a small, randomized, open-label trial of adjunctive lamotrigine, risperidone, or inositol in participants who had depression despite trials of two consecutively administered standard antidepressants of adequate dose and duration was conducted as part of the Systematic Treatment Enhancement Program for Bipolar Disorder (STEP-BD).[32] An equipoise randomization process allowed participants to choose to be randomized to any pair of the study treatments. Although no differences were found in primary pair-wise comparisons in randomized patients ($n = 66$), a secondary, post-hoc analysis found that 8 weeks of sustained recovery was seen in 23.8% of the lamotrigine-treated patients, 17.4% of inositol-treated patients, and 4.6% of risperidone-treated patients. These data must be viewed with caution because they are from a secondary analysis; however, they represent one of few studies for the treatment of refractory bipolar depression.

Carbamazepine

Carbamazepine was the first anticonvulsant studied as a treatment of mania. More than 19 studies (most of which were small case series or open trials) evaluated carbamazepine for the treatment of mania. More recently, carbamazepine (in an extended-release form) was found to be effective for acute mania in two large placebo-controlled trials.[33,34] Multiple treatments meta-analysis of anti-manic drugs showed that carbamazepine was similar to valproate in terms of efficacy and acceptability in the treatment of acute mania; however, all anticonvulsants as a class were outperformed by atypical antipsychotics.[11] Carbamazepine has mixed results regarding efficacy in the rapid cycling subtype and limited evidence regarding efficacy for acute bipolar depression management.[35] No data have directly established carbamazepine as an effective maintenance treatment in BPD. A meta-analysis of four small studies comparing the efficacy of carbamazepine versus lithium in BPD maintenance suggested a possible similarity in relapse rates; however, this was tempered by the finding that carbamazepine use was associated with significantly more study withdrawals because of adverse effects.[36] At present, there are insufficient data to suggest that carbamazepine is more effective than any other treatment in these patients.

PHARMACOKINETICS, PHARMACODYNAMICS, ADVERSE EFFECTS, AND MONITORING

Valproic Acid

Valproic acid (di-n-propylacetic acid) is an anticonvulsant drug chemically unrelated to other psychiatric medications. One of the more commonly used preparations is divalproex sodium (Depakote), a compound of sodium valproate and valproic acid in a one-to-one molar ratio. Valproate is available as tablets (both delayed- and extended-release), capsules, enteric-coated capsules, sprinkles, and syrup. Absorption varies across the different preparations, and it is delayed by the ingestion of food. This may be of some importance when one switches from one preparation to another. Peak plasma levels are achieved between 2 and 4 hours after the ingestion of the direct-release preparation, and its half-life ranges from 6 to 16 hours. More than 90% of plasma valproic acid is protein-bound. The time of dosing is determined by possible side effects, and, if tolerated, a once-a-day dosing could be used. The therapeutic plasma levels generally used for the treatment of mania are the same as those used for anticonvulsant therapy (50–100 µg/mL), and the total daily dosage required to achieve these levels ranges from 500 mg to greater than 1500 mg, although one study suggests a direct relationship between plasma valproate levels and response in acute mania, suggesting optimal levels for acute treatment of greater than 90 µg/mL.[12]

Valproic acid is metabolized by the hepatic cytochrome P (CYP) 2D6 system but, unlike carbamazepine, does not auto-induce its own metabolism. Concomitant administration of carbamazepine decreases plasma levels of valproic acid, and drugs that inhibit the CYP system (e.g., selective serotonin reuptake inhibitors) can cause an increase in valproic acid levels. Valproate is known to increase the plasma levels of lamotrigine; therefore, the lamotrigine dose should be lowered in patients taking valproate. Dose-related and common initial side effects include nausea, tremor, and lethargy. Gastric irritation and nausea can be reduced by dividing the dose or by using enteric-coated preparations. Valproic acid has been associated with potentially fatal hepatic failure, usually occurring within the first 6 months of treatment and most frequently occurring in children younger than age 2 years and in persons with pre-existing liver disease. Transient, dose-related elevations in liver enzymes can occur in up to 44% of patients. Any change in hepatic function should be followed closely, and patients should be told to report symptoms of hepatic failure (such as malaise, weakness, lethargy, edema, anorexia, or vomiting). Multiple cases of valproate-associated pancreatitis have also been reported, as has multi-organ failure. These can occur at any point during treatment.

Valproic acid may produce teratogenic effects, including spina bifida (occurring in 1%) and other neural tube defects. Other potential side effects include weight gain, inhibition of platelet aggregation, hair loss, and severe dermatological reactions (such as Stevens-Johnson syndrome [SJS]).

There is an additional worry that valproate may cause endocrine abnormalities in women. In one study, 230 women were evaluated for polycystic ovarian syndrome (PCOS) as part of an ancillary study during the Systematic Treatment Enhancement Program for Bipolar Disorder (STEP-BD). Criteria for PCOS are met when oligomenorrhea (defined as nine or fewer cycles in the previous year) coincides with at least one feature of hyperandrogenism (including hirsutism, acne, male-pattern alopecia, or elevated serum androgen levels); it can lead to an increased risk of type 2 diabetes mellitus, cardiovascular disease, and some types of cancer.[37] Joffe and associates[37] compared the rate of new-onset PCOS in women with BPD taking valproate compared with the rate in those taking other anticonvulsants and lithium. Nine (10.5%) of the 86 valproate users developed treatment-emergent oligomenorrhea with hyperandrogenism compared with 2 (1.4%) of the 144 valproate non-users. The relative risk for developing PCOS on valproate as opposed to a non-valproate mood stabilizer was 7.5 (95% confidence interval [CI], 1.7–34.1; $P = .02$).[37] The onset of oligomenorrhea usually began within

12 months after beginning valproate treatment.[37] In a recent meta-analysis, women who were treated with valproate had significantly higher rates of PCOS (odds ratio [OR], 6.74; 95% CI, 1.66–27.32; $P = .00$), menstrual disorder (OR, 1.81; 95% CI, 1.02–3.23; $P = .04$), and hyperandrogenism (OR, 1.81; 95% CI, 1.02–3.23; $P = .04$). A later analysis found that discontinuation of valproate in women with valproate-associated PCOS may result in an improvement of the PCOS reproductive features because these symptoms resolved in three of the four women who discontinued valproate but persisted in all three women who continued taking valproate.[38]

Because of the risk of developing PCOS in women of childbearing age who are exposed to valproate-containing products, the use of valproate as a first-line treatment for BPD is not recommended in this population.

Lamotrigine

Lamotrigine was originally developed and approved for use as an anticonvulsant. The mechanism of action of lamotrigine in BPD is not precisely known, although lamotrigine appears to block voltage-gated sodium channels in vitro and decrease presynaptic release of glutamate.[39] Lamotrigine is a weak dihydrofolate reductase inhibitor in vitro and in animal studies, but no effect on folate concentrations has been noted in human studies.[39] It is absorbed within 1 to 3 hours and has a half-life of 25 hours. Non-serious rash can arise in approximately 8% of adults, but serious rash that requires hospitalization is seen in up to 0.5% of lamotrigine-treated individuals.[39] Because of the possibility of SJS, toxic epidermal necrolysis, or angioedema, all rashes should be regarded as potentially serious and monitored closely, and to minimize serious rashes, the dose should be increased at the rate suggested in the package insert. One randomized, open-label trial of rash precautions during the use of lamotrigine found no benefit from taking additional dermatological precautions (e.g., avoiding use of any other new drugs during dosage titration) but found an overall rash rate of approximately 8% while also finding that only 5.3% of participants discontinued lamotrigine because of this adverse effect.[40] Dosing is adjusted upward for patients who are simultaneously taking antiepileptics, such as carbamazepine, that induce the metabolism of lamotrigine and downward for those patients who are simultaneously taking antiepileptics, such as valproate, that may inhibit the clearance of the drug. There is no known relationship between lamotrigine drug levels and response in patients with BPD.

Post-marketing surveillance has revealed an increased risk of fetal anomalies in children born to women exposed to lamotrigine during early pregnancy, specifically oral cleft deformities.[39] One US study found five cases of oral clefts in infants in a study of 684 pregnancies (i.e., 7.3 in 1000 cases) when the mother was taking lamotrigine and no other antiepileptic drugs (AEDs).[41] This is 10.4 times higher (95% CI, 4.3–24.9) than a comparison group of unexposed infants (in whom the prevalence was 0.7 in 1000).[41] Other large-scale studies have not found such an elevated rate, however, and it remains controversial whether the rate elevation is attributable to reporting bias.[42]

Carbamazepine

Carbamazepine, an anticonvulsant drug structurally related to the tricyclic antidepressants (TCAs), has variable absorption and metabolism. Carbamazepine is rapidly absorbed (peak plasma levels within 4–6 hours). Approximately 80% of plasma carbamazepine is protein-bound. Its half-life ranges from 13 to 17 hours. Carbamazepine undergoes extensive oxidative metabolism with its main metabolic pathway mediated by CYP 3A3/4 (40%) followed by CYP 1A2-mediated aromatic hydroxylation (25%) and glucuronidation (15%).[35] Carbamazepine induces the CYP enzymes, causing an increase in the rate of its own metabolism over time (as well as that of other drugs metabolized by the CYP system). Drug monitoring and dose adjustments may be necessary to maintain adequate blood concentrations and therapeutic effects. Extended-release formulations are associated with a lower risk of plasma fluctuations. Carbamazepine metabolism produces an active metabolite with a half-life of about 6 hours.[35]

Concomitant administration of carbamazepine with oral contraceptives, warfarin, theophylline, doxycycline, haloperidol, aripiprazole, TCAs, bupropion, lamotrigine, or valproic acid leads to decreased plasma levels of these other drugs. Concomitant administration of drugs that inhibit the CYP system increases plasma levels of carbamazepine. These drugs include fluoxetine, fluvoxamine, cimetidine, erythromycin, isoniazid, calcium channel blockers, azoles, protease inhibitors, macrolides, and propoxyphene. Concomitant administration of phenobarbital, phenytoin, or primidone causes a decrease in carbamazepine levels through induction of the CYP enzymes. Based on its use as an anticonvulsant, dosages of carbamazepine typically range from 400 mg to 1200 mg/day, and therapeutic plasma levels range from 4 to 12 µg/mL. The relationship between blood levels and the response in mania is unknown.

Carbamazepine frequently causes lethargy, sedation, nausea, tremor, ataxia, and visual disturbances during the acute-treatment phase. Some patients develop mild leukopenia or thrombocytopenia during this phase, although it typically does not progress. Carbamazepine can cause a rare but severe form of aplastic anemia or agranulocytosis—estimated to occur with an incidence of about 2 to 5 per 100,000, which is 11 times the incidence found in the general population. Although most of these reactions occur during the first 3 months of therapy, some cases have been reported as late as 5 years after the start of carbamazepine therapy. If the white blood cell count drops below 3000 cells/mm^3 or the absolute neutrophil count drops below 1000 cells/mm^3, the medication should be discontinued. Patients should seek medical attention if they experience hematological reactions (such as fever, sore throat, oral ulcers, petechiae, easy bruising, or bleeding).

Carbamazepine has also been associated with fetal anomalies, including a risk of spina bifida (occurring in 1%), craniofacial deformities, low birth weight, and small head circumference. It has also been shown to have effects on cardiac conduction, including the slowing of atrioventricular conduction. It remains to be determined if folate supplementation may reduce the risk of these abnormalities. Carbamazepine is present in breast milk at concentrations of about 50% of those in maternal blood. Other reported side effects include inappropriate secretion of antidiuretic hormone with concomitant hyponatremia, decreased thyroid hormone levels without changes in levels of thyroid-stimulating hormone, severe dermatological reactions (such as SJS), and hepatitis.

Because of the cardiac, hematological, endocrine, and renal side effects associated with carbamazepine, patients should have the drug initiated with care. A recent physical examination, complete blood count (CBC) with a platelet count, liver function tests (LFTs), thyroid function tests, and tests of renal function are necessary before starting the drug. The CBC (with platelets) and LFTs should be monitored every 2 to 3 weeks during the initial 3 to 4 months of treatment and yearly after the stabilization of the dose. Any abnormalities in the tests listed should be evaluated, especially decreases in neutrophil counts and sodium levels. As with TCAs, carbamazepine shares the risk of inducing a hypertensive crisis when co-administered with a monoamine oxidase inhibitor, so this combination should be avoided.

OTHER ANTICONVULSANTS

Oxcarbazepine

Oxcarbazepine, a keto-analog of carbamazepine, is purported to have fewer side effects and drug–drug interactions than carbamazepine, but evidence of its efficacy in mania is lacking. There are no published placebo-controlled studies of oxcarbazepine in adults with BPD, and the single published double-blind, placebo-controlled trial of oxcarbazepine in children and adolescents with BPD found no differences in outcome between the drug and placebo.[43] There are a few small studies comparing oxcarbazepine with other anti-manic agents that have not found any difference in efficacy.[44] Because it is now available as a generic drug, it is unlikely that any definitive trials of this drug for BPD will ever be completed.

Gabapentin

Gabapentin was for a time a popular treatment for mania, likely because of perceptions of its tolerability and ease of use and because of aggressive marketing by the drug's manufacturer, Warner-Lambert. Two double-blind studies failed to detect anti-manic or antidepressant effects of gabapentin (one found an antidepressant effect for lamotrigine, however).[45] One double-blind, placebo-controlled study of adjunctive gabapentin in acute mania found that the anti-manic response to placebo was statistically significantly greater than for the drug.[46] Current evidence does not support the use of gabapentin in any phase of BPD.

Levetiracetam

Levetiracetam is an adjunctive treatment for complex partial seizures, and its mechanism of antiepileptic action remains unknown. It has had mixed results in several open-label trials as monotherapy or adjunctive therapy in bipolar mania. In one open-label trial, some of the participants had a marked mood worsening.[47] A randomized, double-blind trial of adjunctive levetiracetam versus placebo in the treatment of acute bipolar depression showed no difference between the two groups in the mean change of HDRS ratings at week 6.[48] A recent double-blind, placebo-controlled study evaluating use of levetiracetam as an adjuvant treatment with lithium in the acute phase of mania reported improvement in the Young Mania Rating Scale (YMRS) and subjective sleep questionnaires in levetiracetam group over placebo.[49] At this time, more evidence is needed to determine the safety and efficacy of the compound before it can be used in patients with BPD.

Pregabalin

Pregabalin binds voltage-gated calcium channels, and it is used in the treatment of fibromyalgia and neuropathic pain. It has also been approved in Europe, but not the United States, for the treatment of anxiety. A recent meta-analysis of randomized controlled trials in generalized anxiety disorder (GAD) showed a small, but statistically significant, effect of pregabalin on the Hamilton Anxiety Rating Scale (HARS) compared with placebo.[50] For BPD, one open-label trial found that the use of adjunctive pregabalin in treatment-refractory patients with BPD improved mood in 41% of patients, as measured by the CGI-BP; however, these data are preliminary.[51] The authors of the study also cited an unpublished double-blind,

placebo-controlled trial by Pfizer, Inc., that showed no difference between pregabalin and placebo in the treatment of acute mania. Thus, further data are needed to support the use of pregabalin in the treatment of patients with BPD, although there is substantial evidence supporting its use in those with GAD.

Tiagabine

Tiagabine is a potent selective inhibitor of the principal neuronal gamma-aminobutyric acid (GABA) transporter (GAT-1) in the cortex and hippocampus, and it is marketed as an AED. There are no published parallel-group trials of tiagabine in BPD. Although there has been hope for this drug as a monotherapy or as an adjunctive treatment for mania, there have been serious concerns about adverse effects in patients treated with it, including syncope and seizures. A recent Cochrane review found little rigorous data for tiagabine in BPD to recommend its use.[52]

Topiramate

Topiramate is an anticonvulsant that inhibits voltage-gated sodium channels, antagonizes kainate and alpha-amino-3-hydroxy-5-methyl-4-isoxazole propionic acid (AMPA) glutamate receptors, and potentiates the $GABA_A$ receptor, although its mechanism of action in the treatment of seizures remains unknown. Although case reports and uncontrolled trials have suggested that topiramate is efficacious in the treatment of acute bipolar mania, controlled trials have not demonstrated this effect.[53] These do not appear to be failed trials (i.e., ones in which the study was not able to demonstrate an effect that was actually there) because the active comparator in some of the trials, lithium, was effective in reducing manic symptoms in these studies.

A randomized, double-blind, placebo-controlled trial that evaluated adjunctive topiramate versus placebo for patients experiencing a manic or mixed episode while on therapeutic levels of valproate or lithium reported no difference in the reduction of YMRS score between the groups.[54]

Zonisamide

The anti-epileptic mechanism of zonisamide is unknown. A randomized, double-blind trial of adjunctive zonisamide in the treatment of acute bipolar mania/hypomania showed no difference in efficacy between the zonisamide and placebo adjunctive groups.[55] In a large, open-label, 56-week trial of zonisamide for acute and continuation treatment in BPD, McElroy and associates[56] found that although some patients may have had improvements in mood, a large proportion of participants dropped out of the study because of adverse effects or worsening of mood. Any beneficial effects of zonisamide on weight loss may be mitigated by concerns about the safety of the drug in those with BPD. A randomized, placebo-controlled study of zonisamide to prevent olanzapine-associated weight gain reported a slower rate of weight gain and statistically significant reduced mean gain in zonisamide group versus placebo, although more cognitive impairment as an adverse event was reported over the placebo group.[57]

CONCLUSION

Three anticonvulsants have proven effective in different phases of BPD (valproate, lamotrigine, and carbamazepine); as outlined in Table 5.1, each has specific (and not broad) efficacy in the disorder. Other anticonvulsants have proved ineffective in rigorous trials or have not been adequately studied.

TABLE 5.1 Anticonvulsants for Bipolar Disorder

	Acute Mania	Acute Depression	Maintenance
Valproate	+	–	–
Carbamazepine	+	–	–
Lamotrigine	–	+/–	+

There is ongoing concern in the epilepsy literature that anticonvulsants, such as zonisamide and topiramate, may induce mood syndromes in patients with seizure disorders.[58] Although BPD is often a life-threatening and disabling illness, anticonvulsants without proven efficacy in BPD must be used with caution in patients with this illness, and it is prudent to wait until firm evidence allows clinicians and patients to make informed decisions regarding defined benefits and known harm before initiating these agents.

REFERENCES

1. Post RM, Uhde TW, Putnam F, et al. Kindling and carbamazepine in affective illness. *J Nerv Ment Dis.* 1982;170(12):717–731.
2. Post RM. Cocaine psychoses: a continuum model. *Am J Psychiatry.* 1975;132(3):225–231.
3. Lenzer J. Pfizer pleads guilty, but drug sales continue to soar. *BMJ.* 2004;328(7450):1217.
4. Bender RE, Alloy LB. Life stress and kindling in bipolar disorders: review of the evidence and integration with emerging biopsychosocial theories. *Clin Psychol Rev.* 2011;31(3):383–398.
5. Turvey CL, Coryell WH, Solomon DA, et al. Long-term prognosis of bipolar I disorder. *Acta Psychiatr Scand.* 1999;99(2):110–119.
6. Bialer M. Why are antiepileptic drugs used for nonepileptic conditions? *Epilepsia.* 2012;53(suppl 7):26–33.
7. Rogawski MA, Loscher W. The neurobiology of antiepileptic drugs for the treatment of nonepileptic conditions. *Nature Med.* 2004;10(7):685–692.
8. Bowden CL, Swann AC, Calabrese JR, et al. A randomized, placebo-controlled, multicenter study of divalproex sodium extended release in the treatment of acute mania. *J Clin Psychiatry.* 2006;67(10):1501–1510.
9. Pope HG, McElroy SL, Keck PE, et al. Valproate in the treatment of acute mania. A placebo-controlled study. *Arch Gen Psychiatry.* 1991;48(1):62–68.
10. Bowden C, Gogus A, Grunze H, et al. A 12-week, open, randomized trial comparing sodium valproate to lithium in patients with bipolar I disorder suffering from a manic episode. *Int Clin Psychopharmacol.* 2008;23(5):254–262.
11. Cipriani A, Barbui C, Salanti G, et al. Comparative efficacy and acceptability of antimanic drugs in acute mania: a multiple-treatments meta-analysis. *Lancet.* 2011;378(9799):1306–1315.
12. Allen MH, Hirschfeld RM, Wozniak PJ, et al. Linear relationship of valproate serum concentration to response and optimal serum levels for acute mania. *Am J Psychiatry.* 2006;163(2):272–275.
13. Bowden CL, Calabrese JR, McElroy SL, et al. A randomized, placebo-controlled 12-month trial of divalproex and lithium in treatment of outpatients with bipolar I disorder. Divalproex Maintenance Study Group. *Arch Gen Psychiatry.* 2000;57:481–489.
14. BALANCE Investigators and Collaborators, Geddes J, Goodwin GM, et al. Lithium plus valproate combination therapy versus monotherapy for relapse prevention in bipolar I disorder (BALANCE): a randomised open-label trial. *Lancet.* 2010;375(9712):385–395.
15. Macritchie K, Geddes J, Scott J, et al. Valproic acid, valproate, and divalproex in the maintenance treatment of bipolar disorder. *Cochrane Database Syst Rev.* 2013;10:CD003196.
16. Hayes JF, Marston L, Walters K, et al. Lithium vs valproate vs olanzapine vs quetiapine as maintenance monotherapy for bipolar disorder: a population-based UK cohort study using electronic health records. *World Psychiatry.* 2016;15(1):53–58.
17. Hirschfeld RMA, Bowden CL, Vigna NV, et al. A randomized, placebo-controlled, multicenter study of divalproex sodium extended-release in the acute treatment of mania. *J Clin Psychiatry.* 2010;71(4):426–432.
18. Calabrese JR, Shelton MD, Rapport DJ, et al. A 20-month, double-blind, maintenance trial of lithium versus divalproex in rapid cycling bipolar disorder. *Am J Psychiatry.* 2005;162:2152–2161.
19. Bond DJ, Lam RW, Yatham LN. Divalproex sodium versus placebo in the treatment of acute bipolar depression: a systematic review and meta-analysis. *J Affect Disord.* 2010;124(3):228–234.
20. Smith LA, Cornelius VR, Azorin JM, et al. Valproate for the treatment of acute bipolar depression: systematic review and meta-analysis. *J Affect Disord.* 2010;124(3):228–234.
21. Calabrese JR, Bowden CL, Sachs GS, et al. A double-blind placebo-controlled study of lamotrigine monotherapy in outpatients with bipolar I depression. Lamictal 602 Study Group. *J Clin Psychiatry.* 1999;60:79–88.
22. Calabrese JR, Suppes T, Bowden CL, et al. A double-blind, placebo-controlled, prophylaxis study of lamotrigine in rapid-cycling bipolar disorder. Lamictal 614 Study Group. *J Clin Psychiatry.* 2000;61:841–850.
23. Calabrese JR, Bowden CL, Sachs G, et al. A placebo-controlled 18-month trial of lamotrigine and lithium maintenance treatment in recently depressed patients with bipolar I disorder. *J Clin Psychiatry.* 2003;64:1013–1024.
24. Judd LL, Akiskal HS, Schettler PJ, et al. The long-term natural history of the weekly symptomatic status of bipolar I disorder. *Arch Gen Psychiatry.* 2002;59:530–537.
25. Judd LL, Akiskal HS, Schettler PJ, et al. A prospective investigation of the natural history of the long-term weekly symptomatic status of bipolar II disorder. *Arch Gen Psychiatry.* 2003;60:261–269.
26. Goodwin GM, Bowden CL, Calabrese JR, et al. A pooled analysis of 2 placebo-controlled 18-month trials of lamotrigine and lithium maintenance in bipolar I disorder. *J Clin Psychiatry.* 2004;65: 432–441.
27. Calabrese JR, Huffman RF, White RL, et al. Lamotrigine in the acute treatment of bipolar depression: results of five double-blind, placebo-controlled clinical trials. *Bipolar Disord.* 2008;10(2):323–333.
28. Geddes JR, Calabrese JR, Goodwin GM. Lamotrigine for treatment of bipolar depression: independent meta-analysis and meta-regression of individual patient data from five randomised trials. *Br J Psychiatry.* 2009;194(1):4–9.
29. van der Loos ML, Mulder PG, Hartong EG, et al. Efficacy and safety of lamotrigine as add-on treatment to lithium in bipolar depression: a multicenter, double-blind, placebo-controlled trial. *J Clin Psychiatry.* 2009;70(2):223–231.
30. van der Loos ML, Mulder P, Hartong EG, et al. Long-term outcome of bipolar depressed patients receiving lamotrigine as add-on to lithium with the possibility of the addition of paroxetine in nonresponders: a randomized, placebo-controlled trial with a novel design. *Bipolar Disord.* 2011;13(1):111–117.
31. Bowden CL, Calabrese JR, Sachs G, et al. A placebo-controlled 18-month trial of lamotrigine and lithium maintenance treatment in recently manic or hypomanic patients with bipolar I disorder. *Arch Gen Psychiatry.* 2003;60:392–400.
32. Nierenberg AA, Ostacher MJ, Calabrese JR, et al. Treatment-resistant bipolar depression: a STEP-BD equipoise randomized effectiveness trial of antidepressant augmentation with lamotrigine, inositol, or risperidone. *Am J Psychiatry.* 2006;163:210–216.
33. Weisler RH, Kalali AH, Ketter TA. SPD417 Study Group. A multicenter, randomized, double-blind, placebo-controlled trial of extended-release carbamazepine capsules as monotherapy for bipolar disorder patients with manic or mixed episodes. *J Clin Psychiatry.* 2004;65(4):478–484.
34. Weisler RH, Keck Jr PE, Swann AC, SPD417 Study Group. Extended-release carbamazepine capsules as monotherapy for acute mania in bipolar disorder: a multicenter, randomized, double-blind, placebo-controlled trial. *J Clin Psychiatry.* 2005;66(3):323–330.
35. Wang PW, Ketter TA. Clinical use of carbamazepine for bipolar disorder. *Exp Opin Pharmacother.* 2005;6(16):2887–2902.
36. Ceron-Litvoc D, Soares BG, Geddes J, et al. Comparison of carbamazepine and lithium in treatment of bipolar disorder: a systematic review of randomized controlled trials. *Hum Psychopharmacol Clin Exp.* 2009;24:19–28.
37. Joffe H, Cohen LS, Suppes T, et al. Valproate is associated with new-onset oligoamenorrhea with hyperandrogenism in women with bipolar disorder. *Biol Psychiatry.* 2006;59(11):1078–1086.
38. Joffe H, Cohen LS, Suppes T, et al. Longitudinal follow-up of reproductive and metabolic features of valproate-associated polycystic

ovarian syndrome features: a preliminary report. *Biol Psychiatry.* 2006;60(12):1378–1381.

39. Lamictal (lamotrigine) package insert, 2006, GlaxoSmithKline.
40. Ketter TA, Greist JH, Graham JA, et al. The effect of dermatologic precautions on the incidence of rash with addition of lamotrigine in the treatment of bipolar I disorder: a randomized trial. *J Clin Psychiatry.* 2006;67(3):400–406.
41. Holmes LB, Baldwin EJ, Smith CR, et al. Increased frequency of isolated cleft palate in infants exposed to lamotrigine during pregnancy. *Neurology.* 2008;70(22):2152–2158.
42. Hunt SJ, Craig JJ, Morrow JI. Comment on: Increased frequency of isolated cleft palate in infants exposed to lamotrigine during pregnancy. *Neurology.* 2009;72(12):1108.
43. Wagner KD, Kowatch RA, Emslie GJ, et al. A double-blind, randomized, placebo-controlled trial of oxcarbazepine in the treatment of bipolar disorder in children and adolescents. *Am J Psychiatry.* 2006;163(7):1179–1186.
44. Vasudev A, Macritchie K, Vasudev K, et al. Oxcarbazepine for acute affective episodes in bipolar disorder. *Cochrane Database Syst Rev.* 2011;7(12):CD004857.
45. Frye MA, Ketter TA, Kimbrell TA, et al. A placebo-controlled study of lamotrigine and gabapentin in refractory mood disorders. *J Clin Psychopharmacol.* 2000;20:607–614.
46. Pande AC, Crockatt JG, Janney CA, et al. Gabapentin in bipolar disorder: a placebo-controlled trial of adjunctive therapy. Gabapentin Bipolar Disorder Study Group. *Bipolar Disord.* 2000;2:249–255.
47. Post RM, Altshuler LL, Frye MA, et al. Preliminary observations on the effectiveness of levetiracetam in the open adjunctive treatment of refractory bipolar disorder. *J Clin Psychiatry.* 2005;66(3):370–374.
48. Saricicek A, Maloney K, Muralidharan A, et al. Levetiracetam in the management of bipolar depression: a randomized, double-blind, placebo-controlled trial. *J Clin Psychiatry.* 2011;72(6):744–750.
49. Keshavarzi A, Sharifi A, Jahangard I, et al. Levetiracetam as an adjunctive treatment for mania: a double-blind, randomized, placebo-controlled trial. *Neuropsychobiology.* 2022;81(3):192–203.
50. Boschen MJ. A meta-analysis of the efficacy of pregabalin in the treatment of generalized anxiety disorder. *Can J Psychiatry.* 2011;56(9):558–566.
51. Schaffer LC, Schaffer CB, Miller AR, et al. An open trial of pregabalin as an acute and maintenance adjunctive treatment for outpatients with treatment resistant bipolar disorder. *J Affect Disord.* 2013;147(1-3):407–410.
52. Vasudev A, Macritchie K, Rao SNK, et al. Tiagabine in the maintenance treatment of bipolar disorder. *Cochrane Database Syst Rev.* 2012;7(12):CD005173.
53. Kushner SF, Khan A, Lane R, et al. Topiramate monotherapy in the management of acute mania: results of four double-blind placebo-controlled trials. *Bipolar Disord.* 2006;8(1):15–27.
54. Chengappa KR, Schwarzman LK, Hulihan JF, et al. Adjunctive topiramate in patients receiving a mood stabilizer for bipolar I disorder: a randomized, placebo-controlled trial. *J Clin Psychiatry.* 2006;67(11):1698–1706.
55. Dauphinais D, Knable M, Rosenthal J, et al. Zonisamide for bipolar disorder, mania, or mixed states: a randomized, double blind, placebo-controlled adjunctive trial. *Psychopharmacol Bull.* 2011;44(1):5–17.
56. McElroy SL, Suppes T, Keck Jr PE, et al. Open-label adjunctive zonisamide in the treatment of bipolar disorders: a prospective trial. *J Clin Psychiatry.* 2005;66(5):617–624.
57. McElroy SL, Winstanley E, Mori N, et al. A randomized, placebo-controlled study of zonisamide to prevent olanzapine-associated weight gain. *J Clin Psychopharmacology.* 2012;32(2):165–172.
58. Mula M, Sander JW. Negative effects of antiepileptic drugs on mood in patients with epilepsy. *Drug Saf.* 2007;30(7):555–567.

6

The Pharmacotherapy of Anxiety Disorders

Eric Bui and Theodore A. Stern

KEY POINTS

- A variety of pharmacological agents effectively treat patients with anxiety disorders.
- Selective serotonin reuptake inhibitors and serotonin–norepinephrine reuptake inhibitors are first-line pharmacological agents for the treatment of anxiety disorders.
- Benzodiazepines are effective, rapidly acting, and well-tolerated, but they are associated with the risk of abuse and dependence, and they lack efficacy for co-morbid depression.
- Anticonvulsants, atypical antipsychotics, adrenergic antagonists, and other classes of agents also play a role in the treatment of anxiety disorders.
- Many patients have persistent symptoms despite use of standard treatments; this necessitates the creative use of available interventions (alone and in combination) and has spurred the development of novel therapeutics.

OVERVIEW AND GENERAL PRINCIPLES

Anxiety disorders are associated with significant distress and dysfunction. This chapter reviews the pharmacotherapy of panic disorder (with or without co-morbid agoraphobia), generalized anxiety disorder (GAD), and social anxiety disorder (SAD). Table 6.1 includes dosing information and common side effects associated with the pharmacological agents that are typically used for the treatment of anxiety.

First-Line Pharmacotherapy for Anxiety Disorders: Selective Serotonin Reuptake Inhibitors and Serotonin–Norepinephrine Reuptake Inhibitors

The selective serotonin reuptake inhibitors (SSRIs) and serotonin–norepinephrine serotonin reuptake inhibitors (SNRIs) are first-line agents for the treatment of panic disorder, SAD, and GAD because of their broad spectrum of efficacy (including benefits for disorders that are commonly co-morbid, such as major depressive disorder), favorable side effect profile, and lack of cardiotoxicity. A meta-analysis (pooled sample of >37,000) of anxiety disorders treatments reported large effect sizes for SNRIs and SSRIs that were greater than those of psychosocial and controlled interventions and comparable to those of tricyclic antidepressants (TCAs) and benzodiazepines, both of which have less favorable side effect and safety profiles.[1]

Because the SSRIs and SNRIs can cause initial restlessness, insomnia, and increased anxiety, and because patients with anxiety disorders are often sensitive to somatic sensations, the starting doses of these agents should be low, typically half (or less) of the usual starting dose (e.g., fluoxetine 5 to 10 mg/d, sertraline 25 mg/d, paroxetine 10 mg/d [or 12.5 mg/d of the controlled-release formulation], controlled-release venlafaxine 37.5 mg/d) to minimize the early anxiogenic effect (see Table 6.1). Doses can typically be increased after about 1 week of acclimation to achieve usual therapeutic levels, with further dose titration based on the clinical response and on side effects, although an even slower upward titration is sometimes necessary in those who are especially sensitive or somatically focused. Doses for patients with anxiety disorders lie in the typical antidepressant range or are sometimes higher, such as fluoxetine 20 to 40 mg/d, paroxetine 20 to 60 mg/d (25 to 72.5 mg/d of the controlled-release formulation), sertraline 100 to 200 mg/d, citalopram 20 to 40 mg/d, escitalopram 10 to 20 mg/d, fluvoxamine 150 to 250 mg/d, and controlled-release venlafaxine 75 to 225 mg/d (although some patients respond at lower doses). In some cases of refractory anxiety disorders, even higher doses may be useful.

Administration of SSRIs and SNRIs has been associated with adverse effects that include sexual dysfunction, sleep disturbance, weight gain, headache, dose-dependent increases in blood pressure (with venlafaxine), gastrointestinal disturbances, the risk of bleeding (with anticoagulants, aspirin, or non-steroidal anti-inflammatory drugs), and provocation of increased anxiety that may make their administration problematic. SSRIs and SNRIs are usually administered in the morning (although for some individuals, paroxetine and other agents may be sedating and better tolerated with bedtime dosing); sleep disruption caused by these agents can usually be managed by the addition of a hypnotic agent. The typical 2- to 3-week lag in therapeutic efficacy for the SSRIs and SNRIs can be problematic for those who are acutely distressed, with some data suggesting that it may take up to 22 weeks for patients to respond.[2] There is also a Food and Drug Administration (FDA) class warning for the risk of thoughts of suicide and suicide attempts based on short-term studies that suggest the need for close monitoring of individuals 24 years or younger, with their use balancing the risk of these adverse effects and clinical need. In addition, data on the dose-dependent QTc prolongation with citalopram in those aged 60 years and older has led to recommendations to limit the dose to 20 mg/d and to monitor electrocardiograms (ECGs) in some populations.

There is no clear evidence of a differential efficacy between the SSRIs and SNRIs to guide selection. On the other hand, differences in their side effect profiles (e.g., the potential for weight gain and discontinuation-related symptomatology), differences in their drug interactions, and the availability of generic formulations may be clinically relevant.[3–5]

TABLE 6.1 Dosing of Selective Serotonin Reuptake Inhibitors and Serotonin–Norepinephrine Reuptake Inhibitors

Agent	Initial Dose (mg/d)	Typical Dose Range (mg/d)	Limitations and Primary Side Effects
Citalopram (Celexa)	10	20–40	Initial jitteriness, GI distress, sedation or insomnia, hypertension (venlafaxine), sexual dysfunction, urinary hesitation (duloxetine), discontinuation syndrome
Duloxetine (Cymbalta)	30	60–90	
Escitalopram (Lexapro)	5–10	10–20	
Fluoxetine (Prozac)	10	20–80	
Fluvoxamine (Luvox)	50	150–300	
Paroxetine (Paxil)	10	20–60	
Paroxetine controlled release (Paxil-CR)	12.5	25–75	
Sertraline (Zoloft)	25	50–200	
Venlafaxine extended release (Effexor-XR)	37.5	75–225	

GI, Gastrointestinal.

PHARMACOTHERAPY OF PANIC DISORDER AND AGORAPHOBIA

The pharmacotherapy of panic disorder targets the prevention of panic attacks, diminishing anticipatory and generalized anxiety, reversing phobic avoidance, improving overall function and quality of life, and treating co-morbid conditions (such as depression). As for all anxiety disorders, the goal of pharmacotherapy is to reduce both the patient's distress and impairment to the point of remission or to facilitate their participation, if necessary, in other forms of treatment (such as cognitive-behavioral therapy [CBT]).

Currently, both paroxetine formulations (immediate [Paxil] and controlled-release [Paxil-CR]), sertraline (Zoloft), fluoxetine (Prozac), and extended-release venlafaxine (Effexor-XR) are approved by the FDA for the treatment of panic disorder. Other SSRIs, including citalopram (Celexa), escitalopram (Lexapro), and fluvoxamine (Luvox) have also demonstrated anti-panic efficacy.

If patients fail to respond to several trials of SSRIs and SNRIs, other pharmacological compounds may be considered, including benzodiazepines and TCAs.

Benzodiazepines

Despite guidelines[6] for the use of antidepressants as first-line anti-panic agents, benzodiazepines are still commonly prescribed for the treatment of panic disorder.[7,8] Two high-potency benzodiazepines, alprazolam (immediate and extended-release forms) and clonazepam, are approved by the FDA for panic disorder; however, other benzodiazepines of varying potency, such as diazepam, and lorazepam,[9] at roughly equipotent doses have demonstrated anti-panic efficacy in randomized controlled trials (RCTs). Benzodiazepines remain widely used for panic (and other anxiety disorders), likely because of their effectiveness, tolerability, rapid onset-of-action, and ability to be used on an "as needed" basis for situational anxiety. It should be noted; however, that "as needed" dosing for the monotherapy of panic disorder is rarely appropriate, as this strategy generally exposes patients to the risks associated with benzodiazepine use without the

benefit of adequate and sustained dosing to achieve and maintain comprehensive efficacy. Furthermore, "as needed" dosing engenders dependency on the medication as a safety cue and interferes with exposure to, and mastery of, avoided situations, especially during CBT.

Side effects of benzodiazepines include sedation, ataxia, and memory impairment (which can be particularly problematic in the elderly and in those with prior cognitive impairment).[10] Despite concerns that ongoing benzodiazepine administration results in the development of therapeutic tolerance (i.e., loss of therapeutic efficacy or dose escalation), studies of their long-term use have suggested that benzodiazepines remain effective for panic disorder[11,12] and do not lead to significant dose escalation.[12] However, even after a relatively brief period (i.e., weeks) of regular dosing, rapid discontinuation of benzodiazepines may result in withdrawal symptoms (including increased anxiety and agitation). Discontinuation of longer-acting agents (such as clonazepam) may lead to fewer and less intense withdrawal symptoms with an abrupt taper. Patients who are sensitive to somatic sensations may find withdrawal-related symptoms particularly distressing, and a slow taper as well as the addition of CBT[13] during discontinuation may help to reduce distress associated with benzodiazepine discontinuation. A gradual taper is recommended for all patients treated with daily benzodiazepines for more than several weeks, to reduce the likelihood of withdrawal symptoms and (rarely) seizures. Although individuals predisposed to substance use disorders (SUDs) are at risk for benzodiazepine abuse, those without this diathesis do not appear to share this risk.[14] However, benzodiazepines and alcohol may act synergistically in combination, and the use of benzodiazepines in those with a current alcohol use disorder (AUD) can be problematic (thus further supporting the use of antidepressants as first-line anti-panic agents in those with an SUD).

Although co-administration of a benzodiazepine improves the rapidity of response when co-initiated with antidepressants, ongoing use may not be necessary after the initial weeks of antidepressant pharmacotherapy.

Tricyclic Antidepressants

Imipramine (Tofranil) was the first pharmacological agent shown to be efficacious for panic disorder, and TCAs were typically the first-line, "gold standard" pharmacological agents for panic disorder until they were supplanted by the SSRIs, SNRIs, and benzodiazepines. Clomipramine may have superior anti-panic properties compared with other TCAs, possibly related to its greater potency for serotonergic uptake. The efficacy of the TCAs is comparable to that of the newer agents for panic disorder, but they are now used less frequently because of their greater side effect burden, including associated anticholinergic effects, orthostasis, weight gain, cardiac conduction delays, and greater lethality in overdose. The side effect profile of the TCAs has also been associated with a high drop-out rate (30%–70%).

Like the recommendations for the use of the SSRIs and SNRIs, treatment with the TCAs should be started at lower doses (e.g., 10 mg/d for imipramine) to minimize the "activation syndrome" (involving restlessness, jitteriness, palpitations, and increased anxiety) that is seen at the onset of treatment (Table 6.2). Typical antidepressant doses (e.g., 100–300 mg/d for imipramine) may ultimately be used to control symptoms of panic. In patients with a poor response to or an intolerability to treatment with standard doses, use of TCA plasma levels, especially for imipramine, nortriptyline (Pamelor), and desipramine (Norpramin), may be informative.

TABLE 6.2 Dosing of Tricyclic Antidepressants and Monoamine Oxidase Inhibitors

Agent	Initial Dose (mg/d)	Typical Dose Range (mg/d)	Limitations and Primary Side Effects
TRICYCLIC ANTIDEPRESSANTS			
Imipramine (e.g., Tofranil)	10–25	100–300	Jitteriness, sedation, dry mouth, weight gain, cardiac conduction
Clomipramine (Anafranil)	25	25–250	effects, orthostasis, variably anticholinergic
MONOAMINE OXIDASE INHIBITORS			
Phenelzine (e.g., Nardil)	15–30	45–90	Diet restrictions, hypertensive reactions, serotonin syndrome
Tranylcypromine (e.g., Parnate)	10	30–60	
BENZODIAZEPINES			
Alprazolam (Xanax)	0.25 QID	2–8	Sedation, discontinuation difficulties, potential for abuse,
Clonazepam (Klonopin)	0.25 at bedtime	1–5	psychomotor and memory impairment, inter-dose rebound
Lorazepam (Ativan)	0.5 TID	3–12	anxiety (for shorter-acting agents)
Oxazepam (Serax)	15	30–60	

QID, Four times a day; *TID*, three times a day.

TABLE 6.3 Dosing of Other Agents

Agent	Initial Dose (mg/d)	Typical Dose Range (mg/d)	Limitations and Primary Side Effects
ANTICONVULSANTS			
Gabapentin (Neurontin)	300	600–6000	Light-headedness, sedation
Pregabalin (Lyrica)	200	300–600	Light-headedness, sedation
Lamotrigine (Lamictal)	25	50–500	GI distress, rash (rare Stevens-Johnson)
Valproic acid (Valproate)	250	500–2000	GI distress, sedation, weight gain (rare polycystic ovary disease, hepatotoxicity, pancreatitis)
ANTIPSYCHOTICS			
Aripiprazole (Abilify)	15	15–45	Extrapyramidal symptoms, metabolic syndrome, weight gain,
Olanzapine (Zyprexa)	2.5	5–15	sedation, akathisia, prolonged QTc, blood pressure changes,
Quetiapine (Seroquel)	25	50–500	neuroleptic malignant syndrome
Risperidone (Risperdal)	0.25	0.5–3	
Trifluoperazine (Stelazine)	2.5	2.5–40	
Ziprasidone (Geodon)	20	40–160	
BETA-BLOCKERS			
Atenolol	25	50–100	Bradycardia, depression, hypotension, light-headedness, seda-
Propranolol (Inderal)	10–20	10–160	tion; monotherapy efficacy limited to performance anxiety
OTHER AGENTS			
Buspirone (BuSpar)	5 TID	15–60/d	Dysphoria; limited efficacy

GI, Gastrointestinal; *TID*, three times a day.

Monoamine Oxidase Inhibitors

Despite their reputation for efficacy, the monoamine oxidase inhibitors (MAOIs) have not been systematically studied in panic disorder as defined by current nomenclature. Reversible inhibitors of monoamine oxidase$_A$ (RIMAs) typically have a more benign side effect profile and a lower risk of hypertensive reactions than irreversible MAOIs (such as phenelzine).

Other Agents

A variety of "other" agents can mitigate SAD (Table 6.3). The data on the potential efficacy of bupropion (a relatively weak reuptake inhibitor of norepinephrine [noradrenaline] and dopamine) for the treatment of panic disorder is mixed. Similarly, there is mixed support for the potential efficacy for panic disorder of another noradrenergic agent, reboxetine.[15,16]

There is suggestive evidence from case reports that buspirone (an azapirone 5-HT$_{1A}$ partial agonist) may be a useful adjunct to antidepressants and benzodiazepines[17] and acutely, although not over the long term, to CBT for panic disorder; however, it appears to be ineffective as a monotherapy. Beta-blockers reduce the somatic symptoms of arousal associated with panic and anxiety; however, they may be more useful as augmentation for an incomplete response rather than as initial monotherapy.[18] Pindolol, a beta-blocker with partial antagonist effects at the 5-HT$_{1A}$ receptor, was effective in a small double-blind RCT[19] of patients with panic disorder.

Atypical antipsychotics, including olanzapine,[20] risperidone,[21] and aripiprazole,[22,23] have demonstrated potential efficacy as monotherapy or as augmentation for the treatment of patients with panic disorder refractory to standard interventions in several small, open-label trials or case series. However, treatment-emergent weight gain, hyperlipidemia, and diabetes with some of the atypical agents, as well as the lack of large RCTs examining their efficacy and safety in panic disorder, do not support the routine first-line use of these agents for panic disorder but rather consideration for patients whose panic disorder has not sufficiently responded to standard interventions.

Based on limited data, some anticonvulsants appear to have a role in the treatment of panic disorder in individuals with co-morbid disorders (such as bipolar disorder [BPD] and SUD), for whom the use of antidepressants and benzodiazepines, respectively, are associated with additional risks. Small studies support the potential efficacy of valproic acid[24,25] but not carbamazepine[26] for the treatment of panic disorder. Gabapentin did not demonstrate significant benefit compared with placebo for patients with panic disorder in a large RCT, but a post-hoc analysis found efficacy for those with at least moderate panic severity.[27] Another related compound, the alpha$_2$ delta calcium channel antagonist pregabalin, demonstrated utility for GAD,[28] but there are no published reports related to panic disorder.

PHARMACOTHERAPY OF GENERALIZED ANXIETY DISORDER

The pharmacotherapy of patients with GAD is aimed at reducing or eliminating excessive and uncontrollable worry, somatic and cognitive symptoms associated with motor tension and autonomic arousal (e.g., muscle tension, restlessness, difficulty concentrating, disturbed sleep, fatigue, and irritability), and common co-morbidities (including depression) that compose the syndrome. The anxiety associated with GAD is typically persistent and pervasive rather than episodic and situational. The severity of GAD, however, may worsen in response to situational stressors. Thus, although the pharmacotherapy of patients with GAD is generally chronic, adjustments may be required in response to worsening during protracted stress.

Like other anxiety disorders, SSRIs and SNRIs are generally considered first-line agents for the treatment of patients with GAD because of their favorable side effect profile compared with older antidepressants (e.g., TCAs), lack of abuse or dependency compared with the benzodiazepines, and a broad spectrum of efficacy for common co-morbidities such as depression. Currently, the SSRIs, paroxetine and escitalopram, and the SNRIs (including the extended-release formulation of venlafaxine [Effexor-XR] and duloxetine [Cymbalta]) have received FDA approval for GAD; however, all agents in these classes, including sertraline, are likely to be effective for GAD but with some differences in their side effect profiles.[29] Long-term trials with SSRIs and SNRIs have demonstrated that treatment for 6 months or longer is associated with significantly lower rates of relapse relative to those who discontinued the drug after acute treatment; furthermore, ongoing treatment appears associated with ongoing gains in the quality of improvement as evidenced by a greater proportion of individuals reaching remission.[30,31]

Benzodiazepines

Benzodiazepines have been widely used for the treatment of patients with generalized anxiety for close to half a century. Although guidelines[32] have emphasized the use of antidepressants for anxiety states (including GAD) particularly when co-morbid depression is present, benzodiazepines remain broadly prescribed, either as co-therapy or monotherapy for GAD, because of their ease of use, rapid and generally reliable anxiolytic effect, and relatively favorable side effect profile.

Given their apparently equivalent efficacy, the selection of a benzodiazepine should be made by matching the pharmacokinetic properties of the agent with the situational parameters and the patient's clinical profile. Agents that are slowly metabolized and have multiple metabolites (such as diazepam and chlordiazepoxide) and those with long half-lives (such as clonazepam) may be easier to taper and are generally associated with fewer symptoms of inter-dose breakthrough compared with shorter-acting and more rapidly metabolized agents (such as oxazepam or lorazepam); the latter agents may be better suited for brief intermittent anxiolysis or for individuals likely to be slower metabolizers (e.g., older adults and those with hepatic disease). The regular use of benzodiazepines for more than 2 or 3 weeks may be associated with physiological dependence and the potential for withdrawal symptoms with rapid discontinuation or a dramatic dose decrease. Discontinuation of benzodiazepines is best done with a gradual taper to minimize withdrawal symptoms. For some patients, switching from a short-acting to a longer-acting agent (e.g., alprazolam to clonazepam) may facilitate discontinuation. The addition of CBT during the tapering process may also facilitate benzodiazepine discontinuation by giving the patient skills to manage recurrent anxiety and withdrawal

and addressing concerns about their ability to function without benzodiazepines. Moreover, the abuse liability of benzodiazepines may be problematic in individuals predisposed to an SUD, although it is less likely to be a concern for most individuals taking benzodiazepines. Pharmacodynamic interactions due the co-administration of benzodiazepines and alcohol or other sedating agents may be problematic because of the additive potential for central nervous system depression.

Buspirone

Buspirone is a 5-HT$_{1A}$ partial agonist belonging to the azapirone class; it is approved by the FDA for use in generalized anxiety. Although it has demonstrated inconsistent efficacy in clinical practice, it may be useful as an adjunct to standard therapies for refractory anxiety disorders[33]; it may also have weak antidepressant effects when used at higher doses.[34] In general, buspirone has a favorable side effect profile, although it has a gradual onset of effect; the average therapeutic dose is in the range of 30–60 mg/d, that is typically administered with twice-a-day dosing.

Anticonvulsants

The alpha-$_2$ delta calcium channel antagonist pregabalin has demonstrated efficacy in large RCTs, including several that showed its efficacy for co-morbid depressive symptoms.[35-37] The typical therapeutic dose range for pregabalin is 300–600 mg/d, with the most common adverse events being somnolence and dizziness. Data suggest that low doses of pregabalin are efficacious and there is additional benefit gained by increasing the dose to 450 mg/d; however, beyond 450 mg, reduction in anxiety symptoms does not continue to improve. Of note, pregabalin is approved in Europe for the treatment of GAD.

The selective gamma aminobutyric acid (GABA) reuptake inhibitor tiagabine demonstrated efficacy for the treatment of GAD in one randomized, placebo-controlled trial at dosages of 4 to 16 mg/d.[38] However, a subsequent series of RCTs failed to confirm this initial observation and did not support the routine use of tiagabine as an anxiolytic.[39,40]

Tricyclic Antidepressants

Several studies have demonstrated the efficacy of imipramine (the prototypical TCA) for the treatment of GAD, with RCTs showing comparable efficacy but a slower rapidity of onset relative to a benzodiazepine comparator and a greater side-effect burden relative to an SSRI comparator.[40] Again, the unfavorable side-effect profile and risk for cardiotoxicity make TCAs a less-than-ideal class of drugs to use.

Antipsychotics

Conventional antipsychotics have long been used in clinical practice for the treatment of anxiety; in fact, based on a large RCT of trifluoperazine (2–6 mg/d),[41] the agent received an FDA indication for the short-term treatment of non-psychotic anxiety. However, concerns regarding the development of extrapyramidal symptoms and tardive dyskinesia limited the use of typical antipsychotics for the treatment of anxiety. Several second-generation antipsychotics (SGAs), including olanzapine,[42] risperidone,[43] aripiprazole, and ziprasidone,[44] have demonstrated efficacy in RCTs, as well as in case series and case reports for the treatment of GAD (although typically not used exclusively as augmentation in individuals refractory to standard interventions). In addition, several RCTs have provided strong support for the efficacy of quetiapine (50–300 mg) monotherapy in the treatment of GAD.[45-47] In addition, the efficacy of the SGAs as mood stabilizers for BPD,[48] their potential efficacy for use in refractory depression, and their lack of abuse potential suggest they may be useful for those with co-morbid anxiety, mood, and SUDs, particularly those refractory to more standard interventions. Decisions regarding the use of SGAs should consider their potential for serious adverse effects as well as sedation, weight gain, and metabolic syndrome.

Vilazodone and Vortioxetine

A meta-analysis of several RCTs found that vilazodone, a serotonergic antidepressant acting as a 5-HT reuptake inhibitor and a 5-HT$_{1A}$ partial agonist, was efficacious (vs placebo), though the effect size was smaller than an SSRI or SNRI or pregabalin. Similarly, a meta-analysis of four RCTs found that vortioxetine, a 5-HT reuptake inhibitor, 5-HT$_{3R}$ antagonist, and 5-HT$_{1R}$ agonist, was efficacious (vs. placebo), though the effect size was small.

Riluzole

The efficacy of riluzole, an anti-glutamatergic agent, often used in the treatment of amyotrophic lateral sclerosis was examined in individuals with GAD in an 8-week, open-label, fixed-dose study of 100 mg/d.[49] Riluzole appeared to be effective and generally well-tolerated. Although its expense makes it unlikely that its use will be widely adopted, the report suggested that there might be a role for anti-glutamatergic agents for the treatment of anxiety.

Chamomile

Chamomile has been used for disturbed sleep for decades. Recently, one of its compounds, apigenin, which may have GABA-ergic actions, has been identified as a potential active agent. A small RCT (chamomile 220–1100 mg, 1.2% apigenin vs. placebo) suggested that chamomile may be useful in the treatment of patients with GAD.[50]

Kava

Similarly, kava roots have been consumed throughout the Pacific Ocean cultures of Polynesia as a drink with sedative and anesthetic properties. Although early reports were inconclusive,[51,52] there is now some support for the efficacy of its active agent kavalactones (120–240 mg) in the treatment of GAD.[53]

PHARMACOTHERAPY OF SOCIAL ANXIETY DISORDER

The pharmacotherapy of SAD is aimed at reducing the patient's anticipatory anxiety before and distress during social interaction and performance situations, thus reducing avoidance of social and performance situations and improving associated impairments in quality of life and function.

The SSRIs and SNRIs have become first-line pharmacotherapy for the treatment of SAD because of their efficacy for this condition, broad-spectrum effects for other anxiety disorders, efficacy for co-morbid depression (in contrast to the benzodiazepines), better tolerability than the TCAs, a more favorable safety profile than the MAOIs, and lack of abuse potential. Currently, the SSRIs, paroxetine and sertraline, as well as the SNRI venlafaxine (extended-release) are approved by the FDA for SAD, although available evidence suggests that other agents from these classes, including fluvoxamine,[54] citalopram,[55] and escitalopram,[56] are efficacious. Finally, some data suggest that

the SNRI duloxetine is efficacious for SAD as well.[57] A meta-analysis of the efficacy of second-generation antidepressants in SAD[58] suggested that escitalopram, paroxetine, sertraline, and venlafaxine produced significantly more responders than placebo and that there were no differences in efficacy among them.

Individuals with SAD are at increased risk for AUD and SUDs, which may in some cases reflect an attempt to "self-medicate" their anxiety in social situations.

Treatment with SSRIs and SNRIs for SAD is typically started at low dosages (e.g., paroxetine 10 mg/d, sertraline 25 mg/d, venlafaxine-extended release 37.5 mg/d) and titrated against a therapeutic response and tolerability (e.g., paroxetine 20–60 mg/d, sertraline 50–200 mg/d, and venlafaxine 75–225 mg/d). There is usually a therapeutic lag in efficacy of 2 to 3 weeks after initiation of SSRI or SNRI therapy for SAD, although a full response can occur after weeks to months, particularly when social anxiety-related avoidance develops, and a return to avoided situations should be encouraged alongside pharmacotherapy to both assess and optimize outcomes.

Beta-Blockers

Beta-blockers, including propranolol (Inderal) and atenolol (Tenormin), are effective for the treatment of non-generalized social anxiety (i.e., "performance anxiety") about public speaking or other performance situations. Beta-blockers blunt the symptoms of physiological arousal associated with anxiety or fear, such as tachycardia and tremor, which are often the focus of an individual's apprehension in performance situations and lead to an escalating cycle of arousal, agitation, and further elevations in social anxiety. Beta-blockers are effective for performance anxiety, at least in part by blocking these physiological symptoms of arousal, interrupting the escalating fear cycle, and mitigating the individual's escalating concern and focus on their anxiety.

Although effective for physiological symptoms of arousal, beta-blockers are not as effective at reducing the emotional and cognitive aspects of social anxiety and thus they are not first-line agents for SAD.

Beta-blockers (e.g., propranolol [10–80 mg/d] or atenolol [50–150 mg/d]) are typically administered "as needed" 1 to 2 hours before a performance situation. Beta-blockers have been associated with orthostatic hypotension, light-headedness, bradycardia, sedation, and nausea. Atenolol is less lipophilic[59] and thus less centrally active than propranolol; therefore, it may be less sedating. In practice, it is best to administer a "test dose" of the beta-blocker before its use in an actual performance-related event to establish the tolerability of an effective dose and to minimize disruptive side effects during a performance that could further increase anxiety.

Monoamine Oxidase Inhibitors

Before they were supplanted by the SSRIs and SNRIs, the MAOIs were the "gold standard" pharmacological treatment for SAD. Interest in their use in SAD grew in part from initial observations of their efficacy for the atypical subtype of depression characterized in part by marked sensitivity to rejection, and they subsequently demonstrated effectiveness in RCTs in SAD.[60]

Although clearly effective, the MAOIs are associated with concerning side effects, including orthostatic hypotension, paresthesias, weight gain, and sexual dysfunction, as well as the need for careful attention to diet and use of concomitant medication because of the risk of potentially fatal hypertensive reactions and serotonin syndrome if the proscriptions are violated. Concerns about the use of MAOIs may have contributed in part to the under-recognition and treatment of SAD that existed until the efficacy of the generally safer and easier-to-use SSRIs and SNRIs was shown. Among the MAOIs, phenelzine has been the best studied for SAD, although tranylcypromine has also been effective.

Phenelzine is typically initiated at 15 mg PO twice a day and is less likely than reuptake inhibitors (such as the TCAs, SSRIs, or SNRIs) to exacerbate anxiety during the initiation of treatment. The usual therapeutic dose range of phenelzine is 60 to 90 mg/d, with some refractory patients responding to higher doses. Careful attention to adherence to a diet free of tyramine-containing foods and avoidance of sympathomimetic and other serotonergic drugs is important to avoid hypertensive or serotonergic crises, and assessment of a patient's ability to maintain these restrictions is a critical component of the risk–benefit analysis of MAOI usage. Because of the need for careful dietary monitoring (including proscriptions against tyramine-containing foods and ingestion of sympathomimetic and other agents) to reduce the risks of hypertensive crises and serotonin syndrome, the MAOIs are often used after a lack of a response to safer and better tolerated agents.

Interest in the RIMAs was stimulated by the significant safety concerns attendant to the administration of the irreversible MAOIs. Because they can be displaced from MAO when a substrate (such as tyramine) is presented, the RIMAs do not require strict dietary prohibitions (and the risk of hypertensive crisis and serotonin syndrome associated with the irreversible MAOIs). There are no systematic data available to date regarding the efficacy of the selegiline transdermal patch for the treatment of SAD (or any other anxiety disorder).

Benzodiazepines

Benzodiazepines are efficacious for SAD, with a response noted as early as 2 weeks in non-depressed individuals with SAD.[61]

Benzodiazepines have the advantage of a relatively rapid onset of action, a favorable side effect profile, and efficacy on an as-needed basis for situational anxiety. The use of benzodiazepines, however, may be associated with adverse effects (including sedation, ataxia, and cognitive and psychomotor impairment), as well as the development of physiological dependence with regular use. Furthermore, they are generally not effective for depression that is often co-morbid with SAD, and they may worsen it. Their potential for abuse in those with a diathesis or a history of an AUD or an SUD, and their potential negative interaction with concurrent alcohol use is relevant given the increased rates of alcohol and substance use amongst those with social phobias. Benzodiazepines are started at low doses (e.g., clonazepam 0.25–0.5 mg every night at bedtime) to minimize adverse effects (such as sedation) and then titrated as tolerated to therapeutic doses (e.g., clonazepam 1–4 mg/d or its equivalent).

For maintenance treatment, to optimize a continuous anxiolytic effect, longer-acting benzodiazepines (such as clonazepam) are associated with less inter-dose rebound anxiety than shorter-acting agents and are generally preferred, whereas a shorter-acting agent with a more rapid onset of effect (such as alprazolam or lorazepam) may be more appropriate if used on an as-needed basis for performance situations. Monotherapy with as-needed dosing of benzodiazepines alone is not, however, recommended for non–"performance only" SAD, and as-needed benzodiazepine use may interfere with the reduction of social anxiety and related avoidance with cognitive-behavioral treatments.

Other Medications

Although TCAs are useful for several anxiety-related disorders, including panic disorder, PTSD, GAD, and, in the case of clomipramine, OCD, results from open and double-blind placebo-controlled trials suggest they are not effective for the treatment of SAD. Small open trials have suggested the efficacy of bupropion in SAD.[62] Although the noradrenergic and serotonergic antidepressant mirtazapine has been reported to be effective for SAD in open-label studies,[63] in a randomized placebo-controlled trial, another study failed to replicate these results in a sample ($n = 60$) that included adults of both genders.[64,65] Small studies and case series suggest the potential efficacy of SGAs, including olanzapine,[66] risperidone, and quetiapine,[67,68] for the treatment of SAD, but their use is generally reserved for patients who remain symptomatic despite more standard interventions. Several anticonvulsants have demonstrated potential efficacy for the treatment of SAD. Gabapentin, a GABA (an alpha-$_2$ delta calcium channel antagonist), demonstrated efficacy for SAD in a double-blind, placebo-controlled, parallel-group trial with doses ranging from 900 to 3600 mg/d, with most patients receiving more than 2100 mg/d.[69] A related compound, pregabalin, currently indicated for the treatment of neuropathic pain and as adjunctive treatment for partial seizures, also demonstrated efficacy for the treatment of SAD at a dosage of 600 mg/d, although the side effect burden at this higher dose was significant.[70] Valproic acid, an anticonvulsant mood-stabilizer, was reported effective for SAD in an open trial with flexible dosing of 500 to 2500 mg/d.[71] Levetiracetam demonstrated promising potential for the treatment of SAD in open trial,[72] but RCT data failed to show any efficacy over placebo. An open-label trial suggested the potential efficacy of topiramate[73] and tiagabine[74] for the treatment of SAD; however, no RCTs have confirmed these findings.

Finally, data from two small RCTs of single IV infusion of the NMDA receptor antagonist ketamine (vs. placebo) suggest it may be efficacious for SAD.

CONCLUSIONS AND FUTURE DIRECTIONS

The increased recognition of the prevalence, early onset, chronicity, and morbid impact of the anxiety disorders has spurred development efforts to find more effective and better-tolerated pharmacotherapies for this condition. Although the SSRIs, SNRIs, and benzodiazepines have demonstrated efficacy and favorable tolerability compared with older classes of agents, many patients remain symptomatic despite standard treatment; only a minority experience full remission. In addition to creative uses of available agents alone and in combination, a variety of other pharmacological agents with novel mechanisms of actions, including fatty acid amide hydrolase inhibitors, corticotropin-releasing factor antagonists, neurokinin–substance P antagonists, metabotropic glutamate receptor agonists, GABA-ergic agents and receptor modulators, and compounds with a variety of effects on serotonin, noradrenergic, and dopaminergic receptors and their subtypes, are in various stages of development. In addition, specific agents targeting ways to enhance outcomes with CBT for anxiety disorders, such as the N-methyl-D-aspartate receptor antagonist, D-cycloserine, remain an active area of translational research. These efforts may provide more effective and better-tolerated agents for the treatment of patients with anxiety.

REFERENCES

1. Bandelow B, Reitt M, Röver C, et al. Efficacy of treatments for anxiety disorders: a meta-analysis. *Int Clinical Psychopharmacol.* 2015;30(4):183–192.

2. Pollack MH, Van Ameringen M, Simon NM, et al. A double-blind randomized controlled trial of augmentation and switch strategies for refractory social anxiety disorder. *Am J Psychiatry.* 2014;171(1):44–53.

3. Andrisano C, Chiesa A, Serretti A. Newer antidepressants and panic disorder: a meta-analysis. *Int Clin Psychopharmacol.* 2013;28(1):33–45.

4. Fava M, Judge R, Hoog SL, et al. Fluoxetine versus sertraline and paroxetine in major depressive disorder: changes in weight with long-term treatment. *J Clin Psychiatry.* 2000;61(11):863–867.

5. Fava M. Prospective studies of adverse events related to antidepressant discontinuation. *J Clin Psychiatry.* 2006;67(suppl 4):14–21.

6. Practice guideline for the treatment of patients with panic disorder Work Group on Panic Disorder. American Psychiatric Association. *Am J Psychiatry.* 1998;155(5 suppl):1–34.

7. Bruce SE, Vasile RG, Goisman RM, et al. Are benzodiazepines still the medication of choice for patients with panic disorder with or without agoraphobia? *Am J Psychiatry.* 2003;160(8):1432–1438.

8. Noyes Jr R, Burrows GD, Reich JH, et al. Diazepam versus alprazolam for the treatment of panic disorder. *J Clin Psychiatry.* 1996;57(8):349–355.

9. Schweizer E, Pohl R, Balon R, et al. Lorazepam vs. alprazolam in the treatment of panic disorder. *Pharmacopsychiatry.* 1990;23(2):90–93.

10. Stewart SA. The effects of benzodiazepines on cognition. *J Clin Psychiatry.* 2005;66(suppl 2):9–13.

11. Pollack MH, Otto MW, Tesar GE, et al. Long-term outcome after acute treatment with alprazolam or clonazepam for panic disorder. *J Clin Psychopharmacol.* 1993;13(4):257–263.

12. Soumerai SB, Simoni-Wastila L, Singer C, et al. Lack of relationship between long-term use of benzodiazepines and escalation to high dosages. *Psychiatr Serv.* 2003;54(7):1006–1011.

13. Otto MW, Pollack MH, Sachs GS, et al. Discontinuation of benzodiazepine treatment: efficacy of cognitive-behavioral therapy for patients with panic disorder. *Am J Psychiatry.* 1993;150(10):1485–1490.

14. Kan CC, Hilberink SR, Breteler MH. Determination of the main risk factors for benzodiazepine dependence using a multivariate and multidimensional approach. *Compr Psychiatry.* 2004;45(2):88–94.

15. Versiani M, Cassano G, Perugi G, et al. Reboxetine, a selective norepinephrine reuptake inhibitor, is an effective and well-tolerated treatment for panic disorder. *J Clin Psychiatry.* 2002;63(1):31–37.

16. Bertani A, Perna G, Migliarese G, et al. Comparison of the treatment with paroxetine and reboxetine in panic disorder: a randomized, single-blind study. *Pharmacopsychiatry.* 2004;37(5):206–210.

17. Gastfriend DR, Rosenbaum JF. Adjunctive buspirone in benzodiazepine treatment of four patients with panic disorder. *Am J Psychiatry.* 1989;146(7):914–916.

18. Munjack DJ, Crocker B, Cabe D, et al. Alprazolam, propranolol, and placebo in the treatment of panic disorder and agoraphobia with panic attacks. *J Clin Psychopharmacol.* 1989;9(1):22–27.

19. Hirschmann S, Dannon PN, Iancu I, et al. Pindolol augmentation in patients with treatment-resistant panic disorder: a double-blind, placebo-controlled trial. *J Clin Psychopharmacol.* 2000;20(5):556–559.

20. Hollifield M, Thompson PM, Ruiz JE, et al. Potential effectiveness and safety of olanzapine in refractory panic disorder. *Depress Anxiety.* 2005;21(1):33–40.

21. Simon NM, Hoge EA, Fischmann D, et al. An open-label trial of risperidone augmentation for refractory anxiety disorders. *J Clin Psychiatry.* 2006;67(3):381–385.

22. Worthington 3rd JJ, Kinrys G, Wygant LE, et al. Aripiprazole as an augmentor of selective serotonin reuptake inhibitors in depression and anxiety disorder patients. *Int Clin Psychopharmacol.* 2005;20(1):9–11.

23. Hoge EA, Worthington 3rd JJ, Kaufman RE, et al. Aripiprazole as augmentation treatment of refractory generalized anxiety disorder and panic disorder. *CNS Spectr.* 2008;13(6):522–527.

24. Woodman CL, Noyes Jr. R. Panic disorder: treatment with valproate. *J Clin Psychiatry.* 1994;55(4):134–136.

25. Lum M, Fontaine R, Elie R. Divalproex sodium's antipanic effect in panic disorder: a placebo-controlled study. *Biol Psychiatry.* 1990;27(suppl 1):164A–165A.

26. Uhde TW, Stein MB, Post RM. Lack of efficacy of carbamazepine in the treatment of panic disorder. *Am J Psychiatry.* 1988;145(9):1104–1109.

27. Pande AC, Pollack MH, Crockatt J, et al. Placebo-controlled study of gabapentin treatment of panic disorder. *J Clin Psychopharmacol.* 2000;20(4):467–471.

28. Rickels K, Pollack MH, Feltner DE, et al. Pregabalin for treatment of generalized anxiety disorder: a 4-week, multicenter, double-blind, placebo-controlled trial of pregabalin and alprazolam. *Arch Gen Psychiatry.* 2005;62(9):1022–1030.

29. Bielski RJ, Bose A, Chang CC. A double-blind comparison of escitalopram and paroxetine in the long-term treatment of generalized anxiety disorder. *Ann Clin Psychiatry.* 2005;17(2):65–69.

30. Montgomery SA, Sheehan DV, Meoni P, et al. Characterization of the longitudinal course of improvement in generalized anxiety disorder during long-term treatment with venlafaxine XR. *J Psychiatr Res.* 2002;36(4):209–217.

31. Stocchi F, Nordera G, Jokinen RH, et al. Efficacy and tolerability of paroxetine for the long-term treatment of generalized anxiety disorder. *J Clin Psychiatry.* 2003;64(3):250–258.

32. Allgulander C, Bandelow B, Hollander E, et al. WCA recommendations for the long-term treatment of generalized anxiety disorder. *CNS Spectr.* 2003;8(8 suppl 1):53–61.

33. Appelberg BG, Syvalahti EK, Koskinen TE, et al. Patients with severe depression may benefit from buspirone augmentation of selective serotonin reuptake inhibitors: results from a placebo-controlled, randomized, double-blind, placebo wash-in study. *J Clin Psychiatry.* 2001;62(6):448–452.

34. Chessick CA, Allen MH, Thase M, et al. Azapirones for generalized anxiety disorder. *Cochrane Database Syst Rev.* 2006;3 CD006115.

35. Boschen MJ. A meta-analysis of the efficacy of pregabalin in the treatment of generalized anxiety disorder. *Can J Psychiatry.* 2011;56(9):558–566.

36. Stein DJ, Baldwin DS, Baldinetti F, et al. Efficacy of pregabalin in depressive symptoms associated with generalized anxiety disorder: a pooled analysis of 6 studies. *Eur Neuropsychopharmacol.* 2008;18(6):422–430.

37. Kasper S, Herman B, Nivoli G, et al. Efficacy of pregabalin and venlafaxine-XR in generalized anxiety disorder: results of a double-blind, placebo-controlled 8-week trial. *Int Clin Psychopharmacol.* 2009;24(2):87–96.

38. Pollack MH, Roy-Byrne PP, Van Ameringen M, et al. The selective GABA reuptake inhibitor tiagabine for the treatment of generalized anxiety disorder: results of a placebo-controlled study. *J Clin Psychiatry.* 2005;66(11):1401–1408.

39. Pollack M, Tiller J, Zie F, et al. Tiagabine in adult patients with generalized anxiety disorder: results from three randomized, double-blind, placebo-controlled, parallel-group studies. *J Clin Psychopharmacol.* 2008;28(3):308–316.

40. Pollack MH, Tiller J, Xie F, et al. Tiagabine in adult patients with generalized anxiety disorder: results from 3 randomized, double-blind, placebo-controlled, parallel-group studies. *J Clin Psychopharmacol.* 2008;28(3):308–316.

41. Mendels J, Krajewski TF, Huffer V, et al. Effective short-term treatment of generalized anxiety disorder with trifluoperazine. *J Clin Psychiatry.* 1986;47(4):170–174.

42. Pollack MH, Simon NM, Zalta AK, et al. Olanzapine augmentation of fluoxetine for refractory generalized anxiety disorder: a placebo-controlled study. *Biol Psychiatry.* 2006;59(3):211–215.

43. Brawman-Mintzer O, Knapp RG, Nietert PJ. Adjunctive risperidone in generalized anxiety disorder: a double-blind, placebo-controlled study. *J Clin Psychiatry.* 2005;66(10):1321–1325.

44. Snyderman SH, Rynn MA, Rickels K. Open-label pilot study of ziprasidone for refractory generalized anxiety disorder. *J Clin Psychopharmacol.* 2005;25(5):497–499.

45. Bandelow B, Chouinard G, Bobes J, et al. Extended-release quetiapine fumarate (quetiapine XR): a once-daily monotherapy effective in generalized anxiety disorder. Data from a randomized, double-blind, placebo- and active-controlled study. *Int J Neuropsychopharmacol.* 2010;13(3):305–320.

46. Katzman MA, Brawman-Mintzer O, Reyes EB, et al. Extended release quetiapine fumarate (quetiapine XR) monotherapy as maintenance treatment for generalized anxiety disorder: a long-term, randomized, placebo-controlled trial. *Int Clin Psychopharmacol.* 2011;26(1):11–24.

47. Khan A, Joyce M, Atkinson S, et al. A randomized, double-blind study of once-daily extended release quetiapine fumarate (quetiapine XR) monotherapy in patients with generalized anxiety disorder. *J Clin Psychopharmacol.* 2011;31(4):418–428.

48. Ketter TA, Nasrallah HA, Fagiolini A. Mood stabilizers and atypical antipsychotics: bimodal treatments for bipolar disorder. *Psychopharmacol Bull.* 2006;39(1):120–146.

49. Mathew SJ, Amiel JM, Coplan JD, et al. Open-label trial of riluzole in generalized anxiety disorder. *Am J Psychiatry.* 2005;162(12):2379–2381.

50. Amsterdam JD, Li Y, Soeller I, et al. A randomized, double-blind, placebo-controlled trial of oral Matricaria recutita (chamomile) extract therapy for generalized anxiety disorder. *J Clin Psychopharmacol.* 2009;29(4):378–382.

51. Connor KM, Payne V, Davidson JR. Kava in generalized anxiety disorder: three placebo-controlled trials. *Int Clin Psychopharmacol.* 2006;21(5):249–253.

52. Connor KM, Davidson JR. A placebo-controlled study of Kava kava in generalized anxiety disorder. *Int Clin Psychopharmacol.* 2002;17(4):185–188.

53. Sarris J, Stough C, Bousman CA, et al. Kava in the treatment of generalized anxiety disorder: a double-blind, randomized, placebo-controlled study. *J Clin Psychopharmacol.* 2013;33(5):643–648.

54. Asakura S, Tajima O, Koyama T. Fluvoxamine treatment of generalized social anxiety disorder in Japan: a randomized double-blind, placebo-controlled study. *Int J Neuropsychopharmacol.* 2007;10(2):263–274.

55. Furmark T, Appel L, Michelgard A, et al. Cerebral blood flow changes after treatment of social phobia with the neurokinin-1 antagonist GR205171, citalopram, or placebo. *Biol Psychiatry.* 2005;58(2):132–142.

56. Kasper S, Stein DJ, Loft H, et al. Escitalopram in the treatment of social anxiety disorder: randomised, placebo-controlled, flexible-dosage study. *Br J Psychiatry.* 2005;186:222–226.

57. Simon NM, Worthington JJ, Moshier SJ, et al. Duloxetine for the treatment of generalized social anxiety disorder: a preliminary randomized trial of increased dose to optimize response. *CNS Spectr.* 2010;15(7):367–373.

58. Hansen RA, Gaynes BN, Gartlehner G, et al. Efficacy and tolerability of second-generation antidepressants in social anxiety disorder. *Int Clin Psychopharmacol.* 2008;23(3):170–179.

59. Conant J, Engler R, Janowsky D, et al. Central nervous system side effects of beta-adrenergic blocking agents with high and low lipid solubility. *J Cardiovasc Pharmacol.* 1989;13(4):656–661.

60. Liebowitz MR, Gorman JM, Fyer AJ, et al. Social phobia. Review of a neglected anxiety disorder. *Arch Gen Psychiatry.* 1985;42(7):729–736.

61. Davidson JR, Potts N, Richichi E, et al. Treatment of social phobia with clonazepam and placebo. *J Clin Psychopharmacol.* 1993;13(6):423–428.

62. Emmanuel NP, Brawman-Mintzer O, Morton WA, et al. Bupropion-SR in treatment of social phobia. *Depress Anxiety.* 2000;12(2):111–113.

63. Van Veen JF, Van Vliet IM, Westenberg HG. Mirtazapine in social anxiety disorder: a pilot study. *Int Clin Psychopharmacol.* 2002;17(6):315–317.

64. Mrakotsky C, Masek B, Biederman J, et al. Prospective open-label pilot trial of mirtazapine in children and adolescents with social phobia. *J Anxiety Disord.* 2008;22(1):88–97.

65. Schutters SI, Van Megen HJ, Van Veen JF, et al. Mirtazapine in generalized social anxiety disorder: a randomized, double-blind, placebo-controlled study. *Int Clin Psychopharmacol.* 2010;25(5):302–304.

66. Barnett SD, Kramer ML, Casat CD, et al. Efficacy of olanzapine in social anxiety disorder: a pilot study. *J Psychopharmacol.* 2002;16(4):365–368.

67. Schutters SI, van Megen HJ, Westenberg HG. Efficacy of quetiapine in generalized social anxiety disorder: results from an open-label study. *J Clin Psychiatry.* 2005;66(4):540–542.

68. Vaishnavi S, Alamy S, Zhang W, et al. Quetiapine as monotherapy for social anxiety disorder: a placebo-controlled study. *Prog Neuropsychopharmacol Biol Psychiatry.* 2007;31(7):1464–1469.

69. Pande AC, Davidson JR, Jefferson JW, et al. Treatment of social phobia with gabapentin: a placebo-controlled study. *J Clin Psychopharmacol.* 1999;19(4):341–348.

70. Pande AC, Feltner DE, Jefferson JW, et al. Efficacy of the novel anxiolytic pregabalin in social anxiety disorder: a placebo-controlled, multicenter study. *J Clin Psychopharmacol.* 2004;24(2):141–149.

71. Kinrys G, Pollack MH, Simon NM, et al. Valproic acid for the treatment of social anxiety disorder. *Int Clin Psychopharmacol.* 2003;18:169–172.

72. Simon NM, Worthington JJ, Doyle AC, et al. An open-label study of levetiracetam for the treatment of social anxiety disorder. *J Clin Psychiatry.* 2004;65(9):1219–1222.

73. Van Ameringen M, Mancini C, Pipe B, et al. An open trial of topiramate in the treatment of generalized social phobia. *J Clin Psychiatry.* 2004;65(12):1674–1678.

74. Dunlop BW, Papp L, Garlow SJ, et al. Tiagabine for social anxiety disorder. *Hum Psychopharmacol.* 2007;22(4):241–244.

7 Pharmacotherapy of Attention-Deficit Hyperactivity Disorder Across the Life Span

Timothy E. Wilens, Jefferson B. Prince, Mira Stone, Joseph Biederman†, Mai Uchida, and Craig B.H. Surman

KEY POINTS

- Attention-deficit hyperactivity disorder (ADHD) is a common disorder in children, adolescents, and adults.
- Although the phenotype of ADHD changes across the life span, ADHD persists in many children, adolescents, and adults.
- Co-morbid psychiatric and learning disorders are common in patients with ADHD across the life span.
- Stimulant and non-stimulant medications are Food and Drug Administration-approved as treatments for ADHD across the life span.

OVERVIEW

ADHD is a common psychiatric condition that occurs in 3% to 10% of school-age children worldwide, in up to 8% of adolescents, and in up to 4% of adults.[1] The classic triad of impaired attention, impulsivity, and excessive motor activity characterizes ADHD, although many patients may manifest only inattentive symptoms. ADHD usually persists, to a significant degree, from childhood through adolescence and into adulthood.[1] Individuals with ADHD who meet the *Diagnostic and Statistical Manual of Mental Disorders* (DSM) definition have significant functional impairment(s) in multiple domains of function.

Attention-deficit hyperactivity disorder is frequently co-morbid with oppositional defiant disorder (ODD), conduct disorder (CD), multiple anxiety disorders (panic disorder, obsessive-compulsive disorder [OCD], tic disorders), mood disorders (e.g., depression, dysthymia, and bipolar disorder [BPD]), learning disorders (e.g., auditory processing problems and dyslexia), and substance use disorders (SUDs). More recently, there has been increasing focus on the overlap of ADHD and autism spectrum disorders (ASDs).[2] In addition to co-morbid psychiatric and SUDs, learning and developmental disorders also need to be assessed in all patients with ADHD and the relationship of these symptoms with ADHD delineated.

As part of the diagnostic evaluation, clinicians should complete a thorough clinical evaluation that establishes whether full ADHD criteria are met, including the current severity, the onset of symptoms by the age of 12 years, impairment in two or more settings because of the symptoms, and a lack of other explanation for the symptoms. A broad differential diagnosis should be considered to rule out other causes of brain dysfunction. A personal and family medical history should be obtained to appreciate the risks relevant to pharmacotherapy. In particular, the clinician should be confident that the patient has a normal cardiovascular (CV) examination and that there is no apparent risk of arrhythmias (e.g., unexplained light-headedness or close relatives with a history of collapse or sudden death). Before treatment with medications, it is also usually important to measure baseline levels of height, weight, blood pressure, and pulse, which should be monitored to evaluate physiological risks during treatment.

Emerging data show the usefulness of cognitive-behavioral therapy (CBT) in the treatment of a largely medicated sample of adolescents and adults with ADHD using both individual and group therapeutic approaches.[3-5] Similar to youth with ADHD, administration of a medication plus CBT appears to be more helpful in the management of adult ADHD and co-morbid symptoms of mood and anxiety than either treatment alone.[3]

STIMULANTS

For more than 70 years, stimulants have been used safely and effectively in the treatment of patients with ADHD, and they are among the most well-established treatments in psychiatry.[6,7] The stimulants used include methylphenidate (MPH) and amphetamines (AMP). The recent development of isomers and various novel delivery systems has significantly advanced the stimulant pharmacotherapy for patients with ADHD (see Table 7.1 for a list of these medications). Longer-term data support the idea that stimulants appear to normalize brain structure and function in growing children with ADHD compared with those without ADHD.[8] Moreover, a recent meta-analysis shows that medication treatment of ADHD over time reverses many of the negative sequelae of ADHD and results in long-term functional improvements in multiple domains.[9]

Pharmacodynamic Properties of Stimulants

Stimulants increase intra-synaptic concentrations of dopamine (DA) and norepinephrine (NE).[10] MPH primarily binds to the DA transporter protein (DAT), blocking the reuptake of DA, increasing intra-synaptic DA.[10] AMP compounds diminish pre-synaptic reuptake of DA by binding to DAT and travel into the DA neuron, promoting release of DA from reserpine-sensitive vesicles in the pre-synaptic neuron.[10] In addition, stimulants (AMP > MPH) increase levels of NE and serotonin (5-HT) in the inter-neuronal space. Although group studies comparing MPH with AMP generally demonstrate similar efficacy,[11] their pharmacodynamic differences may explain why a particular patient may respond to, or tolerate, one stimulant preferentially over another. It is necessary to appreciate that although the efficacy of AMP and MPH is similar, their potency differs, such that 5 mg of AMP is approximately equipotent to 10 mg of MPH. Typically, the isomeric forms of both MPH (e.g., dextro-MPH) and AMP (dextro-AMP) are twice as potent as their racemic counterparts.

---

†deceased

TABLE 7.1 Stimulant Preparations for the Treatment of Attention-Deficit Hyperactivity Disorder[10]

Medication (Brand)	Preparation	Starting Dose	Duration
MPH (Ritalin IR)	5-, 10-, 20-mg tablets	5 mg QD/BID (2 mg/kg/day)	4 hr/BID
MPH XR (Ritalin SR)	20-mg tablets	5 mg QD/BID (2 mg/kg/day)	6 hr
MPH XR (Ritalin LA)	10-, 20-, 30-, 40-mg capsules	20 mg QD	8 hr/once
MPH XR (Concerta)	18-, 27-, 36-, 54-mg capsules	18 mg QD (2 mg/kg/day)	12 hr/once
MPH XR (Metadate CD)	10-, 20-, 30-, 40-, 50-, 60-mg capsules	20 mg QD	8 hr/once
MPH XR (Methylin)	2.5-, 5-, 10-mg chewable tablets; 5-mg/5-cc and 10-mg/5-cc suspension	5 mg BID	4 hr
MPH XR (Daytrana)	10,- 15-, 20-, 30-mg patch	10 mg	6–16 hr
MPH XR (Quillivant)	25-mg/1-tsp suspension	<10 mg QD	12 hr/once
MPH ER (QulliChew ER)	20-, 30-mg chewable tablets	<10 mg QD	8 hr/once
D-MPH (Focalin)	2.5-, 5-, 10-mg tablets	2.5 mg QD/BID (1 mg/kg/day)	4–5 hr/BID–TID
D-MPH XR (Focalin-XR)	5-, 10-, 15-, 20-mg capsules	5 mg QD (1 mg/kg/day)	10–12 hr/QD
MPH (Aptensio XR)	10-mg capsules	10 mg QD (2 mg/kg/day)	12 hr/once
MPH (Adhansia XR)	25-mg capsules	25 mg QD	12 hr/once
MPH (Jornay PM)	20-mg capsules	20 mg QD (100 mg)	12 hr/once
SDX-MPH(Azstarys)	26.1/5.2-mg capsules	26.1/5.2 mg QD (52.3/10.4 mg)	13 hr/once
D-AMP (Dexedrine Tablets)	5-, 10-mg tablets	2.5–5 mg BID (1.5 mg/kg/day)	3–5 hr/BID–QD
D-AMP (Dexedrine Spansule)	5-, 10-, 15-mg capsule	5 mg QD	6 hr/QD–BID
LDX XR (Vyvanse)	20-, 30-, 40-, 50-, 60-, 70-mg capsules	30 mg QD	12–14 hr/QD
MAS (Adderall)	5-, 10-, 15-, 20-, 25-, 30-mg tablets	2.5–5 mg QD (1.5 mg/kg/day)	6 hr/BID
MAS XR (Adderall XR)	5-, 10-, 15-, 20-, 25-, 30-mg capsules	2.5–5 mg QD	12 hr/QD
D-AMP (Mydayis)	12.5-, 25-, 37.5-, 50-mg capsules	12.5 mg QD (50 mg, adults/25 mg, adolescents)	Up to 16 hr/QD
AMP (Evekeo)	2.5-, 5-, 10-, 15-mg tablets	2.5–5 mg BID	3–5 hr/BID–QID
AMP (Dyanavel XR)	2.5-mg/1-mL suspension	2.5–5 mg QD (1.5 mg/kg/day)	13 hr/QD
AMP (Adzenys XR-ODT)	3.1-, 6.3-, 9.4-, 12.5-, 15.7-, 18.8-mg disintegrating tablets	6.3–12.5 mg QD (12.5 mg, adolescents)	12 hr/QD
D-AMP (Xelstrym)	4.5-mg/9-hr patches	4.5 mg	12 hr/QD

AMP, Amphetamine; *BID*, twice a day; *D*, dextro; *ER/XR*, extended release; *IR*, immediate release; *LA*, long acting; *LDX*, lisdexamfetamine; *MAS*, mixed amphetamine salts; *MPH*, methylphenidate; *ODT*, orally disintegrating tablet; *QD*, every day; *SDX*, serdexmethylphenidate; *SR*, sustained release.

Methylphenidate

Behavioral effects of immediate-release MPH peak 1 to 2 hours after administration and tend to dissipate within 3 to 5 hours.[6,7] After oral administration, immediate-release MPH is readily absorbed, reaching peak plasma concentration in 1.5 to 2.5 hours, and has an elimination half-life of 2.5 to 3.5 hours. After oral administration but before reaching the plasma, the enzyme carboxylesterase (CES-1), which is located in the walls of the stomach and liver, extensively metabolizes MPH via hydrolysis and de-esterification, with little oxidation.[6,7] Individual differences in CES-1's hydrolyzing activity may result in variable metabolism and serum MPH levels.[6,7] Several MPH preparations are now available with variable durations of action (see Table 7.1).

Amphetamines

Amphetamine is available in three forms, dextroamphetamine (DEX; Dexedrine), mixed AMP salts (MAS; Adderall), and lisdexamfetamine dimesylate (LDX; Vyvanse). DEX tablets achieve peak plasma levels 2 to 3 hours after oral administration and have a half-life of 4 to 6 hours. Behavioral effects of DEX tablets peak 1 to 2 hours after administration and last 4 to 5 hours. For DEX spansules, these values are somewhat longer. MAS preparations consist of equal portions of d-AMP saccharate, d,l-AMP aspartate, d-AMP sulfate, and d,l-AMP sulfate, and a single dose results in a ratio of approximately 3 : 1 d- to l-AMP.LDL[6,7] An amphetamine sulfate product with 1:1 d- to l-AMP is also available. The two isomers have different pharmacodynamic properties, and some patients with ADHD preferentially respond to one isomer over another.

Clinical Use of Stimulants

Guidelines and recent excellent clinical reviews regarding the use of stimulant medications in children, adolescents, and adults in clinical practice have been published.[6,7] Treatment with immediate-release preparations generally starts at 5 mg of MPH or AMP once daily and is titrated upward every 3 to 5 days until an effect is noted or adverse effects emerge. Typically, the half-life of the short-acting stimulants necessitates at least twice-daily (BID) dosing, with the addition of similar or reduced afternoon doses dependent on break through symptoms. In a typical adult, dosing of immediate-release MPH is generally up to 30 mg three to four times daily or AMP 15 to 20 mg two to three times a day. Currently, most school-age youth and adults with ADHD are treated with a stimulant that has an extended delivery. Often intermediate delivery systems (e.g., having effects that last 8–10 hours) are used in children aged 6 to 12 years with longer-acting extended-release stimulants (e.g., with a duration of effect of 10+ hours) used in youth aged 10 years through adulthood. Because there is no way to determine which stimulant will be best tolerated and most effective, it is wise to consider including trials with preparations of both MPH and AMP, although tolerance is thought to be more common with AMP products.

Side Effects of Stimulants

Although generally well tolerated, stimulants can cause clinically significant side effects (including anorexia, nausea, difficulty falling asleep, obsessiveness, headaches, dry mouth, rebound phenomena, anxiety, nightmares, dizziness, irritability, dysphoria, and weight loss).[6,7] The frequency and types

TABLE 7.2 Pharmacological Strategies in Challenging Cases of Attention-Deficit Hyperactivity Disorder

Symptom	Interventions
Worsening or unchanged ADHD symptoms (inattention, impulsivity, hyperactivity)	Change the medication dose (increase or decrease). Change the timing of the dose. Change the preparation, substitute the racemic to an isomeric preparation, or change the stimulant class. Consider an adjunctive treatment (a noradrenergic agent, stimulant, or cognitive enhancer). If stimulant tolerance is occurring, consider taking planned treatment breaks. Consider adjusting a non-pharmacological treatment (CBT, coaching, or re-evaluating the neuropsychological profile for executive function capacities).
Intolerable side effects	Evaluate if the side effects are medication-induced. Assess the medication response versus tolerability of the side effect. Manage the side effect aggressively (change the timing of the dose, change the preparation of the stimulant, or consider an adjunctive or alternative treatment).
Rebound of ADHD symptoms	Change the timing of the dose. Supplement with a small dose of a short-acting stimulant or α-adrenergic agent 1 hr before symptom onset. Change the preparation. Increase the frequency of the dose.
Development of tics or TS or use with co-morbid tics or TS	Assess the persistence of tics or TS. If tics abate, re-challenge. If tics are clearly worsened with stimulant treatment, discontinue or continue with informed consent. Consider stimulant use with adjunctive anti-tic treatment (α-agonist, haloperidol, pimozide) or use of alternative treatment (α-adrenergic agents, atomoxetine, tricyclics).
Emergence of dysphoria, irritability, acceleration, or agitation	Adjust the dose (upward or downward); examine for toxicity or rebound. Change the stimulant preparation or class. Evaluate for the development or exacerbation of co-morbidity (mood, anxiety, or substance use [including nicotine and caffeine]). Assess sleep and mood. Consider an alternative treatment. Consider the use of an antidepressant or anti-manic agent. Consider non-pharmacological interventions.
Emergence of psychosis or mania	Discontinue the stimulant. Assess for co-morbidity. Assess substance use. Treat the cause of psychosis or mania.

ADHD, Attention-deficit hyperactivity disorder; *CBT*, cognitive-behavioral therapy; *TS*, Tourette's syndrome.

of stimulant side effects appear to be similar in those with ADHD, regardless of their age. In patients with a current co-morbid mood or anxiety disorder, clinicians should consider whether an adverse effect reflects the co-morbid disorder, a side effect of the treatment, or an exacerbation of the co-morbid condition. Moreover, although stimulants can cause these side effects, many individuals with ADHD experience these problems before treatment; therefore, it is important for clinicians to document these symptoms at baseline.[6,7] Recommendations about the management of common side effects are listed in Table 7.2.

Appetite Suppression

Patients treated with stimulants often experience a dose-related reduction in appetite and in some cases weight loss. Although appetite suppression often decreases over time, clinicians should give guidance on how to improve the patient's nutritional options with a higher caloric intake to balance the consequences of reduced food intake. Cyproheptadine, in doses of 4 to 8 mg, has improved appetite in those with ADHD who experience stimulant-associated appetite suppression.

Growth

The impact of stimulant treatment on growth remains a concern, and the data are conflicting. For instance, in the MTA study, youth with ADHD who were treated with a stimulant continuously over a 24-month period experienced a growth deceleration of about 1 cm per year.[12] In contrast, Biederman and colleagues[13] reported on growth trajectories in two

case-control samples of boys and girls with ADHD as compared with control participants. Over 10 to 11 years of follow-up, these authors found no significant impact of ADHD or its treatment on growth parameters except in those with ADHD and depression; girls were larger and boys smaller. Despite reassuring data, to ensure healthy physical development of children with ADHD receiving treatments, monitoring is strongly recommended. The American Academy of Child and Adolescent Psychiatry practice parameters for ADHD recommend routine monitoring of height and weight, including serial plotting of growth parameters.[11] Crossing two percentile lines of height or weight may indicate a clinically significant change in growth that should be addressed clinically. A variety of options may be considered, including a medication holiday, dose adjustment, a change in medication, or consultation. Ultimately, the impact on growth should be balanced with the overall benefits of treatment.

Sleep

Parents often report sleep disturbances in their children with ADHD both before and during treatment.[14] Various strategies (including improving sleep hygiene, making behavioral modifications, adjusting the timing or type of stimulant used, and switching to an alternative ADHD treatment) have been suggested to help make it easier for patients with ADHD to fall asleep.[14] Complementary pharmacological treatments to consider include the following: melatonin (1–3 mg), clonidine (0.1–0.3 mg),[15] diphenhydramine (25–50 mg), trazodone (25–50 mg), mirtazapine (3.75–15 mg), and imipramine (25–50 mg). Melatonin, a hormone secreted by the pineal gland

TABLE 7.3 Non-stimulants Used in the Treatment of Attention-Deficit Hyperactivity Disorder[10]

Medication (Brand)	Dosing Available	Dose Range
Atomoxetine[a,b] (Strattera)	10-, 18-, 25-, 40-, 60-, 80-, 100-mg capsules	1.2 mg/kg/day or 100 mg/day
Viloxazine XR[a,b] (Qelbree)	100-, 200-mg capsules	200 mg (children) to 600 mg (adults)
Guanfacine ER[a] (Intuniv ER Tenex IR)	1-, 2-, 3-, 4-mg tablets (ER)	Up to 7 mg/day
	1-, 2-, 3-, 4-mg tablets (IR)	
Clonidine ER[c] (Kapvay ER, Catapress IR)	0.1-, 0.2-mg tablets (ER)	0.1–0.2 mg twice daily
	0.1-, 0.2-, 0.3-mg tablets (IR)	
Bupropion (Wellbutrin)	75-, 100-mg tablets (IR)	Up to 400 mg (IR or SR) up to 450 mg (XR)
	100-, 200-mg tablets (SR)	
	150-, 300-mg tablets (XR)	
Tricyclic antidepressants (multiple)	10-, 25-, 50-, 100-mg tablets	Nortriptyline up to 2 mg/kg/day; others to 4 mg/kg/day
		Typical adult dosage, 100–200 mg/day
Memantine	10-, 20-mg tablets (IR)	10 mg (children) or 20 mg (adults), given BID (IR) QD (XR)
	7, 14, 21, 28 mg capsules (XR)	
Modafinil	100-, 200-mg tablets	100–200 mg (children); 100–400 mg (adults) QD or BID

BID, Twice a day; *ER/XR*, extended release; *IR*, immediate release; *QD*, every day; *SR*, sustained release.
[a]Approved to treat attention-deficit hyperactivity disorder (ADHD) in patients 6 years of age and older.
[b]Specifically approved for treatment of ADHD in adults.
[c]Approved to treat ADHD in youth 6–17 years old as monotherapy or as adjunctive treatment with stimulant.

that helps regulate circadian rhythms, is often used initially to address sleep problems in children.[16] Melatonin used alone and in conjunction with sleep hygiene techniques or morning bright light therapy may improve sleep patterns in individuals with delayed sleep phase who have ADHD.[17]

Medication Interactions with Stimulants

The interactions of stimulants with other prescription and non-prescription medications are generally mild and not a major source of concern.[6,7] Concomitant use of sympathomimetic agents (e.g., pseudoephedrine) may potentiate the effects of both medications. Likewise, excessive intake of caffeine may compromise the effectiveness of stimulants and exacerbate sleep difficulties. Stimulants have been well tolerated in combination with non-stimulants indicated for ADHD, as well as in combination with serotonin and serotonin–norepinephrine reuptake inhibitors (SNRIs). Co-administration of stimulants with monoamine oxidase inhibitors is contraindicated.

Despite the prominent use of stimulants for ADHD, approximately one-third of individuals may not respond, experience untoward side effects, or manifest co-morbidity that stimulants may exacerbate or be ineffective in treating.[6,7] Several non-stimulants have also been studied for ADHD (Table 7.3).

ATOMOXETINE

Unlike the stimulants, atomoxetine (ATMX; Strattera) is unscheduled; therefore, clinicians can prescribe refills. ATMX acts by blocking the NE reuptake pump on the pre-synaptic membrane, thus increasing the availability of intra-synaptic NE, with little affinity for other monoamine transporters or neurotransmitter receptors. ATMX is rapidly absorbed after oral administration; food does not appear to adversely affect absorption, and the plasma half-life appears to be around 5 hours. ATMX is metabolized primarily in the liver by the cytochrome (CYP) P450 2D6 enzyme.[18] Clinically, ATMX is often initially prescribed for patients not interested in taking a stimulant; it may also have a benefit for co-morbid anxiety disorders. ATMX is often used in conjunction with stimulants, with reports suggesting that this combination is well tolerated and effective.[19]

Atomoxetine can be initiated at doses of 0.5 mg/kg/day, and after 1 week, it can be increased to a target dose of 1.2 mg/kg/day. Although ATMX has been studied in doses of up to 2 mg/kg/day, current dosing guidelines recommend a maximum dosage of 1.4 mg/kg/day, or 100 mg/day. Although some patients have an early response, it may take up to 10 weeks to see the full benefits of ATMX treatment. In the initial trials, ATMX was dosed BID (typically after breakfast and after dinner); however, it may also be used daily.

Atomoxetine may be especially useful when anxiety, mood symptoms, or tics co-occur with ADHD. Moreover, because of its lack of abuse liability, ATMX may be selected for use in adults with recent or current substance use issues.

Although generally well tolerated, the most common side effects seen in children and adolescents taking ATMX include a reduced appetite, dyspepsia, and dizziness, although height and weight in long-term use do not appear to be problematic. In adults, ATMX treatment may be associated with dry mouth, insomnia, nausea, decreased appetite, constipation, decreased libido, dizziness, and sweating.[20] Minor increases in blood pressure and pulse have also been reported. Several strategies can be used to manage ATMX's side effects. When patients experience nausea, the dose of ATMX should be divided and administered with food. Sedation is often transient but may be helped by either administering the dose at night or by dividing the dose.

Patients taking ATMX should also be warned about the risk for liver injury, although the incidence is thought to be rare. However, patients and families should contact their doctors if they develop pruritus, jaundice, dark urine, right upper quadrant tenderness, or unexplained "flu-like" symptoms. As with other psychotropics, thoughts of suicide in patients treated with ATMX have been reported and should be monitored. If maladaptive thinking or mood swings develop, treatment should be stopped and the diagnosis reassessed.

ALPHA-ADRENERGIC AGONISTS

Clonidine is an imidazoline derivative with α-adrenergic agonist properties that stimulate inhibitory, pre-synaptic autoreceptors in the central nervous system.[20] An extended delivery oral formulation of clonidine, clonidine ER (Kapvay) is approved as a treatment for ADHD in youth aged 6 to 17 years and is approved as monotherapy and as an adjunctive treatment with stimulants. Although clonidine reduces the symptoms of ADHD, its overall effect is less than that of the stimulants, and it appears like that of the other non-stimulants. Clonidine may be particularly helpful in patients with ADHD and co-morbid CD or ODD, tic disorders,[21] and ADHD-associated sleep disturbances[15] and may reduce anxiety and hypervigilance in traumatized children.

Clonidine is a relatively short-acting compound with a plasma half-life ranging from approximately 5.5 hours (in children) to 8.5 hours (in adults). Clonidine ER is usually initiated at a dose of 0.1 mg *hora somni* for several days and titrated up to a maximum recommended dose of 0.2 mg BID. Immediate-release clonidine is usually initiated at the lowest manufactured dose of a half or quarter tablet of 0.1 mg. The most common short-term adverse effect of clonidine is sedation, which tends to subside with continued treatment. It can also produce, in some cases, hypotension, dry mouth, vivid dreams, depression, and confusion. Because abrupt withdrawal of clonidine has been associated with rebound hypertension, slow tapering is advised.[20]

Guanfacine, the most selective α_{2A}-adrenergic agonist currently available, appears to act by mimicking NE binding in the pre-frontal cortex.[20] An extended-delivery formulation guanfacine ER (Intuniv) was approved by the US Food and Drug Administration (FDA) for the treatment of ADHD as monotherapy or as an adjunctive treatment with stimulants. Guanfacine ER is usually started at 1 mg/day at bedtime and titrated to a maximum dose of 4 mg. Possible advantages of guanfacine over clonidine include less sedation and a longer duration of action. Like clonidine, guanfacine may be particularly helpful in youth with ADHD and co-morbid tic disorders.[21] Guanfacine treatment is associated with minor, clinically insignificant decreases in blood pressure and pulse rate. The adverse effects of guanfacine include sedation, irritability, and depression. Typically, the α-agonists are used in the treatment of children and adolescents, although recent work demonstrates efficacy at higher doses in older adolescents[22] and adults.[23]

Viloxazine XR

Viloxazine XR is a relatively new agent approved for ADHD in children, adolescents, and adults. Viloxazine XR is a serotonin–norepinephrine modulating agent that is available in an extended-release formulation. Viloxazine modulates serotonergic activity as a selective $5\text{-HT}2_{2B}$ receptor antagonist and 5-HT_{2C} receptor agonist, and it moderately inhibits norepinephrine transporter (NET), thus blocking the reuptake of norepinephrine.[20] Multiple trials have shown that dosing of up to 200 mg in children, 400 mg in adolescents, and 600 mg in adults is effective for all symptom clusters of ADHD.[24] Data also suggest that there is a relatively rapid response to treatment with changes as early as week 2 that predict a complete response at full-dose titration. Currently, studies are largely limited to patients with uncomplicated ADHD; however, given its mechanism of action and its previous use in Europe for depression, it is anticipated that ADHD plus co-morbid mood or anxiety may also be managed with viloxazine XR.

The drug is highly protein-bound (76%–82%), and the mean half-life of viloxazine ER is 7.02 ± 4.74 hours. Viloxazine undergoes metabolism via the CYP P450 enzyme CYP 2D6 and the UDP-glucuronosyltransferase enzymes UGT 1A9 and UGT 2B15.

Patients taking drugs metabolized by the CYP 1A2 enzyme may require dosing reductions because viloxazine is a potent CYP 1A2 inhibitor. Hence, the dosing of agents, such as duloxetine, needs to be adjusted accordingly. Similarly, patients

should be advised to reduce their caffeine intake while taking viloxazine XR.[20]

When initiating viloxazine, dose increases, in 100-mg increments each week in children and adolescents and 100 to 200 mg in adults, appear to help with tolerability. The major side effects of viloxazine XR include sleepiness, appetite suppression, fatigue, nausea or vomiting, irritability, and insomnia. Many of the side effects are time- and dose-related; a slower initial dose escalation of the medication may obviate many of the effects.

ALTERNATIVE (NOT APPROVED BY THE FOOD AND DRUG ADMINISTRATION) TREATMENTS FOR ATTENTION-DEFICIT HYPERACTIVITY DISORDER

Bupropion

Bupropion (Wellbutrin), approved for treatment of depression and as an aid for smoking cessation in adults, has been moderately helpful in reducing ADHD symptoms in children, adolescents,[25] and adults.[26] Bupropion modulates both NE and DA. Although helpful, the magnitude of bupropion's effect is less than that seen with stimulants. Bupropion is often used in patients with ADHD and co-morbidities (such as nicotine use, substance use, and mood disorders).

Dosing for ADHD is like that for depression. The once-daily preparation of bupropion is usually initiated at 150 mg XL once each AM and titrated every 7 to 14 days to a maximum dosage of 450 mg XL/day. Common side effects include insomnia, edginess, and tremor. In addition, there is a risk for seizures that is higher when dosing exceeds 300 mg/day.

Tricyclic Antidepressants

Although effective in youth with ADHD[27] and in adults,[28] tricyclic antidepressants (TCAs), like other non-stimulants, are less effective for ADHD than stimulants. Compared with the stimulants, TCAs have negligible abuse liability; have once-daily dosing; and may be useful in patients with co-morbid anxiety, mood, tics, and SUDs. However, given concerns about potential cardiotoxicity, particularly in overdose, and the availability of other non-stimulants, the use of the TCAs has been significantly curtailed.

Electrocardiograms (ECGs) should be obtained at baseline and when therapeutic dosing has been achieved. Dosing for ADHD appears to be like that for depression.

Common short-term adverse consequences of the TCAs include dry mouth, blurred vision, orthostasis, and constipation. A serious adverse event associated with use of TCAs is overdose. Hence, close supervision of the administration and storage of TCAs is necessary.

Modafinil

Modafinil, a novel stimulant that is distinct from AMP, is approved for the treatment of narcolepsy. In general, whereas pediatric studies were positive for ADHD, modafinil was not effective in adults with ADHD.[6] Anecdotally, clinicians have reported that modafinil is helpful in improving motivation in ADHD. Modafinil has stimulant-like adverse effects as well as a concern for possible Stevens-Johnson syndrome and toxic epidermal necrolysis.

Memantine

Based on its efficacy in Alzheimer's disease, Surman and colleagues[29] openly treated 34 adults who had ADHD with the

N-methyl-D-aspartate (NMDA) receptor antagonist memantine. In this pilot study, memantine, titrated to a maximum dose of 10 mg BID, was generally well tolerated and resulted in improvements in measures of ADHD symptoms and in neuropsychological measures. Similarly, Biederman et al.[30] added memantine to extended-release MPH in adults and found trends toward improvement in cognitive executive functioning. Dosing of memantine of up to 20 mg/day has been used alone or in combination with other treatments for ADHD to support cognitive executive functioning; however, further research is needed to clarify the utility of this agent.

SUGGESTED MANAGEMENT STRATEGIES ACROSS THE LIFE SPAN

Having made the diagnosis of ADHD, a treatment plan should be tailored to mitigate the adverse impact associated with ADHD on psychological, social, and emotional development. The foundations of such planning involve education about which symptoms can be treated with medication and what compensatory strategies can be learned via behavioral therapies (such as parental coaching or CBT). It is also often helpful to steer patients toward environmental accommodations that may be compensatory for personal, social, and work challenges. Under US disability laws, ADHD is recognized as a potential basis for instituting accommodations in school and work settings.

It is useful to explain what an adequate trial of these supportive options will entail and that multiple trials may be necessary to develop an individual treatment plan. It is often helpful to explain that treatment of the core symptoms of ADHD with medication may be necessary for individuals to be able to recall and stick with compensatory behavioral practices. Patients with ADHD who have psychiatric co-morbidity or who demonstrate psychological distress should be directed to complementary treatments.

The stimulants and some of the non-stimulants (ATMX, viloxazine XR) are approved by the FDA and are considered first-line therapy for ADHD across the life span. Data are strongest for the use of stimulants, ATMX, viloxazine XR, bupropion, and TCAs in adults; however, studies with guanfacine XR have also shown efficacy.[23] Although there are no evidence-based guidelines in selecting a first choice of medication for patients with ADHD, it is important to consider issues of co-morbidity, tolerability, efficacy, and duration of action. The European Network of Adult ADHD published a consensus that outlined guidelines regarding ADHD treatment with stimulants. The guidelines recommended that the severity of ADHD and co-morbid disorders should be the first step in selecting treatments, with stimulants being the medication of choice.[31] Long-lasting, extended-release formulations are preferred for reasons of treatment adherence, for protection against misuse, for avoidance of rebound symptoms, and for provision of symptomatic relief throughout the day without the need for multiple doses. When initiating medication trials, the dose may be increased every few days to optimize treatment response. Frequently, patients benefit from adding an immediate-release AMP or MPH in combination with a longer-acting preparation and/or a non-stimulant to extend the duration of coverage to the patient's needs,[32] although the efficacy of this practice has not been well studied.

Consideration of another stimulant or a non-stimulant is recommended when symptoms fail to respond or the patient experiences clinically significant side effects to the initial medication. Given their pharmacodynamic differences, if an MPH product was selected initially, then moving to an AMP-based medication is appropriate. Patients must also be made aware that the full benefits of non-stimulants may not occur for several weeks and they may not "feel" anything like they may have with the stimulants. Monitoring routine side effects, vital signs, and misuse of the medication is warranted.

Cardiovascular Safety of Attention-Deficit Hyperactivity Disorder Treatments

Treatment with stimulants is associated with small increases in heart rate and blood pressure that are weakly correlated with the dose administered. There has been concern about the CV safety and risk in patients receiving stimulants. However, work has shed light on the CV risk of stimulants in adults. Habel and colleagues[33] retrospectively investigated serious CV events in a large group of medication users and non-users ($n = 443,198$ adults aged 25–64 years). The authors reported on 806,182 person-years of follow-up (median, 1.3 years per person) and found no relationship between past or current ADHD medication use and serious CV or stroke outcomes. As highlighted by these authors,[33] among young and middle-aged adults, current or new use of ADHD medications, compared with non-use or remote use, was not associated with an increased risk of serious CV events. These results mirror the findings of a similarly designed study in youth with ADHD and a review of the CV literature related to stimulant exposure in ADHD and seem to suggest that the vital sign changes seen acutely and chronically are usually not clinically significant.

The American Heart Association has commented on CV monitoring of individuals taking psychotropic medications.[34] Despite the generally benign CV effects of these medications, caution is warranted in the presence of a compromised CV system (e.g., untreated hypertension, arrhythmias, and known structural heart defects). Therefore, it is prudent to monitor symptoms referable to the CV system (e.g., syncope, palpitations, shortness of breath, and chest pain) as well as vital signs at baseline and with treatment in all patients with ADHD. It is not necessary to routinely check an ECG at baseline or with treatment. In cases of hypertension, data suggest that if it is well controlled, stimulants may be used safely.[35] Safety remains the paramount concern; thus, in each case, the physician and patient must weigh the risks and the benefits of treatment.

Aggression or Psychosis with Attention-Deficit Hyperactivity Disorder Medications

The FDA has received hundreds of reports of psychosis or manic symptoms, particularly hallucinations, associated with use of ADHD medication in children and adolescents. BPD in children and adolescents, and to a lesser extent in adults, is often co-morbid with ADHD. Current clinical thinking is that stabilization of manic symptoms is necessary before initiating treatment for ADHD. After stabilization, the use of both stimulants and non-stimulants appears safe and effective in individuals with BPD and ADHD.

The importance of aggression should not be underestimated because these patients often have severe psychopathology that adversely affects their families and communities and have high rates of service utilization. Although medications are usually effective in reducing the symptoms of ADHD and impulsive aggression, these patients usually benefit from multi-modal treatment. Medications should initially treat the most severe underlying disorder, after which specific symptoms should be targeted (e.g., irritability, hostility, hypervigilance, impulsivity, fear, or emotional dysregulation).[36] These patients often display aggression before and during the course of treatment, making it imperative to document their aggressive behaviors before the introduction of medications and to make these behaviors an explicit target of treatment. If and when a patient displays a worsening of aggressive behaviors during medication treatment for ADHD, the clinician should make a judgment regarding the tolerability and efficacy of the treatment. Whereas episodes of aggression with all ADHD medications have been reported, aggression in patients with ADHD usually responds to stimulant treatment.[36] During clinical trials, rates of aggression were observed to be similar with active and placebo treatment, and in other trials, less aggression was demonstrated with use of stimulants.

In patients with co-morbid ADHD and ODD or CD, the clinician should first attempt to optimize the pharmacotherapy of ADHD[37] followed by augmentation with behavioral treatments. Supporting this strategy, stimulants significantly reduced both overt and covert aggression as rated by parents, teachers, and clinicians.[36] Youth with ADHD with and without ODD or CD responded robustly and equally well to stimulant medication. Similarly, in youth with ADHD, treatment with a non-stimulant also reduces ODD symptoms. Although these interventions are often sufficient, a significant number of these patients have severe symptoms that necessitate treatment with additional or alternative medications. Neuroleptic use should be limited to individuals with ADHD who have severe aggression or disruptive or mood disorders.

In recent years, the use of atypical antipsychotics in pediatric populations has increased considerably. Clinicians are encouraged to optimize psychosocial and educational interventions followed by appropriate pharmacotherapy of the primary psychiatric disorder followed by use of an atypical antipsychotic medication. Treatment with an atypical antipsychotic warrants careful monitoring because various side effects may be anticipated. Safety remains the paramount consideration, and after a period of remission of the aggressive symptoms, consideration should be given to tapering and discontinuing the atypical antipsychotic. Tapering of atypical antipsychotics should proceed slowly to prevent withdrawal dyskinesias and to allow for an adequate time to adjust to the reduced dose. If there is evidence of severe mood instability, use of other mood stabilizers should be considered.

Attention-Deficit Hyperactivity Disorder Plus Anxiety Disorders

Anxiety disorders, including agoraphobia, panic, over-anxious disorder, simple phobia, separation anxiety disorder, and OCD, occur frequently in children, adolescents, and adults with ADHD.[32] The effect of stimulant treatment in youth with ADHD and anxiety has been variable. Earlier studies found an increased placebo response, increased side effects, and a reduced response to stimulants in patients with both conditions, but others have observed stimulants to be well tolerated and effective; still others showed reductions in anxiety in stimulant-treated individuals.[38] Many youth with ADHD and anxiety experience robust improvements with stimulants and may not experience exacerbations of anxiety.[38] Of interest, ATMX is reported to reduce anxiety in ADHD across the life span.[39] The Texas Medication Algorithm Project Consensus Panel recommends beginning pharmacotherapy for patients with ADHD and a co-morbid anxiety disorder with either ATMX aimed at both the ADHD and anxiety or prescribing a stimulant first to address the ADHD, then adding a selective serotonin reuptake inhibitor (SSRI) or SNRI to address the anxiety, if necessary.[37] Other non-stimulants, such as viloxazine XR and the α-agonists, remain untested in this domain. TCAs have demonstrated efficacy for anxiety and for ADHD, but they have not been tested for anxiety in those with ADHD.[37]

Attention-Deficit Hyperactivity Disorder Plus Obsessive-Compulsive Disorder

Considerable overlap exists between pediatric ADHD and OCD, including rates of ADHD in up to 51% of children and 36% of adolescents with OCD.[40] In general, patients with OCD and ADHD require treatment for both conditions. The SSRIs, especially in combination with CBT, are well-established treatments for pediatric and adult OCD. Although stimulants may exacerbate tics, obsessions, or compulsions, they are frequently used in patients with these conditions, often in combination with SSRIs. Therefore, clinicians should identify and prioritize treatment of the most severe condition first, then address secondary concerns while monitoring for signs of worsening symptoms and recognizing that successfully treated patients have much residual morbidity and that CBT is an essential component of long-term management.

Attention-Deficit Hyperactivity Disorder Plus Tic Disorders

Tics and tic disorders commonly co-occur in patients with ADHD.[21] Tics occur more commonly in males and in youth with combined-type ADHD. Children, adolescents, and adults may suffer from a triad of tics, ADHD, and OCD.[21] Pharmacotherapy of youth with ADHD and tic disorders is challenging. The first-line treatment for tics is education. In most patients, tics are mild to moderate; have a fluctuating course, even when the patient is taking a tic-suppressing medication; and generally decline by early adulthood. Tics may not require treatment unless they are disabling or result in self-esteem issues. Although stimulants may exacerbate tics and are listed as a contraindication to the use of MPH, stimulants have been well tolerated and effective in these patients.[21] Randomized treatments with MPH (26.1 mg/day), clonidine (0.25 mg/day), or MPH plus clonidine (26.1 mg/day plus 0.28 mg/day) were studied in a classic multisite study of children with ADHD and chronic tic disorders.[41] Although MPH treatment improved ADHD and clonidine reduced tics, the greatest effect was observed with the combination treatment. Tic severity diminished with all active treatments and in the following order: clonidine plus MPH, clonidine alone, and MPH alone. No clinically significant CV adverse events were noted. Follow-up of children with ADHD and tics treated with MPH over a 2-year period showed improvement in ADHD symptoms without worsening tics. Given the data on clonidine, interest in guanfacine treatment has grown, and it appears to be effective in reducing symptoms of both ADHD and tics.[21]

Investigations have demonstrated the utility of noradrenergic agents, such as TCAs and ATMX.[42] Although treatment with ATMX was not associated with significant reductions in tics compared with placebo, tic severity did not worsen, and symptoms of ADHD were significantly improved. In patients who do not tolerate or respond to treatment with stimulants, noradrenergic agents, α-adrenergic agents, or their combination, treatment with a neuroleptic should be considered.

Attention-Deficit Hyperactivity Disorder Plus Depression

Depression and dysthymia are commonly co-morbid with ADHD.[32] In patients with ADHD, depression is not an artifact, and it must be distinguished from demoralization, which is commonly seen in ADHD. Although there are no formal evidence-based guidelines, clinicians should, in general, assess the severity of ADHD and depression and direct their initial treatment toward the most impairing condition. In adults with ADHD and depression, bupropion and TCAs remain a reasonable choice and may be helpful for both conditions. Similarly, SSRIs have been helpful with depressive symptoms alone or when used in combination with a stimulant.[43] Although viloxazine XR has been used as an antidepressant in Europe, its utility in adults with ADHD and depression remains unstudied.

Attention-Deficit Hyperactivity Disorder Plus Bipolar Disorder

Although BPD is recognized in ADHD patients, ADHD may complicate the presentation, diagnosis, and treatment of BPD. Differentiating BPD from ADHD can be challenging because these disorders share many features (including symptoms of distractibility, hyperactivity, impulsivity, talkativeness, and sleep disturbance).[44] Clinicians are faced with the challenging and important task of differentiating BPD, ADHD, ADHD with emotional dysregulation, and the diagnosis of disruptive mood dysregulation disorder. Data to guide clinicians in this area are emerging but are often conflicting and confusing. Data show that BPD appears to occur at increased rates in children and adolescents with ADHD; moreover, ADHD is highly co-morbid in children (6%–90%), adolescents (50%), and adults (10%–15%) with BPD.[44]

Given the severe morbidity of pediatric BPD, families and patients usually benefit from an integrated and coordinated treatment plan that includes medications (often more than one is necessary and appropriate), psychotherapies (individual, group, and family), educational and occupational interventions (accommodations or modifications in school or work), and psychoeducation and parent and family support (available through national organizations, such as the National Alliance for the Mentally Ill and the Child and Adolescent Bipolar Foundation).

Medications are usually a fundamental part of the treatment plan of all patients with BPD. Readers are referred to other sections of this text related to the guidelines for both pediatric patients and adults. In treating ADHD in the context of co-morbid BPD, clinicians should first ensure mood stability before the initiation of treatment for ADHD.[45,46] Patients with BPD type I without symptoms of psychosis should receive monotherapy with either a mood stabilizer (e.g., lithium, or carbamazepine) or an atypical antipsychotic. In patients with only a partial response, the initial medication should be augmented with either an additional mood stabilizer or an atypical antipsychotic. Lithium and antipsychotics have substantially reduced symptoms of mania and depression in children, and in patients with BPD type I with psychosis, both a mood stabilizer and an atypical antipsychotic should be started concurrently (following the same augmentation strategy).

In patients with ADHD plus BPD, for example, the risk of mania or hypomania needs to be addressed and monitored during treatment of ADHD. When the mood is euthymic, conservative introduction of anti-ADHD medications along with mood-stabilizing agents should be considered. Systematic study of 2307 patients with BPD and ADHD as part of the Swedish Registry study showed no increase in longer-term mania outcomes with adults treated for their BPD with mood stabilizing medications in concert with MPH whereas those not treated with mood stabilizers were at 6 to 10 times increased risk for a manic episode during the 0- to 3-month and 4- to 6-month follow-up periods, respectively ($P < .001$).[46]

To date, little is known about the use of non-stimulants in treating those with ADHD and BPD. For all classes of medications, clinicians should advise their patients (and perhaps their patients' families) to monitor any induction or exacerbation or worsening of mania or cycling during treatment with ADHD medications. In such situations, it is necessary to prioritize the mood stabilization, which may also necessitate the discontinuation of the ADHD treatment until euthymia has been achieved.

Attention-Deficit Hyperactivity Disorder Plus Substance Use Disorders

Many adolescents and adults with ADHD have either a past or current alcohol or drug use disorder, and co-morbidity within ADHD increases the risk[47] for an SUD. Patients with ADHD frequently misuse a variety of substances (including alcohol, marijuana, cocaine, stimulants, opiates, and nicotine). Children with ADHD start smoking nicotine an average of 2 years earlier than their non-ADHD peers and have increased rates of smoking as adults, more difficulty quitting smoking, and nicotine dependence (achieved more rapidly and lasting longer compared with control participants).[47] Because the rates of SUD in patients with ADHD are increased, concerns persist that stimulant treatment contributes to subsequent substance misuse or use disorders. In a recent review, Wilens and colleagues[48] found a total of 21 studies and revealed that stimulant treatment resulted in a reduction in risk for later SUDs among youth treated with a stimulant for ADHD compared with youths receiving no pharmacotherapy for their ADHD.

A careful history of substance use, misuse, or abuse should be completed as part of the ADHD evaluation in adolescents and adults. When substance misuse, abuse, or dependence is a clinical concern, the clinician should assess the relative severity of the ADHD and the SUD. Furthermore, substance misuse, abuse, or dependence often affects cognition, behavior, sleep, and mood or anxiety, which makes it challenging to assess ADHD symptoms. Stabilizing the substance misuse, abuse, or dependence and addressing co-morbid disorder(s) are generally the priority when treating patients with ADHD and an SUD. Treatment for patients with ADHD and SUD usually includes a combination of substance misuse, abuse, or dependence treatment or psychotherapy and pharmacotherapy along with treatment for ADHD. A recent study in adults with ADHD and an SUD showed a more than three-fold increase in retention in SUD care in those treated pharmacologically for ADHD compared with those not receiving ADHD treatment.[49] Patients with SUD should be considered for treatment of their ADHD in the context of their substance misuse, abuse, or dependence treatments. Structured psychotherapies, such as CBT, that address SUD and ADHD are excellent initial interventions.[48] When selecting medications, clinicians should consider medications that have little likelihood of diversion or low liability, such as non-stimulants, with consideration of progressing to the stimulants. Stimulants have been effective at higher doses when treating ADHD in patients with SUD—even stimulant misuse.[50] When using stimulants in this patient population, it is wise to prescribe an extended-delivery formulation with minimal risk of misuse, such as pro-drug stimulants such as serdexmethylphenidate/MPH or lisdexamfetamine, as well as to agree on a method for monitoring the SUD and adherence to the treatment plan. Moreover, stimulant treatment plan adherence requires careful monitoring because they are controlled substances with addictive potential and are often diverted and misused. Of interest, much of stimulant misuse appears to occur in relation to perceived performance enhancement and not for euphoric effect,[48] although data do not support an objective cognitive enhancement of stimulants.

In these populations, the use of immediate-release stimulants should be avoided. Close monitoring of high-risk groups should also be undertaken to avoid the diversion or further misuse of stimulants.

Attention-Deficit Hyperactivity Disorder Plus Autism Spectrum Disorders

Children, adolescents, and adults with ASD may display a persistent and impairing pattern of hyperactivity, impulsivity, and inattention;[2] when these symptoms can be distinguished from core features of ASD, the *DSM*, Fifth Edition (DSM-5) allows clinicians to diagnose ADHD. In treating this group of patients, clinicians, in collaboration with parents, balance the risks and benefits of treatments. In general, the philosophy is to identify target symptoms and to prioritize impairments. Addressing ADHD in youth with ASD may have a profound impact on improving outcomes in multiple domains.

Interest in the pharmacotherapy of ADHD and ASDs has been emerging; for a review, see Joshi and associates (2021).[51] Although earlier work in small samples supported the use of MPH in doses of 0.3 to 0.6 mg/kg/day, these patients often experienced side effects (such as irritability) that limited stimulant use. What appears to be emerging from the literature[51] is that both stimulants and non-stimulants have an impact on ADHD symptoms in ASD. In particular, one can expect improved attention and reduced distractibility, hyperactivity, and impulsivity, as well as improved behavioral dysregulation. However, particularly in intellectually compromised children with ASD, the effect sizes for medications, according to parent and teacher ratings, were smaller than those usually observed in neurotypically developing children with ADHD. Furthermore, in these children, rates of adverse effects, primarily irritability, appear more frequently and are more dose-related. In contrast, more recent data in intellectually capable children with ASD and ADHD seem to show similar rates of response and side effects relative to children with ADHD without ASD.[51] In terms of non-stimulants, data suggest that ATMX and guanfacine XR, but not clonidine, may be useful in patients with ASD who have ADHD symptoms.[51]

CONCLUSION

The aggregate literature supports the importance of identifying ADHD. A large literature also supports that pharmacotherapy with stimulants and non-stimulants provides an effective treatment for children, adolescents, and adults with ADHD and co-morbid disorders. Structured psychotherapy delivered in individual and group settings is also effective, particularly when used adjunctively with medications. Groups that focus on coping skills, support, and interpersonal psychotherapy may also be very useful for these patients. Further controlled investigations assessing the efficacy of single and combination agents for patients with ADHD are necessary, with careful attention paid to diagnostics, symptoms, and neuropsychological outcome, long-term tolerability, and efficacy, as well as their use in specific ADHD sub-groups.

REFERENCES

1. Barkley RA. International Consensus Statement on ADHD. *J Am Acad Child Adolesc Psychiatry*. 2002;41(12):1389..
2. Kotte A, Joshi G, Fried R, et al. Autistic traits in children with and without ADHD. *Pediatrics*. 2013;132(3):e612–e622.
3. Young S, Khondoker M, Emilsson B, et al. Cognitive-behavioural therapy in medication-treated adults with attention-deficit/hyperactivity disorder and co-morbid psychopathology: a randomized controlled trial using multi-level analysis. *Psychol Med*. 2015;45(13):2793–2804.
4. Sprich SE, Safren SA, Finkelstein D, et al. A randomized controlled trial of cognitive behavioral therapy for ADHD in medication-treated adolescents. *J Child Psychol Psychiatry*. 2016;57(11):1218–1226.
5. Safren SA, Otto M, Sprich S, et al. Cognitive-behavioral therapy for ADHD in medication-treated adults with continued symptoms. *Behav Res and Therapy*. 2005;43(7):831–842.
6. Newcorn JH, Wilens TE. Updates in Pharmacologic Strategies in ADHD, An Issue of Child and Adolescent Psychiatric Clinics of North America. *Vol 31. Elsevier Health Sciences*. 2022.
7. Steingard R, Taskiran S, Connor DF, et al. New formulations of stimulants: an update for clinicians. *J Child Adolesc Psychopharmacol*. 2019;29(5):324–339.
8. Spencer TJ, Brown A, Seidman LJ, et al. Effect of psychostimulants on brain structure and function in ADHD: a qualitative literature review of magnetic resonance imaging-based neuroimaging studies. *J Clin Psychiatry*. 2013;74(9):902–917.
9. Boland H, DiSalvo M, Fried R, et al. A literature review and meta-analysis on the effects of ADHD medications on functional outcomes. *J Psychiatr Res*. 2020;123:21–30.
10. Solanto MV. Neuropsychopharmacological mechanisms of stimulant drug action in attention-deficit hyperactivity disorder: a review and integration. *Behav Brain Res*. 1998;94(1):127–152.
11. Pliszka S. Practice parameter for the assessment and treatment of children and adolescents with attention-deficit/hyperactivity disorder. *J Am Acad Child Adolesc Psychiatry*. 2007;46(7):894–921.
12. Swanson JM, Elliott GR, Greenhill LL, et al. Effects of stimulant medication on growth rates across 3 years in the MTA follow-up. *J Am Acad Child Adolesc Psychiatry*. 2007;46(8):1015–1027.
13. Biederman J, Spencer TJ, Monuteaux MC, et al. A naturalistic 10-year prospective study of height and weight in children with attention-deficit hyperactivity disorder grown up: sex and treatment effects. *J Pediatr*. 2010;157(4):635–640. 640.e1.
14. Cortese S, Brown TE, Corkum P, et al. Assessment and management of sleep problems in youths with attention-deficit/hyperactivity disorder. *Am Acad Child Adolesc Psychiatry*. 2013;52(8):784–796.
15. Prince J, Wilens T, Biederman J, et al. Clonidine for sleep disturbances associated with attention-deficit hyperactivity disorder: a systematic chart review of 62 cases. *J Am Acad Child Adolesc Psychiatry*. 1996;35(5):599–605.
16. Smits MG, van Stel HF, van der Heijden K, et al. Melatonin improves health status and sleep in children with idiopathic chronic sleep-onset insomnia: a randomized placebo-controlled trial. *J Am Acad Child Adolesc Psychiatry*. 2003;42(11):1286–1293.
17. Surman CBH, Walsh DM. Managing sleep in adults with ADHD: from science to pragmatic approaches. *Brain Sci*. 2021;11(10):1361.
18. Sauer JM, Ponsler GD, Mattiuz EL, et al. Disposition and metabolic fate of atomoxetine hydrochloride: the role of CYP2D6 in human disposition and metabolism. *Drug Metab Dispos*. 2003;31(1):98–107.
19. Wilens TE, Hammerness P, Utzinger L, et al. An open study of adjunct OROS-methylphenidate in children and adolescents who are atomoxetine partial responders: I. Effectiveness. *J Child Adolesc Psychopharmacol*. 2009;19(5):485–492.
20. F.D.A. Drugs @FDA: FDA-approved drugs. Accessed July 22, 2024. https://www.accessdata.fda.gov/scripts/cder/daf/index.cfm.
21. Jaffe RJ, Coffey BJ. Pharmacologic treatment of comorbid attention-deficit/hyperactivity disorder and Tourette and tic disorders. *Child Adolesc Psychiatr Clin N Am*. 2022;31(3):469–477.
22. Wilens TE, Bukstein O, Brams M, et al. A controlled trial of extended-release guanfacine and psychostimulants for attention-deficit/hyperactivity disorder. *J Am Acad Child Adolesc Psychiatry*. 2012;51(1):74–85 e2.
23. Iwanami A, Saito K, Fujiwara M, et al. Safety and efficacy of guanfacine extended-release in adults with attention-deficit/hyperactivity disorder: an open-label, long-term, phase 3 extension study. *BMC Psychiatry*. 2020;20(1):485.
24. Nasser A, Hull JT, Chaturvedi SA, et al. A phase III, randomized, double-blind, placebo-controlled trial assessing the efficacy and safety of viloxazine extended-release capsules in adults with attention-deficit/hyperactivity disorder. *CNS Drugs*. 2022;36(8):897–915.
25. Conners CK, Casat CD, Gualtieri CT, et al. Bupropion hydrochloride in attention deficit disorder with hyperactivity. *J Am Acad Child and Adolesc Psychiatry*. 1996;35(10):1314–1321.
26. Wilens TE, Spencer TJ, Biederman J, et al. A controlled clinical trial of bupropion for attention deficit hyperactivity disorder in adults. *Am J Psychiatry*. 2001;158(2):282–288.
27. Biederman J, Baldessarini RJ, Wright V, et al. A double-blind placebo controlled study of desipramine in the treatment of ADD: I. Efficacy. *J Am Acad Child Adolesc Psychiatry*. 1989;28(5):777–784.

28. Wilens T, Biederman J, Prince J, et al. Six-week, double blind, placebo-controlled study of desipramine for adult attention deficit hyperactivity disorder. *Am J Psychiatry*. 1996;153:1147–1153.

29. Surman CB, Hammerness PG, Petty C, et al. A pilot open label prospective study of memantine monotherapy in adults with ADHD. *World J Biol Psychiatry*. 2013;14(4):291–298.

30. Biederman J, Fried R, Tarko L, et al. Memantine in the treatment of executive function deficits in adults with ADHD. *J Atten Disord*. 2017;21(4):343–352.

31. Kooij SJ, Bejerot S, Blackwell A, et al. European consensus statement on diagnosis and treatment of adult ADHD: the European Network Adult ADHD. *BMC Psychiatry*. 2010;10:67.

32. Faraone SV, Banaschewski T, Coghill D, et al. The World Federation of ADHD International Consensus Statement: 208 evidence-based conclusions about the disorder. *Neurosci Biobehav Rev*. 2021;128:789–818.

33. Habel LA, Cooper WO, Sox CM, et al. ADHD medications and risk of serious cardiovascular events in young and middle-aged adults. *JAMA*. 2011;306(24):2673–2683.

34. Gutgesell H, Atkins D, Barst R, et al. Cardiovascular monitoring of children and adolescents receiving psychotropic drugs: A statement for healthcare professionals from the Committee on Congenital Cardiac Defects, Council on Cardiovascular Disease in the Young, American Heart Association. *Circulation*. 1999;99(7):979–982.

35. Wilens T, Zusman RM, Hammerness PG, et al. An open-label study of the tolerability of mixed amphetamine salts in adults with ADHD and treated primary essential hypertension. *J Clin Psychiatry*. 2006;67(5):696–702.

36. Blader JC, Pliszka SR, Jensen PS, et al. Stimulant-responsive and stimulant-refractory aggressive behavior among children with ADHD. *Pediatrics*. 2010;126(4):e796–e806.

37. Pliszka SR, Crismon ML, Hughes CW, et al. The Texas Children's Medication Algorithm Project: revision of the algorithm for pharmacotherapy of attention-deficit/hyperactivity disorder. *J Am Acad Child Adolesc Psychiatry*. 2006;45(6):642–657.

38. Soul O, Gross R, Basel D, et al. Stimulant treatment effect on anxiety domains in children with attention-deficit/hyperactivity disorder with and without anxiety disorders: a 12-week open-label prospective study. *J Child Adolesc Psychopharmacol*. 2021;31(9):639–644.

39. Adler LA, Liebowitz M, Kronenberger W, et al. Atomoxetine treatment in adults with attention-deficit/hyperactivity disorder and comorbid social anxiety disorder. *Depress Anxiety*. 2009;26(3):212–221.

40. Geller DA, Biederman J, Faraone S, et al. Developmental aspects of obsessive compulsive disorder: findings in children, adolescents, and adults. *J Nerv Ment Dis*. 2001;189(7):471–477.

41. Tourette's Syndrome Study Group. Treatment of ADHD in children with tics: a randomized controlled trial. *Neurology*. 2002;58:527–536.

42. Allen AJ, Kurlan RM, Gilbert DL, et al. Atomoxetine treatment in children and adolescents with ADHD and comorbid tic disorders. *Neurology*. 2005;65(12):1941–1949.

43. Weiss M, Hechtman L. A randomized double-blind trial of paroxetine and/or dextroamphetamine and problem-focused therapy for attention-deficit/hyperactivity disorder in adults. *J Clin Psychiatry*. 2006;67(4):611–619.

44. Joshi G, Wilens T. Comorbid conditions in youth with and at risk for bipolar disorder. In: Strakowski SM, DelBello MP, Adler CM, eds. *Bipolar Disorder in Youth: Presentation, Treatment and Neurobiology* Oxford University Press; 2014:0.

45. Findling RL, Short EJ, McNamara NK, et al. Methylphenidate in the treatment of children and adolescents with bipolar disorder and attention-deficit/hyperactivity disorder. *J Am Acad Child Adolesc Psychiatry*. 2007;46(11):1445–1453.

46. Viktorin A, Rydén E, Thase ME, et al. The risk of treatment-emergent mania with methylphenidate in bipolar disorder. *Am J Psychiatry*. 2017;174(4):341–348.

47. Taubin D, Wilson JC, Wilens TE. ADHD and substance use disorders in young people: considerations for evaluation, diagnosis, and pharmacotherapy. *Child and Adolesc Psychiatric Clin N Am*. 2022;31(3):515–530.

48. Wilens TE, Woodward DW, Ko JD, et al. The impact of pharmacotherapy of childhood-onset psychiatric disorders on the development of substance use disorders. *J Child Adolesc Psychopharmacol*. 2022;32(4):200–214.

49. Kast KA, Rao V, Wilens TE. Pharmacotherapy for attention-deficit/hyperactivity disorder and retention in outpatient substance use disorder treatment: a retrospective cohort study. *J Clin Psychiatry*. 2021;82(2): 20m13598.

50. Levin FR, Mariani JJ, Specker S, et al. Extended-release mixed amphetamine salts vs placebo for comorbid adult attention-deficit/hyperactivity disorder and cocaine use disorder: a randomized clinical trial. *JAMA Psychiatry*. 2015;72(6):593–602.

51. Joshi G, Wilens T, Firmin ES, et al. Pharmacotherapy of attention deficit/hyperactivity disorder in individuals with autism spectrum disorder: a systematic review of the literature. *J Psychopharmacol*. 2021;35(3):203–210.

8 Natural Medications in Psychiatry

Felicia A. Smith, Ana Ivkovic, and David Mischoulon

KEY POINTS

- Complementary and integrative medical therapies are made up of a diverse spectrum of practices (including natural medications) that often overlap with more traditional medical practice.
- The use of natural medications is growing considerably in the United States and around the world, and patients often do not report use of natural medications to their physicians.
- Historical lack of scientific research in this area has contributed to deficiencies in knowledge with respect to safety and efficacy of many of the natural remedies on the market today.
- Natural medications are often used for the psychiatric indications of mood disorders, anxiety, insomnia, menstrual and menopausal symptoms, and dementia (among others).

OVERVIEW

Complementary and alternative medical therapies are made up of a diverse spectrum of practices that often overlap with current medical practice. Typically, the descriptor *alternative medicine* is reserved for situations in which a non-mainstream approach is used in place of conventional medicine, whereas *complementary medicine* and *integrative medicine* are the preferred terms when non-mainstream approaches are used along with conventional medicine. *Alternative medicine* has largely been replaced by *integrative medicine* to emphasize the more typical merging of conventional and complementary approaches in clinical practice.[1] The National Center for Complementary and Integrative Health (NCCIH) is the federal government's lead agency responsible for scientific research on complementary and integrative medicine. This chapter focuses on natural medications derived from natural products and not approved by the US Food and Drug Administration (FDA) for their proposed indication.[2] Natural medications include a wide variety of products, such as hormones, vitamins, plants, herbs, fatty acids, amino acid derivatives, and homeopathic preparations. Whereas natural medications have been used in Asia for thousands of years, their use in the United States has been much more recent, with a dramatic increase over the past three decades. Surveys suggest that about 40% of the United States population uses some sort of complementary therapy.[3] Ethnic considerations also impact usage, with African Americans being the group least likely in the United States to try natural remedies and Hispanics being the most prone to their use.[4] Given the considerable portion of the US population trying natural remedies, it is increasingly important for clinicians to be knowledgeable about these medications so that they can provide comprehensive patient care. This chapter provides an overview of natural medications used for psychiatric indications. General safety and efficacy are discussed first. This is followed by an examination of primary natural remedies used for disorders of mood, anxiety, and sleep, as well as menstrual disorders and dementia.

EFFICACY AND SAFETY

Although governmental agencies (including the National Institutes of Health and NCCIH) and the pharmaceutical industry are sponsoring clinical research that involves natural medications, data regarding their efficacy lags. The actual benefits of natural remedies are often unclear because relatively few systematic studies have been conducted. Because the FDA does not routinely regulate natural medications, questions of safety remain unaddressed. Consumers often believe that because a remedy is "natural," it is safe. Moreover, because these products are most often purchased as over-the-counter (OTC) remedies, there is no clear mechanism for reporting toxicity and for informing the public about their adverse effects. Another significant problem lies in the limited information regarding the safety and efficacy of combining natural medications with more conventional ones. In cases in which interactions are known, psychiatrists face the reality that patients frequently do not disclose their use of integrative therapies to their physicians. Asking specific questions about a patient's use of both prescribed and OTC medications may improve disclosures. Finally, because natural medications are not regulated as are more conventional ones, significant variability exists among different preparations. Preparations often vary in purity, quality, potency, and efficacy and have myriad side effects. The increase in government- and industry-sponsored studies may serve to clarify the potential uses, safety, and efficacy of these medications; until such results are available, caution should be used in recommending interventions that are less well understood. The remainder of this chapter outlines our current understanding of several primary natural medications and their potential psychiatric indications.

MOOD DISORDERS

Numerous natural medications have been used to treat mood disorders, including omega-3 fatty acids, St. John's wort (SJW), *S*-adenosylmethionine (SAMe), folic acid, vitamin B_{12}, inositol, and *N*-acetyl cysteine (NAC) (Table 8.1). The efficacy, possible mechanisms of action, dosing, adverse effects, and drug interactions of each of these medications are discussed in the following section.

Omega-3 Fatty Acids

Omega-3 fatty acids are polyunsaturated lipids derived from fish oil, algae, and certain land-based plants (e.g., flax). Omega-3 fatty acids have been shown to have benefits in numerous medical conditions, including rheumatoid arthritis, Crohn's disease, ulcerative colitis, psoriasis, immunoglobulin A (IgA) nephropathy, systemic lupus erythematosus, multiple sclerosis, and migraine headache, among others.[5] Cardioprotective benefits have also been demonstrated, although recent studies and systematic reviews have been less supportive of their role as preventive agents for cardiovascular disease.[6] From a psychiatric standpoint, omega-3 fatty acids may have a role in the treatment of unipolar depression, post-partum depression, bipolar disorder, schizophrenia, and attention-deficit hyperactivity disorder (ADHD).[7] The most promising data are for the

TABLE 8.1 Natural Medications for Mood Disorders

Medication	Active Components	Possible Indications	Possible Mechanisms of Action	Suggested Dosage	Adverse Events
Omega-3 fatty acids	Essential fatty acids (primarily EPA and DHA)	Depression, bipolar disorder, schizophrenia, ADHD	Effects on neurotransmitter signaling receptors; inhibition of inflammatory cytokines; lowering plasma norepinephrine (noradrenaline)	1000–4000 mg/day	Fishy taste and odor, GI upset, theoretical risk of bleeding
Folic acid	Vitamin	Depression, dementia	Neurotransmitter synthesis	400–800 mcg/day; 15 mg/day 5-MTHF (Deplin)	Masking of vitamin B_{12} deficiency, lowers seizure threshold in high doses, and adverse interactions with other drugs
Inositol	Six-carbon ring natural isomer of glucose	Depression, panic, OCD, and possibly bipolar disorder	Second messenger synthesis	12–18 g/day	Mild GI upset, headache, dizziness, sedation, and insomnia
NAC	Biological compound functioning as mitochondrial modulator involved in GSH synthesis	Depression, bipolar disorder (including in children), OCD, spectrum disorders, schizophrenia, substance use disorders, PTSD	Increases GSH synthesis, reduces oxidative stress in mitochondrial electron transport chain, protects brain cells, may function similarly to lithium and valproate	600–3600 mg/day	Dry mouth, nausea, vomiting, diarrhea
SAMe	Biological compound involved in methylation reactions	Depression	Neurotransmitter synthesis	300–3200 mg/day	Mild anxiety, agitation, insomnia, dry mouth, GI disturbance; also possible switch to mania and serotonin syndrome
St. John's wort (Hypericum perforatum L.)	Hypericin, hyperforin, polycyclic phenols, pseudohypericin	Depression	Inhibition of cytokines, decreased serotonin receptor density, decreased neurotransmitter reuptake, MAOI activity	900–1800 mg/day	Dry mouth, dizziness, GI disturbance, and phototoxicity; also possible serotonin syndrome when taken with SSRIs and adverse interactions with other drugs
Vitamin B_{12}	Vitamin	Depression	Neurotransmitter synthesis	500–1000 mcg/day	None

ADHD, Attention-deficit hyperactivity disorder; DHA, docosahexaenoic acid; EPA, eicosapentaenoic acid; GI, gastrointestinal; GSH, glutathione; MAOI, monoamine oxidase inhibitor; MTHF, methyltetrahydrofolate; NAC, N-acetyl cysteine; OCD, obsessive-compulsive disorder; PTSD, post-traumatic stress disorder; SAMe, S-adenosylmethionine; SSRI, selective serotonin reuptake inhibitor.
Adapted from Mischoulon D, Nierenberg AA. Natural medications in psychiatry. In: Stern TA, Herman JB, Rubin DH, eds. Psychiatry Update and Board Preparation. 4th ed. Boston: MGH Psychiatry Academy Publishing; 2018.

treatment of both unipolar and bipolar depression, yet recent meta-analyses have been more reserved in their enthusiasm about the antidepressant efficacy of the omega-3s.[8] In countries with higher fish consumption, lower rates of depression and bipolar disorder provide a clue that omega-3 fatty acids may play a protective role in these disorders. Although there are three main omega-3 fatty acids, eicosapentaenoic acid (EPA) and docosahexaenoic acid (DHA) (sometimes referred to as the marine-based omega-3s) are the two primarily studied for psychiatric indications. The third omega 3-fatty acid, alpha-linolenic acid, is also thought to have neurotropic and other health-promoting effects. Although their mechanisms of action are not completely clear, several have been proposed. These run the gamut from effects on membrane-bound receptors and enzymes that regulate neurotransmitter signaling, to the regulation of calcium ion influx through calcium channels, to the lowering of plasma norepinephrine (noradrenaline) levels, or possibly to anti-inflammatory effects leading to decreased corticosteroid release from the adrenal gland.[9] Omega-3 fatty acids may be consumed naturally from a variety of sources, including fatty fish (e.g., salmon), algae, flax seeds, chia seeds, hemp seeds, walnuts, and enriched eggs. Commercially available preparations of omega-3 fatty acids vary in composition, and the suggested EPA:DHA ratio is at least 3:2 in favor of EPA.[8] Psychotropically active doses are generally thought to be at least 1 to 2 g/day, although higher doses may also be effective. Dose-related gastrointestinal (GI) distress is the major side effect. There is also a theoretical risk of increased bleeding, so concomitant use with high-dose non-steroidal anti-inflammatory drugs or anticoagulants is not recommended. Thus far, there are no known interactions with other mood stabilizers or antidepressants.

In sum, the use of omega-3 fatty acids is promising, particularly given the range of potential benefits and the relative low toxicity observed thus far. However, larger and more definitive studies are still needed.

St. John's Wort

St. John's wort (Hypericum perforatum) is one of the biggest-selling natural medications on the market. It has been shown to be more effective than placebo in the treatment of mild to moderate depression.[10] Studies have further suggested that SJW is as effective as low-dose tricyclic antidepressants (TCAs). When compared with selective serotonin reuptake inhibitors (SSRIs) such as sertraline and fluoxetine, the efficacy of SJW has been comparable to, but not always better than, placebo.[11] Hypericum is thought to be the main antidepressant ingredient in SJW, and polycyclic phenols, pseudohypericin, and hyperforin are also thought to be active ingredients. Several theories regarding the mechanism of action of SJW have been proposed. These include the inhibition of cytokines, a decrease in serotonin (5-HT) receptor density, a decrease in reuptake of neurotransmitters, and monoamine oxidase inhibitor (MAOI) activity.[9] Because SJW has MAOI activity, it should not be combined with SSRIs because of the possible development of serotonin syndrome.

Suggested doses range from 900 to 1800 mg/day depending on the preparation. Adverse effects include dry mouth, dizziness, constipation, and phototoxicity. Care should be taken in patients with bipolar disorder because of the possibility of a switch to mania. Finally, there are several important drug–drug interactions with SJW of note. Hyperforin is metabolized through the liver and it induces CYP 3A4 expression, which may reduce the therapeutic activity of several common medications, including warfarin, calcineurin inhibitors, oral contraceptives, theophylline, digoxin, and indinavir.[12] Transplant recipients should not use SJW because transplant rejections have been reported as a result of interactions between SJW, cyclosporine, and tacrolimus. Individuals with human immunodeficiency virus infection who are taking protease inhibitors also should avoid taking SJW because of drug interactions.

In sum, SJW appears to be better than placebo and equivalent to low-dose TCAs for the treatment of mild depression. Emerging data indicate that SJW also compares favorably to SSRIs for mild depression. On the other hand, studies suggest that SJW may not be effective for more severe forms of depression. Drug–drug interactions should also be considered, as noted earlier.

S-Adenosylmethionine

S-Adenosylmethionine, a compound found in all living cells, is involved in essential methyl group transfers. It is the principal methyl donor in the one-carbon cycle with SAMe levels being dependent on levels of folate and vitamin B_{12} (Figure 8.1). SAMe is involved in the methylation of neurotransmitters, nucleic acids, proteins, hormones, and phospholipids; its role in the production of norepinephrine, serotonin, and dopamine may explain SAMe's antidepressant properties.[13] SAMe has been shown to elevate mood in depressed patients when doses of 300 to 3200 mg/day are used. Studies support antidepressant efficacy of SAMe both when compared with placebo and TCAs (i.e., as monotherapy) and when used to augment SSRI- and SNRI-partial response. Oral preparations of SAMe are somewhat unstable, making high doses required for adequate bioavailability. Because the medication is relatively expensive (and not covered by conventional medical insurance plans), its high cost may be prohibitive for many individuals.

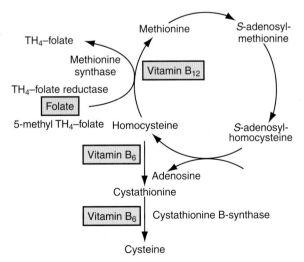

Figure 8.1 One-carbon cycle with S-adenosylmethionine, folate, and vitamin B_{12}. (Redrawn from Dinavahi R, Bonita Falkner B. Relationship of homocysteine with cardiovascular disease and blood pressure. *J Clin Hypertens*. 2004;6:495. © 2004 Le Jacq Communications, Inc.)

Potential adverse effects are relatively minor; these include anxiety, agitation, insomnia, dry mouth, bowel changes, and anorexia. Sweating, dizziness, palpitations, and headaches have also been reported. Psychiatrists should also watch for a potential switch to mania. Finally, significant drug–drug interactions or hepatotoxicity have not yet been reported with SAMe.

Therefore, SAMe is a natural medication that appears to be relatively safe and shows promise as an antidepressant. Further study will help clarify its efficacy and safety.

Folate and Vitamin B_{12}

Folate and vitamin B_{12} are dietary vitamins that play a key role in one-carbon metabolism in which SAMe is formed[14] (see Figure 8.1). SAMe donates methyl groups that are crucial for neurological function and play important roles in the synthesis of central nervous system (CNS) neurotransmitters (e.g., serotonin, dopamine, norepinephrine). Deficiency states of vitamin B_{12} may cause or contribute to a variety of neuropsychiatric and general medical conditions (e.g., macrocytic anemia, neuropathy, cognitive dysfunction or dementia, depression). Folate deficiency has several potential etiologies (e.g., inadequate dietary intake, malabsorption, inborn errors of metabolism, an increased demand [e.g., as seen with pregnancy, infancy, bacterial overgrowth, rapid cellular turnover]). Drugs (e.g., anticonvulsants, oral contraceptives, sulfasalazine, methotrexate, triamterene, trimethoprim, pyrimethamine, and alcohol) may also contribute to folate deficiency. Like folate deficiency, vitamin B_{12} deficiency may also be caused by an inadequate dietary intake, malabsorption, impaired utilization, and interactions with certain drugs (e.g., colchicine, H_2 blockers, metformin, nicotine, oral contraceptive pills, cholestyramine, K-Dur, and zidovudine). From a psychiatric standpoint, deficiency of both folate and vitamin B_{12} has been linked with depression, though the association with folate seems to be greater.[15] Low folate levels have been associated with the delayed onset and degree of clinical improvement of depression. Additionally, folate supplementation may be a beneficial adjunct for treatment of SSRI-refractory depression. The folate form 5-methyltetrahydrofolate (5-MTHF; Deplin) crosses the blood–brain barrier directly, without requiring enzymatic inter-conversion, and may deliver more active product to the brain. As such, this form may be particularly effective as augmentation therapy for the treatment of depression. Metabolically significant vitamin B_{12} deficiency, in turn, has been associated with a greater risk of depression (including psychotic depression) and poor cognitive status, especially in older adults.[16] Recent reviews support B-vitamin supplementation for mood disorders.[17] Adequate levels of each of these is thought to optimize neurotransmitter synthesis, which may aid in reversing depression. One caveat is that supplementation with folate alone may "mask" vitamin B_{12} deficiency by correcting macrocytic anemia while neuropathy persists; therefore, vitamin B_{12} levels should be routinely measured when high doses of folate are given. Folate may also reduce the efficacy of other medications (e.g., phenytoin, methotrexate, and phenobarbital) and has been reported to lower the seizure threshold because high doses disrupt the blood–brain barrier.

In summary, correction of folate deficiency (and perhaps vitamin B_{12} deficiency) may improve depression or at least augment therapy with other medications. Folate (and maybe vitamin B_{12}) supplementation may also shorten the latency of response and enhance the treatment response for depressed patients even when blood levels of these vitamins are normal. Although overall data are inconclusive, psychiatrists should be on the lookout for vitamin deficiency states by checking serum levels in individuals at risk for vitamin deficiencies and in those who have not responded to antidepressant treatment.

Inositol

Inositol is a natural isomer of glucose that is present in many foods. Inositols are cyclic carbohydrates with a six-carbon ring, with the isomer myo-inositol being the most common in the CNS of mammals. Myo-inositol is thought to modulate interactions between neurotransmitters, receptors, cell-signaling proteins, and drugs through its activity in the cell-signaling pathway and is the putative target of the mood-stabilizing drug lithium.[18] Inositol has been effective in several small treatment studies of depression, panic disorder, obsessive-compulsive disorder, and bipolar depression.[19,20] Although promising findings have been noted, negative monotherapy trials with inositol have been conducted in a variety of psychiatric illnesses, including schizophrenia, dementia, ADHD, premenstrual dysphoric disorder, autism, and electroconvulsive-therapy–induced cognitive impairment. Effective dosages are thought to be in the range of 12 to 18 g/day. Adverse effects are generally mild and include GI upset, headache, dizziness, sedation, and insomnia. At present, toxicity and drug interactions are absent.

In summary, treatment with inositol for psychiatric conditions treated with SSRIs and mood stabilizers appears to be safe and promising.

N-Acetyl Cysteine

NAC is a naturally occurring "mitochondrial modulator" with increasing applications in psychiatry. It appears to function by increasing glutathione synthesis, which in turn reduces oxidative stress in the mitochondrial electron transport chain. This may give NAC a protective effect for metabolically active brain cells, like the neuroprotective effects of lithium and valproate. A recent review by Bradlow and colleagues[21] reported promising data in various conditions, including major depressive disorder (two trials), bipolar disorder (eight trials, including one in children aged 5–17 years), obsessive-compulsive spectrum disorders (10 trials), schizophrenia (eight trials), substance use or addiction disorders (15 trials covering tobacco, methamphetamine, gambling, cannabis, and cocaine, including one study with co-morbid post-traumatic stress disorder [PTSD]). Overall, the data are promising. Typical dosages range from 600 to 3000 mg/day. Safety and tolerability are reported as very good, with dry mouth, nausea, vomiting, and diarrhea as the main side effects.

ANXIETY AND INSOMNIA

Valerian

Valerian (*Valeriana officinalis*) is a flowering plant extract that has been used to promote sleep and to reduce anxiety for more than 2000 years. Common names also include *all heal* and *garden heliotrope*. Typical preparations include capsules, liquid extracts, and teas made from roots and underground stems.[22] Valerian is thought to promote natural sleep after several weeks of use by decreasing sleep latency and by improving overall sleep quality; however, methodological problems in most studies conducted limit making firm conclusions in this area. A recent systematic review and meta-analysis[23] covering 60 studies found inconsistent outcomes regarding insomnia and anxiety, although safety and tolerability were deemed good, even in older adults. A proposed mechanism involves decreasing gamma-aminobutyric acid (GABA) breakdown. Sedative effects are dose-related within the usual dose range of 450 to 600 mg, administered about 2 hours before bedtime. Dependence and daytime drowsiness have not been problematic. Adverse effects, including blurry vision, GI symptoms, and headache, seem to be uncommon. Although data are limited,

valerian should probably be avoided in those with liver dysfunction (because of potential hepatic toxicity).[22] Major drug interactions have not been reported.

In summary, valerian has been used as a hypnotic for centuries with relatively few reported adverse effects.

Melatonin

Melatonin is a hormone made in the pineal gland that has helped travelers avoid jet lag and decrease sleep latency for those with insomnia. It may be particularly beneficial for night-shift workers. Melatonin is derived from serotonin (Figure 8.2) and is thought to play a role in the organization of circadian rhythms via interaction with the suprachiasmatic nucleus.[24] Low-dose melatonin treatment has increased circulating melatonin levels to those normally observed at night and thus facilitates sleep onset and sleep maintenance without changing sleep architecture. Melatonin generally facilitates falling asleep within 1 hour, independent of when it is taken. Although several studies have supported use of melatonin as an effective hypnotic, a recent review and meta-analysis suggested limited efficacy in adults but greater efficacy in children and adolescents, with co-morbid and non-co-morbid chronic insomnia.[25] Optimal dosages are thought to be in the range of 0.25 to 0.30 mg/day. Nevertheless, many preparations contain as much as 5 to 10 mg of melatonin.[24] Higher doses can cause daytime sleepiness and confusion; other adverse effects include decreased sex drive, retinal damage, hypothermia, and fertility problems. Melatonin is contraindicated in pregnancy and in those who are immunocompromised.[24] There are few reports of drug–drug interactions.

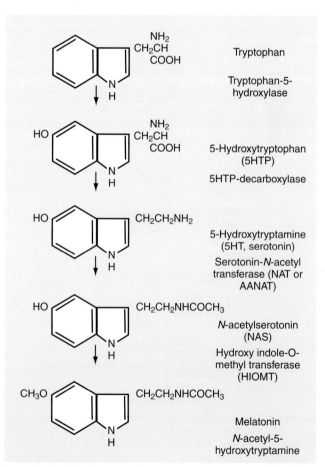

Figure 8.2 Melatonin synthesis.

Melatonin seems to be a relatively safe hypnotic and an organizer of circadian rhythms when taken in appropriate doses. Caution should be taken in at-risk populations and with use of higher doses.

Kava

Kava (*Piper methysticum*) is derived from a root originating in the Polynesian islands, where it is used as a social and ceremonial herb.[22] Although it is thought to have mild anxiolytic and hypnotic effects, study results have been mixed, and recent reviews suggest that kava use leads to limited benefits.[10,26] The mechanism of action is attributed to kavapyrones, which are central muscle relaxants that are thought to be involved in blockade of voltage-gated sodium ion channels, enhanced binding to $GABA_A$ receptors, diminished excitatory neurotransmitter release, reduced reuptake of norepinephrine, and reversible inhibition of MAO_B. The suggested dosage is 60 to 120 mg/day. Major side effects include GI upset, headaches, and dizziness. Toxic reactions, including ataxia, hair loss, respiratory problems, yellowing of the skin, and vision problems, have been seen at high doses or with prolonged use.[22] In the early 2000s, numerous reports of severe hepatotoxicity worldwide were published, including some cases that required liver transplantation.[22,26] For this reason, several countries withdrew kava from the market. Recent investigations suggest that kava is safe to use with proper precautions.[27]

Although kava appears to be somewhat efficacious in the treatment of mild anxiety, concerns about safety reduce our enthusiasm about its use, particularly for long-term treatment. If used, it should be done under medical supervision and with regular monitoring of liver function tests.

Lavender

Lavender (*Lavandula angustifolia*) is an aromatic plant long recognized anecdotally for its calming properties. Lavender essential oil can be taken by mouth, by inhalation (i.e., as aromatherapy), or topically. Its anxiolytic effect is thought to occur through inhibition of voltage-gated calcium channels, reduction of $5\text{-}HT_{1A}$ receptor activity, and increased parasympathetic nervous system activation. Most studies on lavender have examined its anxiolytic effect when administered as aromatherapy. Silexan is a standardized, pharmaceutical quality capsule form containing 80 mg of lavender essential oil per capsule. In a 10-week study of 539 adults with generalized anxiety disorder, Silexan outperformed placebo and paroxetine (determined by reduction of Hamilton Anxiety Scale scores) and was better tolerated than paroxetine (and it did not differ from placebo in terms of adverse effects).[28] Silexan and other forms of lavender are generally well tolerated and do not appear to cause dependency or withdrawal. Lavender's efficacy for insomnia is mixed.

Table 8.2 summarizes the natural medications discussed for the treatment of insomnia and anxiety.

Cannabidiol

Cannabidiol (CBD), the cannabinoid constituent of cannabis has been growing in popularity in the United States and worldwide in view of its increasing legalization and availability. It is often supplied as an oil containing only CBD (no tetrahydrocannabinol [THC]), a full-plant CBD-dominant hemp extract oil, capsules, dried cannabis, or liquid solution.[29] CBD is approved for multiple sclerosis–related pain in Canada and Sweden and in the United States for certain childhood epilepsy disorders.[29] CBD is thought to work via multiple mechanisms, including serotonergic and antioxidant activity.[29] Potential clinical applications are broad. A recent review by Sarris and colleagues[30] found possible reductions of social anxiety, mixed (but mainly positive) evidence for adjunctive use in schizophrenia, and limited evidence in insomnia and PTSD. There was no apparent benefit for depression from high-THC therapeutics or for CBD in mania, but some potential efficacy for an oral cannabinoid/terpene combination in ADHD. Side effects have included sleepiness, decreased appetite, diarrhea, fatigue,

TABLE 8.2 Natural Medications for Anxiety and Insomnia

Medication	Active Components	Possible Indications	Possible Mechanisms of Action	Suggested Dosage	Adverse Events
CBD	Cannabidiol	Social anxiety, schizophrenia, insomnia, PTSD, ADHD, MS-related pain, childhood seizure disorders	Serotonergic; antioxidant	Varies, depending on preparation and condition	Sleepiness, decreased appetite, diarrhea, fatigue, malaise, weakness, insomnia
Kava (*Piper methysticum*)	Kavapyrones	Anxiety	Central muscle relaxant, enhanced $GABA_A$ receptor binding, reversible inhibition of MAO_B	60–120 mg/day	GI disturbance, headaches, dizziness, ataxia, hair loss, visual problems, respiratory problems, rash, severe liver toxicity
Lavender (*Lavandula angustifolia*)	Terpenoids linalool and linalyl acetate	GAD, anxiety-related restlessness	Inhibition of voltage-gated calcium channels; decreased $5\text{-}HT_{1A}$ receptor activity; enhanced vagal tone	Silexan 80–160 mg/day	Nausea, dyspepsia (oral form); dermatitis (topical)
Melatonin	Hormone made in pineal gland	Insomnia	Regulates circadian rhythm in suprachiasmatic nucleus	0.25–0.3 mg/day (may increase up to 5 mg/day if needed)	Sedation, confusion, hypothermia, retinal damage, decreased sex drive, infertility
Valerian (*Valeriana officinalis*)	Valepotriates (from roots and underground stems)	Insomnia	Decrease GABA breakdown	450–600 mg/day	Blurry vision, headache, and possible hepatotoxicity

$5\text{-}HT_{1A}$, Serotonergic $_{1A}$ receptor; *ADHD*, attention-deficit hyperactivity disorder; *CBD*, cannabidiol; *GABA*, gamma-aminobutyric acid; *GAD*, generalized anxiety disorder; *GI*, gastrointestinal; *MAO*, monoamine oxidase; *MS*, multiple sclerosis; *PTSD*, post-traumatic stress disorder.
Adapted from Mischoulon D, Nierenberg AA. Natural medications in psychiatry. In: Stern TA, Herman JB, Rubin DH, eds. *Psychiatry Update and Board Preparation*. 4th ed. Boston: MGH Psychiatry Academy Publishing; 2018.

malaise, weakness, and insomnia but not significant intoxicating effects. Dosages and dosing strategies vary depending on the formulation used, but slow titration is recommended. Caution is recommended with its use in younger individuals as well as in individuals with anxious or psychotic disorders. Likewise, individuals with cardiovascular or respiratory disorders should use CBD cautiously, and CBD should probably be avoided during pregnancy and breast-feeding.[30] Occupational safety should also be considered with this yet-unproven treatment.

PREMENSTRUAL AND MENOPAUSAL SYMPTOMS
Black Cohosh

Black cohosh (Cimicifuga racemosa) is a member of the buttercup family native to the northeastern United States. The available natural supplement, derived from the root of the plant, at a dosage of 40 mg/day or higher has reduced physical and psychological menopausal symptoms, as well as dysmenorrhea.[31,32] Active ingredients are thought to be triterpenoids, isoflavones, and aglycones, which may participate in suppression of luteinizing hormone in the pituitary gland, though studies in humans have shown mixed results. Anti-cancer effects are also inconsistent.[32] Headache, dizziness, GI upset, and weight gain are among its generally mild side effects. Limited data have not revealed specific toxicity or drug interactions. Black cohosh is not recommended for individuals who are pregnant or breast-feeding or who have heart disease or hypertension. Those with adverse reactions to aspirin should also avoid black cohosh because it contains salicylates.

Chaste Tree Berry

Chaste tree berry (Vitex agnus castus) is derived from the dried fruit of the chaste tree; it has been used since ancient Greeks used it to help alleviate female reproductive complaints.[33,34] Its name comes from its earlier use to help monks keep their vow of chastity through decreasing their sex drive. The mechanism in both instances is thought to be via prolactin inhibition by binding dopamine receptors in the anterior pituitary, although this remains under investigation. It is most commonly used to alleviate premenstrual syndrome in dosages of 200 to 400 mg/day.[33,34] Side effects such as nausea, headaches, GI disturbances, menstrual disturbance, acne, pruritus, and rashes seem to be minor.[35] Although there are no clear drug–drug interactions, there is a theoretical risk of decreased efficacy of birth control because of its effects on prolactin. Because it is thought to be a dopamine agonist, there may also be interactions with other dopamine agonists or antagonists.[35] A summary of the natural medications discussed here for premenstrual and menopausal symptoms is found in Table 8.3.

COGNITION AND DEMENTIA
Ginkgo Biloba

Ginkgo biloba has been used in Chinese medicine for thousands of years. This natural medication comes from the seed of the gingko tree, and it has generally been used for the treatment of impaired cognition and affective symptoms in dementias[36]; however, a possible new role has also emerged in the management of antidepressant-induced sexual dysfunction.[37] As far as its role in cognition is concerned, target symptoms in those with dementia include memory and abstract thinking. Studies have shown modest but significant improvements in cognitive performance and social function with dosages of 120 mg/day.[36] Evidence suggests that progression of cognitive dysfunction may be delayed by 6 to 12 months, but those with mild dementia show greatest improvement, and those with more severe disease may stabilize at best. Recent studies have suggested that ginkgo may be effective in combination with registered nootropic agents, the cholinesterase inhibitors.[38-40] Studies of healthy young volunteers taking Ginkgo biloba have shown mixed results regarding cognitive enhancement.[41-43] Flavonoids and terpene lactones are thought to be the active components, which may work by stimulating still functional nerve cells. They may also play a role in protecting cells from pathological effects (such as hypoxia and ischemia). Ginkgo has been shown to inhibit platelet-activating factor, which suggests an increased bleeding risk, but a recent meta-analysis did not bear this out.[44] Nonetheless, it should probably be avoided in those at high risk of bleeding until further data are available. Other noted side effects include headache, GI distress, seizures in epileptics, and dizziness. The suggested dosage of Ginkgo biloba is 120 to 240 mg/day, with a minimum 8-week course of treatment; however, it may take up to 1 year to appreciate its full benefit.

Ginkgo biloba appears to be a safe and efficacious cognition-enhancing medication. It may have an additional role in reducing antidepressant-induced sexual dysfunction. Further studies are needed to fully understand its complete and long-term effects. A summary of Ginkgo biloba as discussed here for cognition and dementia is found in Table 8.4.

CONCLUSION

Complementary and integrative medical therapies are becoming increasingly popular in the United States and around the world. The spectrum of such therapies is quite diverse and often has significant overlap with more traditional medical practice. Lack of scientific research in this area historically has contributed to deficiencies in knowledge with respect to safety and efficacy of many of the natural remedies on the market today. The past three decades have generated new randomized clinical

TABLE 8.3 Natural Medications for Premenstrual and Menopausal Symptoms

Medication	Active Components	Possible Indications	Possible Mechanisms of Action	Suggested Dosage	Adverse Events
Black cohosh (Cimicifuga racemosa)	Triterpenoids, iso-flavones, aglycones	Menopausal and premenstrual symptoms	Suppression of LH in the pituitary gland	40 mg/day	GI upset, headache, weight gain, and dizziness; unclear effects on breast cancer proliferation
Chaste tree berry (Vitex agnus castus)	Unknown	Premenstrual symptoms	Prolactin inhibition by binding to dopaminergic receptors in the anterior pituitary	200–400 mg/day	Minor GI disturbance, increased acne, increased menstrual flow, possible decreased efficacy of birth control

GI, Gastrointestinal; LH, luteinizing hormone.
Adapted from Mischoulon D, Nierenberg AA. Natural medications in psychiatry. In: Stern TA, Herman JB, Rubin DH, eds. Psychiatry Update and Board Preparation. 4th ed. Boston: MGH Psychiatry Academy Publishing; 2018.

TABLE 8.4 Natural Medications for Cognition and Dementia

Medication	Active Components	Possible Indications	Possible Mechanisms of Action	Suggested Dosage	Adverse Events
Ginkgo biloba	Flavonoids, terpene lactones	Dementia and sexual dysfunction	Nerve cell stimulation and protection and free radical scavenging	120–240 mg/day	Mild GI disturbance, headache, irritability, dizziness, seizures in patients with epilepsy

GI, Gastrointestinal.
Adapted from Mischoulon D, Nierenberg AA. Natural medications in psychiatry. In: Stern TA, Herman JB, Rubin DH, eds. *Psychiatry Update and Board Preparation*. 4th ed. Boston: MGH Psychiatry Academy Publishing; 2018.

trials, meta-analyses, and systematic reviews that have allowed for more specific recommendations. For example, the Canadian Network for Mood and Anxiety Treatments recently published a series of guidelines for use of complementary therapies in depressive disorders.[45] SJW, omega-3 fatty acids, and SAMe were the most highly recommended, including a first-line recommendation for SJW for mild to moderate depression. Folic acid received a second-line indication, and inositol was not recommended because of limited evidence. Many of the therapies discussed in this chapter may prove to be valuable additions to the psychopharmacologic armamentarium of psychiatrists. However, caution is needed regarding their potential drug–drug interactions and side effects. A general knowledge of these therapies and routine questioning about their use is an essential part of comprehensive care by psychiatrists.

REFERENCES

1. National Center for Complementary and Integrative Health. *Complementary, alternative, or integrative health: what's in a name?* April 2021. Accessed October 12, 2022. https://www.nccih.nih.gov/health/complementary-alternative-or-integrative-health-whats-in-a-name

2. Mischoulon D, Nierenberg AA. Natural medications in psychiatry. In: Stern TA, Herman JB, Rubin DH, eds. *Psychiatry Update and Board Preparation*. McGraw-Hill; 2018. 4th ed.

3. Hassen G, Belete G, Carrera KG, et al. Clinical implications of herbal supplements in conventional medical practice: a US perspective. *Cureus*. 2022;14:e26893.

4. Kelly JP, Kaufman DW, Kelley K, et al. Use of herbal/natural supplements according to racial/ethnic group. *J Altern Complement Med*. 2006;12:555–561.

5. Simopoulos AP. Omega-3 fatty acids in inflammation and autoimmune diseases. *J Am Coll Nutr*. 2002;21:495–505.

6. Ferrari R, Censi S, Cimaglia P. The journey of omega-3 fatty acids in cardiovascular medicine. *Eur Heart J Suppl*. 2020;22(suppl J):J49–J53.

7. Mischoulon D, Freeman MP. Omega-3 fatty acids in psychiatry. *Psychiatr Clin North Am*. 2013;36:15–23.

8. Appleton KM, Voyias PD, Sallis HM, et al. Omega-3 fatty acids for depression in adults. *Cochrane Database Syst Rev*. 2021;11CD004692.

9. Mischoulon D. Update and critique of natural remedies as antidepressant treatments. *Psychiatr Clin North Am*. 2007;30:51–68.

10. Sarris J, Marx W, Ashton MM, et al. Plant-based medicines (phytoceuticals) in the treatment of psychiatric disorders: a meta-review of meta-analyses of randomized controlled trials. *Can J Psychiatry*. 2021;66:849–862.

11. Haller H, Anheyer D, Cramer H, Dobos G. Complementary therapies for clinical depression: an overview of systematic reviews. *BMJ Open*. 2019;9:e028527.

12. Lippert A, Renner B. Herb-drug interaction in inflammatory diseases: review of phytomedicine and herbal supplements. *J Clin Med*. 2022;11:1567.

13. Sharma A, Gerbarg P, Bottiglieri T, et al. S-Adenosylmethionine (SAMe) for neuropsychiatric disorders: a clinician-oriented review of research. *J Clin Psychiatry*. 2017;78:e656–e667.

14. Maruf AA, Poweleit EA, Brown LC, et al. Systematic review and meta-analysis of l-methylfolate augmentation in depressive disorders. *Pharmacopsychiatry*. 2022;55:139–147.

15. Papakostas GI, Petersen T, Mischoulon D, et al. Serum folate, vitamin B12, and homocysteine in major depressive disorder, part 1: predictors of clinical response in fluoxetine-resistant depression. *J Clin Psychiatry*. 2004;65:1090–1095.

16. Reynolds EH. Folic acid, ageing, depression, and dementia. *BMJ*. 2002;324:1512–1515.

17. Borges-Vieira JG, Cardoso CKS. Efficacy of B-vitamins and vitamin D therapy in improving depressive and anxiety disorders: a systematic review of randomized controlled trials. *Nutr Neurosci*. 2023;26(3):187–207.

18. Williams RS, Cheng L, Mudge AW, et al. A common mechanism of action for three mood-stabilizing drugs. *Nature*. 2002;417:292–295.

19. Belmaker RH, Levine J. Inositol in the treatment of psychiatric disorders. In: Mischoulon D, Rosenbaum J, eds. *Natural Medications for Psychiatric Disorders: Considering the Alternatives*. 2nd ed. Lippincott Williams & Wilkins; 2008.

20. Mukai T, Kishi T, Matsuda Y, et al. A meta-analysis of inositol for depression and anxiety disorders. *Hum Psychopharmacol*. 2014;29:55–63.

21. Bradlow RCJ, Berk M, Kalivas PW, et al. The potential of N-acetyl-L-cysteine (NAC) in the treatment of psychiatric disorders. *CNS Drugs*. 2022;36:451–482.

22. Mischoulon D. Herbal remedies for anxiety and insomnia: kava and valerian. In: Mischoulon D, Rosenbaum J, eds. *Natural Medications for Psychiatric Disorders: Considering the Alternatives*. 2nd ed. Lippincott Williams & Wilkins; 2008.

23. Shinjyo N, Waddell G, Green J. Valerian root in treating sleep problems and associated disorders-a systematic review and meta-analysis. *J Evid Based Integr Med*. 2020;252515690X20967323.

24. Zhdanova V, Friedman L. Melatonin for treatment of sleep and mood disorders. In: Mischoulon D, Rosenbaum J, eds. *Natural Medications for Psychiatric Disorders: Considering the Alternatives*. 2nd ed. Lippincott Williams & Wilkins; 2008.

25. Choi K, Lee YJ, Park S. Efficacy of melatonin for chronic insomnia: systematic reviews and meta-analyses. *Sleep Med Rev*. 2022;66:101692.

26. Soares RB, Dinis-Oliveira RJ, Oliveira NG. An updated review on the psychoactive, toxic and anticancer properties of kava. *J Clin Med*. 2022;11:4039.

27. Thomsen M, Schmidt M. Health policy versus kava (Piper methysticum): anxiolytic efficacy may be instrumental in restoring the reputation of a major South Pacific crop. *J Ethnopharmacol*. 2021;268:113582.

28. Kasper S, Gastpar M, Müller WE, et al. Lavender oil preparation Silexan is effective in generalized anxiety disorder—a randomized, double-blind comparison to placebo and paroxetine. *Int J Neuropsychopharmacol*. 2014;17:859–869.

29. Levine MT, Gao J, Satyanarayanan SK, et al. S-adenosyl-l-methionine (SAMe), cannabidiol (CBD), and kratom in psychiatric disorders: clinical and mechanistic considerations. *Brain Behav Immun*. 2020;85:152–161.

30. Sarris J, Sinclair J, Karamacoska D, et al. Medicinal cannabis for psychiatric disorders: a clinically-focused systematic review. *BMC Psychiatry*. 2020;20:24.

31. McKenna DJ, Jones K, Humphrey S, et al. Black cohosh: efficacy, safety, and use in clinical and preclinical applications. *Altern Ther Health Med*. 2001;7:93–100.

32. Mohapatra S, Iqubal A, Ansari MJ, et al. Benefits of black cohosh (*Cimicifuga racemosa*) for women's health: an up-close and in-depth review. *Pharmaceuticals (Basel)*. 2022;15:278.

33. Tesch BJ. Herbs commonly used by women: an evidence-based review. *Am J Obstet Gynecol*. 2002;188(5 suppl):S44–S55.

34. van Die MD, Burger HG, Teede HJ, et al. Vitex agnus-castus (Chaste-Tree/Berry) in the treatment of menopause-related complaints. *J Altern Complement Med*. 2009;15:853–862.

35. Daniele C, Thompson Coon J, et al. Vitex agnus castus: a systematic review of adverse events. *Drug Saf*. 2005;28:319–332.

36. Tomino C, Ilari S, Solfrizzi V, et al. Mild cognitive impairment and mild dementia: the role of *Ginkgo biloba* (EGb 761®). *Pharmaceuticals (Basel)*. 2021;14:305.

37. Niazi Mashhadi Z, Irani M, Kiyani Mask M, et al. A systematic review of clinical trials on Ginkgo (*Ginkgo biloba*) effectiveness on sexual function and its safety. *Avicenna J Phytomed*. 2021;11:324–331.

38. Yancheva S, Ihl R, Nikolova G, GINDON Study Group *Ginkgo biloba* extract Egb 761®, donepezil or both combined in the treatment of Alzheimer's disease with neuropsychiatric features: a randomized, double-blind, exploratory trial. *Aging Ment Health*. 2009;13:183–190.

39. Cornelli U. Treatment of Alzheimer's disease with a cholinesterase inhibitor combined with antioxidants. *Neurodegener Dis*. 2010;7:193–202.

40. Canevelli M, Adali N, Kelaiditi E, et al. Effects of Gingko biloba supplementation in Alzheimer's disease patients receiving cholinesterase inhibitors: data from the ICTUS study. *Phytomedicine*. 2014;21:888–892.

41. Stough C, Clarke J, Lloyd J, et al. Neuropsychological changes after 30-day *Ginkgo biloba* administration in healthy participants. *Int J Neuropsychopharmacol*. 2001;4:131–134.

42. Elsabagh S, Hartley DE, Ali O, et al. Differential cognitive effects of Ginkgo biloba after acute and chronic treatment in healthy young volunteers. *Psychopharmacology (Berl)*. 2005;179:437–446.

43. Kennedy DO, Jackson PA, Haskell CF, et al. Modulation of cognitive performance following single doses of 120 mg Ginkgo biloba extract administered to healthy young volunteers. *Hum Psychopharmacol*. 2007;22:559–566.

44. Kellermann AJ, Kloft C. Is there a risk of bleeding associated with standardized Ginkgo biloba extract therapy? A systematic review and meta-analysis. *Pharmacotherapy*. 2011;31:490–502.

45. Ravindran AV, Balneaves LG, Faulkner G, et al. Canadian Network for Mood and Anxiety Treatments (CANMAT) 2016 Clinical Guidelines for the Management of Adults with Major Depressive Disorder: Section 5. Complementary and Alternative Medicine Treatments. *Can J Psychiatry*. 2016;61:576–587.

9 Antipsychotic Drugs

Shreedhar Paudel, Carol Lim, and Oliver Freudenreich

KEY POINTS

- All currently available antipsychotics (except for pimavanserin, which is approved by the US Food and Drug Administration [FDA] for the treatment of psychosis in Parkinson disease) share dopamine$_2$ blockade as the presumed main mechanism of action. Primary symptom targets of antipsychotics are positive symptoms (disorganization, delusions, and hallucinations) and agitation. Antipsychotics are mostly ineffective for negative symptoms and the cognitive deficits of schizophrenia and may even worsen them. Increasingly, antipsychotics are used also for the treatment of mood disorders.

- Historically, antipsychotics have been grouped into first-generation antipsychotics (typical or conventional antipsychotics, which are all characterized by their risk of extrapyramidal symptoms [EPSs]) and second-generation antipsychotics (with a reduced risk of EPSs; hence, they are called "atypical" antipsychotics). However, antipsychotics within each class are not necessarily interchangeable. Newer partial dopamine agonist–antagonist antipsychotics are sometimes referred to as third-generation antipsychotics.

- Currently available antipsychotics have variable efficacy and tolerability. They need to be selected based on individualized risk–benefit assessments (i.e., balancing the degree of symptomatic response with day-to-day tolerability and long-term medical morbidity, particularly cardiovascular risk).

- The two main risks associated with taking antipsychotics are neurological side effects (e.g., dystonias, akathisia, parkinsonism, tardive dyskinesia) and metabolic problems (e.g., weight gain, dyslipidemia, hyperglycemia). Antipsychotics differ in their risks for these side effects.

- First-line antipsychotics are equally effective for non-refractory schizophrenia. For patients with treatment-resistance, olanzapine and especially clozapine have been the most efficacious.

- Clozapine has minimal or no risk of inducing EPSs and is the most effective antipsychotic. However, its clinical use is limited to treatment-resistant patients because of serious side effects (including metabolic problems and agranulocytosis, which requires absolute neutrophil count monitoring).

INTRODUCTION

This chapter reviews the basic pharmacology of antipsychotics, emphasizing the differential efficacy and side effect profiles among antipsychotics, including clozapine, based on the schizophrenia literature. Although antipsychotics are used primarily for the treatment of schizophrenia, antipsychotic agents have received FDA approval for additional indications, particularly for the treatment of mood disorders for which they are used routinely. Specific treatment considerations regarding the choice of an antipsychotic for major psychiatric syndromes (e.g., schizophrenia, bipolar disorder, depression, autism) can be found in the chapters on these conditions.

HISTORY

Chlorpromazine and the Early Agents

In 1952, Henri Laborit, a French naval surgeon, experimented with combinations of preoperative medications to reduce the autonomic stress of surgical procedures. He tried a newly synthesized antihistamine, chlorpromazine, and was impressed by its calming effect. He noted that patients seemed indifferent about their impending surgery, yet they were not overly sedated. Convinced that the medication had potential for the care of psychiatric patients, Laborit urged his colleagues to test his hypothesis. Eventually, a surgical colleague told his brother-in-law, the psychiatrist Pierre Deniker, about Laborit's discovery.

Pierre Deniker and Jean Delay, who was the chairman of his department at the Hôpital Sainte-Anne in Paris, experimented with chlorpromazine and found remarkable tranquilizing effects in their most agitated and psychotic patients.[1] By 1954, Delay and Deniker had published six papers on their clinical experience with chlorpromazine. They noted in 1955 that both chlorpromazine and the dopamine-depleting agent reserpine shared antipsychotic efficacy and neurological side effects that resembled Parkinson disease. They coined the term *neuroleptic* to describe these effects. Side effects became apparent quickly. In 1956, Frank Ayd[2] described acute dystonia and fatal hyperthermia with chlorpromazine. Sigwald and colleagues[3] published the first reports of tardive dyskinesia (TD) in 1959.

Smith Kline purchased chlorpromazine from the French pharmaceutical company Rhône-Poulenc, and in 1954, chlorpromazine received approval from the FDA for the treatment of psychosis. The care of patients with psychosis was transformed almost overnight, in parallel with new optimism and funding about community-based treatments, away from lifelong "warehousing" of individuals with schizophrenia in large state psychiatric hospitals. An additional 10 antipsychotic compounds were rapidly synthesized and approved for clinical use. These included a series of phenothiazines, the thioxanthenes (that were derived from phenothiazines), and haloperidol, which was synthesized from meperidine by Paul Janssen in 1958. In 1967, haloperidol, the last of the classic "neuroleptics," was approved by the FDA, and because of its relative selectivity for dopamine$_2$ (D$_2$) receptors and paucity of non-neurological side effects, it became the market leader.

By 1964, several multi-center trials sponsored by the Veterans Administration and the National Institutes of Mental Health (NIMH) were completed comparing the rapidly growing list of antipsychotic agents. These landmark studies each enrolled several hundred patients and were the first large clinical trials to be conducted in the new field of psychopharmacology. The phenothiazines were found to be highly effective and superior to placebo, barbiturates, and reserpine. In the NIMH collaborative study of more than 400 acutely ill patients, 75% of patients were at least moderately improved with chlorpromazine, thioridazine, or fluphenazine compared with only 23% with placebo.[4] Although reports of their stand-alone efficacy were impressive, the goal of identifying differences in efficacy among drugs that might allow the matching of specific drugs with subgroups of patients was not realized.

In 1963, Carlsson and Lindqvist[5] discovered that chlorpromazine increased the turnover of dopamine in the brain. This led them to hypothesize that dopamine receptor blockade was responsible for antipsychotic effects. In 1976, Creese and colleagues[6] confirmed this hypothesis by demonstrating that the antipsychotic potency of a wide range of agents correlated closely with affinity for the D$_2$ receptor. This explained the equivalency of efficacy among agents because all were acting via the same mechanism. The dopamine hypothesis led to a reliance on animal models sensitive to D$_2$ blockade as a screen for discovering potentially antipsychotic drugs. The result of this was that new mechanisms were not intentionally explored.

Clozapine, the First Atypical Antipsychotic

The discovery of the first antidepressant, imipramine, led to the synthesis of related heterocyclic compounds, among which clozapine, a dibenzodiazepine derivative, was synthesized in 1958 by the Swiss company Wander. Clozapine was initially a disappointment because it did not produce in animal models the behavioral effects associated with an antidepressant or the neurological side effects associated with an antipsychotic. Clinical trials proceeded in Europe but were halted in 1975 after reports of 17 cases of agranulocytosis in Finland, 8 of which were fatal.[7] However, the impression among researchers that clozapine possessed unique clinical characteristics led the manufacturer Sandoz to sponsor a pivotal multicenter trial comparing clozapine and chlorpromazine in neuroleptic-resistant patients prospectively shown to be refractory to haloperidol. The dramatic results reported by Kane and colleagues in 1988[8] demonstrated the superiority of clozapine for essentially all domains of symptoms and a relative absence of neurological side effects (i.e., "atypical"), prompting a second revolution in the pharmacotherapy of schizophrenia. To this date, clozapine remains the most effective antipsychotic for treatment-resistant schizophrenia.

Risperidone and Other Atypical Agents

Starting in the mid-1980s, Paul Janssen and colleagues began experimenting with serotonin 5-HT$_2$ antagonism added to D$_2$ blockade after demonstrating that this combination reduced the neurological side effects of haloperidol in rats. When the 5-HT$_2$ antagonist ritanserin was added to haloperidol in

patients with schizophrenia, neurological symptoms, specifically extrapyramidal symptoms (EPSs), were diminished, and negative symptoms improved.[9] This led to development of risperidone, a D$_2$ and 5-HT$_{2A}$ antagonist, the first agent designed to follow clozapine's example as an "atypical antipsychotic" with the goal of reduced EPSs and enhanced efficacy. Multicenter trials comparing multiple fixed doses of risperidone with haloperidol at a single, relatively high dosage of 20 mg/day demonstrated reduced EPSs, improved negative symptoms, and, in a subset of relatively resistant patients, greater antipsychotic efficacy.[10] Olanzapine, a chemical derivative of clozapine, similarly demonstrated reduced EPSs and superior efficacy compared with haloperidol. Risperidone and olanzapine rapidly replaced the first generation of neuroleptics, particularly after clinicians became convinced that the risk of TD was substantially lower. However, it soon became apparent that risperidone markedly elevated serum prolactin levels and that olanzapine produced weight gain in some patients to a degree previously seen only with clozapine. In the decades after risperidone's approval, many antipsychotics were approved in the United States based largely on reduced EPSs; these agents did not convincingly demonstrate superior efficacy compared with older neuroleptics. Collectively, the atypical antipsychotics beginning with risperidone are often referred to as second-generation antipsychotics (SGAs) to distinguish them from the original group of typical (conventional) antipsychotics, which are correspondingly also known as first-generation antipsychotics (FGAs).

The CATIE Study

In 1999, the NIMH, recognizing that almost all information regarding the new antipsychotics had come from industry-supported efficacy trials of uncertain generalizability, awarded a competitive contract to Dr. Jeffrey Lieberman to conduct a large multi-center trial to assess the effectiveness and tolerability of the newer, second-generation agents under more representative treatment conditions. Results of this seminal Clinical Antipsychotic Trials of Intervention Effectiveness (CATIE) study were first published in 2005 (Figure 9.1).[11] The study was conducted at 57 sites across the United States and included 1493 representative patients with schizophrenia who were randomly assigned to risperidone, olanzapine, quetiapine, ziprasidone, or the conventional comparator, perphenazine, for an 18-month double-blind trial. Dosing was flexible; the range of doses for each drug was selected based on patterns of clinical use (in consultation with the manufacturers). Ziprasidone became available and was added after the study was roughly 40% completed. Patients with TD at study entry were not randomized to perphenazine, and their data were excluded from analyses comparing the atypical agents with perphenazine. Patients who failed treatment with their first assigned agent could be randomized again in subsequent phases. One re-randomization pathway featured open-label clozapine for treatment-resistant patients, and another pathway featured ziprasidone for treatment-intolerant patients. The secondary randomization pathway did not include perphenazine.

One striking finding of the CATIE study was that only 26% of participants completed the 18-month trial still taking their originally assigned antipsychotic. The primary measure of effectiveness, "all-cause discontinuation," significantly favored olanzapine over the other agents. Olanzapine's superior effectiveness was also reflected in significantly fewer hospitalizations and fewer discontinuations because of lack of efficacy. Although risperidone-treated patients were numerically less likely to discontinue because of intolerance, this difference was not statistically significant. In addition to greater effectiveness,

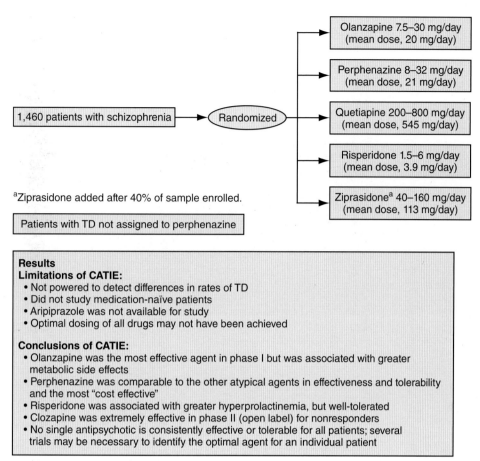

Figure 9.1 Clinical Antipsychotic Trials of Intervention Effectiveness (CATIE) phase 1: double-blind, randomized 18-month trial. *TD*, Tardive dyskinesia.

olanzapine was associated with greater cardiovascular risk. Patients treated with olanzapine demonstrated more weight gain and elevation of hemoglobin A1c, total cholesterol, and triglycerides. The other atypical agents did not significantly differ from perphenazine in either efficacy or tolerability. Overall, the results suggested that no single antipsychotic is likely to be optimal for all, or for most, patients. The duration of the CATIE trial was not long enough to detect differences among agents in the incidence of TD.

Third-Generation and Newer Antipsychotics

Beginning with aripiprazole, drugs were developed that differed from the other atypical or SGAs by possessing partial agonist activity at the D_2 receptor rather than full antagonism (e.g., cariprazine, brexpiprazole). The most recently FDA-approved antipsychotic, lumateperone, has an even more complex receptor profile that defies an easy categorization (Table 9.1). The next drugs approved for the treatment of schizophrenia may no longer be based on direct dopamine blockade, with the hope of eliminating motor side effects, particularly TD. Pimavanserin, which is devoid of dopamine blockade, has been shown to be effective for psychosis in the setting of Parkinson disease but not for the treatment of schizophrenia.

Recent meta-analytic studies have found substantial differences in side effects as well as small, but statistically significant, differences in efficacy among currently available antipsychotics.[12] This argues against a simple categorization of antipsychotics as typical or atypical or first or second generation (or third generation, for partial agonist antipsychotics)[13]

even though this terminology continues to be used (for lack of a better one).

GENERAL CLINICAL CONSIDERATIONS

For schizophrenia, the primary target symptoms for antipsychotic agents fall into three categories: psychotic symptoms (e.g., hallucinations, delusions, disorganization), agitation (e.g., distractibility, affective lability, tension, increased motor activity), and negative symptoms (e.g., apathy, diminished affect, social withdrawal, poverty of speech). Although cognitive deficits are an important contributor to disability in schizophrenia, cognitive deficits usually are not considered a target for antipsychotic agents because they are not very responsive to current agents. Agitation responds to most antipsychotics rapidly and often fully, whereas response of psychotic symptoms is quite variable, and negative symptoms rarely exhibit more than modest improvement (Figure 9.2).

Timing of the antipsychotic response can also be quite variable. In the 1970s, physicians recommended the use of relatively large doses of intramuscular (IM) haloperidol for the treatment of psychosis, a strategy known as "rapid neuroleptization." This was based on the clinical impression that agitation and psychosis responded quickly to this aggressive treatment approach. For the next two decades, the consensus shifted to the view that psychotic symptoms require weeks of antipsychotic treatment before responding. More recently, Kapur and colleagues[14] analyzed data from studies of IM administration of atypical antipsychotics and documented antipsychotic effects within hours of administration, independent of tranquilization. It is likely that tranquilization or

TABLE 9.1 Affinity of Antipsychotic Drugs for Human Neurotransmitter Receptors (Ki, nM)

Receptor	Clozapine	Risperidone	Olanzapine	Quetiapine	Ziprasidone	Aripiprazole	Iloperidone	Haloperidol	Lurasidone	Brexpiprazole	Cariprazine	Lumateperone
D_1	290	580	52	1300	130	410	320	120	—	≤1000	—	52
D_2	130	2.2	20	180	3.1	0.52	6.3	1.4	1.68	0.3	0.49	32
D_3	240	9.6	50	940	7.2	9.1	7.1	2.5	—	1.1	0.085	—
D_4	47	8.5	50	2200	32	260	25	3.3	—	—	—	≤100
$5\text{-}HT_{1A}$	140	210	2100	230	2.5	—	93	3600	6.75	0.12	3	—
$5\text{-}HT_{1D}$	1700	170	530	>5100	2	—	—	>5000	—	—	—	—
$5\text{-}HT_{2A}$	8.9	0.29	3.3	220	0.39	20	5.6	120	2.03	0.47	19	0.54
$5\text{-}HT_{2C}$	17	10	10	1400	0.72	—	43	4700	—	≤100	134	—
$5\text{-}HT_6$	11	2000	10	4100	76	160	63	6000	—	—	—	—
$5\text{-}HT_7$	66	3	250	1800	9.3	15	110	1100	0.495	3.7	112	—
α_1	4	1.4	54	15	13	57	1.4	4.7	47.9	—	155	—
α_2	33	5.1	170	1000	310	—	160	1,200	40.7	—	—	—
H_1	1.8	19	2.8	8.7	47	—	470	440	1000	≤100	23	—
m_1	1.8	2800	4.7	100	5100	—	—	1600	1000	—	—	—

Adapted from Miyamoto S, Duncan GE, Goff DC, et al. Therapeutics in schizophrenia. In Meltzer H, Nemeroff C, eds. *Neuropsychopharmacology: The Fifth Generation of Progress*. Lippincott Williams & Wilkins; 2002. The binding affinities for lurasidone were adapted from Ishibashi T, Horisawa T, Tokuda K, et al. Pharmacological profile of lurasidone, a novel antipsychotic agent with potent 5-hydroxytryptamine 7 (5-HT₇) and 5-HT₁ₐ receptor activity. *J Pharmacol Exp Ther*. 2010;334(1):171–181. The binding affinities for brexpiprazole, cariprazine, and lumateperone were adapted from Orsolini L, De Berardis D, Volpe U. Up-to-date expert opinion on the safety of recently developed antipsychotics. *Expert Opin Drug Saf*. 2020;19(8):981–998.

the improvement of agitation and irritability occurs rapidly with most agents, whereas psychotic symptoms may begin to improve quickly in some patients and only after a delay of several weeks in others. Maximal response to antipsychotic treatment can require months. The pharmacological treatment of psychotic symptoms is like the treatment of infection with antibiotics—the clinician needs to choose a proper dose and then await therapeutic results while monitoring side effects.

The degree of antipsychotic efficacy ranges from complete resolution of psychosis in a substantial number of patients to minimal or no benefit in others. In between, some patients experience diminished delusional conviction or may persist in their delusional conviction but no longer interpret new experiences within the delusional framework. Other patients continue to hear voices (but muted), or less frequently, or with greater insight. Some patients are surprisingly stable and functional despite chronic, attenuated psychotic symptoms. A major benefit of antipsychotics is the prevention of relapse by maintenance treatment.

Negative symptoms of schizophrenia may improve with psychiatric treatment, although a full resolution of negative symptoms is rare. It remains controversial whether "primary" negative symptoms improve with pharmacotherapy. Examples of "secondary" negative symptoms include social withdrawal that results from paranoia and apathy that results from depression. The most common etiology of secondary negative symptoms is neuroleptic-induced parkinsonism. The improvement of negative symptoms after a switch to an atypical agent sometimes represents resolution of iatrogenic parkinsonian side effects caused by the previous conventional neuroleptic.

DRUG SELECTION

Selection of an antipsychotic agent is usually guided by the side effect profile and by available formulations (e.g., tablet, rapidly dissolving or sublingual preparation, patch, liquid, IM immediate release). One critical choice is between prescribing oral antipsychotics or using a long-acting injectable (LAI) antipsychotic. Clinicians can choose among several LAI antipsychotics, with dosing intervals that range from 2 weeks to 6 months. For most patients, an LAI antipsychotic is an effective strategy to reduce the relapse risk in the long-term management of schizophrenia.[15] TD remains a concern for FGAs (but not limited to them) even if used at low doses. A drug's metabolic side effect profile (high metabolic risk vs. low metabolic risk) must be accounted for when selecting an agent, especially when using antipsychotics for maintenance treatment.

Because of the considerable heterogeneity in response and susceptibility to side effects, it is not possible to predict the optimal agent for an individual patient, and sequential trials may be needed. As listed in Table 9.2, side effects likely to influence tolerability and compliance include sedation or activation, weight gain, neurological side effects, and sexual dysfunction. With an emphasis on reducing iatrogenic cardiovascular risk factors (i.e., metabolic syndrome), patients may benefit from a high-risk to a low-risk antipsychotic switch. A switch strategy is often more effective than behavioral interventions.[16] Recently developed antipsychotics, including aripiprazole, brexpiprazole, cariprazine, and lumateperone,

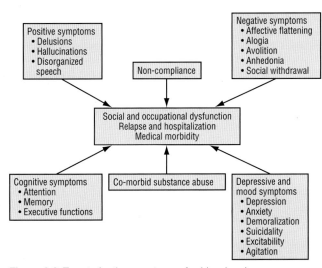

Figure 9.2 Targets for the symptoms of schizophrenia.

TABLE 9.2 Antipsychotic Side Effects								
	EPSs	**Tardive Dyskinesia**	**Prolactin**	**Anticholinergic Side Effects**	**Sedation**	**Weight Gain**	**Diabetes**	**Dyslipidemia**
Chlorpromazine	++	+++	+++	++++	++++	+++	+++	++
Perphenazine	+++	+++	+++	++	++	++	−	+
Haloperidol	++++	+++	+++	−	+	+−−		
Clozapine	−	−	−	++++	++++	++++	++++	++++
Risperidone	++	+	++++	−	++	++	++	+
Olanzapine	+	+	+	+	+++	++++	++++	++++
Quetiapine	−	?	−	++ᵃ	+++	++	+++ᵇ	+++ᵇ
Ziprasidone	+	?	+	−	+	+	−	−
Aripiprazole	+	?	−	−	+	+	−	−
Asenapine	++	?	+	−	++	+	−?	−?
Iloperidone	−	?	−	−	+	++	++?	?
Lurasidone	+/++	?	+	−	+	+/−	−	−?
Brexpiprazole	+/−	?	+	−	+	++	−	−
Cariprazine	++	?	−	−	+	+/−	−	−
Lumateperone	+	?	−	+	++	−	−	−

ᵃElevated urinary hesitancy, dry mouth, or constipation in the Clinical Antipsychotic Trials of Intervention Effectiveness (CATIE) study, probably not mediated via muscarinic acetylcholine receptors.
ᵇPossibly dose related.
EPS, Extrapyramidal symptom.
Adapted from Henderson DC, Copeland PM, Borba CP, et al. Glucose metabolism in patients with schizophrenia treated with olanzapine or quetiapine: a frequently sampled intravenous glucose tolerance test and minimal model analysis. *J Clin Psychiatry*. 2006;67(5):789–797 and Orsolini L, De Berardis D, Volpe U. Up-to-date expert opinion on the safety of recently developed antipsychotics. *Expert Opin Drug Saf*. 2020;19(8):981–998.

may be safer maintenance treatment options with regards to metabolic side effects.[12]

The potential therapeutic benefits of clozapine (including greater efficacy for psychosis, negative symptoms, agitation or tension, suicidal ideation, and relapse prevention) are quite broad.[8] Because of the risk of agranulocytosis, clozapine is reserved for patients who fail to respond to other antipsychotics.

Based on epidemiological studies, all antipsychotics carry a black box warning regarding an increased risk of death when used for behavioral problems in elderly patients with dementia.[17]

FIRST-GENERATION ("TYPICAL") ANTIPSYCHOTICS

Studies that have examined representative FGAs have shown that roughly a 65% occupancy of striatal D_2 receptors is necessary for antipsychotic efficacy, whereas neurological side effects emerge when D_2 occupancy levels exceed approximately 80%. Among the conventional antipsychotics, low-potency agents (such as chlorpromazine) have relatively low affinity for the D_2 receptor and hence require higher doses (~50-fold greater than haloperidol). In addition, they are less selective for D_2 receptors and are thus associated with a wider range of adverse effects, including orthostatic hypotension, anticholinergic side effects, sedation, and weight gain (Box 9.1).

Perphenazine, which was the conventional antipsychotic selected to represent this class in the CATIE study, is a mid-potency agent that requires doses roughly three-fold greater than are necessary with haloperidol. High-potency conventional agents (such as haloperidol and fluphenazine) are more selective for D_2 receptors and more likely to produce EPSs, such as acute dystonias, parkinsonism, and akathisia. Because affinity for the D_2 receptor is readily measured and is inversely correlated with the typical therapeutic dose for each compound, conversion ratios to calculate equivalent dosing between conventional agents, typically expressed in "chlorpromazine equivalents," can be calculated (Table 9.3).

Haloperidol is available for parenteral, including intravenous (IV), administration, and both haloperidol and fluphenazine are available in LAI depot preparations. Although considerable inter-individual variability exists, daily oral doses of haloperidol between 5 and 15 mg are adequate for most chronic patients. Increasing the dose further may only aggravate side effects without improving antipsychotic efficacy. IM and IV administration require roughly half the dosage of oral doses. Great care should be taken with older adults, for whom 0.5 to 2 mg of haloperidol at bedtime may be sufficient. If a patient has not previously received antipsychotic medication, it is best to start at a low dose before arriving at a standard therapeutic dose, which is between 1 and 4 mg orally. Many studies have indicated that an optimal response with haloperidol generally corresponds with trough serum concentrations between 5 and 15 ng/mL,[18] although clinical titration remains the most reliable approach in most situations. In settings of serious medical illness and delirium, especially when other medications with anticholinergic or hypotensive side effects are administered, haloperidol is often used. Patients need to be monitored for torsades de pointes if haloperidol is given IV.[19]

The mid-potency antipsychotic loxapine is available as a rapidly acting aerosolized preparation for inhalation to manage agitation in the setting of psychosis or mania.[20] It shows efficacy within 10 minutes after inhalation and may obviate the need for IM administration of an antipsychotic to patients who need rapid tranquilization.

In the United States, fluphenazine and haloperidol are available as long-acting depot preparations (decanoates) that are administered IM.

EXTRAPYRAMIDAL SYMPTOMS AND TARDIVE DYSKINESIA

Akathisia is an extremely unpleasant sensation of motor restlessness that is primarily experienced in the lower extremities in individuals receiving antipsychotics. Akathisia usually manifests as pacing, although some patients experience akathisia as leg discomfort rather than as restlessness, and it can develop after a single dose. Akathisia increases medication non-adherence and has been associated with self-injurious behaviors, as well as a worsening of psychosis. Untrained staff can mistake akathisia for psychotic agitation, resulting in an unfortunate escalation of the antipsychotic dose. Switching to a different antipsychotic with a lower liability for akathisia usually resolves the problem. Because akathisia is dose dependent, lowering the dose may provide relief. Alternatively, propranolol (10–20 mg two to four times daily) is often helpful.[21] The antidepressant mirtazapine, which has antagonism at serotonin$_{2A}$ receptors that are implicated in the pathophysiology of akathisia, has been shown to reduce akathisia.[21]

Dystonias are sustained spasms that can affect any muscle group. Neuroleptic-induced dystonias usually occur within the first 4 days of initiating a neuroleptic or after a dose increase, and they often affect the neck, tongue, or back. Dystonia may also manifest as a lateral deviation of the eyes

---

BOX 9.1 Side Effects Associated with Low-Potency First-Generation Antipsychotics

- Sedation
- Hypotension
- Weight gain
- Anticholinergic symptoms (dry mouth, urinary retention, constipation, blurred vision)
- Impaired heat regulation (hyperthermia or hypothermia)
- Pigmentary retinopathy (thioridazine > 800 mg/day)
- Cardiac conduction effects (chlorpromazine, thioridazine)

TABLE 9.3 First-Generation Antipsychotic Doses

	Equivalent Dose	Typical Dose Acute/Maintenance
	(mg)[a]	(mg/day)
LOW POTENCY		
Chlorpromazine	100	300–1000/300–600
Thioridazine	100	300–800/300–600
MEDIUM POTENCY		
Loxapine	10	30–100/30–60
Perphenazine	10	12–64/8–32[b]
HIGH POTENCY		
Trifluoperazine	5	15–50/15–30
Thiothixene	5	15–50/15–30
Fluphenazine	2	6–20/6–12
Haloperidol	2	6–20/6–12

[a]Equivalent dose (or "chlorpromazine equivalents") reflects the potency of antipsychotics compared with 100 mg of chlorpromazine as the reference.
[b]Clinical Antipsychotic Trials of Intervention Effectiveness (CATIE) dose range, 8 to 32 mg/day.
Adapted from Buchanan RW, Kreyenbuhl J, Kelly DL, et al. The 2009 schizophrenia PORT psychopharmacological treatment recommendations and summary statements. *Schizophr Bull.* 2010;36(1):71–93.

(opisthotonus), spasmodic movements of the eyeballs into a fixed position (oculogyric crisis), or laryngeal spasm (stridor). Younger patients started on high-potency FGAs are at high risk for developing acute dystonic reactions during the first week of exposure to an antipsychotic medication. The incidence of dystonia decreases by about 4% per year of age until it is almost negligible after age 40 years.

Dystonia can be a frightening and uncomfortable experience. The occurrence of dystonia early in treatment seriously jeopardizes future adherence with antipsychotic medication, so it is important to anticipate and treat this side effect aggressively. The best method of prevention comes from use of an SGA or a newer antipsychotic. When high-potency neuroleptics are initiated, prophylaxis with anticholinergic agents (such as benztropine 1–2 mg twice daily) substantially reduces the likelihood of dystonic reactions in high-risk patients.[22] Prophylaxis with an anticholinergic is risky in older adults because of their sensitivity to adverse effects, although it is usually unnecessary since the elderly are at very low risk for dystonia. Dystonia is uncommon with use of atypical agents and occurs rarely with quetiapine and clozapine.

Antipsychotic-induced parkinsonism mimics the tremor, stiffness, gait disturbance, and diminished facial expression characteristic of idiopathic Parkinson disease. It can be mistaken easily for depression or for the negative symptoms of schizophrenia, although the presence of tremor and rigidity usually distinguishes this side effect. Parkinsonian side effects are most common with use of high-potency FGAs, and they occur in a bi-modal age distribution with maximal risk in the young and in older adults. Symptoms frequently improve with a reduction in the antipsychotic dose or with addition of an antiparkinsonian agent (such as benztropine 1–2 mg twice daily or amantadine 100 mg twice or three times daily).[22] Because anticholinergic agents can produce an array of troublesome side effects (including constipation, dry mouth, dental caries, blurred vision, urinary retention, and memory impairment), particularly in older adults, long-term use of these agents should be avoided. In addition, anticholinergics may impede cognitive gains hoped for when using cognitive-behavioral therapy or cognitive remediation. As a class, the atypical agents produce substantially fewer parkinsonian side effects, and both clozapine and quetiapine are essentially free of EPSs, making them the drugs of choice for patients with idiopathic Parkinson disease complicated by psychosis. Box 9.2 describes EPSs.

Tardive dyskinesia rarely appears when there has been less than 6 months of treatment with an antipsychotic agent, but after it develops, it may be irreversible. TD usually takes the form of involuntary, choreiform (quick, non-rhythmic) movements of the mouth, tongue, or upper extremities, although a dystonic form has also been described. The risk for developing TD with FGAs is about 6.5%, and that with SGAs is about 2.6% per year of exposure.[23] In general, among the SGAs, clozapine, olanzapine, and aripiprazole have a lower TD risk. Older individuals, women, patients taking a higher antipsychotic dose, and those who develop parkinsonian side effects early during the early phase of treatment appear to be at heightened risk for TD. The best treatment of TD is prevention because options are limited after TD develops. Clozapine and quetiapine present minimal risk for TD, and switching a patient who develops TD to these antipsychotics increases the likelihood of spontaneous improvement of TD. Lowering the dose of an FGA or switching to an SGA can occasionally produce "withdrawal dyskinesias," which typically resolve within 6 weeks, or may unmask an underlying dyskinesia that was suppressed by the antipsychotic medication. Tetrabenazine was an option to treat TD until the approval of vesicular monoamine transporter type 2 inhibitors valbenazine and deutetrabenazine,

---

BOX 9.2 Extrapyramidal Symptoms

AKATHISIA

Restlessness in lower extremities; often results in pacing
Can occur after the first dose
Risk factors: use of high-potency first-generation agents in high doses

DYSTONIA

Acute muscle spasm: can be very distressing
Usually occurs within the first 4 days after starting the drug
Risk factors: youth and use of high-potency first-generation antipsychotics

PARKINSONISM

Tremor, bradykinesia, rigidity—often confused with negative symptoms
Usually does not become evident until after several weeks of treatment
Risk factors: use of high-potency first-generation antipsychotics, high doses, youth, and old age

---

BOX 9.3 Tardive Dyskinesia

Late-developing, chronic choreiform (non-rhythmic, quick) movements, most commonly the oral-buccal muscles and tongue

RISK FACTORS

Old age
>6 months of first-generation neuroleptic exposure
History of parkinsonian side effects
Diabetes
Risk is reduced with second-generation agents

---

making the treatment of TD more promising.[24] In severe cases, deep brain stimulation can be tried. Box 9.3 describes risk factors for TD.

NEUROLEPTIC MALIGNANT SYNDROME

Neuroleptic malignant syndrome (NMS) is a rare, potentially lethal complication of neuroleptic treatment that is characterized by hyperthermia, rigidity, confusion, diaphoresis, autonomic instability, elevated creatine phosphokinase (CPK), and leukocytosis (Box 9.4). The symptoms of NMS may evolve gradually, typically starting with mental status changes and culminating in fever and an elevated CPK. NMS probably occurs in fewer than 1% of patients receiving conventional antipsychotic agents, although subsyndromal cases may be much more common.[25] Parallels have been drawn between NMS and malignant hyperthermia (resulting from general anesthesia), largely based on common clinical characteristics. Patients with a history of either NMS or malignant hyperthermia, however, appear to be at no increased risk for developing the other syndrome, and analysis of muscle biopsy specimens has not consistently demonstrated a physiological link between the two conditions. Lethal catatonia is a spontaneously occurring syndrome that may be indistinguishable from NMS and has been described in the absence of neuroleptic treatment. In addition, antipsychotic agents may impair temperature regulation, so they may produce low-grade fever in the absence of other symptoms of NMS. A recent review outlines the importance of pharmacological and non-pharmacological approaches to address NMS.[25] The clinician's immediate response to NMS

BOX 9.4 Neuroleptic Malignant Syndrome

TRIAD

1. Rigidity
2. Fever
3. Altered mental status

PRESENTATION (MAY GRADUALLY EVOLVE, USUALLY IN THE FOLLOWING ORDER)

- Confusion and fluctuating levels of consciousness
- Rigidity (can be less pronounced with clozapine)
- Diaphoresis
- Mutism
- Autonomic instability
- Hyperthermia
- Elevated creatine phosphokinase

Adapted from Guinart D, Misawa F, Rubio JM, et al. A systematic review and pooled, patient-level analysis of predictors of mortality in neuroleptic malignant syndrome. *Acta Psychiatr Scand*. 2021;144(4):329-341.

TABLE 9.4 Second- and Third-Generation Antipsychotic Doses

	Typical Dose (mg/day)	High Dose[a] (mg/day)	Potential Dose-Limiting Side Effects
Risperidone	3–6	6–12	EPSs
Olanzapine	10–20	30–40	Sedation
Quetiapine	300–600	600–1200[b]	Sedation
Ziprasidone	80–160	160–320[c]	Akathisia
Aripiprazole	10–20	20–40	
Clozapine	100–400	400–900[d]	Sedation, orthostatic hypotension, seizures
Iloperidone	12–24	24	Orthostatic hypotension
Asenapine	10–20	20	Sedation; EPSs
Lurasidone	40–80	160	EPSs
Brexpiprazole	1–4	4	
Cariprazine	3–6	6	EPSs
Lumateperone	42	42	Sedation

[a]Evidence for benefit of higher dose available for olanzapine only.
[b]Two controlled trials[28,29] have *not* found benefit from high-dose quetiapine.
[c]One controlled trial[30] has not found benefit from high-dose ziprasidone.
[d]The dose should be guided by clozapine serum levels. An optimal highest dose has not been established.[31]
EPS, Extrapyramidal symptom.

---

should be to discontinue dopamine-blocking medication and hospitalize the patient to provide IV fluids and cooling. Whether bromocriptine or dantrolene facilitates recovery remains the subject of debate.[25] It is important that re-institution of antipsychotic medication be delayed at least 2 weeks until after the episode of NMS has resolved. NMS has been described with all antipsychotics, including clozapine. It has been suggested that a variant of NMS without rigidity may result from use of SGAs, although if such a syndrome occurs, it is probably quite rare: perhaps with the exception of clozapine in which NMS can display few EPSs, SGAs produce the typical clinical picture of NMS with rigidity.

SECOND-GENERATION ("ATYPICAL") AND THIRD-GENERATION ANTIPSYCHOTICS

The SGAs and newest agents (Table 9.4) are generally better tolerated with regard to EPSs, producing fewer neurological side effects (dystonia, akathisia, and parkinsonism) than the FGAs and possibly less TD (see Table 9.3). Although relatively free of EPSs in most patients at dosages of less than 6 mg/day, risperidone (and its metabolite, paliperidone) requires careful titration to avoid EPSs at higher doses and is unique among the atypical agents in producing sustained hyperprolactinemia.[26] However, over the past decade, attention has focused on effects of SGAs on glucose metabolism and lipids and the associated metabolic syndrome. A large number of cases of treatment-emergent diabetes have been reported, which in some cases resolved after discontinuation of the antipsychotic.[27] In the CATIE study, olanzapine produced significantly greater weight gain, impairment of glucose metabolism, and dyslipidemia than the other agents[11]; this has since been confirmed in a meta-analysis that found clozapine and olanzapine to be the drugs with the highest metabolic liability.[25] Nonetheless, intermediate-risk drugs, such as quetiapine, may carry similar risks when used in doses necessary to treat psychotic symptoms. However, newer antipsychotics (e.g., brexpiprazole, cariprazine, lumateperone) may pose less risk for metabolic profiles.[12] Possible differences among SGAs in their risk for causing diabetes may be obscured in part by the considerable variability between individuals for weight gain, the potential delay between initiation of treatment and elevation of glucose levels, and a possible propensity for abnormal glucose metabolism associated with schizophrenia, independent of drug treatment. Therefore, all patients treated with an antipsychotic

should be monitored regularly for weight gain, diabetes, and hyperlipidemia, with attention paid to more frequent monitoring for patients who receive high-risk drugs (i.e., olanzapine and clozapine) (see Table 9.2). Olanzapine and aripiprazole have few or no cardiac effects (including QTc prolongation). Clozapine, risperidone, quetiapine, ziprasidone, and iloperidone have α-adrenergic effects that necessitate dose titration to avoid orthostatic hypotension. Clozapine produces more hypotension and tachycardia than other atypical agents; both are generally easily managed. Ziprasidone's approval was delayed when it became clear that it prolongs the QT interval more than other SGAs (but less than thioridazine).[12]

Clozapine

Clozapine (Box 9.5) is a tricyclic dibenzodiazepine derivative approved for the treatment of treatment-resistant schizophrenia and for the reduction of suicidal behavior in patients with schizophrenia or schizoaffective disorder. Clozapine binds to a wide array of central nervous system receptors (including dopaminergic [all five subtypes], muscarinic cholinergic receptors, histaminergic, noradrenergic, and serotonergic). In addition, it appears to modulate glutamatergic N-methyl-D-aspartate (NMDA) receptor sensitivity and the release of brain-derived neurotropic factor. The absence of neurological side effects has been attributed to serotonin 5-HT_{2A} antagonism, a high D_2 dissociation constant (loose binding) that results in relatively low levels of D_2 receptor occupancy at therapeutic doses, strong anticholinergic activity, and preferential binding to limbic over striatal dopamine receptors. However, the exact mechanism by which clozapine achieves greater efficacy than other agents remains a mystery despite decades of research.

Peak plasma levels of clozapine are attained approximately 2 hours after oral administration. It is metabolized primarily by hepatic microsomal enzymes CYP 1A2 and, to a lesser extent, 3A4 and 2D6, with a mean half-life of 8 hours after a single dose and 12 hours after repeated dosing. Only the desmethyl metabolite is active. Clozapine blood levels are significantly lowered by cigarette smoking and by other hepatic

---

BOX 9.5 Clozapine

CLINICAL EFFICACY

Effective in 30% of treatment-resistant patients at 6 weeks
Prevents relapse
Stabilizes mood
Improves polydipsia and hyponatremia
Reduces hostility and aggression
Reduces suicidality
Possibly reduces cigarette smoking and substance use

ADVERSE EFFECTS

Common Side Effects

Sedation
Tachycardia
Sialorrhea (impairs esophageal motility)
Dizziness
Constipation (can lead to bowel impaction)
Hypotension
Fever (usually within first 3 weeks, lasting a few days)
Weight gain

Serious Side Effects

Agranulocytosis[a]
Seizures[a]
Myocarditis[a]
Orthostatic hypotension with syncope or cardiorespiratory arrest[a]
Pulmonary embolus
Diabetes mellitus

[a] Clozapine-specific black box warnings.

BOX 9.6 Clozapine-Induced Agranulocytosis

- Granulocytes <500/mm^3
- Risk factors: Ashkenazi Jews (HLA-B38, DR4, DQw3) and Finns
- Preservation of other cell lines (platelets and RBCs)
- Maximum risk: 4–18 weeks (77% of cases)
- Recovery usually within 14 days if drug stopped
- No cross-reactivity with other drugs but avoid carbamazepine, captopril, sulfonamides, propylthiouracil, and other drugs that might affect bone marrow or WBCs
- Because of sensitization: Do not rechallenge!

RBC, Red blood cell; *WBC,* white blood cell.

BOX 9.7 Monitoring for Agranulocytosis

ANC ≥1500/μL to initiate clozapine (1000/μL for patients with BEN)
Weekly ANC for 6 months, if all ANCs ≥1500/μL; then biweekly for 6 months; then monthly
Repeat ANC if:
- ANC <1500/μL or
- ANC drops by 1500/μL from previous test or
- Three consecutive weekly drops
If ANC = 1000–1500/μL (500–1000/μL for patients with BEN), proceed with three times weekly ANCs until ≥1500/μL (≥1000 for patients with BEN)
If ANC <1000/μL (<1000/μL for patients with BEN): Hold drug and proceed with daily ANCs until ≥1000/μL (<500/μL for patients with BEN)
If ANC <500/μL: Discontinue drug and proceed with daily ANCs until ≥1000/μL. *Do not rechallenge.*

ANC, Absolute neutrophil count; *BEN,* benign ethnic neutropenia.

---

enzyme inducers (including phenytoin and rifampin) and elevated by CYP 1A2 and 3A4 inhibitors (such as fluvoxamine and erythromycin). Fluvoxamine has been shown to increase clozapine plasma concentrations by as much as four-fold. Some patients double their clozapine blood levels after smoking cessation, with attendant sedation and worsening of other side effects. Inflammation, including COVID-19 and other infections, can reduce CYP 1A2 enzyme activity and increase clozapine drug plasma levels. In such cases, the dose should be reduced by half until the active infection subsides. Several studies have indicated that clozapine is most likely to be effective at trough serum concentrations of 350 ng/mL or greater. In a prospective, double-blind trial, patients randomly assigned to treatment with a clozapine dose adjusted to produce a serum concentration between 200 and 300 ng/mL responded more fully than did patients assigned to lower concentrations; moreover, their response was comparable to patients assigned to higher concentrations.[32]

Approved for treatment-resistant schizophrenia, clozapine has been found to improve positive and negative symptoms of psychosis, aggression, suicidality, depression, anxiety, and refractory symptoms of mania. Clozapine is FDA-approved for the treatment of suicidality in the setting of psychosis. In addition, clozapine may improve polydipsia with hyponatremia, reduce arrest rates, and facilitate a decrease in cigarette smoking or other substance use. Clozapine is the most effective antipsychotic medication, and its response rate in treatment-resistant schizophrenia can be as high as 30% to 60%.

Potentially serious side effects (such as agranulocytosis, seizures, diabetes, and myocarditis) have limited clozapine treatment to the most refractory patients; the more common side effects of weight gain, sialorrhea, orthostatic hypotension, constipation, and sedation further complicate its use (see Box 9.5). Sialorrhea can cause aspiration pneumonia

and become a significant burden for patients on clozapine. Addressing this promptly with medications (e.g., sublingual ipratropium or glycopyrrolate) is critical to improving adherence in many cases.[33] Similarly, proactive treatment of constipation is important in preventing clozapine-associated life-threatening ileus. Because of the risk of agranulocytosis, patients must meet a minimum threshold for their neutrophil count before starting the drug and must continue to meet safety criteria with weekly blood tests during the first 6 months of treatment, biweekly tests for the second 6 months, and then monthly bloods tests for as long as the patient takes the drug (Boxes 9.6 and 9.7). Because clozapine can cause agranulocytosis, the FDA mandates registry-based prescribing, with regular absolute neutrophil count (ANC) monitoring.[34] Severe neutropenia (ANC <500/μL) is rare, affecting 0.9% people started on clozapine, and the case fatality rate is 2.1%.[35] The severe neutropenia has a peak incidence in the first several months after starting clozapine, with a negligible incidence after 1 year. The mechanism of agranulocytosis is likely metabolite toxicity or a hapten-based immune-mediated mechanism. Patients usually recover from clozapine-induced agranulocytosis within 14 to 24 days of stopping the drug, but re-challenge with clozapine is contraindicated because of the very high rate of recurrence.

Some patients have habitually a low ANC count due to their ethnic background (the old term *benign ethnic neutropenia* is sometimes still used). The registry allows for people in this category to be treated using a different monitoring algorithm.

Of additional concern are reports of myocarditis and cardiomyopathy occurring in 3% or more of the patients treated with clozapine, and approximately 20% of the cases can be fatal.[36] These cases commonly manifested within the first month of treatment with fever, dyspnea, a "flu-like illness," and chest pain; abnormal laboratory findings included a reduced ventricular ejection fraction on echocardiogram, T-wave changes on the electrocardiogram, eosinophilia, and an elevated CPK. Weekly monitoring of cardiac enzymes (mainly troponin C) and C-reactive proteins for the first 4 to 6 weeks of clozapine administration can be helpful in identifying and treating myocarditis and cardiomyopathy in a timely manner.[36]

Seizures have been reported in 5% to 10% of patients treated with clozapine. Seizure risk appears to be related to both rapid dose escalation and high plasma concentrations. High rates of obesity, diabetes, and dyslipidemia have also been associated with clozapine. Whereas the striking abdominal adiposity associated with clozapine treatment might explain the elevated rate of diabetes, markedly decreased insulin sensitivity has been documented in non-obese patients treated with clozapine.

Given the rare but serious risks of agranulocytosis and myocarditis and the more common risks of seizures and metabolic complications, clozapine should be reserved for patients who fail at least two antipsychotic trials. However, the potential therapeutic benefits of clozapine often outweigh the risks of medical morbidity in treatment-resistant patients. Because of a nearly 90% reduction in suicide associated with clozapine treatment, mortality rates can increase in patients after ceasing clozapine treatment. Similarly, clozapine-treated patients, compared with those treated with other antipsychotics (or no treatment), may not have increased cardiac deaths despite increased risk of metabolic derangement.

Risperidone and Paliperidone

Risperidone is a benzisoxazole derivative that received FDA approval for the treatment of schizophrenia in 1994 and later for bipolar mania. It is characterized by a very high affinity for the 5-HT$_{2A}$ receptor and by moderate affinity for D$_2$, H$_1$, and α_1- and α_2-adrenergic receptors. Risperidone has essentially no activity at muscarinic acetylcholine receptors. Risperidone has a high affinity and low dissociation constant for the D$_2$ receptor, making it "tightly bound" and thereby more likely to produce EPSs at high doses than some more "loosely bound" agents. At typical clinical doses, risperidone was found to occupy 65% to 69% of D$_2$ receptors 12 to 14 hours after the last dose; a mean occupancy of 79% was found in patients treated with a risperidone dosage of 6 mg/day.[37]

Risperidone is rapidly absorbed after oral administration with peak plasma levels achieved within 1 hour. It is metabolized by hepatic microsomal enzyme CYP 2D6 to form the active metabolite 9-hydroxyrisperidone, which exhibits a pattern of receptor binding that is like that of the parent compound. 9-Hydroxyrisperidone is in turn metabolized by N-dealkylation. The half-life of the "active moiety" (risperidone plus 9-hydroxyrisperidone) is approximately 20 hours. CYP 2D6 activity, which varies dramatically between "rapid" and "poor" metabolizers, determines the ratio of risperidone to 9-hydroxyrisperidone serum concentrations and influences the half-life of the active moiety. Drugs that inhibit CYP 2D6, such as paroxetine and fluoxetine, may increase risperidone levels, thereby increasing the risk of neurological side effects.

Relapse rates with haloperidol compared to risperidone were found to be nearly doubled, but risperidone demonstrated similar efficacy as the FGA perphenazine in the CATIE trial.[11] Increasing the risperidone dosage above 8 mg/day might not improve response in patients who do not fully respond to a treatment with a customary dosage.

Risperidone is well tolerated at doses low enough to avoid EPSs (generally <6 mg/day). In the CATIE trial, risperidone, at a mean dosage of 3.9 mg/day, was the best-tolerated agent, although differences among agents were not statistically significant. Weight gain with risperidone is intermediate compared with other atypical agents and is quite variable. Woerner and colleagues[38] found a cumulative TD rate of 7.2% over 2 years in older, antipsychotic-naïve patients who were treated and prospectively followed. Risperidone causes a small increase in the QTc interval (a mean prolongation of 10 ms at a dosage of 16 mg/day).[12]

Risperidone differs from other SGAs in causing persistent hyperprolactinemia. Side effects tend not to correlate with serum prolactin concentrations. Hyperprolactinemia in patients with pituitary tumors lowers estrogen and testosterone levels, which may secondarily result in osteopenia. Similarly, risperidone-induced hyperprolactinemia might increase the risk for osteoporosis.

The active metabolite of risperidone, 9-hydroxyrisperidone, was re-named paliperidone and approved for the treatment of schizophrenia in 2006. It is equipotent to risperidone with which it shares its receptor and side effect profile, including significant prolactin elevation. Its typical dosage range is 3 to 6 mg/day, although dosages up to 12 mg/day can be given. As the end-product of oxidative metabolism, paliperidone is primarily excreted renally, and it does not rely on P450 metabolism (59% of it is excreted unchanged in the urine).

Both risperidone and paliperidone are available as LAI formulations. The long-acting risperidone formulation consists of polymer microspheres containing risperidone, which, immediately before injection, are suspended in a water-based diluent. After injection, the microspheres begin to release risperidone after a delay of 3 to 4 weeks, after which levels persist for about 4 weeks. Microspheres are administered by gluteal injection every 2 weeks (dose range, 12.5–50 mg); oral dosing of risperidone should continue until the third injection (4 weeks after the first). If an increase in the dose is necessary, oral supplementation should be provided for 3 to 4 weeks after increasing the dose of risperidone microspheres. Paliperidone is also available as a LAI formulation (paliperidone palmitate) for monthly IM injections at a dose between 39 and 234 mg. A loading strategy (i.e., 234 mg once followed by 117 mg 1 week later) produces therapeutic steady-state drug levels rapidly and can be started in inpatient settings. Three-month and 6-month LAI options of paliperidone palmitate are also available and can be used after patients tolerate monthly injections. Before administering any LAI antipsychotic, tolerability of the oral preparation should be established.

Olanzapine

Olanzapine, a thienobenzodiazepine derivative chemically related to clozapine, was approved by the FDA in 1997 for the treatment of schizophrenia and subsequently approved for bipolar mania. Olanzapine binds to dopamine D$_1$, D$_2$, D$_4$, and D$_5$; serotonin 5-HT$_{2A}$ and 5-HT$_{2C}$; muscarinic M$_{1-5}$; histaminergic H$_1$; and α_1-adrenergic receptors.

After oral administration, olanzapine is well absorbed, producing peak concentrations in 4 to 6 hours. Olanzapine is metabolized via glucuronidation and oxidation by CYP 450 1A2 with a mean half-life of 24 to 36 hours. Like clozapine, olanzapine's metabolism is induced by cigarette smoking and slowed by CYP 1A2 inhibitors but to a lesser degree because of alternative metabolic pathways.

In the CATIE study, olanzapine at a mean dosage of 20 mg/day was the antipsychotic with the best efficacy.[11] Since the original designation of 10 mg/day as the recommended dosage at the time of olanzapine's introduction, typical clinical

TABLE 9.5 Recommendations for Monitoring Patients Starting Antipsychotics[a]

	Baseline	4 Weeks	8 Weeks	16 Weeks	Quarterly	Annually
Personal or family history	X					X
Weight (body mass index [BMI])	X	X	X	X	X	
Waist circumference	X			X	X	
Blood pressure	X			X	X	
Fasting plasma glucose[b]	X			X		X[c]
Fasting lipid profile	X			X		X[c]

Consider an intervention (weight reduction program or switch antipsychotic) if:
- ≥5% increase in weight
- 1-point increase in BMI
- 1-inch or greater increase in waist circumference
- Criteria met for metabolic syndrome

[a]The monitoring recommendations are derived from the literature about second-generation antipsychotics. However, the first-generation antipsychotics (particularly low-potency antipsychotics) are not devoid of metabolic problems.
[b]Hemoglobin A1c can be used instead.
[c]More frequent monitoring (e.g., every 3 months until stable; then every 6 months) is indicated for patients taking high-risk drugs (clozapine, olanzapine).
Adapted from Goff DC, Cather C, Evins AE, et al. Medical morbidity and mortality in schizophrenia: guidelines for psychiatrists. *J Clin Psychiatry.* 2005;66(2):183-194; quiz 147, 273-184 and American Psychiatric Association. *The American Psychiatric Association Practice Guideline for the Treatment of Patients with Schizophrenia.* 3rd ed. American Psychiatric Publishing; 2020.

dosages have steadily climbed to the 15 to 20 mg/day range. A dosage higher than 20 mg/day should only be considered for individuals with treatment-resistant psychosis with close monitoring.

Olanzapine may cause sedation, which some patients experience as a welcome treatment for insomnia; others are distressed by difficulty awakening in the morning. Even at high doses, olanzapine is relatively free of EPSs and prolactin elevation. However, weight gain and dyslipidemia and metabolic dysregulation are common and are major long-term concerns. Both olanzapine and clozapine have been linked to insulin resistance and to diabetes—an effect that may occur in the absence of obesity. Patients should be carefully screened for metabolic risk factors before initiating olanzapine and should be monitored according to established guidelines (Table 9.5).

An LAI olanzapine formulation (olanzapine pamoate) can be given every 2 to 4 weeks. Very rarely (~1 event per 1700 injections), the injection can cause confusion, severe drowsiness, or coma because of excessive olanzapine plasma concentrations, resembling alcohol intoxication.[39] Called post-injection delirium/sedation syndrome (PDSS), it requires patients to be observed for 3 hours after receiving the injection, which can only be given by certified prescribers and facilities that are able to manage PDSS.

In 2021, a combination of olanzapine and samidorphan was approved by the FDA for the treatment of schizophrenia. The major benefit of this combination medication is the blunting of weight gain compared with olanzapine monotherapy.[40] Samidorphan is an opioid antagonist that helps reduce the cravings for high-calorie foods, and it comprises a fixed dosage of 10 mg/day combined with different doses of olanzapine. The use of olanzapine–samidorphan can cause opiate withdrawal and increases the risk for opiate overdoses in patients using opiates.

Quetiapine

Quetiapine was approved in 1997 for the treatment of schizophrenia. Quetiapine has a high affinity for serotonin 5-HT$_{2A}$, α_1- and α_2-adrenergic, and histaminergic H$_1$ receptors and a relatively low affinity for D$_2$ receptors. Whereas maximal D$_2$ occupancy levels of approximately 60% are achieved 2 to 3 hours after a single dose, because of quetiapine's high dissociation constant and short half-life, D$_2$ occupancy drops to less than 30% after 12 hours.[41]

Quetiapine is rapidly absorbed after oral administration, with peak plasma concentrations achieved in 1 to 2 hours. It is primarily metabolized via CYP P450 3A4, producing two active metabolites. Quetiapine metabolism is significantly influenced by drugs that inhibit 3A4 (such as ketoconazole) or induce 3A4 (such as carbamazepine). The half-life of quetiapine is approximately 6 hours; despite this short half-life, quetiapine is frequently prescribed as a once-daily dose, at bedtime, with good results. No significant association has been identified between quetiapine blood levels and clinical response.

In controlled clinical trials, quetiapine demonstrated efficacy for global psychopathology, psychotic symptoms, and negative symptoms greater than placebo, and it was comparable to haloperidol or chlorpromazine. In the CATIE study, quetiapine at a mean dosage of 543 mg/day was less effective than olanzapine, but it did not differ statistically from the other antipsychotics in tolerability or effectiveness.[11] Dosages above 800 mg/day have not added therapeutic benefit.

Common side effects reported with quetiapine include somnolence and dizziness. Quetiapine is very sedating; however, because of its short half-life, bedtime dosing may minimize daytime sedation. Mild orthostatic hypotension was observed in trials that followed a conservative schedule of dose titration, starting with quetiapine 25 mg twice daily. Initiation at higher doses may cause significant orthostatic hypotension, particularly in older adults, because of quetiapine's adrenergic effects. Reports of dry mouth are probably attributable to its adrenergic mechanisms because quetiapine is essentially free of muscarinic activity. Quetiapine has consistently demonstrated extremely low levels of EPSs and prolactin elevation, comparable to placebo. Quetiapine is intermediate among the SGAs in producing weight gain and in estimates for risk for producing dyslipidemia and diabetes. Early concerns about a possible link with cataracts have not been supported in postmarketing surveillance, nor was a link detected in the CATIE study. Although QTc prolongation is not clinically significant at typical doses, quetiapine overdoses have been associated with cardiac arrhythmias.[12]

Ziprasidone

Ziprasidone was approved in 2001 for the treatment of schizophrenia. Like other SGAs, it has a favorable ratio of serotonin 5-HT$_2$ to dopamine D$_2$ affinities. In addition, it is an antagonist with high affinity for serotonin 5-HT$_{1D}$ and 5-HT$_{2C}$ receptors and an agonist at the 5-HT$_{1A}$ receptor. Ziprasidone differs from other agents in its moderate reuptake blockade of serotonin and norepinephrine (noradrenaline).

After oral administration, absorption of ziprasidone is significantly more rapid when administered within 1 hour of eating a meal compared with fasting. Ziprasidone is metabolized by several pathways. Approximately two-thirds of ziprasidone's metabolism is via aldehyde oxidase, and the remainder is by CYP450 3A4 and 1A2 hepatic microsomal enzymes. Clinically significant drug–drug interactions have not been reported.

In early trials, ziprasidone exhibited efficacy comparable to haloperidol at dosages above 120 mg/day but with fewer EPSs and without sustained elevation of prolactin. Ziprasidone did not become available for inclusion in the CATIE trial until after approximately 40% of participants had entered and been randomized. At a mean dosage of 113 mg/day ziprasidone was less effective than olanzapine and did not differ from the other antipsychotics.[11] Notably, ziprasidone was associated with a mean weight loss of 0.3 lb per month, normalization of lipids, and a lowering of prolactin levels. Subsequent meta-analyses have consistently confirmed that ziprasidone is the metabolically safest antipsychotic and causes the least amount of weight gain (or no weight gain) in many patients.[42] A ziprasidone dosage greater than 160 mg/day may not improve patient outcomes.

Side effects commonly associated with ziprasidone include insomnia or somnolence, nausea, anxiety, and headache. The finding of a mean QTc prolongation of 15.9 ms raised concerns about the risk of torsades de pointes, particularly when administered to patients with an underlying cardiac conduction defect or another cardiac risk factor. However, QTc intervals greater than 500 ms have been extremely rare, and a large post-marketing surveillance study of more than 18,000 patients (Ziprasidone Observational Study of Cardiac Outcomes [ZODIAC]) did not find an increased rate of non-suicide deaths compared to olanzapine-treated patients.[43] Despite the reassuring safety data, cardiac risk factors should be assessed before initiating this agent.

Iloperidone

Iloperidone was approved for the treatment of schizophrenia in 2009. Like risperidone, it belongs to the class of benzisoxazole antipsychotics. It has high affinity for D$_{2/3}$-HT$_{2A}$ receptors, consistent with other atypical agents, and the D$_3$ and norepinephrine α_1-receptor. In addition, it has moderate affinities for D$_4$, 5-HT$_6$ and 5-HT$_7$ receptors. It is not anticholinergic.

Iloperidone is well absorbed in 2 to 4 hours. Although food slows its absorption, it does not alter overall bioavailability, and it can be given without regard to meals. It is extensively metabolized by 3A4 and 2D6, leading to two active metabolites, P88 and P95.

The effective dosage range for iloperidone is 12 to 24 mg/day, given as twice-daily dosing (half-life, 18 hours). Iloperidone needs to be titrated slowly over the course of at least 1 week or more (e.g., starting with 1 mg twice daily and daily increases by a maximum of 2 mg twice daily [4 mg/day]; to 2 mg, 4 mg, 6 mg, 8 mg, 10 mg, and 12 mg twice daily) to minimize orthostatic hypotension.[44] In registration trials, orthostatic hypotension was observed in 5% of patients given 20 to 24 mg/day of drug versus 1% given placebo. Consistent with iloperidone's prominent α-blocking properties, retrograde ejaculation and priapism have been observed. Other side effects reported in clinical trials include tachycardia, dizziness, dry mouth, nasal congestion, somnolence, and dyspepsia. Headache, insomnia, and anxiety were reported as well. Iloperidone can cause modest prolactin elevation but few EPSs, which might be a relative advantage. It has been associated with dose-dependent weight gain, but its overall propensity for metabolic problems remains to be defined. Iloperidone can increase the QTc interval in a dose-dependent fashion.[12] Its use needs thus to be preceded by an assessment of cardiac safety, including possible drug interactions that could alter iloperidone drug levels. In known poor metabolizers of 2D6, half the dose should be used.

Asenapine

Asenapine was approved in 2009 for the treatment of schizophrenia and the acute treatment of manic or mixed mood episodes of bipolar disorder, either as monotherapy or in conjunction with lithium or valproate. Its chemical structure is unique among antipsychotics (a dibenzo-oxepino pyrrole). It has high affinity for a host of receptors, including dopamine$_{1-4}$, 5-HT$_{1A}$ (partial agonist)/B, 5-HT$_{2A,B,C}$, 5-HT$_{5/6/7}$; and $\alpha_{1/2}$ receptors; it has negligible muscarinic receptor affinity but moderate H$_{1/2}$ receptor affinity.

Because of poor gastrointestinal absorption, asenapine is formulated as a sublingual tablet that gets rapidly absorbed. For 10 minutes after the dose, there should be no eating or drinking; if asenapine is swallowed as an oral tablet, the bioavailability is less than 2%.[45] For schizophrenia and adjunctive treatment of mood episodes, the starting dosage is 5 mg twice daily that can be adjusted to 10 mg twice daily; for mania monotherapy, the recommended starting dosage is 10 mg twice daily. Asenapine is cleared via glucuronidation by UGT$_{1A4}$ and oxidative metabolism, mostly via CYP 1A2.

The most prominent side effects in asenapine registration trials were somnolence and EPSs, dose-related akathisia, and oral hypoesthesia as well as dizziness and dysgeusia. Asenapine is not weight neutral, but its propensity for weight gain and metabolic disturbances remains to be elucidated.[14] Allergic reactions and syncope have been reported as rare but dangerous side effects. Prolactin levels can be increased with asenapine. The registration trials found modest QTc prolongation ranging from 2 to 5 ms for dosages up to 40 mg/day, which should be accounted for before prescribing asenapine.[12] Asenapine is also available as a patch.

Lurasidone

In 2010, the benzisothiazolone antipsychotic lurasidone was approved by the FDA for schizophrenia. It has high affinity binding for dopamine-$_2$ receptors, 5-HT$_{2A}$ receptors, and 5-HT$_7$ receptors. Moderate binding exists for α_{2C}, partial antagonism 5-HT$_{1A}$, and antagonism for α_{2A}. It does not appreciably bind histamine$_1$ and muscarinic M$_1$ receptors. Lurasidone has a half-life of 18 hours. Its total absorption is increased by two-fold with food, and it should be taken with a meal of at least 350 calories (no effect of fat composition). It is mostly metabolized via 3A4, and blood levels of lurasidone may be significantly affected by CYP 3A4 inducers or inhibitors. The recommended starting dosage, which is also an effective dosage, is 40 mg/day given once daily but dosages up to 160 mg/day have been studied. Lurasidone can increase prolactin levels, and it can cause insomnia and EPSs, including akathisia, particularly at higher doses. In contrast, its propensity for weight gain and metabolic disturbances seems to be low, and its effects on the QTc interval are minimal.[12]

THIRD-GENERATION AND NEWEST ANTIPSYCHOTICS

Aripiprazole

Aripiprazole is a dihydroquinoline, structurally unrelated to the other antipsychotics. It was approved for the treatment of schizophrenia in 2002 and subsequently for bipolar or mixed mania. It exhibits a novel mechanism of action as a partial agonist at the D_2 receptor with approximately 30% activity compared to dopamine. In addition, aripiprazole has high affinity as a partial agonist at serotonin $5-HT_{1A}$ and as a full antagonist at $5-HT_{2A}$. Aripiprazole has moderate affinity for α_1-adrenergic and histamine H_1 receptors, as well as the serotonin reuptake site. At typical clinical dosages of 15 to 30 mg/day, aripiprazole exhibits D_2 receptor occupancy greater than 80% and is not associated with EPSs at occupancy levels greater than 90%, presumably the result of partial agonism. Aripiprazole and subsequently approved partial agonist antipsychotics differ in their D_2/D_3 selectivity, which may explain some clinical differences.[46]

Aripiprazole is well absorbed and reaches peak plasma levels within 3 to 5 hours of an oral dose. It is metabolized primarily by CYP 450 2D6 and 3A4 to dehydroaripiprazole, an active metabolite with a pharmacological profile like that of aripiprazole. The half-life of aripiprazole and dehydroaripiprazole are 75 and 94 hours, respectively. Because of this unusually long half-life, approximately 2 weeks is required to achieve steady-state drug levels after a change in dosing. Aripiprazole's metabolism may be altered by inhibitors and inducers of CYP 450 3A4 and 2D6.

In registration studies, aripiprazole at dosages ranging from 15 to 30 mg/day exhibited efficacy comparable to haloperidol (10 mg/day) and risperidone (6 mg/day). Because aripiprazole was not included in the CATIE trial, its relative effectiveness compared with other agents remains unclear.

Aripiprazole has generally been found to be well tolerated, with side effects largely restricted to insomnia, somnolence, headache, agitation, nausea, and anxiety. It has not differed from placebo in prolactin elevation, EPSs, or QTc prolongation. Aripiprazole can lower prolactin (to below the lower normal of prolactin levels in some cases), and it can be used adjunctively to reverse antipsychotic-induced hyperprolactinemia. In a prospective study of first-time users of antipsychotics, aripiprazole caused weight gain, but it does not seem to have major effects on glucose or lipid metabolism.

The first LAI aripiprazole formulation was approved in 2013 for the maintenance treatment of patients with schizophrenia. Whereas aripiprazole monohydrate is available as a monthly injection, aripiprazole lauroxil is available for injections every 4 to 6 weeks.

Brexpiprazole

Brexpiprazole is also a partial agonist of the D_2 receptor and was approved for the treatment of patients with schizophrenia in 2015. In comparison with aripiprazole, brexpiprazole has less intrinsic activity on D_2 receptors and less affinity for the histamine receptor but more potent binding at the $5-HT_{2A}$, $5-HT_{1A}$, and α_{1B} receptors. These differences are designed to make brexpiprazole more tolerable than aripiprazole but with similar clinical benefits. The most effective brexpiprazole dosage is 2 to 4 mg/day, but it should be started at 1 mg/day.

Cariprazine

In 2015, the FDA approved the piperazine antipsychotic cariprazine for the treatment of patients with schizophrenia. It is a partial agonist of dopamine$_{2/3}$ receptors, $5-HT_{1A}$ receptors, and antagonist of $5-HT_{2A}$ receptors. Low-affinity antagonism exists for α_1 but it has no significant affinity to the histamine$_1$ and muscarinic M_1 receptors. Similar to aripiprazole and brexpiprazole, cariprazine has affinity for D_3 receptors and D_2 receptors, with its metabolite having a strong affinity for D_3. Cariprazine has a long half-life of 2 to 4 days, and the active metabolites (desmethylcariprazine and didesmethylcariprazine) have half-lives of up to 3 weeks. It is mostly metabolized via 3A4, and blood levels of cariprazine may be significantly affected by CYP 3A4 inducers or inhibitors. The recommended starting dosage, which is also an effective dosage, is 1.5 mg/day administered once daily, and the maximum recommended dosage is 6 mg/day. Cariprazine may also have significant benefits in counteracting cognitive deficits and the negative symptoms of schizophrenia.[47] However, cariprazine can cause EPSs, including akathisia, particularly at higher doses. Despite this, its propensity for insomnia, weight gain, and metabolic disturbances seems to be low. Its effects on the QTc interval are minimal.

Lumateperone

In 2020, the FDA approved lumateperone, a novel medication to treat schizophrenia by modulating glutamate, serotonin, and dopamine neurotransmission. Like aripiprazole, lumateperone is a presynaptic D_2 agonist and postsynaptic D_2 antagonist. However, its high affinity to the $5-HT_{2A}$ receptor without increasing dopamine receptor affinity differentiates it from aripiprazole. Another unique feature of lumateperone is its clinical efficacy at 40% D_2 receptor occupancy as shown in positron emission tomography studies. Differences in the receptor affinity and activity may be the reason behind its good side effect profile regarding EPSs. In addition, lumateperone acts as a D_1 agonist and may increase glutamate signaling through the NMDA receptor. In multiple trials, lumateperone has shown to improve schizophrenia symptoms with minimal EPSs and metabolic and endocrine side effects.[48] Dose titration of lumateperone is not necessary, and the recommended dosage is 42 mg/day, with or without food. Dose adjustment of lumateperone is necessary while co-administering it with moderate or strong CYP 3A4 inhibitors. The half-life of lumateperone is 13 hours, but the active metabolites have a half-life of up to 21 hours.

Pimavanserin

In 2016, the FDA approved pimavanserin for the treatment of psychosis associated with Parkinson disease. It has inverse agonist and antagonist activity at $5-HT_{2A}$ and, to a lesser extent, at the $5-HT_{2C}$ receptors. Pimavanserin has no appreciable binding affinity for dopamine, histamine, muscarinic, or adrenergic receptors. It also has no significant metabolic side effects or EPSs, although it can prolong the QTc interval. Strong CYP 3A4 inhibitors increase the drug level of pimavanserin, and in severe cases, the dosage may need to be adjusted. The recommended daily dose is 34 mg, and no dose titration is necessary.[49] Of note, pimavanserin has not been shown to be effective in the treatment of schizophrenia.

DRUG INTERACTIONS WITH ANTIPSYCHOTIC AGENTS

Antipsychotic drugs are most likely to interact with other medications as a result of alterations of hepatic metabolism or when combined with drugs that produce additive side effects (such as anticholinergic effects) or when combined with drugs that impair cardiac conduction. Most conventional antipsychotic agents are extensively metabolized by the 2D6 isoenzyme of the hepatic P450 enzyme system, whereas atypical agents generally have more variable hepatic metabolism, typically involving isoenzymes 3A4, 1A2, and 2D6. Fortunately, because the therapeutic index (risk ratio) of antipsychotic drugs is quite large, interactions with agents that inhibit hepatic metabolism are unlikely to be life threatening but may increase side effects. Among the atypical antipsychotics, clozapine can produce the most serious adverse effects when blood levels are dramatically elevated; obtundation and cardiovascular effects have been associated with inhibition of clozapine metabolism by fluvoxamine or erythromycin. Addition of 2D6 inhibitors (e.g., some selective serotonin reuptake inhibitors) to conventional antipsychotics would be expected to increase EPSs, but in one placebo-controlled trial, this was not clinically significant despite substantial increases in blood levels of haloperidol and fluphenazine. Drugs that induce hepatic metabolism (such as certain anticonvulsants [e.g., carbamazepine, phenobarbital, phenytoin]) may lower antipsychotic blood concentrations substantially and cause loss of therapeutic efficacy.

Great care must be taken if low-potency agents (such as chlorpromazine, thioridazine, and clozapine) are combined with other highly anticholinergic drugs because the additive anticholinergic activity may produce confusion, urinary retention, and constipation. In addition, low-potency antipsychotic agents can depress cardiac function and significantly impair cardiac conduction when added to class I antiarrhythmic agents (such as quinidine or procainamide). Ziprasidone and iloperidone also significantly affect cardiac conduction and should not be combined with low-potency phenothiazines or the antiarrhythmic agents.

ONGOING CHALLENGES

Two major challenges remain: antipsychotics are not effective for all patients with psychosis, and they pose significant long-term medical risks to patients who need maintenance treatment. Very little guidance is available from controlled trials for additional interventions if a patient with schizophrenia remains symptomatic despite treatment with an adequate dose of clozapine. Early reports described improvement of positive and negative symptoms with the addition of risperidone to clozapine, consistent with the hypothesis that achieving a higher degree of D_2 blockade might enhance clozapine's effectiveness for some patients. Subsequent placebo-controlled trials produced inconsistent results, and therefore the role of clozapine augmentation in refractory cases remains controversial and poorly substantiated, except for electroconvulsive therapy.[50] As a result, polypharmacy for refractory disease remains a widely used, expensive practice with little support from clinical trials, particularly for patients with serious mental illness. Some forms of secondary psychosis (e.g., psychosis in setting of dementia) show little, if any, benefit from a treatment, which might increase mortality rates.

For patients who benefit sufficiently from treatment, prevention of antipsychotic-induced metabolic problems has become a major clinical focus and creating an integrated treatment setting that allows for appropriate medical management of psychiatric patients who receive antipsychotics is a major health care systems goal. Currently, even simple preventive measures (i.e., guideline-concordant metabolic monitoring) remain a major hurdle in many settings, hindering progress in preventing premature death from iatrogenic contributions. The use of metformin to blunt antipsychotic-induced weight gain and metabolic problems has been shown to be an effective prevention strategy in both the early and chronic course of schizophrenia.[51] Patients can benefit from a switch to antipsychotics with less metabolic liability, and some patients can

safely reduce polypharmacy. Recently, the use of glucagon-like peptide-1 receptor agonists (e.g., semaglutide) has attracted interest in managing antipsychotic-associated weight gain.[52] Such proactive management strategies are necessary to reduce the multi-morbidity that characterizes many patients who are treated with antipsychotics. In addition to metabolic problems, there remain concerns about neurotoxicity from antipsychotics over and above disease-related changes as suggested by brain volume loss in treatment studies of patients with schizophrenia. Recently, a long-term follow-up of a randomized first episode clinical trial comparing early antipsychotic drug discontinuation with maintenance treatment in symptomatically remitted first-episode patients found that the less aggressive approach with early drug discontinuation led to better long-term functional outcomes compared with patients assigned to maintenance treatment.[53] However, this approach may not be possible for many patients, and a personalized approach is necessary to manage the relapse risk, including how to find the minimally effective dose. In acute settings, many patients require the combination of multiple antipsychotics and mood stabilizers to address agitation and other active psychotic symptoms in hospital settings. In such cases, active deprescribing is important in outpatient settings to minimize severe side effects and to improve adherence.[54]

Despite the short-comings of antipsychotics, not treating patients with schizophrenia with an antipsychotic has been shown to have an increased overall mortality rate that needs to be accounted for when considering the risk–benefit equation. For most patients, the biggest risk to their lives is untreated psychosis, which can result in suicide but also affects a person's ability to manage medical illnesses. As the old adage goes, there is no physical health without mental health.

REFERENCES

1. Delay J, Deniker P. Neuroleptic effects of chlorpromazine in therapeutics of neuropsychiatry. *J Clin Exp Psychopathol*. 1955;16 (2):104–112.
2. Ayd Jr. FJ. Fatal hyperpyrexia during chlorpromazine therapy. *J Clin Exp Psychopathol*. 1956;17(2):189–192.
3. Sigwald J, Bouttier D, Raymondeaud C, et al. 4 cases of facio-bucco-linguo-masticatory dyskinesis of prolonged development following treatment with neuroleptics. *Rev Neurol (Paris)*. 1959;100:751–755.
4. Lasky J, Klett C, Caffey E, et al. A comparison evaluation of chlorpromazine, chlorprothixene, fluphenazine, reserpine, thioridazine and triflupromazine. *Dis Nerv Syst*. 1962;23:1–8.
5. Carlsson A, Lindqvist M. Effect of chlorpromazine or haloperidol on formation of 3methoxytyramine and normetanephrine in mouse brain. *Acta Pharmacol Toxicol (Copenh)*. 1963;20:140–144.
6. Creese I, Burt DR, Snyder SH. Dopamine receptor binding predicts clinical and pharmacological potencies of antischizophrenic drugs. *Science*. 1976;192(4238):481–483.
7. Idanpaan-Heikkila J, Alhava E, Olkinuora M, et al. Letter: clozapine and agranulocytosis. *Lancet*. 1975;2(7935):611.
8. Kane J, Honigfeld G, Singer J, et al. Clozapine for the treatment-resistant schizophrenic. A double-blind comparison with chlorpromazine. *Arch Gen Psychiatry*. 1988;45(9):789–796.
9. Duinkerke SJ, Botter PA, Jansen AA, et al. Ritanserin, a selective 5-HT2/1C antagonist, and negative symptoms in schizophrenia. A placebo-controlled double-blind trial. *Br J Psychiatry*. 1993;163:451–455.
10. Chouinard G, Jones B, Remington G, et al. A Canadian multicenter placebo-controlled study of fixed doses of risperidone and haloperidol in the treatment of chronic schizophrenic patients. *J Clin Psychopharmacol*. 1993;13(1):25–40.
11. Lieberman JA, Stroup TS, McEvoy JP, et al. Effectiveness of antipsychotic drugs in patients with chronic schizophrenia. *N Engl J Med*. 2005;353(12):1209–1223.
12. Huhn M, Nikolakopoulou A, Schneider-Thoma J, et al. Comparative efficacy and tolerability of 32 oral antipsychotics for the acute treatment of adults with multi-episode schizophrenia: a systematic review and network meta-analysis [published

correction appears in Lancet]. 2019;394(10202):918. Erratum in. *Lancet*. 2019;394(10202):918.

13. Mailman RB, Murthy V. Third generation antipsychotic drugs: partial agonism or receptor functional selectivity? *Curr Pharm Des*. 2010;16(5):488–501.

14. Kapur S, Arenovich T, Agid O, et al. Evidence for onset of antipsychotic effects within the first 24 hours of treatment. *Am J Psychiatry*. 2005;162(5):939–946.

15. Tiihonen J, Mittendorfer-Rutz E, Majak M, et al. Real-world effectiveness of antipsychotic treatments in a nationwide cohort of 29 823 patients with schizophrenia. *JAMA Psychiatry*. 2017; 74(7):686–693.

16. Siskind D, Gallagher E, Winckel K, et al. Does switching antipsychotics ameliorate weight gain in patients with severe mental illness? A systematic review and meta-analysis. *Schizophr Bull*. 2021;47(4):948–958.

17. Gill SS, Bronskill SE, Normand SL, et al. Antipsychotic drug use and mortality in older adults with dementia. *Ann Intern Med*. 2007;146(11):775–786.

18. Van Putten T, Marder SR, Wirshing WC, et al. Neuroleptic plasma levels. *Schizophr Bull*. 1991;17(2):197–216.

19. Meyer-Massetti C, Cheng CM, Sharpe BA, et al. The FDA extended warning for intravenous haloperidol and torsades de pointes: how should institutions respond? *J Hosp Med*. 2010;5(4):E8–E16.

20. Currier G, Walsh P. Safety and efficacy review of inhaled loxapine for treatment of agitation. *Clin Schizophr Rel Psychoses*. 2013;7(1):25–32.

21. Poyurovsky M, Pashinian A, Weizman R, et al. Low-dose mirtazapine: a new option in the treatment of antipsychotic-induced akathisia. A randomized, double-blind, placebo- and propranolol-controlled trial. *Biol Psychiatry*. 2006;59(11):1071–1077.

22. Ward KM, Citrome L. Antipsychotic-related movement disorders: drug-induced parkinsonism vs. tardive dyskinesia-key differences in pathophysiology and clinical management. *Neurol Ther*. 2018;7(2):233–248.

23. Carbon M, Kane JM, Leucht S, et al. Tardive dyskinesia risk with first- and second-generation antipsychotics in comparative randomized controlled trials: a meta-analysis. *World Psychiatry*. 2018;17(3):330–340.

24. Ricciardi L, Pringsheim T, Barnes TRE, et al. Treatment recommendations for tardive dyskinesia. *Can J Psychiatry*. 2019;64(6):388–399.

25. Tse L, Barr AM, Scarapicchia V, et al. Neuroleptic malignant syndrome: a view from a clinically oriented perspective. *Curr Neuropharmacol*. 2015;13(3):395–406.

26. Kleinberg DL, Davis JM, de Coster R, et al. Prolactin levels and adverse events in patients treated with risperidone. *J Clin Psychopharmacol*. 1999;19(1):57–61.

27. Rummel-Kluge C, Komossa K, Schwarz S, et al. Head-to-head comparisons of metabolic side effects of second-generation antipsychotics in the treatment of schizophrenia: a systematic review and meta-analysis. *Schizophr Res*. 2010;123(2-3):225–233.

28. Lindenmayer JP, Citrome L, Khan A, et al. A randomized, double-blind, parallel-group, fixed-dose, clinical trial of quetiapine at 600 versus 1200 mg/d for patients with treatment-resistant schizophrenia or schizoaffective disorder. *J Clin Psychopharmacol*. 2011;31(2):160–168.

29. Honer WG, MacEwan GW, Gendron A, et al. A randomized, double-blind, placebo-controlled study of the safety and tolerability of high-dose quetiapine in patients with persistent symptoms of schizophrenia or schizoaffective disorder. *J Clin Psychiatry*. 2012;73(1):13–20.

30. Goff DC, McEvoy JP, Citrome L, et al. High-dose oral ziprasidone versus conventional dosing in schizophrenia patients with residual symptoms: the ZEBRAS Study. *J Clin Psychopharmacology*. 2013;33(4):485–490.

31. Remmington G, Agid O, Foussias G, et al. Clozapine and therapeutic drug monitoring: is there sufficient evidence for an upper threshold? *Psychopharmacology*. 2013;225(3):505–518.

32. VanderZwaag C, McGee M, McEvoy JP, et al. Response of patients with treatment-refractory schizophrenia to clozapine within three serum level ranges. *Am J Psychiatry*. 1996;153(12):1579–1584.

33. Bird AM, Smith TL, Walton AE. Current treatment strategies for clozapine-induced sialorrhea. *Ann Pharmacother*. 2011;45(5):667–675.

34. Clozapine REMS? What is the clozapine REMS? Accessed October 30, 2022. http://www.newclozapinerems.com.

35. Myles N, Myles H, Xia S, et al. Meta-analysis examining the epidemiology of clozapine-associated neutropenia. *Acta Psychiatr Scand*. 2018;138(2):101–109.

36. Sandarsh S, Bishnoi RJ, Shashank RB, et al. Monitoring for myocarditis during treatment initiation with clozapine. *Acta Psychiatr Scand*. 2021;144(2):194–200.

37. Kapur S, Zipursky RB, Remington G. Clinical and theoretical implications of 5-HT2 and D2 receptor occupancy of clozapine, risperidone, and olanzapine in schizophrenia. *Am J Psychiatry*. 1999;156(2):286–293.

38. Woerner MG, Correll CU, Alvir JM, et al. Incidence of tardive dyskinesia with risperidone or olanzapine in the elderly: results from a 2-year, prospective study in antipsychotic-naive patients. *Neuropsychopharmacology*. 2011;36(8):1738–1746.

39. McDonnell DP, Detke HC, Bergstrom RF, et al. Post-injection delirium/sedation syndrome in patients with schizophrenia treated with olanzapine long-acting injection, II: investigations of mechanism. *BMC Psychiatry*. 2010;10:45.

40. Monahan C, McCoy L, Powell J, et al. Olanzapine/Samidorphan: new drug approved for treating bipolar I disorder and schizophrenia. *Ann Pharmacother*. 2022;56(9):1049–1057.

41. Kapur S, Zipursky R, Jones C, et al. A positron emission tomography study of quetiapine in schizophrenia: a preliminary finding of an antipsychotic effect with only transiently high dopamine D2 receptor occupancy. *Arch Gen Psychiatry*. 2000;57(6):553–559.

42. Tek C, Kucukgoncu S, Guloksuz S, et al. Antipsychotic-induced weight gain in first-episode psychosis patients: a meta-analysis of differential effects of antipsychotic medications. *Early Interv Psychiatry*. 2016;10(3):193–202.

43. Strom BL, Eng SM, Faich G, et al. Comparative mortality associated with ziprasidone and olanzapine in real-world use among 18,154 patients with schizophrenia: the Ziprasidone Observational Study of Cardiac Outcomes (ZODIAC). *Am J Psychiatry*. 2011;168(2):193–201.

44. Tarazi FI, Stahl SM. Iloperidone, asenapine, and lurasidone: a primer on their current status. *Expert Opin Pharmacother*. 2012;13(13):1911–1922.

45. Citrome L. Role of sublingual asenapine in treatment of schizophrenia. *Neuropsychiatr Dis Treat*. 2011;7:325–339.

46. Frankel JS, Schwartz TL. Brexpiprazole and cariprazine: distinguishing two new atypical antipsychotics from the original dopamine stabilizer aripiprazole. *Ther Adv Psychopharmacol*. 2017;7(1):29–41.

47. Laszlovszky I, Barabássy Á. Németh G. Cariprazine, a broad-spectrum antipsychotic for the treatment of schizophrenia: pharmacology, efficacy, and safety. *Adv Ther*. 2021;38(7):3652–3673.

48. Correll CU, Davis RE, Weingart M, et al. Efficacy and safety of lumateperone for treatment of schizophrenia: a randomized clinical trial [published correction appears in JAMA Psychiatry]. 2020;77(4):349-358. Erratum in. *JAMA Psychiatry*. 2020 Feb 19

49. Espay AJ, Guskey MT, Norton JC, et al. Pimavanserin for Parkinson's disease psychosis: effects stratified by baseline cognition and use of cognitive-enhancing medications. *Mov Disord*. 2018;33(11):1769–1776.

50. Wagner E, Kane JM, Correll CU, et al. Clozapine combination and augmentation strategies in patients with schizophrenia -recommendations from an international expert survey among the Treatment Response and Resistance in Psychosis (TRRIP) working group. *Schizophr Bull*. 2020;46(6):1459–1470.

51. Fitzgerald I, O'Connell J, Keating D, et al. Metformin in the management of antipsychotic-induced weight gain in adults with psychosis: development of the first evidence-based guideline using GRADE methodology. *Evid Based Ment Health*. 2022;25(1):15–22.

52. Rubino DM, Greenway FL, Khalid U, et al. Effect of weekly subcutaneous semaglutide vs daily liraglutide on body weight in adults with overweight or obesity without diabetes: the STEP 8 randomized clinical trial. *JAMA*. 2022;327(2):138–150.

53. Wunderink L, Nieboer RM, Wiersma D, et al. Recovery in remitted first-episode psychosis at 7 years of follow-up of an early dose reduction/discontinuation or maintenance treatment strategy: long-term follow-up of a 2-year randomized clinical trial. *JAMA Psychiatry*. 2013;70(9):913–920.

54. Paudel S, Vyas CM, Stern TA. A prescription for deprescribing antipsychotics: managing polypharmacy in schizophrenia. *Prim Care Companion CNS Disord*. 2020;22(6).

10 Patients with Abnormal Movements

Oliver Freudenreich, Felicia A. Smith, and Alice W. Flaherty

KEY POINTS

- Movement disorders are clinical diagnoses that are based upon the history and physical examination; laboratory tests and brain imaging typically do not facilitate making the diagnosis.
- Movement disorders caused by basal ganglia dysfunction all create difficulty starting or stopping movements. Movement disorders along the hyperkinetic-hypokinetic spectrum (from fast to slow) include chorea, choreoathetosis, athetosis, dystonia, lead-pipe rigidity, bradykinesia, and akinesia.
- Tardive dyskinesia is a late complication of treatment with dopamine-blocking agents, usually antipsychotics.
- Recognizing and correctly labeling motor phenomena in clinical settings helps to create a differential diagnosis that serves as the foundation for optimal treatment.

OVERVIEW

Psychiatrists encounter patients with abnormal movements in a variety of clinical settings. Recognizing and correctly labeling motor phenomena in each setting helps to create a differential diagnosis that serves as the basis for optimal treatment since abnormal movements can be the first indication of an unsuspected medical or neurologic disorder in a patient treated for psychiatric symptoms. A solid understanding of conditions that have prototypical abnormal movements (e.g., Huntington disease, Parkinson disease) or tremors will help psychiatrists to correctly categorize abnormal movements. All movement disorders, whether they are primary or drug induced, contribute to morbidity (with loss of independence) and mortality (e.g., secondary to falls or choking). Many of these disorders are stigmatizing, as abnormal movements are immediately obvious to others.

Movement disorders caused by basal ganglia damage or dysfunction create trouble starting or stopping movements. They differ from cerebellar disorders (that affect movement targeting) and stroke-related weakness. Observing real patients and watching videos are excellent ways to learn to recognize abnormal movements. A word of caution: many of the free videos available on the internet show patients with functional movement disorders (FMDs) who have made videos of themselves and do not depict classic movement disorders; therefore one should select reputable sources, such as a video atlas.[1]

Gathering the History and Performing a Physical Examination

A movement disorder is a clinical diagnosis based on the patient's history and a physical examination; laboratory tests and brain imaging usually do not facilitate making the diagnosis. A family history can be informative if there is a history of a hereditary movement disorder. One should ask about the current and past use of prescribed medications as well as substances of abuse, as these are the most common causes of abnormal movements.

The examination begins with unobtrusive observation when meeting the patient in the waiting area or when approaching the patient's bedside. One should determine if the movements exist when unobserved and if the patient shuffles or writhes when walking. A patient who lies stiffly in bed might be parkinsonian or catatonic. The neurologic examination is focused on establishing deficits beyond their relationship to the motor strip and the basal ganglia; it also includes the assessment of cortical and cerebellar functioning, as well as the elicitation of other motor signs. Muscle tone should be evaluated (e.g., as being rigid, spastic, or hypotonic). If you suspect catatonia, you should perform an examination looking for other signs of catatonia. Some patients cannot relax while their limb is being examined for muscle tone, and as a result they seem to (voluntarily) resist each passive movement. This is called *gegenhalten* or paratonia.

Table 10.1 summarizes common abnormal movements. Overall, it is helpful to determine if your patient moves too much (hyperkinetic) or too little (hypokinetic), or if there are rhythmic tremors or non-rhythmic twitches. Myoclonus or asterixis can initially appear somewhat rhythmic, so one must observe carefully. Asterixis can suggest the presence of a serious metabolic disturbance, whereas myoclonus is non-specific and may be benign. Other phenomena that mimic tremors include focal seizures and cerebellar dysmetria. Some movements defy easy categorization but should be considered in patients with psychiatric conditions (e.g., catatonic symptoms, stereotypies, mannerisms).

When examining a patient with a tremor, the main question is whether the tremor occurs mainly at rest (a resting tremor) or during action (an action tremor). Postural tremors can occur with either action or rest and are not in and of themselves diagnostic. Writing or drawing will reliably evoke an action tremor in the writing hand, whereas rest tremors can intensify with movement of the opposite hand. The phenomenological description of the tremor is followed by a search for other neurologic signs or symptoms to help refine the diagnostic possibilities. This is important since treatment depends on the etiology of tremors, although the treatment of some tremors can be non-specific and based on their severity and the patient's tolerance of them.

Table 10.2 summarizes manifestations of gait disorders. Observing a patient's gait and understanding the etiology of a gait disturbance are particularly important during a patient visit. Gait disturbances not only interfere with a patient's independence, but they can lead to dangerous falls (especially in the elderly). Hypokinetic movement disorders, including parkinsonism associated with the use of antipsychotics, lead to falls because patients react too slowly when they stumble. Those with ataxia or hyperkinetic movement disorders sustain fewer falls. A potentially reversible cause of a gait disturbance

TABLE 10.1 Motor Symptoms

Tremor (Rhythmic Involuntary Alternation of Agonist and Antagonist Muscles)
Action tremor—triggered by voluntary movement
Rest tremor—stops during voluntary movement
Postural tremor—seen with either action or rest tremor, not itself diagnostic
Movements That Can Look Like Tremor But Are Not
Cerebellar dysmetria (intention "tremor")—worsens as limb approaches target
Myoclonus—involuntary non-rhythmic jerk, moves only one joint
Asterixis (negative myoclonus, "flapping tremor")—arrhythmic lapses of sustained posture
Focal seizures—non-rhythmic trains of unilateral twitching, lasting seconds to minutes.
Fasciculations—visible contractions within a muscle that do not move a joint
The Hyperkinetic–Hypokinetic Spectrum—From Fast to Slow, in Descending Order
Chorea—brief, unpredictable, semi-purposeful movements
Choreoathetosis—when you cannot decide if it is chorea or athetosis
Athetosis—slow but continuous movements
Dystonia—abnormal postures held for at least several seconds
Lead-pipe rigidity—constant resistance throughout the range of passive motion
Bradykinesia—slow movements
Akinesia—sustained periods of no movement
Other Hyperkinetic Movements
Hemiballism—violent, unilateral, repetitive but non-rhythmic jerks of proximal limbs
Stereotypies—repetitive self-soothing movements (e.g., tapping foot, biting nails)
Tics—semi-voluntary fast movement, often multi-joint, usually urge driven

TABLE 10.2 Gait Syndromes

Parkinsonian: slow, shuffling, stooping with arms flexed, festinating (unable to stop); many falls
Choreic: posturing, writhing; fewer falls
Ataxic: wide based, lurching; fewer falls
Neuropathic: foot slaps, patient steps high to avoid tripping
Spastic: stiff, circumducted leg, toe walking
Functional (astasia-abasia): wild, seemingly poor balance but no falls

TABLE 10.3 Clinical Symptoms in Parkinson Disease

Motor
Bradykinesia
Masked facies
Stooped posture and festinating gait
Falls, especially backward
Atypical parkinsonism: spasticity, eye movement abnormalities
Neuropsychiatric
Pre-morbid personality (conscientious, inflexible, risk averse)
Depression: may precede motor symptoms
Dementia: if early, is a sign of atypical parkinsonism
Psychosis: if early, is a sign of atypical parkinsonism

is complicated by levodopa-induced dyskinesias that arise due to striatal hyper-responsiveness to acute dopaminergic stimulation. In the later stages of the disease, patients experience periods of immobility that alternate with good symptom control (called "on-off phenomenon"). Some patients with parkinsonism have an *atypical* response to dopamine agonists (i.e., it is poor). Atypical parkinsonian syndromes (e.g., Parkinson-plus) occur in patients who experience not only parkinsonian symptoms but other symptoms as well. Such syndromes include Lewy body dementia (LBD) or multi-system atrophy (MSA), where, as the name implies, other brain systems are affected. Clinicians should consider that they will only know if a patient is poorly responsive to levodopa if it is tried.

PD is, for most patients, a multi-faceted disease; it is more than a pure movement disorder (by virtue of the biological nature of the illness, treatment side effects, or the psychological effects of having a progressive illness). Table 10.3 summarizes its core clinical symptoms.

Some patients who are eventually diagnosed with PD have a pre-morbid (i.e., prior to the onset of abnormal movements) personality style that is characterized by an affinity for high harm avoidance and low novelty.[3] Such patients are temperamentally conscientious, industrious, inflexible, and prone to dysthymia. On the other hand, a complication of PD progression is a dopamine dysregulation syndrome, with impulsive behaviors that can take the form of gambling, hypersexuality, compulsive shopping, or binge eating,[4] all manifestations that were not characteristic of the patient. Punding (i.e., repetitive, prolonged, purposeless behavior) is another late complication that makes life difficult for PD patients and their families.[5] These problems are due, at least in part, to the use of medications and antipsychotics with partial dopamine agonist properties (e.g., aripiprazole) that carry some risk of inducing compulsions and impulsive urges to shop, eat, have sex, or gamble.

Fatigue, apathy, insomnia, and depression are very common in PD. Dementia and psychosis are late-stage problems of PD; when these complications begin early in the illness course, they usually indicate atypical parkinsonism. Autonomic dysfunctions, such as postural hypotension and drooling, are severe in MSA and are often problematic in PD. Muscle rigidity can cause pain, especially in the muscles of the shoulder and back.

At least one-third of patients with PD have depression and apathy (*abulia*). Apathy can be the first symptom of PD; it needs to be differentiated from depression (a treatable psychiatric disorder). Depression often goes undiagnosed due to its symptom overlap with PD, which includes psychomotor retardation, masked facies, poor sleep, and cognitive complaints. As in other medical disorders, depression, when present, is a major contributor to poor quality of life. Depression and motor fluctuations are poorly correlated. In a clinical trial that compared a placebo, paroxetine, and a noradrenergic tricyclic antidepressant, nortriptyline was effective but paroxetine was not.[6] The role of selective serotonin reuptake inhibitors (SSRIs) is therefore thought to be limited, and perhaps best reserved for those with a pseudobulbar affect, as

is normal-pressure hydrocephalus, which is manifest by a triad of (a parkinsonian) gait, incontinence, and dementia (the latter being a late-stage manifestation). Shunt placement can prevent symptom progression, and if this intervention is carried out early in the condition's course, some of the symptoms may even be reversed.

One should also ask about swallowing difficulties, which can result in aspiration pneumonia.

IDIOPATHIC MOVEMENT DISORDERS

Parkinson Disease

Idiopathic Parkinson disease (PD) is a hypokinetic syndrome characterized by the triad of slow movement, rigidity, and tremor. The combination of tremor and rigidity leads to the cogwheeling on examination. Although a resting tremor is often the first sign of PD, up to one-fourth of patients have no tremor. Difficulties initiating movements, like starting to walk, are called freezing, where a patient's feet appear to be glued to the ground.

The mainstay of treatment for PD is the administration of the dopamine precursor levodopa.[2] Bradykinesia responds better to levodopa than does tremor. Unfortunately, while levodopa is highly effective early in the illness course (reversing dopamine loss-related akinesia), its long-term administration

SSRIs can worsen motor symptoms. A recent placebo-controlled trial, however, showed benefit from paroxetine and venlafaxine without exacerbating motor symptoms.[7] Other antidepressants to consider are bupropion or a stimulant; the latter is often used for the treatment of apathy. The dopamine agonist pramipexole has a direct antidepressant effect in patients with PD and is another therapeutic option.[8] In refractory depression, electroconvulsive therapy (ECT) and transcranial magnetic stimulation can be tried, although post-ECT delirium complicates its use. Mirtazapine is a good choice for those with anxiety and poor sleep.

In a large epidemiologic study, almost one-third of patients with PD who were receiving routine outpatient neurologic care met the criteria for dementia; higher rates of sub-syndromal cognitive impairment were found in this group.[9] Over time, most patients with PD develop dementia. In a cohort of newly diagnosed patients, 83% of patients who lived for 20 years with PD had dementia.[10] The dementia associated with PD is a subcortical dementia that is characterized by slowed mentation and processing (bradyphrenia), poor attention, and difficulties with executive function. The Mini-Mental State Examination (MMSE) is insensitive for the detection of these problems, and it should not be used as a screening tool in this population. However, co-morbidities with cortical dementias (e.g., Alzheimer dementia, LBD) lead to mixed cortical/subcortical pictures. On autopsy, LBD and PD with dementia look alike. They may represent the same disease, with dementia preceding motor problems in LBD and the reverse being true in PD dementia. Very poor tolerability of antipsychotics is a hallmark of both LBD[11] and late-stage PD dementia. The mainstay of treatment for PD with dementia is acetylcholinesterase inhibitors, which are also frequently used in LBD. Levodopa is ineffective and poorly tolerated; moreover, it can induce hallucinations in both conditions.

Psychosis is a complication of PD in about half of those with PD. Symptoms (that include vivid dreams, illusions, hallucinations, misidentification syndromes, and paranoid delusions) can result from the treatment of PD and from the disease itself, particularly if dementia develops. Early-onset hallucinations are a predictor of dementia, and they are primarily, but not exclusively, visual. They can be simple (seeing flashes), of the passage variety (i.e., seeing fleeting images in the periphery of vision), or take the form of presence hallucinations (i.e., feeling that someone is close by). More complex hallucinations include seeing small animals or children. Both hallucinations and delusions predict nursing home placement; therefore, attempts to treat these symptoms are important. The first step is to exclude other causes of psychosis, including polypharmacy. Next, modifying the PD regimen by reducing polypharmacy, lowering the levodopa dose, and dosing it more frequently can be helpful. Last, antipsychotics should be trialed, although the tolerability of most antipsychotics, including those with loose binding to the dopamine receptor (e.g., quetiapine), is poor, particularly in later disease stages. Moreover, efficacy has not been clearly established for quetiapine, an agent that is often used because of its perceived better tolerability. Low-dose clozapine (e.g., 6.25 mg or 12 mg/day) might be the best choice, as it can be used when other antipsychotics have not been tolerated.[12] Pimavanserin is a selective 5-HT$_{2A}$ inverse agonist used for the treatment of PD-related psychosis.[13] While effective, its role in the management of psychosis in PD has yet to be established, particularly regarding its efficacy when compared with clozapine.[13]

Sleep disruption from restless legs syndrome (RLS) or obstructive sleep apnea is common in PD, can be debilitating, but is relatively treatable (with gabapentin and continuous positive airway pressure, respectively). Many individuals with PD have rapid eye movement behavior disorder (RBD), which can greatly disrupt their caregivers' sleep and contribute to caregiver stress. Of patients with RBD without PD, 50% will develop PD within a decade, and most of the rest will develop another neurodegenerative disorder.[14]

Huntington Disease

Huntington chorea or Huntington disease (HD) is a rare autosomal dominant progressive neuropsychiatric disorder. It typically begins in the fourth decade of life and leads to death in about a decade. Psychiatrists should keep in mind, however, that 10% of cases of HD (juvenile HD) begin during adolescence, and such patients may be misdiagnosed as having schizophrenia or another psychiatric disorder when neuropsychiatric symptoms precede motor symptoms. The age of onset is inversely correlated with the number of CAG repeat expansions in the pathogenic gene, a phenomenon known as genetic anticipation. Unfortunately, knowledge of the genetic mutation and its mechanism has not yet been translated into disease-modifying treatments for this single-gene disorder.

As the term chorea implies, HD is a hyperkinetic movement disorder with its hallmark choreiform movements. Psychiatrists might encounter patients with stimulant-induced chorea, which is a complication that arises in those with a long history of stimulant misuse; it is also known as "crack dancing," which can develop acutely during cocaine use or with chronic use.[15] The differential diagnosis of choreiform movements is provided in Table 10.4.

Other motor phenomena in HD include dysphagia, parkinsonism, and dystonia, particularly as the illness progresses. In addition, almost all patients with HD experience neuropsychiatric symptoms, ranging from dysphoria and irritability to anxiety and psychosis. Depression is also frequent, and the risk of suicide is high. The end-stage of HD is characterized by increased immobility and dementia. Patients with juvenile HD experience difficult-to-manage seizures and early psychiatric and cognitive symptoms in addition to bradykinesia, dystonia, rigidity, and oropharyngeal dysfunction. Purely behavioral problems, such as aggression, are other early signs. A diagnosis of HD should be suspected if the hallmark imaging findings of caudate and putamen degeneration are seen. Genetic testing confirms the diagnosis.

There are no disease-modifying treatments. Death typically occurs within 10 to 15 years of the initial diagnosis. Symptomatic treatments include the use of SSRIs for depression, low-dose antipsychotics for psychosis, and one of the vesicular monoamine transporter (VMAT)-2 inhibitors (i.e., tetrabenazine, deutetrabenazine, and valbenazine) for chorea.

TABLE 10.4 Differential Diagnosis of Choreiform Movements

Inherited Disorders
Huntington disease
Fahr syndrome (idiopathic basal ganglia calcification)
Neuroacanthocytosis
Wilson disease
Friedreich ataxia
Spinocerebellar ataxia
Acquired Disorders
Focal striatal lesion
Post-infectious: Sydenham chorea, PANDAS (pediatric autoimmune disorders associated with streptococcal infection)
Pregnancy: chorea gravidarum
Lupus erythematosus
Thyrotoxicosis
Acquired immunodeficiency syndrome
Paraneoplastic syndromes
Drug Induced
Tardive dyskinesia
Phenytoin
Cocaine ("crack dance")
Levodopa
Oral contraceptives

All treatments carry a risk of worsening the disease (e.g., worsening dysphagia) and must be adjusted to the disease stage.

A family history allows for early diagnosis, which can be facilitated by pre-symptomatic testing. However, in some families, the history might be unknown, or the parent might not have expressed symptoms yet. Genetic testing poses ethical challenges, particularly the testing of asymptomatic family members who might still be children.[16] The risk of suicide after the diagnosis is made needs to be considered.

Tourette Syndrome

The hallmark of Tourette syndrome (TS) is the presence of tics that start before the age of 18 years and that consist of both multiple motor tics (e.g., eye blinking or shoulder shrugging) and vocal tics (e.g., throat clearing). Chronic tic disorders, with either motor or vocal tics but not both, are likely a *forme fruste* of TS. The male-to-female ratio for tic disorders is 3:1. Many children who develop TS in early childhood have complete resolution of their symptoms by early adulthood. Co-morbid psychiatric disorders, especially obsessive-compulsive disorder and attention-deficit disorder (ADD), are common. Other problems include depression and secondary social phobia that are related to the tics. As with other movements, tics worsen with stress, excitement, or fatigue. Tics are somewhat voluntary and can be suppressed when a patient experiences a premonitory urge, at least for a while. These features differentiate tics from myoclonus. An individual tic may move several joints, unlike myoclonus. Complex tics, like repeating phrases (echolalia) or shouting obscenities (coprolalia), are rare and often misperceived as volitional.

Treatment of tics is usually unnecessary unless they are persistent, impairing, or distressing. Social phobia that has developed in response to tics can be treated directly with therapy and SSRIs. Habit-reversal training is a psychological treatment for tics that can work.[17] ADD, which is highly co-morbid with tics, can probably be treated with stimulants without the risk of worsening tics, contrary to previous recommendations and fears.[18] Tic-suppressing medications include α_2-adrenergic receptor agonists (e.g., clonidine and guanfacine) and antipsychotics.[19] Clonidine or guanfacine should be tried first, as they are safer than, albeit not as effective as, antipsychotics. Antipsychotics can cause tardive dyskinesia (TD) and rebound tics on their withdrawal. While high-potency antipsychotics (e.g., haloperidol or pimozide) have been traditionally used to manage patients with TS, they are apt to induce extrapyramidal symptoms (EPS) (and in the case of pimozide, the QTc interval can be prolonged). Instead, clinicians should try using aripiprazole or risperidone. In severe presentations, patients may consider undergoing deep brain stimulation (DBS).

Wilson Disease

Wilson disease (WD) is a very rare disorder of copper elimination.[20] Its symptoms are the result of insidious copper accumulation in organs, most importantly the liver and the brain. Depending on which organ is affected most, patients may present to hepatologists (because of liver enzyme abnormalities or frank cirrhosis), to neurologists (because of a mix of movement problems, including dysarthria, dysmetria, chorea, and tremor), or to psychiatrists (because of mood and personality changes, or rarely psychosis or catatonia). Kayser-Fleischer rings in concert with a serum ceruloplasmin level of <100 mg/L are diagnostic for WD. However, 50% of patients with WD do not develop eye findings. A 24-hour copper excretion in the urine >100 µg per 24 hours, in the absence of cholestatic liver disease, is strong evidence for WD. Ultimately, the diagnosis of WD hinges not on a single test result but on accounting for all available clinical information.

Timely diagnosis is important since eliminating excess copper from the body by means of chelating and depleting agents, such as penicillamine, while also preventing the addition of copper to the body by means of copper-absorption inhibitors (e.g., zinc) is only effective when initiated early before tissue damage has occurred. Psychiatric treatments are not well studied but are like those of other disorders that affect the basal ganglia; antipsychotics tend to be poorly tolerated. Without treatment, WD is fatal.

Restless Legs Syndrome (Willis-Ekbom Disease)

Restless legs syndrome (RLS) is a common neurologic movement disorder that affects up to 10% of those in the general population. The core feature of RLS is the urge to move the legs in response to an increasingly unpleasant (often described as a "creeping") feeling that builds in the legs when patients are at rest. Moving the legs relieves this sensation. For most patients, RLS is worse at night, making it difficult for them to fall asleep or to sleep soundly. RLS should not be confused with mere positional discomfort, leg pain, or leg cramps. An important differential diagnostic consideration for psychiatrists is akathisia. Periodic limb movements in sleep (PLMS) is distinct from RLS, but almost all patients with RLS show such movements during polysomnography. RLS can be primary or secondary to other medical disorders, most importantly iron deficiency anemia and renal failure.[21] One should consider measuring the ferritin level to rule out iron deficiency in cases of suspected RLS. RLS is frequently co-morbid with depression, which can pose a dilemma since antidepressants can exacerbate RLS.

Treatment typically involves the use of dopamine agonists (e.g., pramipexole or ropinirole) or alpha$_2$ delta calcium-channel ligands (e.g., gabapentin or pregabalin).[22] Benzodiazepines and opiates can help in refractory cases of RLS, but clinicians need to use them judiciously to avoid falls in the elderly and to guard against misuse, respectively.

TREMORS

The frequencies of different types of tremors overlap too much to be helpful unless they are unusually slow (e.g., 4 Hz in PD) or high (e.g., 18 Hz in primary orthostatic tremor). To complicate matters, different types of tremors can co-exist in the same patient. A so-called "intention tremor" (dysmetria) associated with cerebellar disorders is often accompanied by other cerebellar signs (e.g., an ataxic gait or ocular nystagmus); however, as noted earlier, it is not a true tremor. Seizures with retained consciousness would be a very rare cause of bilateral tremor.

Because stress-induced adrenaline itself causes tremors, anxious people often have a tremor, and their awareness of it can worsen their anxiety. It is important to appropriately reassure patients if they perceive a mild tremor to be disabling or a new-onset tremor as a sign of things to come (e.g., a brain tumor or a disabling progressive neurological disease). The psychological responses to tremors need to be managed with support to help cope with the tremor; treatment includes appropriate management of both the tremor and the psychological response to it. A physiologic (i.e., normal) bilateral finger tremor can be made worse by stress, physical work, or anxiety, as well as from stimulants, such as nicotine and caffeine. Professionals with stage fright, for example, can use a beta-blocker prior to a public appearance to suppress their physiological tremors. Some people have a prominent ("enhanced") physiologic tremor independent from stress or another neurological disease.

A so-called "benign essential tremor" is an isolated action tremor in the absence of other neurological movements that almost always involve the upper limbs (as seen in 95% of cases), although the head and voice among other body parts can be affected. The tremor is bilateral and symmetric and is said to respond well to the use of alcohol and to run in families. However, it is usually over-diagnosed because additional neurological signs suggestive of other syndromes, like PD, are overlooked. Moreover, it is increasingly recognized as not "benign" in the sense that it can be progressive and include non-tremor symptoms.[23] Propranolol is the first-line treatment. Primidone can be helpful, but it must be titrated very slowly because of its propensity to induce severe sedation. Up to half of patients with an action tremor will show no clear benefit from pharmacotherapy.

DRUG-INDUCED MOVEMENT DISORDERS

Iatrogenic movement disorders and tremors are secondary to medication treatments, most often, but not always, due to the use of antipsychotics. For psychiatrists, the most important to consider are iatrogenic movement disorders that are related to antipsychotic-induced EPS and drug-induced tremors. These side effects are important because they can be life threatening (e.g., laryngeal dystonia), unpleasant (e.g., akathisia), functionally impairing (e.g., parkinsonism), and socially stigmatizing (e.g., tremor, TD). TD is also problematic, in that it is potentially irreversible, as opposed to the other drug-induced symptoms that usually subside once treatment with the offending agent has been stopped. Finally, current or recent drug use can lead to movement disorders and tremors, either during intoxication or withdrawal, depending on the substance. NMS, which is accompanied by motor abnormalities, is an iatrogenic form of malignant catatonia.

Drug-Induced Tremors

Myriad medications, including but not limited to psychotropics, can cause tremors. A complete review of the patient's medication list, including over-the-counter drugs as well as alcohol and stimulants (e.g., caffeine and nicotine), is therefore critical for patients with a tremor. All major psychiatric medication groups (e.g., antidepressants, antipsychotics, and mood stabilizers [including lithium]) can cause a tremor at usual doses. Sedatives, including benzodiazepines and alcohol, can cause movements during withdrawal states, typically with a coarse tremor.

A resting tremor is almost always parkinsonian, including its drug-induced variant. On the other hand, lithium, many anti-epileptic drugs (e.g., valproate, lamotrigine), and stimulants cause action tremors. The lithium-induced tremor is an exaggerated physiologic tremor (postural tremor)[24]; it is symmetric and related to the dose and blood level of lithium. A more prominent and coarser tremor is the most common symptom of lithium intoxication that should alert clinicians to search for other signs of lithium toxicity (e.g., confusion, dysarthria, diarrhea) and to check the lithium level. If missed, prolonged lithium toxicity can cause an irreversible, poorly treatment-responsive cerebellar tremor.[25] Using the lowest effective lithium dose and removing aggravating factors (e.g., non-steroidal anti-inflammatory drugs, hyponatremia, diuretics) is often enough to manage lithium-induced tremor. The most commonly prescribed beta-blocker, propranolol, at doses between 60 and 320 mg/day, is effective in cases that require treatment. Primidone, gabapentin, or benzodiazepines (to reduce arousal) are other options.

Whenever possible, the tremors should be treated in the context of the psychiatric syndrome. For example, one can switch from most antipsychotics to clozapine in a patient with EPS, or one can avoid medications, such as valproate, that worsen tremors in depressed patients with a tremor.

Antipsychotic-Induced Extrapyramidal Symptoms

Patients who are treated with an antipsychotic can develop one of three types of iatrogenic movement disorders in the form of EPS; each follows a different time course. Early complications, after only a dose or so, include akathisia and acute dystonic reactions. Parkinsonism usually does not become apparent until after several weeks of treatment. By definition, a late-developing ("tardive") problem is TD. Tardive variants have also been described for akathisia and dystonia. The Pisa syndrome is a variant of dystonia that can also be medication induced, and as the name suggests leads to a sideways-leaning patient due to persistent truncal dystonia.[26] In populations with serious mental disorders, patients might display various admixtures of the three main complications from antipsychotic use. In a representative cohort of 99 chronically institutionalized patients with schizophrenia who received mostly first-generation antipsychotics (FGAs), only about 40% were free from motor symptoms when carefully examined, while 60% suffered from one of three side effects.[27] Despite the increased use of second-generation antipsychotics (SGAs) over the past decade, the same group found an almost unchanged number of movement disorder–free patients in their cohort when they were able to repeat their cross-sectional assessment 8 years later.[28] Antipsychotic-induced EPS remains a major clinical concern for any psychiatrist who prescribes antipsychotics, including newer agents, for longer periods. When assessing a patient who is taking an antipsychotic, one should examine for all three main manifestations of EPS, accounting for the possibility of overlap, as graphically depicted in Fig. 10.1.[28]

Acute Dystonic Reactions

Patients can have an acute dystonic reaction after only a single antipsychotic dose, with most cases occurring within a week. Younger male patients are at the highest risk of developing this complication. Classically, it takes the form of an oculogyric crisis (with eyes rolling backward), opisthotonus (body arching), torticollis, or trismus (jaw locking). These acute-onset problems are frightening and painful. Many older patients with schizophrenia still remember and will tell you about the first time they received high-dose FGAs like haloperidol and had a dystonic reaction. High-potency antipsychotics are a poor choice for treatment initiation in antipsychotic-naive, first-episode psychosis patients; it is best to avoid inducing an acute dystonic reaction. While anxiety-provoking, dystonic symptoms are rarely life threatening, except when the dystonia affects the larynx.

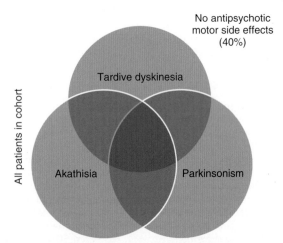

Fig. 10.1 ■ Overlap between antipsychotic-induced extrapyramidal symptoms (EPS) in a cohort of patients treated with antipsychotics. Based on Janno S, Holi M, Tuisku K, et al. Prevalence of neuroleptic-induced movement disorders in chronic schizophrenia inpatients. *Am J Psychiatry*. 2004;161(1):160–163.

One can treat acute dystonic reactions effectively with the use of a parenteral benztropine or diphenhydramine. When patients are sent home, they should receive several days of oral benztropine or diphenhydramine to prevent a return trip to the ED. In addition, one should keep in mind that cocaine and phencyclidine can cause dystonia.

Akathisia

Akathisia is an inability to sit still; afflicted patients fidget and may stand up and walk about during the interview. In mild akathisia, patients describe inner restlessness, but they can, with effort, suppress visible movements. Very severe akathisia can induce suicidal and homicidal behavior. As with acute dystonic reactions, akathisia can occur after a single antipsychotic dose. It is important to distinguish akathisia from anxiety-driven stereotypies and involuntary dyskinesias by asking patients what drives their movements. Dyskinetic patients feel that their movements are involuntary. Akathisic and anxious patients each describe their movements as voluntary, but patients with akathisia often feel irritable or bored, not frightened. If akathisia is misdiagnosed as psychotic anxiety, clinicians can worsen the patient's symptoms by increasing, rather than by decreasing, the antipsychotic.

Treatment of acute akathisia with a benzodiazepine (e.g., 10 mg diazepam) is reasonable, and, if possible, the antipsychotic dose should be lowered. As with RLS, akathisia may respond to the use of dopamine agonists and gabapentin. Although patients with akathisia sometimes tolerate a switch to a more sedating antipsychotic with a lower propensity for akathisia (e.g., quetiapine, clozapine), all antipsychotics, including SGAs and clozapine, can cause akathisia. In mild akathisia, low-dose mirtazapine (7.5 or 15 mg)[29] and high-dose propranolol (at a high-enough dose, starting with 10 mg tid) can suppress akathisia. Of note, anticholinergics—while they are often used in the mistaken belief that they treat all manifestations of EPS—are ineffective for akathisia.

Case 1

John, a 22-year-old college student, was brought to the emergency department (ED) by his friends, who had become increasingly concerned about him. He had been making illogical statements, not attending classes, and staying in his room all day. In the ED, he was found to be psychotic but neither depressed nor manic, and he was psychiatrically admitted. He had no medical problems and there was no substance use. Apparently, he had a similar episode 1 year ago, for which he was briefly admitted and treated with haloperidol.

On the unit, John was initially unwilling to start treatment because he had reacted badly to haloperidol. He remembered from his first hospitalization that he had "neck pulling" and "eyes rolling back into my head," which was frightening and painful. "Nobody warned me that this could happen." His treatment team told him he had an acute dystonic reaction and added benztropine to his haloperidol. He had stopped treatment shortly after being discharged because he "didn't feel right, kind of wired." With some hesitation, he agreed to try a different antipsychotic during this hospitalization. He was discharged on aripiprazole 10 mg/day, greatly improved after a 7-day hospitalization.

When John's outpatient psychiatrist saw him a week after discharge, John appeared visibly uncomfortable, and he was unable to sit still during the interview. He described general restlessness, and anxiety "all over," but he was not clearly psychotic. Walking helped transiently, but the restlessness was otherwise constant. His neurologic examination was normal, except for psychomotor agitation. He displayed no abnormal movement, had normal

muscle tone and muscle strength, and there was no tremor. There were no signs of catatonia.

To manage acute akathisia, the psychiatrist prescribed 5 mg of diazepam twice daily and stopped aripiprazole. The patient's sensitivity to EPS suggested that he would need an antipsychotic with a very low risk of akathisia, that is, quetiapine, as opposed to trying to manage akathisia symptomatically with propranolol or low-dose mirtazapine. If quetiapine turned out to be insufficient to control his psychosis, he might need clozapine to manage his illness. Unfortunately, adherence might already be compromised by having had an acute dystonic reaction and acute akathisia.

Parkinsonism

Antipsychotic-induced parkinsonian symptoms should be managed if they are functionally impairing (e.g., increasing the fall risk or leading to difficulties swallowing) or distressing (e.g., tremors). Parkinsonian symptoms overlap with negative symptoms (the expressivity cluster) and can easily be mistaken for depression. The drug-induced parkinsonian tremor is a coarse, low-frequency, resting tremor that is indistinguishable from the idiopathic resting tremor of PD. Although psychiatrists often try to distinguish idiopathic parkinsonism from drug-induced parkinsonism by the predominance of a unilateral tremor, in the former, their main treatment response should be the same in either case: lower any dopamine blockers, if possible. Parkinsonism can cause a lip tremor—sometimes called a "rabbit tremor" because of its resemblance to a rabbit who is eating—and is more rhythmic than the orobuccal dyskinesia of TD. Unless a patient also has underlying PD, withdrawing the antipsychotic resolves drug-induced parkinsonism, but it may take months for the symptoms to resolve completely. Anticholinergics, such as benztropine (1 or 2 mg twice daily), can suppress parkinsonism in patients with EPS who are unable to tolerate levodopa. Because anticholinergics can cause delirium in the elderly, some clinicians try to use the milder drug, amantadine (100 mg twice daily)[30]; it is an N-methyl-D-aspartate receptor antagonist related to memantine. The risk of exacerbating psychosis is low in patients treated with antipsychotics.

Tardive Dyskinesia

TD is a late complication from treatment with dopamine-blocking agents, usually antipsychotics. One should remember that metoclopramide and prochlorperazine, used widely to manage nausea and migraine headaches, are dopamine antagonists that can cause TD. Risk factors for TD include cumulative antipsychotic exposure, advanced age, and previous experience of EPS. The risk of developing TD from exposure to FGAs is estimated to be 5% per year in young adults.[31] While somewhat lower for SGAs, the risk of TD remains a clinical concern given its usually irreversible nature.[32] Older adults have a much higher risk (25%) per year of developing this complication. Patients with a mood disorder are more likely than those with schizophrenia to develop TD.

The classical movements of TD are involuntary and choreiform; they begin insidiously. Sometimes, a dystonic element can be present. As noted earlier, TD can also co-exist with residual parkinsonian EPS. Movements of TD typically affect the face, but they can also affect the limbs and trunk. Symptoms of TD fluctuate with one's level of arousal. Although TD often does not worsen after the first few months, even mild TD movements can cause social stigma. Voluntary movement can temporarily suppress mild TD; this should not be mistaken for the "distractibility" of a psychosomatic

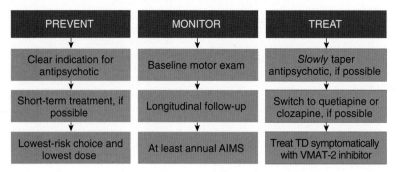

Fig. 10.2 ■ Prevention and treatment of tardive dyskinesia (TD). *AIMS*, Abnormal Involuntary Movement Scale.

movement disorder. Severe TD is so disabling that its constant movements make patients unable to sit in a chair, feed themselves, or hold a book. TD can affect the diaphragm, thereby interrupting breathing.

The best treatment for TD is prevention. A clear indication for the use of antipsychotics should exist, and a low-risk antipsychotic should be chosen. Increasingly, SGAs are used in the management of treatment-resistant depression. The risk-benefit analysis of using this medication class for (non-psychotic) mood disorders must include consideration of TD.[33] Antipsychotics should also be used judiciously in elderly individuals with psychosis, particularly those with dementia where the risk-benefit may be unfavorable. The American Psychiatric Association has published guidelines regarding the use of antipsychotics to treat agitation or psychosis in a patient with dementia.[34] Key recommendations included a quantitative assessment of agitation and psychosis and a periodic assessment of the need for ongoing treatment. Patients who receive antipsychotics in acute care settings to manage delirium should not leave the hospital with an order for an antipsychotic unless ongoing treatment is indicated. Patients who are treated with a maintenance antipsychotic need to be appropriately monitored.[35] Clinicians must examine for TD at every visit, as part of the mental status examination. In addition, a formal examination for TD with the Abnormal Involuntary Movement Scale (AIMS) should be documented periodically. The AIMS should be administered at least annually in routine care and more often to high-risk antipsychotic-treated patients. Instructions for the use of the AIMS are nicely summarized in a classic paper by Munetz and Benjamin.[36] One should obtain a baseline assessment for abnormal motor abnormalities before starting an antipsychotic to document either the presence or absence of any pre-existing motor abnormalities.

The best treatment for TD, once it is recognized, is to stop the offending drug—and to do so slowly. Abrupt discontinuation of an antipsychotic can induce withdrawal dyskinesia that can be severe and even involve respiratory muscles. Any patient with mild TD can convert to having fulminant TD, with respiratory muscle involvement, because the clinician panicked and stopped the drug suddenly, causing a serious rebound.

If ongoing antipsychotic treatment is required, clozapine is the best choice, followed by quetiapine. The treatment of choice for TD is the use of the newer VMAT-2 inhibitors (i.e., valbenazine, deutetrabenazine) that have been shown in clinical trials to reduce the symptoms of TD.[37] However, this class of dopamine-depleting agents can be sedating, worsen mood, and cause parkinsonism. Patients should be monitored for thoughts of suicide if depression develops. VMAT-2 inhibitors do not cure TD; once stopped, the abnormal movements return. Vitamin E used to be given in the hope of preventing TD; however, its use has fallen out of favor as the promising

response seen in initial trials failed to show benefit in subsequent larger trials.[38] For some patients with TD, particularly if there is a dystonic component or focal involvement (e.g., blepharospasm), botulinum toxin injections can help, but they need to be repeated every 3 months.[39] DBS is a treatment of last resort for TD.[40] The basic management principles for TD are summarized in Fig. 10.2.[40]

FUNCTIONAL MOVEMENT DISORDERS

Up to 20% of patients in movement disorder clinics have functional movement disorders (FMDs). Such movements can mimic any of the known movement disorders but appear willful or motivated. The diagnosis of FMD is problematic. All movement disorders affect willed action and the motivation to move—the line between "real" and "psychogenic" disorders is not especially clear. While the *Diagnostic and Statistical Manual of Mental Disorders, Fourth Edition* (DSM-IV) definition of somatoform disorders included having a "non-organic" cause that reflected the intuitive dualism that even trained neuroscientists find hard to resist, the DSM-5 definition of somatic symptom disorder avoids this error.[41]

Observers typically suspect that patients with FMDs are malingering or acting to obtain unconscious secondary gain. However, patients with FMDs do not benefit from their symptoms; they are typically more disabled, more depressed, and more stigmatized than those whose symptoms have a clear physical cause. Patients who malinger typically have symptoms that are more traditional and convincing than the apparently willful symptoms of functional disorders. Classic clues of "psychogenicity," such as *la belle indifference* (lack of concern for the medical problem) are highly unreliable. Clinicians should also not depend on the perceived "bizarreness" of the movements. Sudden unexplained onsets and full remissions suggest an FMD. Not falling despite wild flailing movements (astasia-abasia) suggests a functional disorder. Improvement of the symptom with distraction is often misdiagnosed since most movement disorders are highly influenced by attention, anxiety, and movement of other body parts. A more reliable sign is the entrainment of a tremor to the voluntary tapping of another body part at a new frequency.

Mass psychogenic illness (also referred to as mass sociogenic illness) is an interesting phenomenon that can produce epidemics of FMDs. Such outbreaks are not only of historical interest (e.g., Saint Vitus dance in the Middle Ages during the Black Death or hysterical illnesses in the Salem witch trials) but continue to occur. For example, a recent outbreak affected about 20 teenagers in Le Roy, New York.[41] Mass psychogenic illnesses show us the importance of role expectations, social learning, and social networks, including social media.[42] In the specific context of a modern Western society, fears of toxins combined with distrust of industry and a cover-up by the state (all not necessarily unfounded) combine to produce psychogenic illness in a susceptible group, where an initial index case allows for spread to those in the social network. Recognizing mass psychogenic illness is as difficult at the level of a group as it is for individual patients, as one can "never be sure" that there is no toxin. Endless investigations can never clearly settle the case, just like more laboratory tests can never put to rest the idea that one might have a yet-to-be-discovered illness. Mass psychogenic illness requires recognition and prevention of spread. In many cases, opinion leaders need to be separated from the larger group. Media attention and rapid spread through social media unfortunately make containment next to impossible.

Neurologists typically perform exhaustive tests to rule out rare disorders that can cause abnormal movements and wait until all are negative to discuss psychiatric factors that may contribute to the symptoms. It is better for both neurologists and psychiatrists to be involved from the start if a functional disorder is likely. Neurology needs to be involved since it is difficult to ascertain the functional character of movements unless clinical experience is there to recognize functional unsteadiness (astasia-abasia). Psychiatry, on the other hand, can identify treatable psychiatric disorders and work with patients' psychological responses to their symptoms and build coping skills. However, quite frequently, patients resist referral to psychiatric practitioners, and one could argue that roughly 50% of those without psychiatric psychopathology or distress have a point (i.e., there does not seem to be a conversion from psychological conflict to bodily expression). Unfortunately, these patients get stuck if neurologists feel that they have little else to offer beyond offering a diagnosis.

When and how should you tell a patient that their movements are "functional?" One should not wait until "every possible test" has been done; instead, one should discuss anxiety and other psychiatric aspects of their symptoms at the beginning of their neurologic work-up. Most patients are firmly committed to finding a traditional medical explanation whose severity explains their subjective sense that there is something terribly wrong with their body. Rather than telling a patient "Don't worry, your tremor is just anxiety," consider re-framing your description physiologically, for example, "past stress has raised your adrenaline levels, and adrenaline causes tremors." Explain that their symptoms have "real" brain correlates (i.e., altered neurocircuitry) in functional neuroimaging studies. The term "psychogenic" is best avoided as patients feel dismissed. Direct the patients to www.neurosymptoms.org, an excellent self-help website for patients who want to educate themselves about FMDs.[43]

Doctors become frustrated by patients with functional symptoms when they do not know how to help them and if they believe that the patient does not truly want to get better. Cognitive-behavioral therapy, however, is one psychological treatment modality that can help.[44] Specialized physical and occupational therapies have been developed.[45] Psychotropics can be used judiciously to address distress. A solid doctor-patient relationship that conveys sincere caring and a hopeful approach with symptom remission as a goal can prevent chronicity.

REFERENCES

1. Bhidayasiri R, Tarsy D. *Movement Disorders: A Video Atlas.* Humana Press; 2012.
2. Reich SG, Savitt JM. Parkinson's disease. *Med Clin North Am.* 2019;103:337–350.
3. Menza M. The personality associated with Parkinson's disease. *Curr Psychiatry Rep.* 2000;2:421–426.
4. O'Sullivan SS, Evans AH, Lees AJ. Dopamine dysregulation syndrome: an overview of its epidemiology, mechanisms and management. *CNS Drugs.* 2009;23:157–170.
5. Evans AH, Stegeman JR. Punding in patients on dopamine agonists for restless leg syndrome. *Mov Disord.* 2009;24:140–141.
6. Menza M, Dobkin RD, Marin H, et al. A controlled trial of antidepressants in patients with Parkinson disease and depression. *Neurology.* 2009;72:886–892.
7. Richard IH, McDermott MP, Kurlan R, et al. A randomized, double-blind, placebo-controlled trial of antidepressants in Parkinson disease. *Neurology.* 2012;78:1229–1236.
8. Ji N, Meng P, Xu B, et al. Efficacy and safety of pramipexole in Parkinson's disease with anxiety or depression: a meta-analysis of randomized clinical trials. *Am J Transl Res.* 2022;14:1757–1764.
9. Riedel O, Klotsche J, Spottke A, et al. Cognitive impairment in 873 patients with idiopathic Parkinson's disease. Results from the German Study on Epidemiology of Parkinson's Disease with Dementia (GEPAD). *J Neurol.* 2008;255:255–264.
10. Hely MA, Reid WG, Adena MA, et al. The Sydney multicenter study of Parkinson's disease: the inevitability of dementia at 20 years. *Mov Disord.* 2008;23:837–844.
11. Walker Z, Possin KL, Boeve BF, et al. Lewy body dementias. *Lancet.* 2015;386:1683–1697.
12. Kyle K, Bronstein JM. Treatment of psychosis in Parkinson's disease and dementia with Lewy Bodies: a review. *Parkinsonism Relat Disord.* 2020;75:55–62.
13. Mansuri Z, Reddy A, Vadukapuram R, et al. Pimavanserin in the treatment of Parkinson's disease psychosis: meta-analysis and meta-regression of randomized clinical trials. *Innov Clin Neurosci.* 2022;19:46–51.
14. Howell MJ, Schenck CH. Rapid eye movement sleep behavior disorder and neurodegenerative disease. *JAMA Neurol.* 2015;72:707–712.
15. Brust JC. Substance abuse and movement disorders. *Mov Disord.* 2010;25:2010–2020.
16. Baig SS, Strong M, Rosser E, et al. 22 years of predictive testing for Huntington's disease: the experience of the UK Huntington's Prediction Consortium. *Eur J Hum Genet.* 2016;24:1396–1402.
17. Dutta N, Cavanna AE. The effectiveness of habit reversal therapy in the treatment of Tourette syndrome and other chronic tic disorders: a systematic review. *Funct Neurol.* 2013;28:7–12.
18. Tourette's Syndrome Study Group. Treatment of ADHD in children with tics: a randomized controlled trial. *Neurology.* 2002;58:527–536.
19. Pringsheim T, Okun MS, Muller-Vahl K, et al. Practice guideline recommendations summary: treatment of tics in people with Tourette syndrome and chronic tic disorders. *Neurology.* 2019;92:896–906.
20. Schilsky ML, Roberts EA, Bronstein JM, et al. A multidisciplinary approach to the diagnosis and management of Wilson disease: executive summary of the 2022 Practice Guidance on Wilson disease from the American Association for the Study of Liver Diseases. *Hepatology.* 2023;77:1428–1455.
21. Trenkwalder C, Allen R, Hogl B, et al. Restless legs syndrome associated with major diseases: a systematic review and new concept. *Neurology.* 2016;86:1336–1343.
22. Manconi M, Garcia-Borreguero D, Schormair B, et al. Restless legs syndrome. *Nat Rev Dis Primers.* 2021;7:80.
23. Louis ED, Okun MS. It is time to remove the 'benign' from the essential tremor label. *Parkinsonism Relat Disord.* 2011;17:516–520.
24. Baek JH, Kinrys G, Nierenberg AA. Lithium tremor revisited: pathophysiology and treatment. *Acta Psychiatr Scand.* 2014;129:17–23.
25. Niethammer M, Ford B. Permanent lithium-induced cerebellar toxicity: three cases and review of literature. *Mov Disord.* 2007;22:570–573.
26. Barone P, Santangelo G, Amboni M, et al. Pisa syndrome in Parkinson's disease and parkinsonism: clinical features, pathophysiology, and treatment. *Lancet Neurol.* 2016;15:1063–1074.
27. Janno S, Holi M, Tuisku K, et al. Prevalence of neuroleptic-induced movement disorders in chronic schizophrenia inpatients. *Am J Psychiatry.* 2004;161:160–163.
28. Parksepp M, Ljubajev U, Taht K, et al. Prevalence of neuroleptic-induced movement disorders: an 8-year follow-up study in chronic schizophrenia inpatients. *Nord J Psychiatry.* 2016;70:498–502.
29. Poyurovsky M, Weizman A. Treatment of antipsychotic-induced akathisia: role of serotonin 5-HT(2a) receptor antagonists. *Drugs.* 2020;80:871–882.
30. McEvoy JP. A double-blind crossover comparison of antiparkinson drug therapy: amantadine versus anticholinergics in 90 normal volunteers, with an emphasis on differential effects on memory function. *J Clin Psychiatry.* 1987;48(suppl):20–23.

31. Jeste DV, Caligiuri MP. Tardive dyskinesia. *Schizophr Bull.* 1993;19:303–315.
32. Carbon M, Hsieh CH, Kane JM, et al. Tardive dyskinesia prevalence in the period of second-generation antipsychotic use: a meta-analysis. *J Clin Psychiatry.* 2017;78:e264–e278.
33. Jha MK, Mathew SJ. Pharmacotherapies for treatment-resistant depression: how antipsychotics fit in the rapidly evolving therapeutic landscape. *Am J Psychiatry.* 2023;180:190–199.
34. Reus VI, Fochtmann LJ, Eyler AE, et al. The American Psychiatric Association Practice Guideline on the Use of Antipsychotics to Treat Agitation or Psychosis in Patients With Dementia. *Am J Psychiatry.* 2016;173:543–546.
35. Caroff SN, Citrome L, Meyer J, et al. A modified Delphi consensus study of the screening, diagnosis, and treatment of tardive dyskinesia. *J Clin Psychiatry.* 2020;81..
36. Munetz MR, Benjamin S. How to examine patients using the Abnormal Involuntary Movement Scale. *Hosp Community Psychiatry.* 1988;39:1172–1177.
37. Solmi M, Pigato G, Kane JM, et al. Treatment of tardive dyskinesia with VMAT-2 inhibitors: a systematic review and meta-analysis of randomized controlled trials. *Drug Des Devel Ther.* 2018;12:1215–1238.
38. Adler LA, Rotrosen J, Edson R, et al. Vitamin E treatment for tardive dyskinesia. Veterans Affairs Cooperative Study #394 Study Group. *Arch Gen Psychiatry.* 1999;56:836–841.
39. Anandan C, Jankovic J. Botulinum toxin in movement disorders: an update. *Toxins (Basel).* 2021;13(1):42..
40. Szczakowska A, Gabryelska A, Gawlik-Kotelnicka O, et al. Deep brain stimulation in the treatment of tardive dyskinesia. *J Clin Med.* 2023;12(5):1868..
41. Mink JW. Conversion disorder and mass psychogenic illness in child neurology. *Ann N Y Acad Sci.* 2013;1304:40–44.
42. Muller-Vahl KR, Pisarenko A, Jakubovski E, et al. Stop that! It's not Tourette's but a new type of mass sociogenic illness. *Brain.* 2022;145:476–480.
43. *Functional Neurological Disorders.* Available from: https://neuro-symptoms.org/en/
44. Sharpe M, Walker J, Williams C, et al. Guided self-help for functional (psychogenic) symptoms: a randomized controlled efficacy trial. *Neurology.* 2011;77:564–572.
45. Maggio JB, Ospina JP, Callahan J, et al. Outpatient physical therapy for functional neurological disorder: a preliminary feasibility and naturalistic outcome study in a U.S. cohort. *J Neuropsychiatry Clin Neurosci.* 2020;32:85–89.

11 Pathophysiology, Psychiatric Co-morbidity, and Treatment of Pain

Menekse Alpay, Shamim H. Nejad, and Gregory Alexander Acampora

KEY POINTS

- Psychiatric co-morbidity is common among patients with pain syndromes.
- Specific terminology is used to characterize pain and pain syndromes.
- Pain is transmitted in pathways involving the peripheral and central nervous systems.
- Psychiatric treatment can effectively treat pain and its common co-morbidities.
- Multi-modal and multi-disciplinary treatment facilitates relief from chronic pain.

OVERVIEW

Pain, defined in 1979 by the International Association for the Study of Pain as "an unpleasant sensory and emotional experience associated with actual or potential tissue damage or described in terms of such damage," was revised in 2020 and now centers on an individual's experience of pain.[1] This chapter describes pain terminology, pain assessment, and the physiological aspects of pain and discusses the major classes of medications used to relieve pain; in addition, the diagnosis and treatment of psychiatric conditions that affect patients with chronic pain are reviewed.

EPIDEMIOLOGY

Psychiatric co-morbidity (e.g., anxiety, depression, personality disorders, post-traumatic stress disorder [PTSD], and substance use disorders [SUDs]) affects those with both cancer-related pain and non–cancer-related pain. Epidemiological studies indicate that roughly 30% of those in the general population with chronic musculoskeletal pain also experience depression or an anxiety disorder.[2] Similar rates exist in those with cancer pain.[3] In clinic populations, roughly 50% to 80% of patients with pain have co-morbid psychopathology, including problematic personality traits. The personality (i.e., the characterological or temperamental) component of negative affect had been termed *neuroticism*, in which patients experience anger, disgust, sadness, anxiety, and a variety of other negative emotions.[4] It can lead to maladaptive behaviors that have an adverse impact on the response to pain.[5]

Rates of SUDs (15%–26%) involving illicit drugs or prescription medications are elevated in those with chronic pain relative to those in the general population.[6] Opioid use disorders (OUDs) are an increasing prevalent problem among those who are prescribed repeated opioid prescriptions for chronic pain. This chapter concentrates on individuals with an underlying mood disorder or somatic disorder in the context of chronic pain.

PATHOPHYSIOLOGY OF PAIN TRANSMISSION

Detection of noxious stimuli (i.e., nociception) starts with the activation of peripheral nociceptors (that results in somatic pain) or with the activation of nociceptors in bodily organs (that leads to visceral pain).

Tissue injury stimulates the nociceptors by the liberation of adenosine triphosphate (ATP), kinins, and arachidonic acid from injured cells; histamine, serotonin, prostaglandins, and bradykinin from mast cells; and cytokines and nerve growth factor from macrophages. These substances and a decreased pH cause a decrease in the threshold for activation of nociceptors, a process called *peripheral sensitization*. Subsequently, axons transmit the pain signal to the spinal cord and to cell bodies in the dorsal root ganglia (Figure 11.1). Three different types of axons are involved in the transmission of pain from the skin to the dorsal horn. A-β fibers are the largest and most heavily myelinated fibers that transmit the awareness of light touch. A-Δ fibers and C fibers are the primary nociceptive afferents. A-Δ fibers are 2 to 5 μcm in diameter and are thinly myelinated. They conduct "first pain," which is immediate, rapid, and sharp, with a velocity of 20 m/s. C fibers are 0.2 to 1.5 μcm in diameter and are unmyelinated. They conduct "second pain," which is prolonged, burning, and unpleasant, at a speed of 0.5 m/s. A-Δ and C fibers enter the dorsal root and ascend or descend one to three segments before synapsing with neurons in the lateral spinothalamic tract (in the substantia gelatinosa in the gray matter) (see Figure 11.1). Second pain transmitted with C fibers is integrally related to chronic pain states. Repetitive C-fiber stimulation can result in a progressive increase of electrical discharges from second-order neurons in the spinal cord. *N*-methyl-D-aspartate receptors play a role when prolonged activation occurs. This pain amplification is related to a temporal summation of the second pain or "wind-up." This hyperexcitability of neurons in the dorsal horn contributes to central sensitization, which can occur as an immediate or delayed phenomenon. In addition to wind-up, central sensitization involves several factors: activation of A-β fibers and lowered firing thresholds for spinal cord cells that modulate pain (i.e., they trigger pain more easily); neuroplasticity (a result of functional changes, including recruitment of a wide range of cells in the spinal cord so that touch or movement causes pain); convergence of cutaneous, vascular, muscle, and joint inputs (where one tissue refers pain to another); or aberrant connections (electrical short-circuits between the sympathetic and sensory nerves that produce causalgia). Inhibition of nociception in the dorsal horn is quite important. Stimulation of the A-Δ fibers not only excites some neurons but also inhibits others. This inhibition of nociception

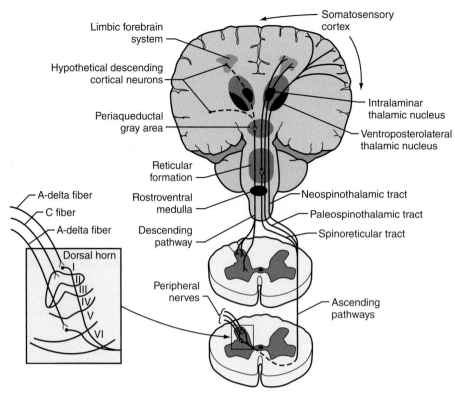

Figure 11.1 Schematic diagram of neurological pathways for pain perception. (From Hyman SH, Cassem NH. Pain. In: Rubenstein E, Federman DD, eds. *Scientific American Medicine: Current Topics in Medicine*. Subsection II. Scientific American; 1989. Originally from Stern TA, Herman JB, eds. *Psychiatry Update and Board Preparation*. McGraw-Hill; 2004.)

through A-Δ fiber stimulation may explain the effects of acupuncture and transcutaneous electrical nerve stimulation.

The lateral spinothalamic tract crosses the midline and ascends toward the thalamus. At the level of the brainstem, more than half of this tract synapses in the reticular activating system (in an area called the spinoreticular tract), in the limbic system, and in other brainstem regions (including centers of the autonomic nervous system). Another site of projections at this level is the periaqueductal gray (PAG) (Figure 11.2), which plays an important role in the brain's system of endogenous analgesia. After synapsing in the thalamic nuclei, pain fibers project to the somatosensory cortex, located posterior to the Sylvian fissure in the parietal lobe, in Brodmann's areas 1, 2, and 3. Endogenous analgesic systems involve endogenous peptides with opioid-like activity in the central nervous system (CNS) (e.g., endorphins, enkephalins, and dynorphins). Different opioid receptors (μ, κ, and δ receptors) are involved in different opiate effects. The centers involved in endogenous analgesia include the PAG, the anterior cingulate cortex (ACC), the amygdala, the parabrachial plexus (in the pons), and the rostral ventromedial medulla.

The descending analgesic pain pathway starts in the PAG (which is rich in endogenous opiates), projects to the rostral ventral medulla, and from there descends through the dorsolateral funiculus of the spinal cord to the dorsal horn. The neurons in the rostral ventral medulla use serotonin to activate endogenous analgesics (enkephalins) in the dorsal horn. This effect inhibits nociception at the level of the dorsal horn because neurons that contain enkephalins synapse with spinothalamic neurons. Additionally, there are noradrenergic neurons that project from the locus coeruleus (the main noradrenergic center in the CNS) to the dorsal horn and inhibit the response of dorsal horn neurons to nociceptive stimuli. The analgesic effect of tricyclic antidepressants (TCAs) and the

serotonin–norepinephrine reuptake inhibitors (SNRIs) is thought to be related to an increase in serotonin and norepinephrine (noradrenaline) that inhibits nociception at the level of the dorsal horn, through their effects on enhancing descending pain inhibition from above.

CORTICAL SUBSTRATES FOR PAIN AND AFFECT

Advances in neuroimaging have linked the function of multiple brain areas with pain and affect. These areas (e.g., the ACC, the insula, and the dorsolateral prefrontal cortex [DLPFC]) form functional units through which psychiatric co-morbidity may amplify pain and disability (see Figure 11.2). These areas are part of the spinolimbic (also known as the medial) pain pathway,[7] which runs parallel to the spinothalamic tract and receives direct input from the dorsal horn of the spinal cord. The interactions among these areas, pain perception, and psychiatric illness are still being investigated. The spinolimbic pathway is involved in descending pain inhibition (that involves cortical and subcortical structures), whose function may be negatively affected by the presence of psychopathology. This in turn could lead to heightened pain perception. Coghill[8] has shown that differences in pain sensitivity between patients can be correlated with differences in activation patterns in the ACC, the insula, and the DLPFC. The anticipation of pain is also modulated by these areas, suggesting a mechanism by which anxiety related to pain can amplify pain perception. The disruption or alteration of descending pain inhibition is a mechanism of neuropathic pain, which can be described as *central sensitization* that occurs at the level of the brain, a concept supported by recent neuroimaging studies of pain processing in the brains of patients with fibromyalgia.[9] The ACC, the insula, and the DLPFC are also laden with opioid receptors, which are less responsive to endogenous opioids in pain-free

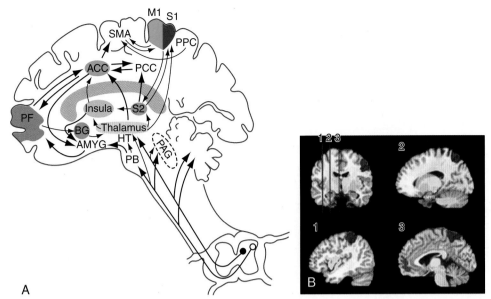

Figure 11.2 Pain processing in the brain. Locations of brain regions involved in pain perception are color coded in a schematic (A) and in an example magnetic resonance imaging (MRI) scan (B). **A**, Schematic shows the regions, their inter-connectivity, and afferent pathways. **B**, The areas corresponding to those in (A) are shown in an anatomical MRI, on a coronal slice, and on three sagittal slices as indicated on the coronal slice. The six areas used in meta-analysis are primary and secondary somatosensory cortices (S1 and S2, *red* and *orange*), anterior cingulated (*ACC, green*), insula *(blue)*, thalamus *(yellow)*, and prefrontal cortex (*PF, purple*). Other regions indicated include primary and supplementary motor cortices (*M1* and *SMA*), posterior parietal cortex (*PPC*), posterior cingulated (*PCC*), basal ganglia (*BG, pink*), hypothalamic (*HT*), amygdala (*AMYG*), parabrachial nuclei (*PB*), and periaqueductal gray (*PAG*). (Redrawn from Apkarian AV, Bushnell MC, Treede RD, et al. Human brain mechanisms of pain perception and regulation in health and disease. *Eur J Pain*. 2005;9:463-484.)

participants with high negative affect.[10] Thus, negative affect may diminish the effectiveness of endogenous and exogenous opioids through direct effects on supraspinal opioid binding.

INTERACTIONS BETWEEN PAIN AND PSYCHOPATHOLOGY

Most patients with chronic pain and psychiatric conditions have a physical basis for their pain. However, the perception of pain is amplified by co-morbid psychiatric disorders, which predispose people to develop chronic pain. This is commonly referred to as the *diathesis-stress model*, also called the vulnerability-stress model, in which the combination of physical, social, and psychological stresses associated with pain induces significant psychiatric co-morbidity.[5] This can occur in those with or without a pre-existing vulnerability to psychiatric illness (e.g., a genetic or temperamental risk factor). Patients with chronic pain and psychopathology report greater pain intensity, more pain-related disability, and a greater affective component to their pain than those without psychopathology. Overall, it is not the specific qualities or symptomatology of depression, anxiety, or neuroticism that predict poor outcomes but the overall levels of psychiatric symptoms.[11] Depression, anxiety, and neuroticism are the psychiatric states that most often co-occur in those with chronic pain; those with several conditions are predisposed to the worst outcomes.

PAIN TERMINOLOGY

Acute pain is usually related to an identifiable injury or to a disease; it is self-limited and resolves over hours to days or in a time frame that is associated with injury and healing. Acute pain is usually associated with objective autonomic features (e.g., tachycardia, hypertension, diaphoresis, mydriasis, or pallor).

Chronic pain (i.e., pain that persists beyond the normal time of healing or lasts longer than 6 months) involves different mechanisms in local, spinal, and supraspinal levels. Characteristic features include vague descriptions of pain and an inability to describe the pain's timing and localization. It is usually helpful to determine the presence of a dermatomal pattern (Figure 11.3), to determine the presence of neuropathic pain, and to assess pain behavior.

Neuropathic pain is a disorder of neuromodulation. It is caused by an injured or dysfunctional central or peripheral nervous system; it is manifest by spontaneous, sharp, shooting, or burning pain, which may be distributed along dermatomes. Deafferentation pain, phantom limb pain, complex regional pain syndrome, diabetic neuropathy, central pain syndrome, trigeminal neuralgia, and postherpetic neuralgia are examples of neuropathic pain. Qualities of neuropathic pain include hyperalgesia (an increased response to stimuli that are normally painful); hyperesthesia (an exaggerated pain response to noxious stimuli [e.g., pressure or heat]), allodynia (pain with a stimulus not normally painful [e.g., light touch or cool air]), and hyperpathia (pain from a painful stimulus with a delay and a persistence that is distributed beyond the area of stimulation). Both acute and chronic pain conditions can involve neuropathic processes in addition to nociceptive causes of pain.

Idiopathic pain, previously referred to as *psychogenic pain*, is poorly understood. The presence of pain does not imply or exclude a psychological component. Typically, there is no evidence of an associated organic etiology or an anatomical pattern consistent with symptoms. Symptoms are often grossly out of proportion to an identifiable organic pathology.

Myofascial pain can arise from one or several of the following problems: hypertonic muscles, myofascial trigger points, arthralgias, and fatigue with muscle weakness. Myofascial pain is generally used to describe pain from muscles and connective tissue. Myofascial pain results from a primary

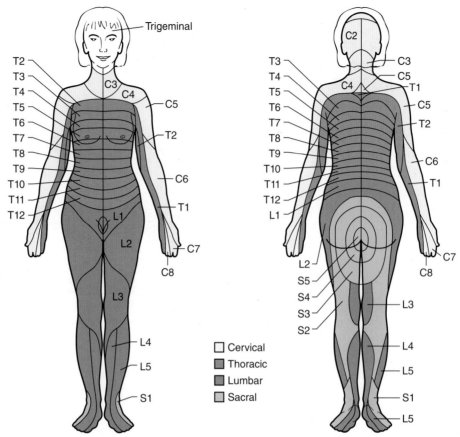

Figure 11.3 Schematic diagram of segmental neuronal innervation by dermatomes. (From Hyman SH, Cassem NH. Pain. In: Rubenstein E, Federman DD, eds. *Scientific American Medicine: Current Topics in Medicine.* Subsection II, Scientific American; 1989.)

condition (e.g., fibromyalgia) or, as more often is the case, a co-morbid process (e.g., with vascular headaches or with a psychiatric diagnosis).

ASSESSMENT OF PAIN

The evaluation of pain initially focuses on five questions: (1) Is the pain intractable because of nociceptive stimuli (e.g., from the skin, bones, muscles, or blood vessels)? (2) Is the pain maintained by non-nociceptive mechanisms (i.e., have the spinal cord, brainstem, limbic system, and cortex been recruited as reverberating pain circuits)? (3) Is the complaint of pain primary (as occurs in disorders such as major depression or delusional disorder)? (4) Is there a more efficacious pharmacological treatment? (5) Have pain behavior and disability become more important than the pain itself? Answering these questions allows the mechanism(s) of the pain and suffering to be pursued. A psychiatrist's physical examination of the patient in pain typically includes examination of the painful area, muscles, and response to pinprick and light touch (Table 11.1).

The experience of pain is always subjective. However, several sensitive and reliable clinical instruments for the measurement of pain are available. These include the following:

1. The *pain drawing* that involves having the patient draw the anatomical distribution of the pain as it is felt in his or her body
2. The visual analog scale (VAS) and numerical rating scales that use a VAS from "no pain" to "pain as bad as it could possibly be" on a 10-cm baseline or a 0 to 10 scale on which the patient can rate pain on a scale of 1 to 10. It is also exquisitely sensitive

TABLE 11.1 General Physical Examination of Pain by a Psychiatrist

Physical Finding	Purpose of Examination
Motor deficits	Does the patient give way when checking strength?
	Does the person try?
	Is there a pseudoparesis, astasia-abasia, or involuntary movement that suggests a somatoform disorder?
Trigger points in head, neck, shoulder, and back muscles	Are common myofascial trigger points present that suggest myofascial pain?
	Is there evoked pain (such as allodynia, hyperpathia, or anesthesia) that suggests neuropathic pain?
Evanescent, changeable pain, weakness, and numbness	Does the psychological complaint pre-empt the physical?
Abnormal sensory findings	Does lateral anesthesia to pinprick end sharply at the midline?
	Is there topographical confusion?
	Is there a non-dermatomal distribution of pain and sensation that suggests either a somatoform or CNS pain disorder?
	Is there an abnormal sensation that suggests neuropathy or CNS pain?
Sympathetic or vascular dysfunction	Is there swelling, skin discoloration, or changes in sweating or temperature that suggests a vascular or sympathetic element to the pain?
Uncooperativeness, erratic responses to the physical examination	Is there an interpersonal aspect to the pain, causing abnormal pain behavior, as in somatoform disease?

CNS, Central nervous system.

3. The Pain Intensity Scale that is a categorical rating scale that consists of three to six categories for the ranking of pain severity (e.g., no pain, mild pain, moderate pain, severe pain, very severe pain, worst pain possible).

CORE PSYCHOPATHOLOGY AND PAIN-RELATED PSYCHOLOGICAL SYMPTOMS

In patients with chronic pain, heightened emotional distress, negative affect, and elevated pain-related psychological symptoms (i.e., those that are a direct result of chronic pain, and when the pain is eliminated, the symptoms disappear) can all be considered as forms of psychopathology and psychiatric co-morbidity because they represent impairments in mental health and involve maladaptive psychological responses to medical illness (Figure 11.4). This approach combines classification methods from psychiatry and behavioral medicine to describe the scope of psychiatric disturbances in patients with chronic pain. In those with pain, the most common manifestations of psychiatric co-morbidity involve one or more core psychopathologies in combination with pain-related psychological symptoms. Unfortunately, not all patients and their symptoms fit precisely into the *Diagnostic and Statistical Manual of Mental Disorders* (DSM) categories of illness.

Pain-related anxiety, which includes state and trait anxiety related to pain, is the form of anxiety most germane to pain.[12] Elevated levels of pain-related anxiety, such as fear of pain, also meet *Diagnostic and Statistical Manual of Mental Disorders, Fifth Edition* (DSM-5), criteria for an anxiety disorder due to a general medical condition. Because anxiety is present in both domains of core psychopathology and pain-related psychological symptoms, the assessment of anxiety in a patient with chronic pain (as detailed below) must include a review of manifestations of generalized anxiety as well as pain-specific anxiety symptoms (e.g., physiological changes associated with the anticipation of pain).

Limited coping skills are often linked to pain-related psychological symptoms and behaviors that include passive responses to chronic pain (e.g., remaining bed-bound), catastrophizing (including cognitive distortions centered around pain and mistakenly assuming chronic pain is indicative of ongoing tissue damage), and low self-efficacy (i.e., with a low estimate by the patient of what he or she is capable of doing).[13] Patients with limited coping mechanisms use few self-management strategies (such as using ice, heat, or relaxation strategies). A tendency to catastrophize often predicts poor outcomes and disability, independent of other psychopathologies, such as major depression. The duration of chronic pain and psychiatric co-morbidity are each independent predictors of pain intensity and disability. High levels of anger, which tend to occur more often in men, can also explain a significant variance in pain severity.[14]

PAIN AND CO-MORBID PSYCHIATRIC CONDITIONS

Virtually all psychiatric conditions are treatable in individuals with chronic pain, and most patients who are provided with appropriate treatment improve significantly. Many physicians who treat pain often do not realize that this is the case. Major depressive disorder (MDD) and anxiety disorders are the disorders that most often affect patients with chronic pain; however, they have the best response to medications. Whenever possible, medications that are effective for psychiatric illness and that have independent analgesic properties should be used. *Independent analgesia* refers to the efficacy of a pain medication such as a TCA or an SNRI for neuropathic pain, which is independent of its effect on mood.[15]

Regardless of the type of psychopathology present, improvement in psychiatric symptoms may result in the reduction of pain levels, greater acceptance of the pain's chronicity, improved function, and improved quality of life. Chronic pain may precipitate or worsen psychopathology, and psychopathology may worsen pain. It is important for physicians who treat patients with pain to recognize psychiatric illness early in the course of pain and to treat both conditions. In general, as with most psychiatric illnesses, a combination of pharmacological and psychotherapeutic treatments is more effective in treating depression and anxiety in those with pain than with pharmacological treatment alone. There is good evidence that psychiatric co-morbidity can be successfully treated even if the pain does not improve.

Major Depression

The diagnosis and treatment of MDD in a patient with chronic pain is not significantly different from the approach to MDD in an individual with co-morbid medical illness. The combination of medications and cognitive-behavioral therapy (CBT) yields the best outcome.

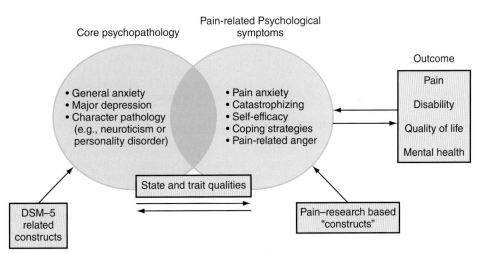

Figure 11.4 Common psychiatric symptoms in patients with chronic pain. *DSM-5, Diagnostic and Statistical Manual of Mental Disorders*, Fifth Edition.

Symptoms

Major depressive disorder can be diagnosed, using DSM-5 or similar research criteria, in approximately 15% of those who have chronic pain and in 50% of individuals evaluated in chronic pain clinics. Recurrent affective illness, a family history of depression, and other psychiatric conditions (e.g., anxiety or SUDs) are often present. MDD can be distinguished from situational depression (also termed *demoralization* or an *adjustment disorder with depressed mood*) by the triad of persistently low mood, neurovegetative symptoms, and changes in self-attitude that last at least 2 weeks.[16] It may be important to distinguish which neurovegetative signs (such as disturbed sleep) are the result of pain and which are the result of depression. However, given the high rate of co-morbid depression in patients with chronic pain, it is prudent to err on the side of attributing neurovegetative symptoms to depression, particularly if they are accompanied by changes in mood or self-attitude. MDD is a serious complication of persistent pain; if not treated effectively, it will likely reduce the effectiveness of all pain treatments. Even low levels of depression ("subthreshold depression") may worsen the physical impairment associated with chronic pain, and it should be treated.

Medication Treatment

Patients with pain and MDD tend to be more treatment-resistant, particularly when their pain is not effectively managed.[17] In general, the first-line agent for a patient in pain is an agent with independent analgesic properties. Among the antidepressants, these include TCAs and SNRIs (duloxetine and venlafaxine). Each has shown efficacy in a variety of neuropathic pain conditions. The details of prescribing a specific antidepressant are covered elsewhere in this text.

Selective Serotonin Reuptake Inhibitors. Since the introduction of fluoxetine (Prozac) in 1987, many selective serotonin reuptake inhibitors (SSRIs) have been developed. The antidepressant efficacy and low side effect profile of SSRIs have made them the most widely prescribed class of antidepressants. Patients with pain whose depression responds to an SSRI may experience less pain, a finding that is attributable to improvements in the affective components of their pain; however, there is little evidence to support the independent analgesic activity of SSRIs. SSRIs should not be prescribed in conjunction with tramadol because of the heightened risk of seizures.

Other Antidepressants. Bupropion and mirtazapine are atypical antidepressants with unique mechanisms of action. Some preliminary evidence indicates that they have analgesic properties, but further study is required. Bupropion is particularly useful in those with pain because of its activating effects that lessen fatigue. Mirtazapine is helpful in patients with impaired sleep, anxiety, and depression. It may be helpful in those with myofascial pain disorders, such as fibromyalgia.

Coping and Psychotherapy

Improving coping skills is a mainstay of the treatment for any psychiatric condition associated with chronic pain. In addition to improving psychological distress, the use of active coping strategies improves pain and function (e.g., remaining active despite the pain). Coping involves using adaptive defense mechanisms to negotiate maladaptive thoughts and feelings that arise in response to pain.

The psychodynamic aspects of coping often involve conflicts over autonomy and care. Regression can be manifest as non-adherence, help-rejecting complaining, and behaviors akin to the metaphorical "cutting off your nose to spite your face." Pain may make both patients and physicians appear hateful;

psychiatrists are well served by clarifying how these problems get played out in the physician–patient relationship. To help their patients cope, psychiatrists must be sensitive to the unconscious feelings of their patients; in addition, denial must be managed, and family counseling, relaxation, exercise, physical rehabilitation, and pharmacotherapy should be considered.

Cognitive-behavioral therapy in conjunction with antidepressant therapy is the most efficacious treatment for MDD, including MDD that is exacerbated in the setting of chronic pain. Typically, CBT improves coping skills and self-efficacy and diminishes catastrophizing. When CBT is used, the patient must be motivated, have sufficient insight, and have the ego strength to tolerate challenges to his or her beliefs. CBT for patients in pain focuses on the thoughts and cognitive distortions that surround chronic pain (such as fear of re-injury, the belief that the only meaningful life is one without pain, and thoughts that the patient's pain is not taken seriously by others).

Anxiety Disorders

Symptoms

Anxiety disorders encompass a broad spectrum of disorders (including generalized anxiety disorder [GAD], panic disorder, obsessive-compulsive disorder, and PTSD). In addition, pain-related anxiety is the most common manifestation of anxiety in those with chronic pain.[12] Anxiety is prevalent in patients who attend chronic pain clinics, with 30% to 60% of patients experiencing pathological anxiety.[18] Among the anxiety disorders, GAD is the condition that most often affects patients in pain. More than 50% of patients with anxiety disorders also have MDD or a history of MDD or another psychiatric disorder. Alcohol use disorders and SUDs commonly accompany chronic pain; consequently, recognition and treatment of co-morbid depression and substance abuse are critical to long-term treatment outcomes.

In individuals with pain, situational (state) anxiety may be centered on the pain itself and its negative consequences (pain anxiety). Patients may have conditioned fear, believing that activities will cause uncontrollable pain, causing avoidance of those activities. Pain may also activate thoughts that a person is seriously ill.[12] Several questions can be helpful: "Does the pain make you panic? If you think about your pain, do you feel that your heart is beating fast? Do you have an overwhelming feeling of dread or doom? Do you experience a sense of sudden anxiety that overwhelms you?"

Anxiety amplifies both the perception and complaints of pain through several bio-psycho-social mechanisms (e.g., sympathetic arousal that lowers the nociceptive threshold, increased firing of ectopically active pain neurons, excessive focusing on pain symptoms, and implementation of poor coping skills). Patients with pathological anxiety are often restless, fatigued, irritable, and concentrate poorly. They may also have muscle tension and sleep disturbances.

Treatment

Overall, CBT demonstrates the best treatment outcomes for anxiety disorders, including pain-specific anxiety in patients with chronic pain. Further improvement can be obtained with relaxation therapy, meditation, and biofeedback. Physical therapy by itself, with no other psychological treatment, is effective for addressing the fear of pain (termed *kinesiophobia*, the fear of movement because of pain). A flexibility program that addresses muscle disuse (which by itself creates pain) and imparts several psychological insights: activity and function can be improved, despite high pain levels. It is more meaningful to be active with pain than to remain inactive with pain, and the fear of pain and re-injury can be diminished. Antidepressants are also effective, but they may need to be used at higher doses than are typically prescribed for depression. Anxiolytics (such as benzodiazepines and buspirone) are most useful in the initial stages of treatment. However, the side effects and potential for physiological dependency make them a poor choice over the long term.

Antidepressants

Antidepressants may take 2 to 4 weeks until improvement is noted. To improve adherence, dose escalation must be slow because anxious patients tolerate side effects poorly. Antidepressants reduce the overall anxiety level and prevent anxiety or panic attacks, but they have no role in the treatment of acute anxiety. Among antidepressants, SSRIs are the most effective. Effective doses are often higher than those used for depression. Of the SNRIs, both venlafaxine and duloxetine have demonstrated efficacy in GAD.[19,20]

Somatic Symptom Disorders

Classification

Somatic symptom disorder (SSD) is characterized by somatic symptoms that are either very distressing or result in significant disruption of functioning and are accompanied by excessive and disproportionate thoughts, feelings, and behaviors regarding those symptoms.[16] Historically, pain-related psychological symptoms were shown to amplify pain perception and disability, leading to an overlap between the somatoform component of chronic pain and other psychiatric co-morbidities. The DSM, Fourth Edition, Text Revision (DSM-IV-TR), defined four somatoform disorders: somatization disorder, conversion disorder, hypochondriasis, and pain disorder (with or without a physical basis for pain). The new SSD criteria no longer require a specific number of complaints from among four symptom groups; however, somatic symptoms must be significantly impactful on daily activities and be excessive. Notably, with SDD, the condition may be associated with a medical condition.

GENERAL PRINCIPALS OF MULTI-MODAL ANALGESIA

In the medication management of chronic pain, multi-modal analgesia is the preferred method because frequently, multiple receptor systems must be targeted to achieve optimal pain control. By logical extension, successful treatment of chronic pain typically involves the use of more than one medication, nerve blocks, physical therapy, and relaxation or biofeedback techniques (i.e., treatment is conducted by a multi-disciplinary team or by an inter-disciplinary pain medicine program). In general, treatment goals are reports of pain that are less than 5 of 10 and an improvement in function. Typically, this corresponds to a 30% to 50% long-term improvement in chronic pain and improved quality of life. At a level of 4 of 10 or below, most patients can perform most of their activities of daily living satisfactorily. A 30% improvement in pain has been viewed as clinically meaningful and at a level at which most patients feel significantly better. Many nerve blocks (such as epidural steroid injections) are effective for acute exacerbations of chronic pain. However, their relatively short duration of efficacy (2–6 weeks on average) makes them inadequate for the long-term management of chronic pain if they are the sole treatment modality. Interventional procedures with longer-term efficacy include spinal cord stimulation, radiofrequency lesioning, and intrathecal pump implantation.

Major Medication Classes

Non-steroidal Anti-inflammatory Drugs

Non-steroidal anti-inflammatory drugs (NSAIDs) are useful for acute and chronic pain (such as pain due to inflammation, muscle pain, vascular pain, or post-traumatic pain). NSAIDs are usually equally efficacious (whether they are non-selective or cyclooxygenase-2 [COX-2] inhibitors), and they have similar side effects, but there is great individual variability in response across the different NSAIDs (Table 11.2). Ketorolac (up to 30 mg every 6 hours) intramuscularly (IM) or intravenously (IV) followed by oral dosing has a rapid onset and a high potency, enabling it to be substituted for morphine

TABLE 11.2 Properties of Aspirin and Non-steroidal Anti-inflammatory Drugs

Drug	Dosage (mg)	Dosage Interval (h)	Daily Dose (mg/day)	Peak Effect (h)	Half-Life (h)
Aspirin	81–975	4	2400	0.5–1	0.25
Celecoxib	100–200	12	400	1	11
Diclofenac	25–75	6–8	200	2	1–2
Diflunisal	250–500	12	1500	1	13
Etodolac acid	200–400	6–8	1200	1–2	7
Meloxicam	7.5–15	24	15	2	15–20
Flurbiprofen	50–100	6–8	300	1.5–3	3–4
Ibuprofen	200–800	6–8	2400	1–2	2
Indomethacin	25–75	6–8	150	0.5–1	2–3
Ketoprofen	25–75	6–8	300	1–2	1.5–2.0
Ketorolac[a]					
Oral	10	6–8	40	0.5–1	6
Parenteral	60 load; then 30	6–8	120	0.5	6
Choline magnesium trisalicylate	500–1000	12	3000	1	2–12
Nabumetone	1000–2000	12–24	2000	3–5	22–30
Naproxen	500 load; then 250–375	6–8	1000	2–4	12–15
Oxaprozin	60–1200	24	1200	2	3–3.5
Piroxicam	40 load; then 20	24	20	2–4	36–45
Sulindac	150–200	12	400	1–2	7–18
Tolmetin	200–600	8	1800	4–6	2

[a]Use no longer than 5 days.

Adapted from *Tarascon Pocket Pharmacopoeia.* Tarascon Publishers; 2006.

(30 mg of ketorolac is equivalent to 10 mg of morphine). It should be used for no more than 5 days.

Side Effects. Most NSAIDs can cause bronchospasm in aspirin-sensitive patients, induce gastric ulcers, interact with angiotensin-converting enzyme inhibitors (thereby contributing to renal failure), precipitate lithium toxicity, and impair renal function with long-term use. NSAIDs can elevate blood pressure in patients treated with beta-blockers and diuretics. The COX-2 inhibitors (e.g., celecoxib) have a lower incidence than non-selective NSAIDs of ulcer disease in the first year of treatment but not necessarily beyond this time frame.

Muscle Relaxants

Muscle relaxants are useful for the treatment of acute and chronic musculoskeletal pain. Their exact mechanism of action is unknown, and their mechanisms likely differ among the various compounds. In general, they are thought to enhance the inhibition of descending pain pathways. Some of the most frequently prescribed muscle relaxants include baclofen (an anti-spasticity agent), cyclobenzaprine, metaxalone, orphenadrine, and tizanidine.

Tricyclic Antidepressants

The TCAs are some of the primary medications used to treat neuropathic pain; TCAs have independent analgesic properties and work as adjuvant agents. A series of studies[15] has illustrated the analgesic properties of TCAs, which are independent of their effects on improving depression. TCAs have been effective for the pain associated with diabetic neuropathy, chronic regional pain syndromes, chronic headache, post-stroke pain, and radicular pain. Although early studies of TCAs were done with amitriptyline and desipramine, subsequent studies have confirmed that other TCAs have equivalent analgesic properties. Of note, the typical doses for the analgesic benefit of TCAs (25–75 mg) are lower than the doses generally used for antidepressant effects (150–300 mg). Nevertheless, there is a dose–response relationship for analgesia, and some patients benefit from a TCA used in the traditional antidepressant dose range, in conjunction with blood level monitoring. A TCA and an antiepileptic drug (AED) are often combined for the treatment of chronic pain, and this combination facilitates the treatment of mood disorders. Because individuals with pain are frequently treated with a variety of medications that may increase TCA serum levels, the value of blood level monitoring, even at low doses, cannot be understated.

Serotonin-Norepinephrine Reuptake Inhibitors

The SNRIs are a newer group of antidepressants, which, like the TCAs, act by inhibiting serotonin and norepinephrine reuptake. Venlafaxine and duloxetine are the most familiar drugs in this category; they have less alpha$_1$, cholinergic, and histamine inhibition than TCAs. This results in fewer side effects than the TCAs, with equivalent antidepressants and potentially equal analgesic benefits. Placebo-controlled studies have demonstrated the efficacy for neuropathic pain with both venlafaxine and duloxetine.

Structurally, venlafaxine is similar to tramadol, and in mice, venlafaxine demonstrates opioid-mediated analgesia that is reversed by naloxone. Duloxetine has a Food and Drug Administration (FDA) indication for both diabetic peripheral neuropathic (DPN) pain and for MDD. Thus, it is an excellent choice for those in pain with psychiatric co-morbidity who have failed to respond to a TCA. It has also been efficacious in fibromyalgia and GAD. It is started at 30 mg/day for 1 week (or 20 mg in older adults) and then increased to 60 mg/day. Up to 120 mg/day can be prescribed for DPN. The most common side effects are nausea and sedation. Its metabolism is like that of venlafaxine. Many patients are unable to tolerate TCAs' side effects, so both venlafaxine and duloxetine are promising agents in those with co-morbid MDD and chronic pain.

Antiepileptic Drugs

Blocking abnormally high-frequency and spontaneous firing in afferent neurons, in the dorsal horn, and in the thalamus is the putative mechanism for the efficacy of anticonvulsants regarding pain. The consequence of blocking the hyperexcitability of low threshold mechanoreceptive neurons in the brain is pain relief. AEDs are used in this population primarily for the treatment of neuropathic pain. Patients with co-morbid psychiatric illnesses (such as bipolar disorder, schizoaffective disorder, and impulse control problems) are treated with AEDs.

Phenytoin has alleviated pain associated with various neuropathies, particularly trigeminal, diabetic, and post-stroke pain, as well as with sharp, shooting, and lancinating pain. It has a narrow therapeutic index with a higher likelihood of drug toxicity, and it is less effective than carbamazepine for analgesia, and it is not indicated for psychiatric disorders. Carbamazepine is generally more effective than phenytoin for pain. The effect of carbamazepine on pain suppression is likely mediated by central and peripheral mechanisms. The analgesic properties of carbamazepine for patients with trigeminal neuralgia was first noted in 1962. Carbamazepine has been effective for post-herpetic pain, post-sympathetic pain, diabetic neuropathy, multiple sclerosis, and assorted neuralgias; it is used in higher doses.

Valproic acid (VPA) was used in neuropathic pain in the early 1980s. VPA has been shown to decrease post-herpetic neuralgia, episodic and chronic cluster headaches, migraine, and post-operative pain, as well as various neuralgias. The efficacy in pain reduction is in addition to the traditional place for VPA in the treatment of psychiatric disorders (bipolar and schizoaffective disorders). VPA sprinkles are well tolerated and can substitute for carbamazepine and lithium in the treatment of pain.

Gabapentin is a part of a new generation of AEDs; it is used for the treatment of neuropathic pain. Gabapentin relieves pain and associated symptoms in patients with both peripheral diabetic neuropathy, post-herpetic neuralgia, human immunodeficiency virus–related neuropathy, and cancer-related neuropathic pain. Other AEDs used in pain disorders include topiramate, oxcarbazepine, pregabalin, and lamotrigine.[21]

Opioids

Acute, severe, and unremitting pains in patients with cancer, as well as in non–cancer-related chronic pain, which has been refractory to other medication modalities, typically requires treatment with opioids. At times, opioids are the most effective treatment for chronic, non-malignant pain, such as the pain associated with post-herpetic neuralgia, degenerative disorders, and vascular conditions. Nociceptive pain and the absence of any co-morbid substance use have been associated with long-term opioid treatment efficacy. Morphine is often the opioid of choice for acute and chronic pain because it is well-known to most physicians and has a good safety profile. Beyond these starting points, the basic principles of opioid treatment are outlined in Box 11.1 and Table 11.3.

Tramadol deserves special mention because it has weak μ-opioid receptor activity, but it is not classified as a controlled substance in the United States. It also has SNRI properties. Its analgesic mechanism is unknown, but it is thought to enhance descending pain inhibition. Tramadol should be prescribed cautiously when used along with an SSRI, TCA, or SNRI because of a unique interaction that results in an increased risk for seizure and the development of serotonin syndrome. Caution should also be taken when prescribing it with other medications (such as bupropion, TCAs, and dopamine antagonists) that may lower the seizure threshold.

Recent evidence suggests that patients should be screened for risk factors for opioid misuse (e.g., current use of a history of an SUD, a family history of an SUD, a significant legal history, and a significant mood disorder) before prescribing them so that the physician can prescribe and monitor the use of opiates appropriately. State and nationwide databases have been helpful to decrease the misuse of these medications. After oral doses have been initiated and titrated to a satisfactorily level, the analgesic effect needs to be sustained by minimizing fluctuations in blood levels and the variable effects of dosing schedules. Long-acting or controlled-release formulations are ideal for this homeostasis because they are released more slowly than short-acting opioids.

For the treatment of chronic pain, dosing with short-acting medications only on an as-needed basis should be avoided because this makes steady relief impossible. It also predisposes the patient to drug-respondent conditioning and to subsequent behavior problems. Typically, long-lasting formulations are combined with short-acting agents for breakthrough pain. In those at risk for opioid misuse or with demonstrated aberrant substance use, longer-acting agents (i.e., methadone, fentanyl patch) are preferred to avoid inappropriate self-medication. Other chapters in this text discuss strategies for the prescription of opiates to those with SUDs. The most frequently reported side effects of opioid therapy are constipation, dry mouth, and sedation.

Buprenorphine. Buprenorphine is a partial agonist with high binding affinity at μ-opioid receptors, an agonist with low binding affinity at the nociceptin opioid receptor (NOP), and an antagonist with high binding affinity at κ- and δ-opioid receptors. The term "partial agonist" has been used owing to a partial effect on stimulating the receptor with in vitro assays. This does not necessarily translate to a partial analgesic efficacy in vivo or in clinical practice because the analgesic signaling pathway can be sufficiently activated by a partial agonist. Partial agonism at the μ-opioid receptor by buprenorphine yields effective analgesia and a ceiling effect on respiratory depression and euphoria and reduces other adverse events commonly observed with conventional full agonist opioids. Because buprenorphine does not occupy all μ-opioid receptors, this allows for efficacy of concomitant full μ-opioid receptor agonists. Antagonism at the δ- and κ-opioid receptors may limit constipation, respiratory depression, dysphoria, and substance abuse. In addition, κ-opioid receptor antagonists are

---

BOX 11.1 Guidelines for Opioid Maintenance

- Maintenance opioids should be considered only after other methods of pain control have been proven unsuccessful. Alternative methods (which typically include use of NSAIDs, anticonvulsants, membrane-stabilizing drugs, monoaminergic agents, local nerve blocks, and physical therapy) vary from case to case.
- Opioids should be avoided for patients with addiction disorders unless there is a new major medical illness (e.g., cancer or trauma) accompanied by severe pain. In such cases, a second opinion from another physician (a pain medicine or addiction specialist) is suggested.
- If opioids are prescribed for longer than 3 months, the patient should have a second opinion plus a follow-up consultation at least once per year. Monitoring with a urine toxicology screen at least yearly is also recommended.
- One pharmacy and one prescriber should be designated as exclusive agents.
- Dosages of opioids should be defined, as should expectations of what will happen if there are deviations from it. For example, abuse will lead to rapid tapering of the drug and entry into a detoxification program. There should be no doubt that the physician will stop prescribing the drug.
- Informed consent as to the rationale, risks, benefits, and alternatives should be documented.
- The course of treatment (in particular, the ongoing indications, changes in the disease process, efficacy, and the presence of abuse, tolerance, or addictive behavior) should be documented.

TABLE 11.3 Opioid Potencies and Special Features

Drug	Parenteral (mg equivalent)	Oral (mg)	Duration (h)	Special Features
Morphine	10	30	4	Morphine sulfate controlled-release has 12-h duration
Codeine	120	200	4	Ceiling effect as dose increases, low lipophilic
Oxycodone	4.5	30	4	Every 12 h Oxycontin (10, 20, 40 slow- release mg)
Hydromorphone	2	8	5	Suppository 6 mg = 10 mg parenteral morphine
Levorphanol	2	4	4	Low nausea and vomiting, low lipophilic
Methadone	5	10	2–12	Cumulative effect; day 3–5 decreased respirations; equi-analgesic ratio varies considerably
Meperidine	100	300	3	κ, proconvulsant metabolite, peristaltic slowing and sphincter of Oddi decrease
Fentanyl	0.1	25 μg SL	1 (patch 72 h)	50-μg patch = 30 mg/day morphine IM or IV
Sufentanil	Not recommended	15 μg SL	1	High potency with low volume of fluid
Propoxyphene	Not available	325	4	High dose leads to psychosis
Pentazocine	60	150	3	κ, σ agonist–antagonist, nasal 1 mg q1–2h
Butorphanol	2	Not available 3 (IM), 2 (NS)	μ, κ, σ, agonist-antagonist, nasal 1 mg q1–2h	
Buprenorphine	0.3	4	4–6	Partial agonist
Tramadol	Not available	150	4	μ agonist, decreased reuptake 5-HT and NE, P450 metabolism
Nalbuphine	10	Not available	3	Agonist-antagonist

5-HT, 5-Hydroxytryptamine; *IM,* intramuscular; *IV,* intravenous; *NE,* norepinephrine; *NS,* nasal; *SL,* sublingual.

currently being considered as promising therapeutics for psychiatric conditions, including depression, anxiety, and SUDs. Agonism at NOP contributes to spinal analgesia and may limit the potential for substance misuse and tolerance commonly observed with full μ-opioid receptor agonists.

Buprenorphine is approved by the FDA for acute pain, chronic pain, OUD, or opioid dependence, depending on the formulation. Buprenorphine formulations exist as either a combination therapy with naloxone (used to minimize IV misuse of buprenorphine) or as stand-alone products.

Clinical safety and efficacy data suggest that buprenorphine may be a tolerable alternative with equivalent or superior analgesia to conventional opioids for patients with pain. IV buprenorphine has been the most extensively studied formulation, and it is approved by the FDA for acute pain; the transdermal patch and buccal film are approved by the FDA for patients with chronic pain. The transdermal patch has demonstrated efficacy for chronic pain with once-weekly dosing; however, clinicians may find that the buprenorphine buccal film formulation has favorable bioavailability, available doses, efficacy, adverse event profile, and benefit-to-risk assessments for the treatment of chronic pain.

Because of buprenorphine's partial agonist properties, historical concerns have arisen as to preferred strategies for their use in the peri-operative period. Although there is no risk of precipitated withdrawal when opioids are used in patients already on buprenorphine, there is a risk of inducing precipitated withdrawal in patients receiving full agonist opioids (FAO) and have buprenorphine newly introduced.[22] In the case of patients who are already receiving buprenorphine for medications for opioid use disorder (MOUD) and require FAO for surgery or a significant procedure, continuation and/or reduction in buprenorphine dosing is recommended with use of FAO as-needed for optimal analgesia. Buprenorphine is maintained at lower dosing until the increased pain event has passed, FAO is tapered down, and buprenorphine is returned toward the patient's baseline dose.[22,23] The concept of stopping buprenorphine pre-operatively, with a washout period before introducing FAO has been abandoned and replaced by this blended approach.

Treatment of Neuropathic Pain

Neuropathic pain is responsive to multiple medication classes, including TCAs, AEDs, and opioids when used at higher doses than those that are typically prescribed for chronic musculoskeletal pain. Multiple medications are often combined with physical therapy and with coping skills training for comprehensive inter-disciplinary care.

Sympathetically Maintained Pain

Sympathetically maintained pain is a type of neuropathic pain. Regardless of its etiology (e.g., complex regional pain syndrome, inflammation, post-herpetic neuralgia, trauma, or facial pain) sympathetically maintained or mediated pain can respond to sympathetic blockade. Medications often used in the sympathetic blockade are alpha-blocking drugs, such as phentolamine; alpha-blocking antidepressants; and clonidine. Intrathecal, epidural, and systemic administration of a local anesthetic or clonidine also produces analgesia and may be useful in some types of vascular or neuropathic pain with a sympathetic component. Beta-blockers are not efficacious in the treatment of sympathetically maintained pain except for their use in the alleviation of migraine headaches. Guanethidine, bretylium, reserpine, and phentolamine have also been used to produce a chemical sympathectomy.

Headaches

Headaches affect people's quality of life and ability to participate in work, family, and social events. Migraines, tension headaches, and cluster headaches are major types of headaches, and they cause significant disability. People with headaches need to be screened for anxiety disorders, including PTSD and mood disorders and their ability to cope with stress because co-morbidity is common. Treatment of headaches and psychiatric conditions should be combined for successful outcomes.

Migraine headaches tend to be hemi-cranial and throbbing, and they may be associated with nausea, hyperacusis, and photophobia. Tension-type headaches are bilateral, dull, and usually not associated with other symptoms. Cluster headaches occur in groups of one to eight times a day and are sharp, non-throbbing pains that bore into one eye and adjacent areas. There may be eye tearing, conjunctival injection, nasal congestion, and a partial Horner's syndrome with cluster headaches. Common treatments for headaches include IV fluids, anti-dopaminergic agents with diphenhydramine, steroids, divalproex, NSAIDs, IV dihydroergotamine, and nerve blocks. Other therapies (e.g., ketamine and lidocaine) are used despite limited evidence. Transcranial magnetic stimulation may also be efficacious when pain is co-morbid with a depressive disorder.

Triptans (including almotriptan, eletriptan, frovatriptan, rizatriptan, lasmiditan, sumatriptan, and zolmitriptan) can abort migraines and treat them. Significant progress has been made in the treatment of migraines recently. Migraine is a leading cause of disability worldwide, and 15% of Americans experience migraines.

A new class of medication, calcitonin gene-related peptide (CGRP) antagonists, has been approved for migraine prevention in adults. The newly approved CGRP antagonists include erenumab, fremanezumab, galcanezumab, and eptinezumab. Lasmiditan, ubrogepant, and rimegepant are currently emerging acute migraine therapies that may be added to the arsenal of migraine management. These medications come in injectable forms as well as tablet forms. Many patients with severe debilitating headaches and high levels of anxiety and depression have been helped with these medications.[24,25]

When co-morbid migraines and depression occur, the use of SSRIs, SNRIs, TCAs, and monoamine oxidase inhibitors (MAOIs) with triptans is an important topic. There is an increased risk of serotonin syndrome (with fever, autonomic instability, hyperreflexia, nausea, vomiting, diarrhea, tremor, flushing, confusion, seizures, and coma). Patients need to be informed, advised, and followed closely if these medications are combined.

Fibromyalgia

Fibromyalgia is a common condition characterized by widespread chronic pain, physical exhaustion, cognitive difficulties, depressed mood, sleep problems, and deteriorated quality of life with a prevalence of 2% to 4% in the general population. Its exact pathogenesis remains unclear, but it is involved with neural over-sensitization and decreased conditioned pain modulation, combined with cognitive dysfunction, memory impairment, and altered information processing. Psychological trauma and PTSD are co-morbid conditions with fibromyalgia as are personality traits. Three drugs are approved by the FDA for fibromyalgia: pregabalin, duloxetine, and milnacipran. In addition, amitriptyline, a TCA, was also found to be efficacious in treating symptoms of fibromyalgia.[26,27]

TREATMENT OF PAIN BEHAVIOR AND THE USE OF MULTI-DISCIPLINARY PAIN CLINICS

Medicare guidelines offer a broad set of criteria to qualify for structured multi-disciplinary pain management. The pain must last at least 6 months (and result in significant life disturbance and limited function), it must be attributable to a physical cause, and it must be unresponsive to the usual methods of treatment. Quality control guidelines developed by the Commission on Accreditation of Rehabilitation Facilities (CARF) have led to the certification of more than 100 multi-disciplinary chronic pain management programs nationwide. Behavioral treatments are a key component of these programs, and they can be effective for the relief of pain and can help extinguish the behaviors associated with pain.

Inpatient or outpatient multi-disciplinary pain treatment should be considered early in the course of chronic pain. This is particularly important when intensive observation is necessary (e.g., to rule out malingering); no single modality of outpatient treatment is likely to work; the patient has already obtained maximum benefit from outpatient treatments (such as NSAIDs, nerve blocks, antidepressants, and simple physical and behavioral rehabilitation); intensive daily interventions are required, usually with multiple concurrent types of therapy (such as nerve blocks, physical therapy, and behavior modification); and the patient exhibits abnormal pain behavior and agrees to the goals of improved coping, work rehabilitation, and psychiatric assessment.

REHABILITATION

Successful rehabilitation of those with chronic pain syndromes may require some combination of psychiatry, physiatry, and behavioral psychology. These treatments include exercise, gait training, spinal manipulation, orthoses, traction therapy, psychotherapy, and yoga. Successful rehabilitation aims to decrease symptoms, increase independence, and allow the patient to return to work. A positive, rapid return to light-normal activities and work is essential if the disability is to be minimized. Psychologically, this is the key to coping with acute trauma. There is no evidence that a return to work adversely affects the course of most chronic pain syndromes.

CONCLUSIONS

Pain is an exciting and burgeoning discipline for psychiatrists. Whether the psychiatrist is treating the pain or its psychological sequelae, it is critical to have a firm understanding of the physical basis for the pain complaints in conjunction with a thorough appreciation of how psychiatric co-morbidity interacts with perceptions of pain. Patients who attend pain clinics have significant psychiatric pathology. This co-morbidity worsens their pain and disability, and this mental distress is an independent source of suffering, further reducing the quality of life. More emphasis is being placed on the individual's experience of pain. Fortunately, with the boom in psychotherapeutic medications over the past 15 years and with more effective psychotherapies, significant multi-modal improvement in pain treatment has been advanced.

REFERENCES

1. International Association for the Study of Pain (IASP) Updates the Definition of Pain Saurab Sharma. August 12, 2020. https://www.iasp-pain.org. Accessed August 30, 2023.
2. Lerman SF, Rudich Z, Brill S, et al. Longitudinal associations between depression, anxiety, pain, and pain-related disability in chronic pain patients. *Psychosom Med.* 2015;77(3):333–341.
3. Unseld M, Zeilinger EL, Fellinger M, et al. Prevalence of pain and its association with symptoms of post-traumatic stress disorder, depression, anxiety and distress in 846 cancer patients: a cross sectional study. *Psychooncology.* 2021;30(4):504–510.
4. Widiger TA, Oltmanns JR. Neuroticism is a fundamental domain of personality with enormous public health implications. *World Psychiatry.* 2017;16(2):144–145.
5. Yang S, Chang MC. Chronic pain: structural and functional changes in brain structures and associated negative affective states. *Int J Mol Sci.* 2019;20:3130.
6. Strain EC. Assessment and treatment of comorbid psychiatric disorders in opioid-dependent patients. *Clin J Pain.* 2002;18(4 suppl):S14–S27.
7. Sprenger T, Valet M, Boecker H, et al. Opioid-ergic activation in the medial pain system after heat pain. *Pain.* 2006;122:63–67.
8. Coghill RC. Individual differences in the subjective experience of pain: new insights into mechanisms and models. *Headache.* 2010;50(9):1531–1535.
9. Lim M, Roosink M, Kim JS, et al. Augmented pain processing in primary and secondary somatosensory cortex in fibromyalgia: a magnetoencephalography study using intra-epidermal electrical stimulation. *PLoS One.* 2016;11(3):e0151776.
10. Nummenmaa L, Tuominen L. Opioid system and human emotions. *Br J Pharmacol.* 2018;175(14):2737–2749.
11. Woo AK. Depression and anxiety in pain. *Rev Pain.* 2010;4(1):8–12.
12. Mittinty MM, McNeil DW, Brennan DS, et al. Assessment of pain-related fear in individuals with chronic painful conditions. *J Pain Res.* 2018;11:3071–3077.
13. Keefe FJ, Rumble ME, Scipio CD, et al. Psychological aspects of persistent pain: current state of the science. *J Pain.* 2004;5(4):195–211.
14. Meints SM, Edwards RR. Evaluating psychosocial contributions to chronic pain outcomes. *Prog Neuropsychopharmacol Biol Psychiatry.* 2018;87(Pt B):168–182.
15. Baltenberger EP, Buterbaugh WM, Martin S, et al. Review of antidepressants in the treatment of neuropathic pain. *Mental Health Clinician.* 2015;5(3):123–133.
16. American Psychiatric Association.Text rev. *Diagnostic and Statistical Manual of Mental Disorders.* 5th ed. American Psychiatric Publishing; 2022.
17. Bonilla JH, Sánchez-Salcedo JA, Estevez-Cabrera MM, et al. Depression and pain: use of antidepressants. *Curr Neuropharmacol.* 2022;20(2):384–402.
18. Kosson D, Malec-Milewska M, Gałązkowski R, et al. Analysis of anxiety, depression and aggression in patients attending pain clinics. *Int J Environ Res Public Health.* 2018;15(12):2898.
19. Thase ME, Entsuah AR, Rudolph RL. Remission rates during treatment with venlafaxine or selective serotonin reuptake inhibitors. *Br J Psychiatry.* 2001;178(3):234–241.
20. Goldstein DJ, Lu Y, Detke MJ, et al. Duloxetine vs. placebo in patients with painful diabetic neuropathy. *Pain.* 2005;116:109–118.
21. Nejad SH, Chuang K, Hirschberg R, et al. The use of antiepileptic drugs in acute neuropsychiatric conditions: focus on traumatic brain injury, pain, and alcohol withdrawal. *Int J Clin Med.* 2014;5:724–736.
22. Acampora GA, Nisavic M, Zhang Y. Perioperative buprenorphine continuous maintenance and administration simultaneous with full opioid agonist: patient priority at the interface between medical disciplines. *J Clin Psychiatry.* 2020;81(1):19com12810.
23. Greenwald MK, Herring AA, Perrone J, et al. A neuropharmacological model to explain buprenorphine induction challenges. *Ann Emerg Med.* 2022;80(6):509–524.
24. Peters GL. Migraine overview and summary of current and emerging treatment options. *Am J Manag Care.* 2019;25(2 suppl):S23–S34.
25. Robblee J, Grimsrud KW. Emergency department and inpatient management of headache in adults. *Curr Neurol Neurosci Rep.* 2020;20(4):7.
26. Farag HM, Yunusa I, Goswami H, et al. Comparison of amitriptyline and US Food and Drug Administration-approved treatments for fibromyalgia: a systematic review and network meta-analysis. *JAMA Netw Open.* 2022;5(5):e2212939.
27. Afari N, Ahumada SM, Wright LJ, et al. Psychological trauma and functional somatic syndromes: a systematic review and meta-analysis. *Psychosom Med.* 2014;76(1):2–11.

12 Psychiatric Illness During Pregnancy and the Post-partum Period

Rebecca Leval, Ruta Nonacs, Betty Wang, Adele C. Viguera, and Lee S. Cohen

KEY POINTS

Epidemiology

- Pregnancy does not protect against psychiatric disorders.

Clinical Findings

- A growing body of information exists regarding the course of psychiatric illness during pregnancy and the reproductive safety of psychotropic medications.

Complications

- Except for one anticonvulsant, sodium valproate, most psychotropics are *not* major teratogens.

- Post-partum depression is the most common complication in modern obstetrics; its definitive treatment is essential to minimize maternal morbidity.

OVERVIEW

Care of pregnant and post-partum women involves the evaluation and treatment of a wide array of psychiatric problems. Clinical lore previously held that the state of pregnancy conferred a positive mood to women; however, more recent data suggest that subpopulations of patients are at risk for new-onset illness or recurrence of prior psychiatric illness during pregnancy. There is now a far greater appreciation of the contribution that untreated mental illness has on adverse outcomes in pregnancy, delivery, and the post-partum period.

Psychiatric evaluation of pregnant and post-partum women requires a thorough assessment of the severity of symptoms and their impact on functioning. Clinicians must assess whether symptoms are normative or pathological, manifestations of a new psychiatric disorder, or an exacerbation of an existing psychiatric disorder. Pregnancy is an emotionally laden time that naturally evokes anxiety and increased mood reactivity. Intermittent mild psychological stress, which may promote healthy fetal development, must be distinguished from moderate to severe psychological stress that may adversely impact fetal growth and development.

Screening for psychiatric disorders during pregnancy and the post-partum period is often conducted inconsistently, and even when a depressed pregnant woman is identified, definitive treatment is not always forthcoming. Screening for depression during pregnancy, followed by prudent and timely treatment, may minimize maternal morbidity and the negative downstream effects that maternal mental illness has on the mother, her child, and the family.

Given the prevalence of mood and anxiety disorders in women during the childbearing years and the growing number of women who receive treatment for these disorders, women increasingly present before conception for consultation regarding the use of psychotropics during pregnancy. Outside of the peri-natal period, there is increasing evidence of high rates of relapse after discontinuation of psychotropics; thus, it is not surprising that many women who discontinue their medications either before or after conception develop recurrent symptoms.

Treatment during the peri-natal period involves weighing the individualized risks of the untreated illness against the risks of any intervention. Maternal psychiatric illness is not benign and it may cause significant morbidity in both the mother and her child; thus, discontinuing or withholding medication during pregnancy is not always the safest option. At the same time, in contrast to other times in a woman's life, the threshold for treatment of psychiatric disorders during pregnancy tends to be higher, typically reserved for situations in which the disorder interferes, to a high degree, with maternal and fetal well-being.

There is variability in women's attitudes toward pharmacological treatment in pregnancy, and women often receive conflicting information from psychiatrists, obstetricians, family, friends, and the media. It is common for women with similar illness histories to make vastly different decisions regarding treatment. Whichever treatment course a woman pursues, non-pharmacological supports and interventions should be optimized.

This chapter provides a broad overview of peri-natal mood and anxiety disorders and their treatment in pregnant, post-partum, and nursing women.

PRECONCEPTION CONSIDERATIONS

Whenever pharmacological interventions are initiated in women with childbearing potential, the reproductive safety of the medications must be considered. According to the Centers for Disease Control and Prevention, nearly half of pregnancies in the United States are unplanned. Unintended pregnancy rates are higher in those who are younger and unmarried and who have a lower income, a lower educational level, and a substance use disorder, as well as those from ethnic minorities.[1] Thus, every psychiatric interview of a woman of reproductive age should include a reproductive history, including current method of contraception and family planning, and a discussion of the reproductive safety of medications early in the course of treatment.

Knowing that organogenesis occurs early during pregnancy, often before a woman is even aware that she is pregnant, the US Preventive Services Task Force (USPSTF) strongly recommends ("Grade A") that all women capable of pregnancy, regardless of pregnancy planning, take a daily supplement containing 400 to 800 μg of folic acid. The critical period for supplementing folic acid, both to prevent neural tube defects and other congenital malformations, as well as to reduce the risk for neurodevelopmental disorders, begins at least 1 month before conception up until 2 to 3 months of pregnancy.[2]

SCREENING AND DIAGNOSIS OF DEPRESSION AND ANXIETY DURING PREGNANCY

Early identification of both at-risk women and women experiencing depression and problematic anxiety prevents and reduces disease burden and permits more effective management. Diagnosing a mood disorder during pregnancy, however, may prove challenging. It is important to distinguish between normative psychological experiences and pathological ones, recognizing and appreciating that women and their partners may have misconceptions about pregnancy or cognitive distortions surrounding how they "should" feel or behave in pregnancy.

Many common somatic pregnancy symptoms overlap with depressive symptoms, such as sleep and appetite disturbances and decreased libido. Screening tools, such as the Edinburgh Postnatal Depression Scale (EPDS), a brief 10-item self-report questionnaire validated for use during pregnancy and the post-partum period, excludes common constitutional symptoms of pregnancy. The EPDS may also be used to identify women with an anxiety disorder; however, screeners more specific to anxiety disorders, such as the Perinatal Anxiety Screening Scale (PASS), a 31-item self-report questionnaire, are also available.

Peri-natal Risk Assessment

When considering treatment options, a thorough risk assessment should be conducted. Regardless of the treatment plan, an element of risk remains with all treatment decisions made during the peri-natal period. Electing to treat illness poses a risk, and electing to withhold treatment or modify treatment poses a risk. The concept of "safety" in this period is relative and individualized, in that what might be "safest" for one woman, in that it mitigates certain risks while exposing her to other potential risks, might not be the "safest" for another woman.

Although the focus of the psychiatric risk assessment weighs the risks of the mental illness, including those outlined in the literature and those observed in an individual patient, against the risk of pharmacological and non-pharmacological interventions, it is also worth considering other risks to the pregnancy. These risks include the general risks to any pregnancy, or the "background risk" (such as congenital malformations), other medical risks (such as a history of illness or medical treatments), and psychosocial risks (such as accessibility to care or social support).

Untreated or sub-optimally treated moderate to severe psychological stress of mood and anxiety disorders has been associated with numerous adverse pregnancy outcomes. Pregnant women with an untreated psychiatric illness are more likely to use tobacco, alcohol, and recreational drugs, behaviors that may negatively impact outcomes. In addition, they are less likely to use prenatal vitamins, to receive prenatal care, and to adhere to recommendations regarding nutrition and weight gain during pregnancy. Psychiatric illness in the mother has been associated with higher rates of complications, including pre-eclampsia, gestational diabetes, preterm birth, operative delivery, lower birth weight, lower Apgar scores, and a smaller head circumference. Infants born to mothers with a psychiatric illness may spend more time in the special care nursery and have lower rates of breast-feeding and impaired bonding or attachment to their mothers.[3]

Although these adverse outcomes are concerning, these conditions also increase the risk of long-term emotional, behavioral, and neurodevelopmental adverse outcomes in children.[4]

Antidepressant Use During Pregnancy

Selective serotonin reuptake inhibitors (SSRIs) are the first-line agents for the treatment of depression and anxiety and are the best characterized antidepressants in pregnancy and lactation. The prevalence of antidepressant use is roughly 10% to 15% in reproductive-aged women and 7% in pregnant women.[5]

Prospectively gathered data are available for all SSRIs; however, more limited data are available for less commonly prescribed SSRIs, such as fluvoxamine, and newer SSRIs, such as vortioxetine. SSRIs do not increase the risk of major congenital malformations above the baseline incidence ("background risk") present in any pregnancy. The background risk of major congenital malformations in US-born newborns is estimated at 2% to 4%, and in most cases, the cause of the malformation is unknown. Past reports of an increased risk of cardiac malformations with paroxetine have not been duplicated in newer studies.[6]

More limited data are available on the use of serotonin–norepinephrine reuptake inhibitors (SNRIs), such as venlafaxine and duloxetine. Recent reports are reassuring, in that they have not demonstrated an increased risk of congenital malformations in infants exposed to duloxetine (>4700 exposures)[7,8] or venlafaxine (>3100 exposures)[9] above background risk.

Bupropion may be an attractive option for women who have not optimally responded to other antidepressants, either as monotherapy or for augmentation, or for use with smoking cessation. Data remain limited, but overall are reassuring. However, there have been several studies that observed a small increase in the risk of cardiovascular defects, specifically left ventricular outflow tract obstructions and ventricular septal defects. These studies have had several limitations, including potential confounding by indication, but it appears that the absolute risk is still relatively low (2.1–2.8 per 1000 births).[10]

Three prospective and more than ten retrospective studies have examined the risk of organ malformation in more than 400 cases of first-trimester exposure to tricyclic antidepressants (TCAs). Both when evaluated on an individual basis and when pooled as a class, these studies have not found a significant association between fetal exposure to TCAs (except for clomipramine, which may increase the risk of cardiac defects) and the risk for any major congenital anomaly.[11] Among the TCAs, desipramine and nortriptyline are often preferred because they are less anticholinergic and the least likely to exacerbate the orthostatic hypotension that may occur during pregnancy.

Limited information is available on other antidepressants, including trazodone, vortioxetine, vilazodone, and esketamine. It is estimated that at least 600 to 800 exposures must be collected to demonstrate a two-fold increase in the risk for a malformation over what is observed in the general population. When possible, women taking these medications should, in general, switch to an antidepressant with a better characterized reproductive safety profile.

Scant information is available regarding the reproductive safety of monoamine oxidase inhibitors, and these agents are generally not used during pregnancy because they may produce a hypertensive crisis when combined with tocolytic medications, such as terbutaline.

Other potential adverse outcomes with in utero antidepressant exposure, outside of teratogenicity, include the risk of post-partum hemorrhage, poor neonatal adaptation, and persistent pulmonary hypertension of the newborn (PPHN).

With in utero SSRI exposure, the risk of post-partum hemorrhage, or cumulative blood loss of 1000 mL or greater within 24 hours after delivery, with signs and symptoms of hypovolemia, has been inconsistently reported. A recent Swedish registry study looking at more than 30,000 pregnant women found an increased risk of post-partum hemorrhage in women treated with SSRIs at any point during their pregnancy and among women with a current or past psychiatric illness. The clinical significance of this finding remains unclear. Although obstetricians/gynecologists should be aware of this risk, post-partum hemorrhage may be managed effectively.

Multiple studies have reported an increased risk of a transient poor neonatal adaptation in 25% to 30% of infants exposed prenatally to antidepressants near the time of delivery. Symptoms include tachypnea, increased muscle tone, restlessness, irritability, and jitteriness. There are no standardized scales or guidelines for monitoring, reporting, or managing symptoms. The pathophysiology is poorly understood, but it is likely that multiple factors contribute to the constellation of symptoms and it is unclear to what degree maternal illness itself contributes. A study in which SSRIs were discontinued at least 2 weeks before delivery did not show a decrease in symptoms.[12] Thus, discontinuation of antidepressants proximate to delivery to reduce the risk of poor neonatal adaptation may prove ineffective. Discontinuation of an antidepressant late in pregnancy would poorly position a woman to face the post-partum period, a time of heightened risk for affective illness, essentially leaving her unprotected. Reassuringly, the symptoms of poor neonatal adaptation appear to be relatively benign and short-lived, resolving within 1 to 4 days after delivery without any specific medical intervention.[13] The TCA clomipramine has been associated with more severe and prolonged symptoms of poor neonatal adaptation.[11]

Another concern has been the association of maternal SSRI use with PPHN, a condition wherein pulmonary vascular resistance remains elevated after birth.[14–18] In the initial report published in 2006, the use of an SSRI after the 20th week of gestation was significantly associated with a six-fold greater risk of PPHN. In that first study, PPHN was estimated to occur in 1% of infants with late pregnancy exposure to SSRIs. Since this initial report, three studies have found no association between antidepressant use during pregnancy and PPHN, and one study showed a much lower risk than the originally reported 1%. These findings, taken together, bring into question whether there is any association between SSRIs and PPHN; however, if there is a risk, it is much lower than the rate reported in 2006. In 2018, the Food and Drug Administration (FDA) revised its warning on the subject, stating that there was insufficient evidence to conclude that there is a causative relationship between SSRIs and PPHN.[14]

Evaluating the risk for long-term neurodevelopmental outcomes in children exposed in utero to antidepressants has been the focus of increasing attention. Although previous studies had yielded conflicting, albeit overall reassuring findings, a recent study of more than 145,500 exposed children did not find an increased risk of neurodevelopmental disorders (e.g., autism spectrum disorder [ASD], attention-deficit hyperactivity disorder [ADHD], specific learning disorders, developmental speech/language disorder, developmental coordination disorder, intellectual disability, or behavioral disorders).[19]

TREATMENT OF DEPRESSION DURING PREGNANCY: CLINICAL GUIDELINES

Despite the growing number of reviews on the subject, the management of patients with antenatal depression is still largely guided by practical experience, with few definitive data and no controlled studies to inform treatment. In the absence of well-defined guidelines, clinicians must work collaboratively with their patients to arrive at the lowest risk decision based on available information. A patient's psychiatric history, current symptoms, and attitude toward the use of psychiatric medications during pregnancy must be carefully assessed and factored into any decision.

In patients with mild depression, it may be appropriate to consider discontinuation of pharmacological therapy during pregnancy. Although data on the use of cognitive-behavioral therapy (CBT) and interpersonal therapy (IPT) to facilitate antidepressant discontinuation before conception are not available, it makes clinical sense to pursue such treatment in women who seek to discontinue antidepressants as they plan pregnancy. These treatment modalities may reduce the risk of recurrent depressive symptoms during pregnancy, although, as noted previously, this has not been studied systematically. Close monitoring of affective status during pregnancy is essential, even if all medications are discontinued and there is no readily apparent need for re-introduction of an antidepressant. Early detection and treatment of recurrent illness may significantly reduce the morbidity associated with recurrent illness during pregnancy.

Women may also experience the new onset of depressive symptoms during pregnancy. For women who present with minor depressive symptoms, non-pharmacological treatment strategies should be explored first. CBT or IPT may be beneficial for reducing the severity of depressive symptoms and may either limit or obviate the need for antidepressants. Recent studies evaluating the effectiveness of digital CBT (using technological elements such as text messages, videos, gaming, or peer group discussions) for the treatment of depression during pregnancy have demonstrated efficacy, albeit with varying effect sizes.[20] In general, pharmacological treatment is pursued when non-pharmacological strategies have failed or when it is thought that the risks associated with psychiatric illness during pregnancy outweigh the risks of fetal exposure to a particular medication.

Many women who discontinue antidepressant treatment during pregnancy experience recurrent depressive symptoms. In one study, women who discontinued their medications were five times more likely to relapse than women who maintained their antidepressant treatment across their pregnancy.[21] Thus, women with recurrent or refractory depressive illness may decide in collaboration with their clinician that the safest option is to maintain pharmacological treatment during pregnancy to minimize the risk for recurrent illness.

When prescribing medications during pregnancy, every attempt should be made to simplify the medication regimen using the fewest number of agents at the lowest effective dose. It is important to ensure that every medication affords benefit to the patient and is necessary to maintain euthymia and to use or optimize medications that might treat multiple symptom domains. For instance, a more sedating TCA may be used for a woman who presents with depression and a sleep disturbance instead of using an SSRI and a sleep aid.

The dose of the medication must be effective, but care must be taken to ensure that the dose is not unnecessarily high and that the benefit was derived from the last dose increase. Decreasing the dose of a medication below an effective dose to limit risk to the fetus may increase the risk of illness recurrence because dose requirements during pregnancy will likely increase in response to pregnancy-related metabolic changes. During pregnancy, changes in plasma volume and increases in hepatic metabolism and renal clearance may result in medication blood levels that decrease below the therapeutic threshold, particularly in the later stages of pregnancy. Several investigators have described a reduction of up to 65% in serum levels of

TCAs during pregnancy.[22] Because sub-therapeutic levels may be associated with depressive relapse, an increase in daily TCA or other psychotropics may be clinically indicated.

The question of whether to switch from a newer medication with less reproductive safety data to an older medication with greater reproductive safety data is one that ideally should be considered preconception. Consideration of risks might include the potential of relapse should the older medication prove ineffective and the risk of unknown adverse effects. Switching medications during pregnancy is best avoided, if possible.

Clinicians should attempt to use, to the greatest extent possible, medications with the "safest" reproductive profile while factoring in the woman's history of medication trials. What is "safest" for one woman may not necessarily be "safest" for another. Although SSRIs, such as fluoxetine and sertraline, have been well characterized as having reassuring safety data, these medications may not be ideal for women who previously failed to respond to these agents. In some situations, one may recommend an antidepressant with less information on reproductive safety. As an example, consider a woman who has a history of multiple severe depressive episodes and suicide attempts who tried and failed multiple SSRIs, SNRIs, and atypical antidepressants but who was ultimately stabilized on vortioxetine. Although there are less available safety data, the provider and patient may determine that this newer antidepressant is indeed the "safer" option for the patient because it is the medication that has kept her well.

When considering the reproductive safety of a medication, the Pregnancy and Lactation Labeling Rule (PLLR) has replaced the FDA Pregnancy Risk Categories (A, B, C, D, and X), which had been used for more than 30 years. The FDA Pregnancy Risk Categories were overly simplistic and often misleading. The new PLLR, which took effect in 2015, includes more clearly described, comprehensive information regarding the potential risks and benefits throughout pregnancy and lactation (to the mother and her baby).

ELECTROCONVULSIVE THERAPY DURING PREGNANCY

The use of electroconvulsive therapy (ECT) during pregnancy often raises considerable anxiety among clinicians and patients despite its well-documented safety record over the past 50 years. Fears that treatment might pose harm to fetuses often precludes its use. Anderson and Reti[23] reviewed 339 cases of ECT in pregnancy, predominantly for the treatment of depression. They identified 11 complications, including 2 fetal deaths, not directly related to ECT. The most common fetal complication was bradyarrhythmia (2.7%) and the most common maternal complication was induction of premature labor (3.5%), although it was not clearly increased by ECT.[23]

Electroconvulsive therapy may be considered in women whose symptoms (e.g., impulsivity, self-harm, suicidality, agitation, psychosis), signs, and conditions (e.g., catatonia, life-threatening physical status) pose a risk to the safety of the pregnancy, as may be seen in depression or mania. ECT should also be considered in women who have responded well to ECT, who wish to avoid extended exposure to psychotropics during pregnancy or lactation, and who fail to respond to standard antidepressant treatments. A limited course of treatment may be sufficient, concurrent with, or followed by treatment with one or a combination of psychotropics. A multi-disciplinary treatment team, including an anesthesiologist, psychiatrist, and obstetrician/gynecologist, is recommended.[24]

MOOD STABILIZERS DURING PREGNANCY

Although the effect of pregnancy on the natural course of bipolar disorder (BPD) is poorly understood, a recent study found that just greater than 20% of women without a psychiatric history and almost 55% of women with a history of BPD will experience an episode of bipolar illness during the perinatal period.[25] The risk for chronicity and relapse after discontinuation of mood stabilizers is high. At the same time, among the psychotropic medications, it is the mood stabilizing agents that convey the greatest reproductive safety risks. Given these data, clinicians, and women with BPD who are either pregnant or planning pregnancy find themselves between a "teratologic rock and a clinical hard place." Consequently, given the apparent need for pharmacological therapy with mood stabilizers, women with BPD may be counseled against becoming pregnant or advised to terminate their pregnancies after exposure to a mood stabilizer.

The use of the mood stabilizer lithium has received a great deal of negative attention because of the known risk of cardiovascular malformations, specifically of Ebstein anomaly (a malformation of the leaflets of the tricuspid valve), with use during the first trimester of pregnancy. Recent data, however, suggest the risk is much lower than previously estimated. In one study, the risk of any type of cardiac malformation was 1.15% in unexposed fetuses and rose to 1.9% in lithium-exposed fetuses.[26] There appears to be a dose–response relationship between lithium and Ebstein anomaly. The risk of cardiac malformations at doses above 900 mg/day is three times higher than with doses below 600 mg/day, although not every woman's illness may be effectively managed at such low doses.

Women may elect to proceed in various ways given this risk. Potential options include continuing lithium, discontinuing lithium with the potential for re-introducing lithium after the first trimester or at delivery, or switching to an alternative mood stabilizing agent. In weighing these options, the illness severity and prior mediation trials must be considered. If lithium is used during the first trimester, fetal echocardiography and a level II ultrasound examination should be performed. No clear consensus has been reached as to lithium blood level monitoring during pregnancy, although it should be noted that lithium levels decline during pregnancy. Although some providers elect to adjust lithium only if symptoms emerge, others choose to follow levels closely and to keep lithium levels within the therapeutic range.

Of the mood stabilizers, lamotrigine has the strongest reproductive safety profile. Lamotrigine has emerged as a preferred agent in reproductive-aged women with BPD, although it has limited benefits in treating or preventing manic episodes. Although early data from the North American Anti-Epileptic Drug registry indicated a six-fold increase in the risk of oral clefts in infants exposed to lamotrigine in the first trimester, this finding has not been supported by other large registry-based studies (International Registry of Antiepileptic Drugs and Pregnancy [EURAP] and European Concerted Action on Congenital Anomalies and Twins [EUROCAT] registries).[27] No significant increase in risk of other malformations has been found in any registry study.

Dosing of lamotrigine must be carefully considered because rising levels of estrogen in pregnancy decrease lamotrigine levels by up to 50%. Levels may begin to decline as early as 5 weeks of gestation and continue to decrease up to 32 weeks of gestation.[28] Levels return to pre-pregnancy levels within 3 to 4 weeks after delivery. Consensus has not been reached as to how to best manage these changing levels in pregnancy and postpartum. Although lamotrigine levels are closely monitored during pregnancy and doses adjusted accordingly in patients with epilepsy,[29] there are no established therapeutic ranges for lamotrigine in the treatment of BPD. Although some clinicians choose to obtain a lamotrigine level before conception and to adjust dosage accordingly during pregnancy, there is no evidence to indicate that specific blood levels of lamotrigine heighten the risk of BPD relapse during pregnancy.[29] Close monitoring of symptoms throughout pregnancy is essential, and dose changes may be made based on clinical indication.

Compared with lithium and lamotrigine, valproic acid, and to a lesser extent carbamazepine have been associated with a high risk of congenital malformations. Exposure to valproic acid in the first 2 months of gestation increases the risk of neural tube defects (with an adjusted odds ratio of 19.4), ventricular and atrial septal defects, pulmonary valve atresia, hypoplastic left heart syndrome, cleft palate, anorectal atresia, and hypospadias.[30] Outside of major congenital malformations, valproic acid use in pregnancy is associated with an increased risk of ASD and ADHD and a worse overall neurodevelopmental outcome.[31] No significant increase in neurodevelopmental disorders was found among children exposed to carbamazepine or lamotrigine.

Given the teratogenicity of valproic acid and considering the high percentage of unintended pregnancies, as well as its propensity to induce polycystic ovarian syndrome, consideration of alternative agents to treat BPD in reproductive-aged women is strongly advised. Valproic acid should never be a first-line treatment in reproductive-aged women; rather, it should be reserved for situations when other agents with superior reproductive safety data have failed. If unable to use alternative options in a woman of reproductive age, one should consider use of an antipsychotic and a dual contraceptive method, preferably with one method being either an intrauterine device or an implant.

TREATMENT OF BIPOLAR DURING PREGNANCY: CLINICAL GUIDELINES

The treatment algorithm for managing reproductive-age women during pregnancy depends on the severity of illness. Patients with a history of a single episode of mania and a brisk and full recovery followed by sustained well-being may tolerate discontinuation of mood stabilizers proximate to conception. Unfortunately, even among women with a history of prolonged well-being and sustained euthymia, discontinuation of prophylactic treatment may be associated with subsequent relapse. For women with BPD and a history of multiple and frequent recurrences of mood episodes, several options may be considered.

For women who tolerate discontinuation of maintenance treatment, the decision of when to resume treatment is a matter for clinical judgment. Some patients and clinicians prefer to avoid exposure entirely and elect to re-start medications after delivery; others prefer to limit the risk of recurrence by re-starting treatment at the start of the second trimester.

For women with severe forms of BPD, such as those with multiple severe episodes, especially those who present with psychosis and suicidal ideation, maintenance treatment with a mood stabilizer before and throughout the pregnancy may be the most prudent option. In such a setting, accepting the relatively small absolute increase in teratogenic risk with first-trimester exposure to lithium or another mood stabilizing agent may be justified. Please refer to Table 12.1 for adverse pregnancy outcomes associated with commonly prescribed anti-epileptic mood stabilizing agents.

Regardless of the treatment plan, pregnancy in the context of BPD should be considered high risk, and close monitoring is warranted. For women who elect to proceed with a mood stabilizing agent, prenatal screening for congenital malformations (including cardiac anomalies) with a fetal ultrasound at 16 to 18 weeks of gestation is recommended. The possibility of neural tube defects should be evaluated with maternal serum alpha-fetoprotein levels and ultrasonography. High-dose folic acid supplementation (4 mg/day) before conception and throughout the first trimester for women receiving anticonvulsants is frequently recommended. However, it should be noted that supplemental use of folic acid to attenuate the risk of neural tube defects in the setting of anticonvulsant exposure has not been systematically evaluated.

PSYCHOTIC DISORDERS DURING PREGNANCY

Psychosis during pregnancy may interfere with a woman's ability to care for herself, obtain appropriate and necessary prenatal care, and cooperate with caregivers during delivery. Psychosis during pregnancy is associated with adverse pregnancy outcomes, including a higher risk of operative delivery, ante- or post-partum hemorrhage, placental abruption, preterm delivery, premature rupture of membranes, poor fetal growth, fetal distress, and stillbirth.[34] Acute psychosis during pregnancy is both an obstetric and psychiatric emergency.

Treatment of psychosis during pregnancy may include use of typical high-potency antipsychotic medications, such as haloperidol, which have not been associated with an increased risk of congenital malformations when used in pregnancy.[35]

There is growing, albeit more limited, data on the reproductive safety of the second-generation, "atypical" antipsychotic (SGA) medications. A recent review, including a meta-analysis, two large observational studies, and nearly 14,000 infants with prenatal SGA exposure, is reassuring. Thus far, no consistent increased risk for major congenital malformations has been observed. However, these studies included mostly exposures to risperidone, olanzapine, quetiapine, and aripiprazole; there are much fewer data on the newer, less commonly prescribed agents such as lurasidone, asenapine, and cariprazine.[36]

Atypical antipsychotics have been associated with an increased risk of metabolic syndrome and a small but statistically significant increased risk in gestational diabetes and large-for-gestational age babies, most notably with the use of olanzapine, clozapine, and quetiapine.[37] There has not been a similarly increased risk shown with aripiprazole and risperidone. It is unclear if discontinuation of these agents diminishes risk.

A 2022 study using data from two large medical databases evaluated neurodevelopmental outcomes in more than 10,500 children exposed to SGAs in utero. After controlling for potential confounding factors, no association was found between prenatal antipsychotic exposure and the risk of neurodevelopmental disorders, except for aripiprazole; however, in the case of aripiprazole, a causal link was not established.[38] Although these preliminary data are reassuring, more research is required to better understand the reproductive safety of specific SGAs.

Given the limited data regarding the reproductive safety of SGAs, some patients taking an antipsychotic drug may choose to discontinue this medication; however, in those with severe illness (e.g., a primary psychotic disorder, BPD), this approach may be associated with an unacceptable risk of recurrent illness. One may consider switching to a better-characterized first-generation antipsychotic (FGA), such as haloperidol. However, many women do not respond as well to an FGA or who have such severe illness that making any change in their regimen places them at significant risk of illness recurrence. Thus, women and their clinicians may choose to use an SGA during pregnancy to sustain functioning while acknowledging that information regarding their reproductive safety remains incomplete.

TABLE 12.1 Anti-epileptic Mood Stabilizers During Pregnancy

Drug	Teratogenicity	Other Associated Adverse Outcomes
Carbamazepine[26]	Neural tube defects (spina bifida), cleft lip or palate, cardiac defects	Vitamin K deficiency
Gabapentin[32]	No consistent evidence of teratogenicity	Preterm delivery (association, unclear causation), low birth weight, small for gestational age, NICU admissions, neonatal withdrawals
Lamotrigine[26]	No consistent evidence of teratogenicity; early studies demonstrating cleft lip or palate not subsequently reproduced	
Lithium[33]	Overall increased risk of major malformations in the first trimester, including Ebstein anomaly	NICU admissions or readmissions
Oxcarbazepine[15]	No consistent evidence of teratogenicity	Vitamin K deficiency, small for gestational age, increased elective cesarean section deliveries
Pregabalin[16]	No consistent evidence of teratogenicity	
Topiramate[15,29]	Cleft lip with or without cleft palate, hypospadias	Preterm delivery, low birth weight, small for gestational age, neurodevelopmental abnormalities
Valproic acid[26,32]	Neural tube defects	Neurodevelopmental problems: autism spectrum disorders, attentional problems, pervasive developmental disorders, disorders of psychological development, intellectual disabilities

NICU, Neonatal intensive care unit.

ANXIETY DISORDERS DURING PREGNANCY

Although some degree of anxiety is often experienced during pregnancy, especially the first pregnancy, some women have more severe and disabling anxiety disorders, including generalized anxiety disorder (GAD), obsessive-compulsive disorder (OCD), and panic disorder.

The course of anxiety disorders in pregnancy is variable. Pregnancy may ameliorate symptoms of anxiety and panic in some patients and may provide an opportunity to discontinue medication. For other women, the persistence or worsening of anxiety symptoms may develop during pregnancy. Of concern is the finding that anxiety symptoms during pregnancy may be associated with worse obstetric outcomes, including increased rates of premature labor, lower birth weight, lower Apgar scores, and placental abruption.[39]

The use of non-pharmacological treatment, such as CBT and supportive psychotherapy, may be of great value in attenuating symptoms of anxiety, helping patients to discontinue medications and potentially prolonging the time to relapse.

For other patients, especially those with panic disorder, OCD, or severe GAD, pharmacological intervention during pregnancy may be necessary. Pharmacotherapy of those with severe anxiety during pregnancy may include treatment with SSRIs, SNRIs, TCAs, and benzodiazepines. These classes of drugs each have demonstrated efficacy in the management of patients with anxiety disorders and well-characterized reproductive safety profiles.

Although some patients respond well to an antidepressant alone, others benefit from benzodiazepines for the management of residual symptoms and insomnia. The consequences of prenatal exposure to benzodiazepines have been debated for more than 20 years. Although older studies of diazepam indicated an increased risk of oral clefts, newer data have not shown an association between benzodiazepines and an increased risk of congenital malformations.[40] There are some data surrounding an increased risk of preterm birth, low birth weight, and small-for-gestational-age infants with benzodiazepines; however, here as well, findings are inconsistent.[41] There are inadequate data on the reproductive safety of buspirone.

With respect to the third-trimester use of benzodiazepines, reports of infant hypotonia, neonatal apnea, neonatal withdrawal syndromes, and temperature dysregulation have prompted recommendations to consider tapering or discontinuing benzodiazepines as delivery nears.[42] Consideration should be given to the potential risk of relapse or worsening of anxiety symptoms in so doing.

Early studies suggested worse neurodevelopmental outcomes in children exposed to benzodiazepines during pregnancy; however, recent large studies have not supported an association between prenatal exposure to benzodiazepines and developmental disorders in children.[43]

ATTENTION-DEFICIT HYPERACTIVITY DISORDER AND PREGNANCY

An increasing number of women seek consultation to better understand the reproductive safety data of psychostimulants used for the management of ADHD, as well as for adjunctive treatment of mood disorders. Several recent studies have evaluated the reproductive safety profile of psychostimulants when taken as prescribed. Two studies have demonstrated a small increase in the risk of ventricular septal defects with methylphenidate use in pregnancy. In contrast, with more than 5500 exposures, amphetamines have not demonstrated such a risk.[44,45] In a fashion consistent with the risk posed outside of pregnancy, stimulant use has been associated with gestational hypertension.[46] No other obstetric complications during pregnancy, such as preterm delivery or low birth weight, have thus far been identified as having an increased risk with either stimulant class.

There is a paucity of data evaluating the longitudinal course of ADHD throughout pregnancy. Presently, untreated ADHD does not appear to pose a risk to pregnancies; however, secondary effects of untreated ADHD might. For example, women with ADHD may experience a higher risk of physical accidents or injuries because of inattention, with special concern for the risk of motor vehicle collisions. Inattention may also result in profound impairment in functioning at work, school, or at home, which may result in adverse financial, occupational, academic, and relational outcomes, in turn causing or worsening mood and anxiety symptoms. Finally, the indication for stimulant use extends outside of ADHD, and this must be factored into any decision regarding continued stimulant use in pregnancy because the medication might be used for treatment-resistant depression or may confer benefits from a mood standpoint.

If their use is non-essential, ideally, these medications would be discontinued during pregnancy. Optimizing non-pharmacological interventions, such as workplace or school accommodations, executive coaching, and use of public transportation, may be appropriate. Non-stimulant options have not been as well studied as stimulants.

If medication continuation is considered as essential, the lowest effective dose of shorter-acting formulations is recommended, with potential drug holidays on days when use is non-essential, with potential discontinuation as delivery nears to minimize the risk of neonatal withdrawal symptoms. Before conception, for women concerned about the risks of methylphenidate, a trial of amphetamines may be warranted.

In the post-partum period, shorter-acting stimulant formulations may be preferred to extended-release formulations to permit sleep protection. Shorter-acting formulations may afford the mother greater flexibility to sleep when her baby sleeps. Additionally, shorter-acting formulations may further mitigate the risk with breast-feeding, in that a woman may elect to breast-feed right before taking the stimulant or after the medication's concentration peaks. These potential benefits must be weighed against the higher abuse potential of shorter-acting formulations and the potential changes in the efficacy of the medication in symptom management.

CANNABIS USE DURING PREGNANCY

There has been a growing rise in marijuana use during pregnancy. Some women report using marijuana for mood or anxiety symptoms or for the management of pregnancy-related nausea and vomiting.

It is difficult to study marijuana because it contains hundreds of chemicals, and some preparations are contaminated with other drugs and pesticides. Based on the growing body of literature on the subject, data indicate a vulnerability of the fetus to the effects of marijuana. Thus far, evidence indicates that peri-natal use of marijuana is associated with a low birth weight, small-for-gestational-age babies, preterm delivery, neonatal intensive care unit admissions, lower Apgar scores (at 1 minute), and smaller head circumferences.[47] Preterm and low-birth-weight babies are at risk for higher rates of learning problems and other disabilities in childhood. Several studies have suggested a small increase in the risk of gastroschisis, a birth defect in which an opening develops in the abdominal wall.

A long-term association has been found between marijuana use in pregnancy and in adolescence with an increased vulnerability to psychiatric illness, including depressive disorders, psychotic disorders, and sleep disturbances.[48] Several studies have also shown an association with increased impulsivity, hyperactivity, aggression, and memory impairments, leading to poorer academic achievement.[49]

Consequently, complete abstinence from marijuana is advised during pregnancy and breast-feeding. Alternative options for the management of mood, anxiety, and sleep disturbances with more favorable reproductive safety profiles should be considered.

POST-PARTUM MOOD AND ANXIETY DISORDERS: DIAGNOSIS AND TREATMENT

During the post-partum period, roughly 85% of women experience some mood disturbance. For most women, the symptoms are mild; however, 13% to 19% of women develop clinically significant symptoms.[50] Post-partum psychiatric disorders are typically divided into three categories: (1) post-partum blues, (2) non-psychotic major depression, and (3) post-partum psychosis. Because of the significant overlap between these three categories, it is unclear if they represent three distinct disorders or a diagnostic continuum, with post-partum blues as the mildest form and post-partum psychosis as the most severe form of the illness.

Post-partum blues is common and occurs in approximately 25% to 85% of women after delivery.[51] Symptoms include mood reactivity, tearfulness, and irritability; it typically remits by the 10th post-partum day. Because post-partum blues is not associated with a significant impairment in functioning and is time-limited, no specific treatment is indicated. Symptoms that persist beyond 2 weeks require further evaluation and may suggest an evolving depressive disorder. When severe, post-partum blues is a risk factor for post-partum depression and, especially in women with a history of a recurrent mood disorder, may herald the onset of a post-partum major depressive episode.

Post-partum Depression

Risk factors for post-partum depression include depression or anxiety during pregnancy and a history of major depressive disorder before pregnancy. The signs and symptoms of post-partum depression usually appear over the first 2 to 3 months after delivery and generally are indistinguishable from depressive episodes that occur at other times in a woman's life, including depressed mood and loss of interest in usual activities. Insomnia, prominent fatigue, and a loss of appetite are also frequently described. Post-partum depressive symptoms may co-mingle with anxiety and obsessional symptoms, and women may present with generalized anxiety, panic disorder, or anxiety related to illness. Intrusive, ego-dystonic thoughts about harming the baby occur commonly in women with post-partum depression and may be very distressing.

Although it may be difficult to diagnose depression in the acute post-partum period given the normal occurrence of symptoms suggestive of depression, it is an error to dismiss neurovegetative symptoms (such as severe decreased energy, profound anhedonia, and guilty ruminations) as normal features of the post-partum period.

A wealth of literature indicates that post-partum depression, especially when left untreated, has a significant impact on infants' development and well-being. Treatment should be guided by the nature and severity of the symptoms and by the degree of functional impairment. However, before initiating psychiatric treatment, medical causes of mood disturbance, such as thyroid dysfunction and anemia, must be excluded. Initial evaluation should include a thorough history, physical examination, and routine laboratory tests.

Non-pharmacological therapies, such as short-term CBT and IPT, may be useful in the treatment of patients with mild to moderately severe post-partum depression, and several preliminary studies have yielded encouraging results. These non-pharmacological interventions may be particularly attractive to patients (such as women who are breast-feeding) who are reluctant to use psychotropics or for patients with milder forms of depressive illness. Further investigation is required to determine the efficacy of these treatments in women with more severe forms of post-partum mood disturbances.

Women with more severe post-partum depression may choose to use pharmacological treatment, either in conjunction with or in place of non-pharmacological therapies. To date, only a few studies have systematically assessed the pharmacological treatment of post-partum depression. Conventional antidepressant medications at standard antidepressant doses have shown efficacy in the treatment of post-partum depression. The choice of an antidepressant should be guided by the patient's prior response to antidepressant medication, the medication's side effect profile, and available lactation safety data. SSRIs and SNRIs are ideal first-line agents because they confer non-sedating, anxiolytic, and antidepressant properties and are generally well tolerated. Bupropion and TCAs may also be considered. TCAs may be more sedating, which may be helpful for women experiencing sleep disturbances; however, it is important that excessive sedation not occur, so that the patient may rouse with the baby. Adjunctive use of a benzodiazepine may help in the management of anxiety and insomnia, especially during the first weeks after initiating an antidepressant.

Neurosteroids, brexanolone, and zuranolone, which are allopregnanolone analogs and positive allosteric modulators of gamma aminobutyric acid A receptors, have emerged as novel treatments for post-partum depression. Brexanolone, approved by the FDA in 2019 for the treatment of patients with post-partum depression, has demonstrated a rapid onset of action, with initial studies indicating remission of depressive symptoms within 24 to 48 hours after intravenous administration. Because of potentially serious adverse effects, specifically excessive sedation and loss of consciousness, the FDA requires Risk Evaluation and Mitigation Strategies at facilities that administer brexanolone, requiring hospitalization and medical supervision. Zuranolone, an oral version of brexanolone, was approved by the FDA in August 2023 as the first oral medication for the treatment of post-partum depression, and has shown promise in the treatment of patients with post-partum depression, albeit with a slower onset of action (3 days) than brexanolone. Both options, however, are still much more rapidly acting than conventional antidepressants.[52]

Electroconvulsive therapy is another option for women with severe post-partum illness, both post-partum depression and psychosis. This option should be considered early in treatment given its proven efficacy. In choosing this treatment strategy, the maternal psychological impact of a potentially prolonged hospitalization with separation from the infant, and the potential adverse impacts of protracted treatment on infant development and attachment should be considered. ECT may be an attractive option given that improvement may occur more promptly than with conventional antidepressants or antipsychotics.

Post-partum Psychosis

The third and most severe category of post-partum affective and psychotic disorders is post-partum psychosis. Post-partum psychosis is a psychiatric emergency. The clinical picture is most often consistent with mania or a mixed mood state and may include waxing and waning symptoms of restlessness, agitation, sleep disturbances, paranoia, delusions, disorganized thinking, and impulsivity. Associated symptoms and behaviors place the mother and the infant at imminent risk. The typical onset of symptoms is within the first 2 weeks after delivery, but in some cases, symptoms may appear as early as during delivery itself or immediately after delivery. Although investigators have debated whether post-partum psychosis is a discrete diagnostic entity or a manifestation of BPD, treatment should follow the same algorithm as treatment of acute manic psychosis, including obtaining laboratory tests to rule out medical causes (e.g., autoimmune thyroiditis, infection, substance use); hospitalization; and potentially using mood stabilizers, antipsychotic agents, benzodiazepines, or ECT alone or in combination.

PREVENTION OF POST-PARTUM PSYCHIATRIC DISORDERS

Although it is difficult to predict which women will experience a post-partum affective or psychotic episode, identification of certain sub-groups of women who are at increased risk, such as women with a personal or family history of post-partum depression or psychosis, is possible. For women with an episode of post-partum depression or an isolated post-partum psychosis, rates of recurrence in subsequent post-partum periods is as high as 50% and 31%, respectively.[53,54] Women with BPD are at increased risk for post-partum relapse of depression and mania, as well as for post-partum psychosis. Women with a history of depression are vulnerable to post-partum psychosis, whether they take medications prophylactically or are medication-free during pregnancy. Prophylactic treatment, specifically with lithium, either before or immediately after delivery significantly decreases their risk.

Watchful waiting may be an appropriate strategy for women with no history of post-partum psychiatric illness; however, women with BPD or a history of post-partum psychosis should be monitored closely. To reduce the risk of illness in those at high risk for recurrent illness, prophylactic treatment with a mood stabilizer, such as lithium or an SGA, is recommended.

Finally, although symptoms of post-partum panic attacks and OCD are frequently subsumed within descriptions of post-partum mood disturbances, a growing literature supports the likelihood that post-partum anxiety disorders represent discrete diagnostic entities. Several investigators have described post-partum worsening of panic disorder and OCD in women with a pre-gravid history of these anxiety disorders in the absence of co-morbid depressive illness. Symptoms of post-partum OCD include ego-dystonic infant-harming intrusions (thoughts or images); may be passive (e.g., what if the baby stopped breathing?) or active (e.g., what if I smothered the baby?); and may lead to time-consuming ritualistic behaviors, such as checking or avoidance. These intrusive thoughts and compulsive behaviors are distressing and interfere with mother–baby bonding. Psychoeducation, CBT, and use of anti-obsessional agents (e.g., SSRIs or clomipramine) have proven effective. Reassuringly, compared with post-partum depression and post-partum psychosis, no increased risk of harsh parenting or violence has been demonstrated in women experiencing these ego-dystonic infant-harming intrusions.[55]

BREAST-FEEDING AND PSYCHOTROPIC DRUG USE

The psychological and physical health benefits of breast-feeding to both mothers and infants have been well established. Given the prevalence of psychiatric illness during the post-partum period, a significant number of women require pharmacological treatment while nursing.

The data indicate that all psychotropics, including antidepressants, antipsychotics, mood stabilizers, and benzodiazepines, are secreted into breast milk. However, concentrations of these agents within breast milk vary considerably. The amount of medication to which an infant is exposed depends on the drug (e.g., its molecular weight, protein binding, lipid solubility), as well as maternal and infant factors.

Maternal factors include the dosage of the medication, the frequency of dosing, and the rate of drug metabolism. Typically, peak concentrations in the breast milk are attained approximately 6 to 8 hours after the medication has been ingested. Thus, the frequency and timing of feedings can influence the amount of drug to which the nursing infant is exposed. By restricting breast-feeding to times during which breast milk drug concentrations are at their lowest (either shortly before or immediately after dosing medication), exposure may be reduced; however, this approach may not be practical for newborns who typically feed every 2 to 3 hours.

Infant factors include the quantity of breast milk ingested and how well the ingested medication is metabolized. In the first few days post-partum, because of wider gaps between alveolar cells, there is increased transmission of medications into the colostrum; however, given the low volume of colostrum, the absolute dose the infant receives remains limited. Likewise, if an infant is not being exclusively breast-fed, a lower volume of medication-containing milk is ingested, lessening exposure.

As to infant metabolism, most psychotropics are metabolized by the liver. During the first few weeks of a term infant's life, there is a lower capacity for hepatic drug metabolism, which is about one-third to one-fifth that of the adult capacity. Over the next few months, the capacity for hepatic metabolism increases significantly, and by about 2 to 3 months of age, it surpasses that of adults. In premature infants and in infants with signs of compromised hepatic metabolism (e.g., hyperbilirubinemia), breast-feeding is typically deferred because these infants are less able to metabolize drugs and are more likely to experience toxicity.

Consultation surrounding the safety of psychotropic use in breast-feeding should include a discussion of the known physical and psychological benefits of breast-feeding, the potential risks of breast-feeding (such as sleep interruption), the risks of untreated maternal mental illness, the known safety of the individual medication in lactation, the limitations of data, and the infant's status (e.g., age, weight, behaviors, stability). Although routine monitoring of infant serum drug levels was recommended in earlier treatment guidelines, this procedure is likely not warranted.

Much of the data on psychotropic use in breast-feeding pertain to antidepressants. The available data, particularly on SSRIs, during breast-feeding have been encouraging and suggest that the relative infant dose is low and that significant complications related to neonatal exposure to SSRIs in breast milk appear to be rare. Typically, very low or undetectable levels of drug have been detected in the infant serum, and one recent report indicated that exposure during nursing did not result in clinically significant blockade of serotonin reuptake in infants. Among the SSRIs, sertraline and paroxetine, and of the TCAs, nortriptyline and imipramine, are the best characterized.[56]

Given the prevalence of anxiety symptoms during the post-partum period, anxiolytics are often used. Data regarding the use of benzodiazepines have been limited; however, the available data also suggest a relatively low infant dose. Shorter-acting benzodiazepines, taken intermittently, at the lowest effective dose are preferred. Case reports of sedation, poor feeding, and respiratory distress in nursing infants have been published; however, when pooled, the data suggest a relatively low incidence of adverse events.[57]

For women with BPD, breast-feeding may pose more significant challenges. On-demand breast-feeding may significantly

disrupt the mother's sleep, which may increase her vulnerability to relapse during the acute post-partum period. Additionally, there have been reports of toxicity in nursing infants exposed to mood stabilizers, including lithium and carbamazepine. In mothers nursing while taking lithium, infant serum levels are about one-third of those observed in the mother.[32] Signs of lithium toxicity include cyanosis, hypotonia, and hypothermia. Most women taking lithium elect to forgo breast-feeding; however, if breast-feeding is pursued, lithium blood levels, renal function (e.g., blood urea nitrogen, creatinine), and thyroid function (thyroid-stimulating hormone) in the infant should be determined routinely. Collaboration with the infant's pediatrician is necessary because the child needs to be assessed closely for signs of lithium toxicity and blood levels monitored.

Several studies have suggested that lamotrigine exposure may be relatively high in nursing infants; higher infant serum levels of lamotrigine may be explained by poor neonatal metabolism of lamotrigine.[33] In addition, maternal serum levels of lamotrigine increased significantly after delivery, which may have contributed to the high levels found in nursing infants. A longstanding concern with lamotrigine is the risk for Stevens-Johnson syndrome (SJS), a rare, severe, potentially life-threatening rash, most commonly resulting from a hypersensitivity reaction to a medication. Thus far, there have been no reports of SJS in infants exposed to lamotrigine in breast milk. Nonetheless, if a rash develops in an infant exposed to lamotrigine, breast-feeding should be stopped until the infant is medically evaluated and a cause determined.

Similarly, concerns have arisen regarding the use of carbamazepine and valproic acid. These mood stabilizers have been associated with hepatic dysfunction and fatal hepatotoxicity in adults. Although the American Academy of Pediatrics has deemed that both carbamazepine and valproic acid are compatible with breast-feeding, few studies have assessed the impact of these agents on infant well-being, particularly in mothers without epilepsy. For women who choose to use valproic acid or carbamazepine while nursing, routine monitoring of both the mother's and infant's drug levels, liver function test results, and complete blood count is recommended. Ongoing collaboration with the child's pediatrician is crucial.

Limited information is available regarding the use of other medications, including stimulants, newer antidepressants, and SGAs. In most instances, low or undetectable infant serum drug levels have been documented, and serious adverse side effects have been reported infrequently. Although routine blood testing of the infant is not typically recommended, testing is indicated when neonatal toxicity related to drug exposure is suspected.

REFERENCES

1. Finer LB, Zolna MR. Declines in unintended pregnancy in the United States, 2008-2011. *N Engl J Med.* 2016;374(9):843–852.
2. Cheng Z, Gu R, Lian Z, Gu HF. Evaluation of the association between maternal folic acid supplementation and the risk of congenital heart disease: a systematic review and meta-analysis. *Nutr J.* 2022;21(1):20.
3. Creeley CE, Denton LK. Use of prescribed psychotropics during pregnancy: a systematic review of pregnancy, neonatal, and childhood outcomes. *Brain Sci.* 2019;9(9):235.
4. Kong L, Chen X, Liang Y, et al: Association of preeclampsia and perinatal complications with offspring: neurodevelopmental and psychiatric disorders. *JAMA Netw Open.* 2022;5(1):e2145719.
5. Anderson KN, Lind JN, Simeone RM, et al. Maternal use of specific antidepressant medications during early pregnancy and the risk of selected birth defects. *JAMA Psychiatry.* 2020;77(12):1246–1255.
6. Huybrechts KF, Palmsten K, Avorn J, et al. Antidepressant use in pregnancy and the risk of cardiac defects. *N Engl J Med.* 2014;370(25):2397–2407.
7. Ankarfeldt MZ, Petersen J, Andersen JT, et al. Exposure to duloxetine during pregnancy and risk of congenital malformations and

stillbirth: a nationwide cohort study in Denmark and Sweden. *PLoS Med.* 2021;18(11):e1003851.

8. Huybrechts KF, Bateman BT, Pawar A, et al. Maternal and fetal outcomes following exposure to duloxetine in pregnancy: cohort study. *BMJ.* 2020;368:m237.

9. Lassen D, Ennis ZN, Damkier P. First-trimester pregnancy exposure to venlafaxine or duloxetine and risk of major congenital malformations: a systematic review. *Basic Clin Pharmacol Toxicol.* 2016;118(1):32–36.

10. Turner E, Jones M, Vaz LR, Coleman T. Systematic review and meta-analysis to assess the safety of bupropion and varenicline in pregnancy. *Nicotine Tob Res.* 2019;21(8):1001–1010.

11. Gentile S. Tricyclic antidepressants in pregnancy and puerperium. *Expert Opin Drug Saf.* 2014;13(2):207–225.

12. Warburton W, Hertzman C, Oberlander TF. A register study of the impact of stopping third trimester selective serotonin reuptake inhibitor exposure on neonatal health. *Acta Psychiatr Scand.* 2010;121(6):471–479.

13. Ornoy A, Koren G. Selective serotonin reuptake inhibitors in human pregnancy: on the way to resolving the controversy. *Semin Fetal Neonatal Med.* 2014;19(3):188–194.

14. Huybrechts KF, Bateman BT, Palmsten K, et al. Antidepressant use late in pregnancy and risk of persistent pulmonary hypertension of the newborn. *JAMA.* 2015;313(21):2142–2151.

15. Chambers CD, Hernandez-Diaz S, Van Marter LJ, et al. Selective serotonin-reuptake inhibitors and risk of persistent pulmonary hypertension of the newborn. *New Engl J Med.* 2006;354(6):579–587.

16. Andrade SE, McPhillips H, Loren D, et al. Antidepressant medication use and risk of persistent pulmonary hypertension of the newborn. *Pharmacoepidemiol Drug Saf.* 2009;18(3):246–252.

17. Wichman C, Moore K, Lang T, et al. Congenital heart disease associated with selective serotonin reuptake inhibitor use during pregnancy. *Mayo Clin Proc.* 2009;84(1):23–27.

18. Källén B, Olausson PO. Maternal use of selective serotonin reuptake inhibitors and persistent pulmonary hypertension of the newborn. *Pharmacoepidemiol Drug Saf.* 2008;17:801–806.

19. Suarez EA, Bateman BT, Hernández-Díaz S, et al. Association of antidepressant use during pregnancy with risk of neurodevelopmental disorders in children. *JAMA Intern Med.* 2022;182(11):1149–1160.

20. Wan Mohd Yunus WMA, Matinolli HM, Waris O, et al. Digitalized cognitive behavioral interventions for depressive symptoms during pregnancy: systematic review. *J Med Internet Res.* 2022;24(2):e33337.

21. Cohen LS, Altshuler LL, Harlow BL, et al. Relapse of major depression during pregnancy in women who maintain or discontinue antidepressant treatment. *JAMA.* 2006;295(5):499–507.

22. Wisner K, Perel J, Wheeler S. Tricyclic dose requirements across pregnancy. *Am J Psychiatry.* 1993;150:1541–1542.

23. Anderson EL, Reti IM. ECT in pregnancy: a review of the literature from 1941 to 2007. *Psychosom Med.* 2009;71(2):235–242.

24. Ward HB, Fromson JA, Cooper JJ, et al. Recommendations for the use of ECT in pregnancy: literature review and proposed clinical protocol. *Arch Womens Ment Health.* 2018;21:715–722.

25. Masters GA, Hugunin J, Xu L, et al. Prevalence of bipolar disorder in perinatal women: a systematic review and meta-analysis. *J Clin Psychiatry.* 2022;83(5):21r14045.

26. Patorno E, Huybrechts KF, Bateman BT, et al. Lithium use in pregnancy and the risk of cardiac malformations. *N Engl J Med.* 2017;376(23):2245–2254.

27. Kaplan YC, Demir O. Use of phenytoin, phenobarbital, carbamazepine, levetiracetam, lamotrigine and valproate in pregnancy and breastfeeding: risk of major malformations, dose-dependency, monotherapy vs polytherapy, pharmacokinetics and clinical implications. *Curr Neuropharmacology.* 2021;19(11):1805–1824.

28. Pennell PB, Newport DJ, Stowe ZN, et al. The impact of pregnancy and childbirth on the metabolism of lamotrigine. *Neurology.* 2004;62:292–295.

29. Clark CT, Klein AM, Perel JM, et al. Lamotrigine dosing for pregnant patients with bipolar disorder. *Am J Psychiatry.* 2013;170(11):1240–1247.

30. Blotière PO, Raguideau F, Weill A, et al. Risks of 23 specific malformations associated with prenatal exposure to 10 antiepileptic drugs. *Neurology.* 2019;93(2):e167–e180.

31. Wiggs KK, Rickert ME, Sujan AC, et al. Antiseizure medication use during pregnancy and risk of ASD and ADHD in children. *Neurology.* 2020;95(24):e3232–e3240.

32. Viguera AC, Newport DJ, Ritchie J, et al. Lithium in breast milk and nursing infants: clinical implications. *Am J Psychiatry.* 2007;164(2):342–345.

33. Goldsmith DR, Wagstaff AJ, Ibbotson T, Perry CM. Spotlight on lamotrigine in bipolar disorder. *CNS Drugs.* 2004;18(1):63–67.

34. Zhong QY, Gelaye B, Fricchione GL, et al. Adverse obstetric and neonatal outcomes complicated by psychosis among pregnant women in the United States. *BMC Pregnancy Childbirth.* 2018;18:120.

35. Huybrechts KF, Hernández-Díaz S, Patorno E, et al. Antipsychotic use in pregnancy and the risk for congenital malformations. *JAMA Psychiatry.* 2016;73(9):938–946.

36. Andrade C. Major congenital malformations associated with exposure to second-generation antipsychotic drugs during pregnancy. *J Clin Psychiatry.* 2021;82(5):21f14252.

37. Heinonen E, Forsberg L, Nörby U, et al. Antipsychotic use during pregnancy and risk for gestational diabetes: a national register-based cohort study in Sweden. *CNS Drugs.* 2022;36(5):529–539.

38. Straub L, Hernández-Díaz S, Bateman BT, et al. Association of antipsychotic drug exposure in pregnancy with risk of neurodevelopmental disorders: a national birth cohort study. *JAMA Intern Med.* 2022;182(5):522–533.

39. Grigoriadis S, Graves L, Peer M, et al. Maternal anxiety during pregnancy and the association with adverse perinatal outcomes: systematic review and meta-analysis. *J Clin Psychiatry.* 2018;79:e1–e22.

40. Okun ML, Ebert R, Saini B. A review of sleep-promoting medications used in pregnancy. *Am J Obstet Gynecol.* 2015;212(4):428–441.

41. Shyken JM, Shilpa B, Babbar S, et al. Benzodiazepines in pregnancy. *Clin Obst Obstet Gynecol.* 2019;62(1):156–167.

42. Tripathi BM, Majumder P. Lactating mother and psychotropic drugs. *Mens Sana Monogr.* 2010;8(1):83–95.

43. Chen VC, Wu SI, Lin CF, et al. Association of prenatal exposure to benzodiazepines with development of autism spectrum and attention-deficit/hyperactivity disorders. *JAMA Netw Open.* 2022;5(11):e2243282.

44. Huybrechts KF, Bröms G, Christensen LB, et al. Association between methylphenidate and amphetamine use in pregnancy and risk of congenital malformations: a cohort study from the International Pregnancy Safety Study Consortium. *JAMA Psychiatry.* 2018;75(2):167–175.

45. Kolding L, Ehrenstein V, Pedersen L, et al. Associations between ADHD medication use in pregnancy and severe malformations based on prenatal and postnatal diagnoses: a Danish registry-based study. *J Clin Psychiatry.* 2021;82(1):20m13458.

46. Newport DJ, Hostetter AL, Juul SH, et al. Prenatal psychostimulant and antidepressant exposure and risk of hypertensive disorders of pregnancy. *J Clin Psychiatry.* 2016;77(11):1538–1545.

47. Marchand G, Masoud AT, Govindan M, et al. Birth outcomes of neonates exposed to marijuana in utero: a systematic review and meta-analysis. *JAMA Netw Open.* 2022;5(1):e2145653.

48. Paul SE, Hatoum AS, Fine JD, et al. Associations between prenatal cannabis exposure and childhood outcomes: results from the ABCD Study. *JAMA Psychiatry.* 2021;78(1):64–76.

49. Grant KS, Conover E, Chambers CD. Update on the developmental consequences of cannabis use during pregnancy and lactation. *Birth Defects Res.* 2020;112(15):1126–1138.

50. Shorey S, Chee CYI, Ng ED, et al. Prevalence and incidence of postpartum depression among healthy mothers: a systematic review and meta-analysis. *J Psychiatr Res.* 2018;104:235–248.

51. O'Hara MW, Wisner KL. Perinatal mental illness: definition, description and aetiology. *Best practice & research. Clin Obstet Gynaecol.* 2014;28(1):3–12.

52. Deligiannidis KM, Meltzer-Brody S, Gunduz-Bruce H, et al. Effect of zuranolone vs placebo in postpartum depression: a randomized clinical trial. *JAMA Psychiatry.* 2021;78(9):951–959.

53. Kupfer DJ, Frank E. Relapse in recurrent unipolar depression. *Am J Psychiatry.* 1987;144(1):86–88.

54. Bergink V, Rasgon N, Wisner KL. Postpartum psychosis: madness, mania, and melancholia in motherhood. *Am J Psychiatry.* 2016;173(12):1179–1188.

55. Brok EC, Lok P, Oosterbaan DB, et al. Infant-related intrusive thoughts of harm in the postpartum period: a critical review. *J Clin Psychiatry.* 2017;78(8):e913–e923.

56. Lanza Di Scalea T, Wisner KL. Antidepressant medication use during breastfeeding. *Clin Obstet Gynecol.* 2009;52(3):483–497.

57. Burt VK, Suri R, Altshuler L, et al. The use of psychotropic medications during breast-feeding. *Am J Psychiatry.* 2001;7:1001–1009.

13 Side Effects of Psychotropic Medications

Henry K. Onyeaka, Scott R. Beach, Jeff C. Huffman, and Theodore A. Stern

KEY POINTS

Background

- A systematic approach to side effects of medications should include consideration of the nature, severity, and timing of symptoms to facilitate optimal management of such side effects.

History

- Many medications (e.g., nefazodone) previously used in psychiatric disorders but shown to have serious adverse side effects have been removed from the market over the years.

Clinical and Research Challenges

- Rates of medication side effects may be difficult to quantify.
- Although some side effects may be class effects, others are specific to individual agents.
- It is difficult to predict who will have side effects; some side effects are idiosyncratic.

Practical Pointers

- Tricyclic antidepressants are associated with cardiac effects and can be dangerous in overdose.
- Use of monoamine oxidase inhibitors requires education about dietary limitations and drug–drug interactions.
- Selective serotonin reuptake inhibitors (SSRIs) and newer antidepressants are generally well tolerated and safer in overdose than older agents but still may cause clinically significant side effects. Some SSRIs, such as citalopram, have been associated with an increased risk for arrhythmias.
- Some selective norepinephrine (noradrenaline)–serotonin reuptake inhibitors have been associated with increased blood pressure (e.g., venlafaxine) and liver dysfunction (e.g., duloxetine).

- Some antidepressants have been associated with an elevated risk for suicide, particularly among young populations.
- Bupropion is known to lower the seizure threshold and has also been associated with an increase in panic symptoms.
- Mirtazapine is associated most commonly with sedation and weight gain.
- Lithium and anticonvulsant mood stabilizers are associated with a variety of side effects, including cognitive slowing, weight gain, and neurological symptoms.
- Lamotrigine is the mood stabilizer most closely associated with the development of Stevens-Johnson syndrome, a rare but life-threatening skin disease.
- Typical antipsychotics are associated with tardive dyskinesia, and, of them, the high-potency typical antipsychotics commonly cause extrapyramidal symptoms.
- Several atypical antipsychotics are linked to weight gain and metabolic side effects.
- Most antipsychotics can cause QTc interval prolongation, which may increase the risk for lethal ventricular arrhythmias.
- Stimulants predispose to an increase in heart rate and blood pressure, and their use is not recommended for patients with underlying ventricular arrhythmias.
- Benzodiazepines are associated with a variety of side effects (including falls, dizziness, and ataxia).
- Short-acting sedative-hypnotic agents, such as zolpidem, have been associated with various sleep-related behaviors, including eating and driving.

OVERVIEW

Side effects of psychotropics, which can range from minor nuisances to life-threatening conditions, can seriously affect the quality of a patient's life and his or her ability to adhere to psychopharmacological treatment regimens. For these reasons, it is important for clinicians who prescribe psychotropic medications to be knowledgeable about their potential side effects and how such side effects can be managed.

Determining which medication is causing a specific side effect and whether *any* medication is to blame for a given adverse effect can be difficult. A stepwise approach to the assessment of a potential side effect can help to ensure that true side effects are quickly addressed, and knee-jerk reactions that result in the discontinuation of well-tolerated treatments can be avoided. This approach (Box 13.1) involves an assessment of the nature and severity of the effect, a thoughtful investigation into the causality of the effect, and the appropriate management of the symptom.

In this chapter, the most common and most dangerous side effects of psychotropics are discussed to guide clinicians to treatment decisions and management of adverse effects. For each agent or class of agents, the chapter reviews common initial side effects, frequent long-term side effects, severe but rare adverse events, consequences of overdose, and (where applicable) withdrawal symptoms.

ANTIDEPRESSANTS

Selective Serotonin Reuptake Inhibitors

SSRIs are generally well tolerated. The most common side effects of SSRIs include gastrointestinal (GI) side effects (e.g., nausea, diarrhea, heartburn) that likely result from interactions with serotonin receptors (primarily 5-HT$_3$ receptors that line the gut), central nervous system (CNS) activation (e.g., anxiety, restlessness, tremor, insomnia), and sedation that appear within the first few days of treatment. GI side effects may be the most common with sertraline and fluvoxamine, CNS activation with fluoxetine, and sedation with paroxetine, although individual patients may react differently to different agents. Headache and dizziness can also occur soon after treatment begins. These symptoms often improve or resolve within the first few weeks of

---

BOX 13.1 A Systematic Approach to Medication Side Effects

NATURE OF THE SIDE EFFECT

- What exactly are the signs and symptoms? In some cases (e.g., drug rash), this can be easily ascertained, but in others (e.g., a severely demented patient with worsening agitation, possibly consistent with akathisia, restlessness, or constipation), it may be difficult.
- When did the symptom start?
- Has this ever happened before?
- Are there associated symptoms?

SEVERITY OF THE SIDE EFFECT

- What subjective distress does the symptom cause?
- What impact is it having on function and quality of life?
- What medical dangers are associated with the side effect?

CAUSALITY OF THE SIDE EFFECT

- Did the side effect start in the context of a new medication or a dosage change?
- What other medications or remedies are being taken?
- Have there been other changes in medication, medical issues, diet, environment, or psychiatric symptoms?
- Are the current signs and symptoms consistent with known side effects of a given medication?

MANAGEMENT OF THE SIDE EFFECT

- If it appears that a specific medication is causing the side effect, options for management include:
  - Discontinue the medication.
  - Decrease the dose.
  - Change the dosing schedule (e.g., splitting up dose, taking medication during meals).
  - Change the preparation (e.g., to a longer-lasting formulation).
  - Add a new medication to treat the side effect (e.g., propranolol for akathisia).

---

treatment. Rarely, akathisia or other extrapyramidal symptoms (EPSs) may occur. Although sertraline, paroxetine, and fluoxetine have been reported to be the major offenders, it appears that EPSs and movement disorders may occur with any SSRI.[1]

Longer-term side effects associated with SSRIs include sexual dysfunction, which occurs in 30% or more of SSRI-treated patients; SSRI-induced sexual dysfunction occurs in both men and women, affecting both libido and orgasms. Weight gain, fatigue, and apathy are infrequent long-term side effects; weight gain may occur more frequently with paroxetine. The syndrome of inappropriate antidiuretic hormone secretion (SIADH) can occur with all SSRIs.[2] Finally, SSRIs may increase the risk of bleeding, primarily due to the effects of these agents on serotonin receptors of platelets, resulting in decreased platelet activation and aggregation; it appears that the bleeding risk associated with use of SSRIs is similar to that of low-dose non-steroidal anti-inflammatory drugs.[3] SSRIs are relatively safe in overdose. A serotonin syndrome can occur when these agents are combined with other serotonergic compounds, or, very rarely, when used alone.

Selective serotonin reuptake inhibitors are generally considered safe in terms of cardiovascular side effects. Concern has arisen regarding the possibility of SSRIs leading to QTc interval prolongation and increasing the risk for torsades de pointes (TdP), a potentially lethal ventricular arrhythmia (Figure 13.1). In fact, all SSRIs except paroxetine have been associated in case reports with QTc prolongation at therapeutic doses and in overdose.[4] In particular, citalopram has been shown to have a modest QTc-prolonging effect, which resulted in a recommendation from the Food and Drug Administration (FDA) in 2011 to limit the maximum daily dose of citalopram to 40 mg (20 mg in patients with hepatic impairment and in those older than 60 years) because of the increased risk of QTc prolongation at higher doses and to declare its use contraindicated in patients with congenital long-QT syndrome. Less stringent recommendations were issued in 2012, but citalopram remains "not recommended" for use at doses greater than 40 mg/day. Nonetheless, individual patients may benefit greatly from doses greater than 40 mg without a significantly increased risk, and prescribers are encouraged to conduct a careful risk-to-benefit analysis for all decisions related to QTc prolongation with psychiatric medications.[5] No QTc-related recommendations have been issued by the FDA for other SSRIs, though escitalopram appears to have a slight, dose-dependent effect on QTc interval prolongation.

Finally, abrupt cessation of SSRIs can lead to a withdrawal syndrome characterized by several somatic symptoms. The

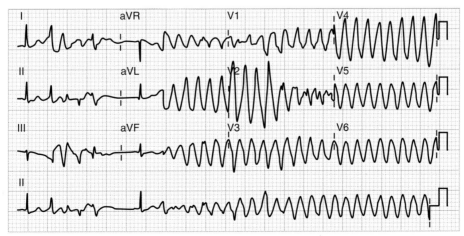

Figure 13.1 Torsades de pointes ventricular arrhythmia. (Redrawn from Khan IA. Twelve-lead electrocardiogram of torsades de pointes. *Tex Heart Inst J.* 2001;28:69.)

syndrome includes dysequilibrium (dizziness, vertigo, and ataxia), flu-like symptoms (headache, lethargy, myalgias, rhinorrhea, and chills), GI symptoms (nausea, vomiting, and diarrhea), sensory disturbances (paresthesias and sensations of electrical shock), and sleep disturbances (insomnia, fragmented sleep, and vivid, often frightening, dreams). In addition, several psychological symptoms (e.g., agitation, irritability, anxiety, crying spells) are associated with SSRI discontinuation.

Symptoms of the discontinuation syndrome typically begin 1 to 3 days after withdrawal of an SSRI. Symptoms usually resolve within 2 weeks. If the original antidepressant is restarted or a longer-acting SSRI is substituted, the symptoms resolve, usually within 24 hours of re-initiation. This syndrome is most common with SSRIs having shorter half-lives (paroxetine and fluvoxamine); it rarely occurs with fluoxetine, whose metabolite has a half-life of more than 1 week.

Serotonin–Norepinephrine Reuptake Inhibitors

Serotonin–norepinephrine reuptake inhibitors (SNRIs) include venlafaxine, duloxetine, and levomilnacipran. All have side effects (including nausea and CNS activation) like those of SSRIs, given their significant serotonergic activity. Sexual dysfunction occurs at rates like those of SSRIs. More serious side effects, including SIADH and serotonin syndrome, have also been reported with all SNRIs. A discontinuation syndrome has been associated with all SNRIs, although it may be less common with duloxetine.

Venlafaxine

Dry mouth and constipation may be associated with venlafaxine use despite its lack of effects on muscarinic cholinergic receptors. Increased blood pressure, presumably related to its effects on norepinephrine (noradrenaline), can occur with immediate-release venlafaxine, with 7% of patients taking 300 mg/day or less and 13% taking doses greater than 300 mg/day having elevated blood pressure; this resolves spontaneously in approximately half of cases.[6] The extended-release (XR) formulation appears to be associated with lower rates of hypertension. Venlafaxine does not appear to have substantial adverse effects on the cardiovascular system.

Overdose of venlafaxine generally causes symptoms like those of SSRI overdose. Although one large epidemiological study suggested that there was a high rate of death in overdose (possibly via seizure and cardiovascular effects),[7] other (smaller) studies have not found an increased lethality with overdose. Some reports of QTc prolongation in the setting of overdose have occurred.

Duloxetine

Nausea, dizziness, headache, and insomnia may be somewhat more frequent in association with use of duloxetine than with SSRIs, but overall this agent is well tolerated. Duloxetine does not appear to have significant effects on blood pressure or other cardiovascular parameters, including the QTc interval. Sexual dysfunction may be less common with duloxetine than with use of SSRIs, such as paroxetine.[8] Duloxetine has not shown significant affinity for histaminic or cholinergic receptors, and thus sedation, weight gain, and anticholinergic effects are uncommon.

Increased levels of hepatic transaminases develop in a small percentage of patients taking duloxetine; this is usually asymptomatic, but patients with chronic liver disease or cirrhosis have developed elevated levels of bilirubin, alkaline phosphatase, and transaminases, and as a result, duloxetine should not be given to patients who consume substantial amounts of alcohol or who exhibit evidence of chronic liver

disease.[9] Duloxetine does not appear to increase death rates in cases of overdose.

Levomilnacipran

Unique GI effects include a mild elevation in alanine aminotransferase and aspartate aminotransferases in a small fraction of patients. However, levomilnacipran can be used safely, without dosage adjustments, in patients with chronic liver disease or cirrhosis.[10] Levomilnacipran is weight neutral and does not appear to cause weight gain as occurs with some SSRIs.

With respect to its cardiovascular profile, levomilnacipran appears to cause modest elevations in blood pressure and heart rate but not the duration of the QTc interval.[10] Additionally, urinary hesitancy is seen more frequently with use of levomilnacipran; it is thought to be caused by a levomilnacipran-induced increase in peripheral noradrenergic tone.[10] Levomilnacipran does not appear to raise the risk of death from overdose.

Tricyclic Antidepressants

Tricyclic antidepressants (TCAs) have several common side effects that require careful management. Anticholinergic effects (including dry mouth, blurry vision, urinary hesitancy, constipation, tachycardia, and delirium) that result from the blockade of muscarinic cholinergic receptors occur with the use of TCAs. In addition, anticholinergic effects can be dangerous to patients with pre-existing glaucoma (leading to acute angle-closure glaucoma), benign prostatic hypertrophy (BPH) (leading to acute urinary retention), and dementia (leading to acute confusional states). TCAs also cause sedation that results from blockade of H₁ histamine receptors, and orthostatic hypotension (OH) caused by blockade of alpha₁ receptors on blood vessels. All three of these side effect clusters are more common with tertiary amine TCAs (e.g., amitriptyline, doxepin, clomipramine, imipramine) than with secondary amine TCAs (e.g., nortriptyline, desipramine, protriptyline). TCAs may also cause increased sweating. Longer-term side effects of TCAs include weight gain (related to histamine receptor blockade) and sexual dysfunction. Box 13.2 describes the management of common side effects related to TCAs and other antidepressants.

In addition to these common initial and long-term side effects, TCAs may induce more serious but uncommon side effects; many of them are cardiac in nature. These agents are structurally similar to class I antiarrhythmics that are proarrhythmic in roughly 10% of the population; approximately 20% of patients with pre-existing conduction disturbances have cardiac complications while taking TCAs.[11] TCAs are associated with cardiac conduction disturbances, and their use can lead to prolongation of the PR, QRS, and QT intervals on the electrocardiogram (ECG), and they have been associated with all manner of heart block. Some TCAs have also been associated with Brugada syndrome, which increases the risk for sudden cardiac death. TCAs most closely linked to Brugada syndrome include amitriptyline, nortriptyline, clomipramine, and desipramine.[12] Furthermore, these agents have been associated with an increased risk of myocardial infarction (MI) compared with SSRIs.[13] In addition to their cardiac effects, other serious adverse events include serotonin syndrome that occurs most often when TCAs are combined with other serotonergic agents. This syndrome can include confusion, agitation, and neuromuscular excitability (including seizures).

Adverse effects associated with TCA overdose include the exacerbation of common side effects (e.g., severe sedation, hypotension, anticholinergic delirium). Ventricular arrhythmias and seizures can also result from TCA overdose. TCA overdose

BOX 13.2 Management of Antidepressant Side Effects

GENERAL PRINCIPLES

- Carefully consider whether the side effect is from the antidepressant.
- Consider the timing, dosing, and the nature of effect, as well as the impact of concomitant medications, environmental changes, and medical conditions.
- Consider drug–drug interactions as the cause of the adverse effects rather than the effects of the antidepressant acting in isolation.
- If an antidepressant appears to be causing non-dangerous side effects, consider lowering the dose (temporarily or permanently), dividing the dose, adjusting the timing (daily or nightly), or changing medications.

MANAGEMENT OF SPECIFIC SIDE EFFECTS

- Anticholinergic effects (e.g., dry mouth, urinary hesitancy, constipation): provide symptomatic treatment (use hard candies for dry mouth, use laxatives for constipation); use bethanechol (25–50 mg/day) for refractory symptoms.
- Sedation: move the dose to bedtime, divide the dose, or add a psychostimulant (e.g., methylphenidate, 5–15 mg each morning) or modafinil (100–200 mg each morning).
- Orthostatic hypotension: increase fluid intake, divide the dose or move it to bedtime, or add a stimulant/mineralocorticoid.
- Gastrointestinal side effects: divide the dose, take it with meals, give it at bedtime, or use an H_2 blocker (e.g., ranitidine 150 mg twice daily).
- Insomnia: move the dose to the morning or add trazodone (25–100 mg), a sedative–hypnotic (e.g., zolpidem 5–10 mg), or another sedating agent.
- Weight gain: use diet and exercise and consider addition of an H_2 blocker, or topiramate. Other agents include metformin and glucagon-like peptide analogs. Can also consider switching to lesser weight gain–inducing medications such as aripiprazole.
- Sexual dysfunction: options include switching to another agent (to bupropion, mirtazapine, or another agent less associated with sexual dysfunction), using a drug holiday (often ineffective), or augmenting with a variety of agents (e.g., sildenafil, methylphenidate, bupropion, amantadine, buspirone, or yohimbine).

BOX 13.3 Medications to Be Avoided by Patients Taking Monoamine Oxidase Inhibitors

INCREASED RISK OF SEROTONIN SYNDROME

- SSRIs
- TCAs
- Mirtazapine
- Nefazodone
- Vilazodone
- Trazodone
- Buspirone
- Lithium
- Dextromethorphan
- Tramadol
- Methadone
- Carbamazepine
- Sumatriptan and related compounds
- Cocaine
- MDMA
- St. John's wort
- SAMe
- Linezolid

INCREASED RISK OF HYPERADRENERGIC CRISIS

- Dopamine
- L-dopa
- Psychostimulants
- Bupropion
- Amphetamine
- Cold remedies or weight loss products containing pseudoephedrine, phenylpropanolamine, phenylephrine, or ephedrine
- Meperidine (may cause seizures and delirium)

MDMA, 3,4-methylenedioxy-N-methylamphetamine; SAMe, S-adenosylmethionine; SSRI, selective serotonin reuptake inhibitor; TCA, tricyclic antidepressant.

is frequently lethal, with death most often occurring via its cardiovascular effects. A withdrawal syndrome (manifested by malaise, nausea, muscle aches, chills, diaphoresis, and anxiety) can also arise after abrupt discontinuation of TCAs.

Monoamine Oxidase Inhibitors

Tranylcypromine and phenelzine are oral, irreversible, monoamine oxidase inhibitors (MAOIs). Whereas tranylcypromine is associated with anxiety, restlessness, insomnia, and tremor, phenelzine is more closely associated with sedation, mild anticholinergic effects, and OH (although this last effect can occur with both agents). Both agents are associated with headache, dry mouth, and GI side effects. Long-term side effects, including weight gain and sexual dysfunction, can occur with all MAOIs, although they are perhaps more common with phenelzine. MAOIs can lead to symptoms of pyridoxine deficiency, including paresthesias and weakness. Finally, MAOIs have been associated with elevated liver transaminases, although true hepatotoxicity is exceedingly rare.

Hyperadrenergic crises, characterized by occipital headache, nausea, vomiting, diaphoresis, tachycardia, and severe hypertension, can develop in patients taking MAOIs. These occur most often when tyramine-containing foods are consumed or when adrenergic agonists (such as sympathomimetics) are taken in combination with an MAOI. Serotonin syndrome can also occur with MAOIs when these agents are taken with SSRIs, TCAs, or other serotonergic agents. (Box 13.3 lists medications that should be avoided by patients who are taking MAOIs.) MAOI overdose is quite dangerous, with rates of death higher than those for SSRIs and other newer antidepressants[7]; with serotonin syndrome, neuromuscular excitability, seizures, arrhythmias, and cardiovascular collapse are all possible.

The transdermal MAOI (selegiline) patch does not require dietary modification at its lowest dose. At this lowest dose (6 mg/24 hours), transdermal selegiline appears to have an incidence of OH, GI side effects, weight gain, and sexual dysfunction that is greater than with placebo but lower than with orally ingested MAOIs; skin irritation at the patch site has been its most common adverse effect. At dosages above 6 mg/24 hours, dietary modification is required, and at all dosages, concomitant use of medications that increase levels of catecholamines or serotonin should be avoided, as is the case with oral MAOIs.

Other Antidepressants

Bupropion

Bupropion, an agent that does not directly affect serotonin neurotransmission, has initial side effects that differ from those of SSRIs and dual-action agents. Its most common and important initial side effects include headache, dizziness, dry mouth, anxiety, restlessness, anorexia, nausea, and insomnia. Long-term side effects are rare; rates of sexual dysfunction and weight gain are as common as those of placebo (weight loss can occur in some patients), and this agent has minimal cardiovascular effects, even in overdose. The most serious side effect associated with bupropion use is seizure. The risk of seizure with the immediate-release preparation is 0.1% at doses below 300 mg/day, and 0.4% at doses from 300 to 400 mg/day; the risk of seizure may be lower with longer-acting preparations, but guidelines to keep the total daily dose at or below 450 mg/day remain. In addition, maximum single doses should not exceed 150 mg for the immediate-release form, 200 mg for the sustained-release form, and 450 mg for the XL form. Because of its increased risk of seizure, bupropion should not be used in individuals with a history of seizures or in those at an increased risk of seizures (e.g., those with eating disorders, head trauma, or alcohol abuse). Overdose is infrequently life-threatening, although seizures, arrhythmias, and death have occurred in association with overdose. There is no withdrawal syndrome associated with abrupt discontinuation of bupropion.

Mirtazapine

The most common initial side effects associated with use of mirtazapine include sedation and increased appetite due to histamine receptor blockade; sedation may be less prevalent at higher doses (i.e., ≥30 mg/day) than at lower doses because of recruitment of noradrenergic effects at higher doses. Less frequently, dry mouth, constipation, and dizziness have been associated with mirtazapine use; OH can also occur. GI side effects, anxiety, insomnia, and headache are all less common with use of mirtazapine than with use of most other antidepressants. Weight gain is the most common long-term side effect, and elevated lipids develop in approximately 15% of patients who use mirtazapine. Rare, but more serious, side effects have included an increase in liver transaminases (seen in ~2% of patients), and neutropenia (seen in 0.1%). Mirtazapine appears to be associated with less sexual dysfunction than with the SSRIs, and it has minimal cardiovascular effects; it has no withdrawal syndrome. There is also a low mortality rate when taken in overdose.

Trazodone

Trazodone was developed as an antidepressant, but its use for depression was limited by sedation; it is now commonly used as a sleep aid. Common initial side effects include dry mouth, nausea, dizziness, and OH. Weight gain and sexual dysfunction are rare, and trazodone is not associated with hepatotoxicity. Trazodone has rarely been associated with cardiac arrhythmias and mild QTc prolongation. Priapism occurs in approximately 1 in 6000 male patients who take trazodone; this effect usually occurs within the first month of treatment.[14] In overdose, sedation and hypotension are the most common adverse effects; isolated trazodone overdose is rarely fatal. There is no discontinuation syndrome.

Vilazodone

Vilazodone has diarrhea, nausea, and headache as its most common side effects, all of which are typically transient. The dose is typically titrated incrementally to avoid GI side effects. Dry mouth, dizziness, insomnia, and abnormal dreams have also been reported. Vilazodone has not been shown to have adverse cardiac effects, and it appears to have minimal effects on weight gain. Although it is purported to cause less sexual dysfunction than other antidepressants, the FDA reported that vilazodone does not meet the minimal criteria to make this claim.[15]

Vortioxetine

Vortioxetine is a novel medication with multi-modal activity on the serotonin receptors that is approved by the FDA for depression. The most common side effects of vortioxetine are vomiting, nausea, dizziness, headaches, and constipation. These are typically transitory and dose dependent. Vortioxetine has not been shown to adversely impact cardiovascular function, and it appears to be weight neutral. Despite its unique serotonergic receptor activity, earlier reports of lesser sexual side effects when compared with the SSRI have not been substantiated by the FDA.[16] With the exception of hyponatremia, which occurs at comparable rates to the SSRIs, vortioxetine has no clinically relevant effects on renal, hepatic, or hematological indices. In overdose, vortioxetine may result in adverse events (nausea, dizziness, somnolence, flushing), but it is rarely fatal.

Brexanolone

Brexanolone is a neuro-steroid and an analog of allopregnanolone with modulatory action on GABA-A receptors; it is approved by the FDA as an intravenous (IV) infusion for the management of post-partum depression. Brexanolone is generally well tolerated. Common side effects are headaches, dizziness, and fatigue. In most cases, each of these adverse effects is mild and self-limited. Because it is administered intravenously, brexanolone has been associated with discomfort, erythema, pain, and localized rash at the infusion site; these effects are typically mild and transient. Serious side effects of brexanolone include an increased risk of profound sedation, loss of consciousness, and syncope. To mitigate the risk of these serious side effects, the FDA mandates that brexanolone's use be limited to health care facilities enrolled in a Risk Evaluation and Management Strategy (REMS) program.[17] Brexanolone is currently classified as a Schedule IV substance, and although it modulates the GABA receptors, data regarding its impact on dependence or withdrawal remain limited.

MOOD STABILIZERS

Lithium

Lithium has many associated adverse effects, summarized in Box 13.4. GI and neurological side effects (e.g., sedation, tremor), along with increased thirst, often arise early in therapy; effects on thyroid and renal function occur more chronically. Box 13.5 summarizes potential treatments for lithium-induced side effects; change in dosing and formulation can reduce GI side effects, but other side effects require additional therapies. Lithium has some effects on sinoatrial node transmission and (less commonly) on atrioventricular conduction. However, other effects on the cardiovascular system, including QTc prolongation, are not common; cardiac disease (aside from sick sinus syndrome) is not an absolute contraindication for lithium use. Lithium has a low therapeutic index, and lithium toxicity (whether intentional or unintentional) can lead to a variety of symptoms, including neurological (e.g., severe sedation, tremor, dysarthria, delirium, anterograde amnesia, myoclonus, seizure), GI (e.g., nausea, vomiting), and cardiovascular (e.g., arrhythmia) effects; renal function often is impaired, and dialysis may be required

BOX 13.4 Common Adverse Effects of Lithium

NEUROLOGICAL

- Sedation
- Tremor (fine action tremor)
- Ataxia or incoordination
- Cognitive slowing

GASTROINTESTINAL

- Nausea and vomiting
- Diarrhea
- Abdominal pain
- Weight gain

RENAL

- Polydipsia or polyuria
- Nephrogenic diabetes insipidus
- Interstitial nephritis

DERMATOLOGICAL

- Acne
- Psoriasis
- Edema

CARDIOVASCULAR

- T-wave inversion on electrocardiogram
- Sinoatrial node slowing
- Atrioventricular blockade

OTHER

- Hypothyroidism
- Leukocytosis
- Hypercalcemia

BOX 13.5 Management of Selected Lithium Side Effects

TREMOR

- Propranolol (10–30 mg twice or three times daily); primidone is a second-line option (25–100 mg/day)

GASTROINTESTINAL

- Change the formulation to a longer-lasting oral preparation or lithium citrate syrup

POLYDIPSIA OR POLYURIA

- Amiloride (5–20 mg/day); hydrochlorothiazide (50 mg/day) is a second-line option (halve the lithium dose and follow lithium levels closely)

EDEMA

- Spironolactone (25 mg/day); follow lithium levels closely

HYPOTHYROIDISM

- Treat with thyroid hormone and continue lithium therapy

---

to treat lithium toxicity if supportive measures and IV normal saline (to aid lithium excretion) are ineffective. Lithium does not have a characteristic discontinuation syndrome, but rapid withdrawal of lithium therapy has been associated with higher rates of relapse than when lithium is tapered.[18]

Lamotrigine

Initial side effects of lamotrigine include neurological side effects (e.g., dizziness, ataxia, visual changes [diplopia and blurred vision], sedation, and headache); nausea, vomiting,

and uncomplicated rash may also occur. Each of these initial effects, however, is uncommon, at least in part because of the slow dose escalation required to reduce the risk of dangerous dermatological conditions. Lamotrigine does not have significant long-term side effects; weight gain is rare, and neither hepatoxicity nor cardiovascular effects have been described when used at usual doses. However, the best-known and most important adverse effects associated with lamotrigine are dermatological conditions related to serious rash. Both Stevens-Johnson syndrome (SJS) and toxic epidermal necrolysis have occurred in association with lamotrigine use; the risk appears to be greater in pediatric patients, when the dose has been escalated rapidly, and with concomitant use of valproic acid (which inhibits lamotrigine metabolism). The risk of life-threatening rash appears to be between 0.1% and 0.3% (as opposed to an ~10% prevalence of benign rash), and it has been on the lower end of this continuum in trials of lamotrigine for psychiatric illness. Any patient who develops rash while taking lamotrigine should be evaluated promptly by a medical professional; furthermore, rash with significant facial involvement, mucous membrane involvement (e.g., dysuria, tongue or mouth lesions), or systemic symptoms (such as fever or lymphadenopathy) should generate great concern for a life-threatening rash that requires immediate emergency evaluation.

Finally, in 2020, the FDA issued a warning regarding the risk of arrhythmias with lamotrigine based on in vitro data. A systematic review of the literature concluded that lamotrigine is largely safe but may lead to modest QRS widening and rarely to Brugada syndrome.[19] Lamotrigine overdose can be fatal; the most common symptoms include stupor, convulsions, and intraventricular conduction delay; treatment is largely supportive.

Valproic Acid

Common initial side effects of valproate therapy include GI side effects (e.g., nausea, vomiting, diarrhea, and abdominal cramps), sedation, tremor, and alopecia; GI side effects are less frequent with divalproex sodium (Depakote) than with other preparations, and tremor can be treated with propranolol, as can lithium-induced tremor. Alopecia is sometimes transient and may be reduced by using a multi-vitamin with zinc and selenium. Longer-term side effects include weight gain and cognitive slowing. More serious adverse effects associated with valproic acid therapy include pancreatitis (which occurs in ~1 in 3000 patients), elevated transaminases (leading rarely to liver failure), hyperammonemia (which may induce confusion), thrombocytopenia, platelet dysfunction, and leukopenia. These effects are all rare, except for elevated hepatic transaminase levels. There is some controversy regarding whether valproic acid is associated with polycystic ovarian syndrome (PCOS) in women[20]; some studies have indicated that bipolar disorder itself may be associated with menstrual irregularities. Practitioners are advised to watch for hirsutism, acne, menstrual irregularities, and weight gain in their female patients who take valproic acid; an evaluation of PCOS should be conducted if such symptoms arise. Valproate overdose can lead to CNS depression, but it is rarely fatal; dialysis has been used to facilitate removal of valproate. Abrupt withdrawal might increase the risk of seizure, especially in individuals on long-term therapy or with a seizure disorder, but there is no withdrawal syndrome.

Carbamazepine

The initial side effects of carbamazepine include GI side effects (e.g., nausea, vomiting), neurological side effects (e.g., sedation, ataxia, vertigo, diplopia, and blurry vision), and rash. The rash is often benign, but carbamazepine should be discontinued if the rash is widespread or if SJS is suspected. More serious side effects, in addition to SJS, include hyponatremia (from SIADH), elevated liver transaminases (although this appears less often than with valproic acid), and aplastic anemia and other blood dyscrasias (which occur in approximately 1 in 10,000 to 1 in 150,000 treated patients). Carbamazepine also slows cardiac conduction and it should be avoided in patients with high-grade atrio-ventricular block and sick sinus syndrome. Low levels of free triiodothyronine (T_3) and thyroxine (T_4) can develop with carbamazepine use. Overdose of carbamazepine results in exacerbation of neurological side effects, the potential for high-grade atrio-ventricular block, and stupor or CNS depression; supportive care is required, and hemodialysis is ineffective. When possible, carbamazepine should be tapered rather than discontinued abruptly to minimize lowering of the seizure threshold.

Oxcarbazepine

Initial side effects from the related compound, oxcarbazepine, are like those of carbamazepine, with GI and neurological side effects being the most common. Rash is much less common with oxcarbazepine than with carbamazepine, but it occurs more frequently than with placebo. The neurological side effects (including cognitive difficulties, incoordination, visual changes, and sedation) associated with oxcarbazepine are less frequent than with carbamazepine, but they occur substantially more frequently than in patients who take placebo. Like carbamazepine, it appears to be associated with less weight gain than with lithium or valproic acid. Regarding more serious effects, oxcarbazepine can lead to elevated transaminase levels, and it is thought to be associated with higher rates of SIADH than with carbamazepine. Patients taking oxcarbazepine are at an elevated risk of SJS and other serious dermatological syndromes; low T_4 values can also occur in isolation. However, oxcarbazepine has not been associated with blood dyscrasias. Overdose with oxcarbazepine has been managed supportively and symptomatically.

ANTIPSYCHOTICS

Typical Antipsychotics

Table 13.1 shows the relative frequencies of the common adverse effects of antipsychotics; chlorpromazine (low-potency), perphenazine (mid-potency), and haloperidol (high-potency) are listed as the prototypic agents in the classes of typical antipsychotics. Initial side effects of the low-potency typical agents are like those of the TCAs: sedation (caused by H_1 receptor blockade), anticholinergic effects (e.g., dry mouth, urinary hesitancy, constipation, blurred vision, tachycardia, and risk of confusion) caused by the blockade of muscarinic receptors, and OH (caused by alpha$_1$-receptor blockade); these effects can occur to a lesser degree with mid-potency agents and are relatively uncommon with high-potency agents. In contrast, EPSs are common in patients taking high-potency typical antipsychotics, and their incidence decreases with decreasing potency (Box 13.6; see also Table 13.1). Common long-term side effects of typical antipsychotics include weight gain (which is greatest with low-potency agents), photosensitivity (perhaps greatest with chlorpromazine), sexual dysfunction (caused by effects on alpha$_2$-receptors), and hyperprolactinemia (which can lead to amenorrhea, galactorrhea, infertility, and osteoporosis). Tardive dyskinesia (TD) (see Box 13.6) is another long-term side effect associated with use of all typical antipsychotics, occurring at a rate of approximately 5% per year.[21]

Rarer, but serious, side effects of low-potency antipsychotics include neuroleptic malignant syndrome (NMS; see Box 13.6), QTc prolongation, and TdP (especially with use of thioridazine, the antipsychotic most commonly associated with TdP). Although IV haloperidol has long been associated with QTc prolongation and TdP, a systematic review found that IV haloperidol is not typically associated with greater QTc prolongation than placebo or other antipsychotic agents and that the risk of TdP is low.[22] Monitoring is therefore not recommended except in patients with multiple risk factors or when using dosages above 5 mg/day. In addition, chlorpromazine has been associated with cholestatic jaundice (at a rate of ~0.1%), and thioridazine has been associated with irreversible pigmentary retinopathy (at doses >800 mg/day) that can lead to blindness. Overdose of typical antipsychotics has been associated with lethargy, delirium, cardiac arrhythmias, hypotension, EPSs, seizures, and death; symptomatic treatment is required, and dialysis is not beneficial.

Atypical Antipsychotics

Most atypical antipsychotics (i.e., second-generation antipsychotics [SGAs]) have significantly lower rates of TD and

TABLE 13.1 Selected Side Effects of Antipsychotic Medications

Agent	Sedation	Orthostasis	Ach	EPSs	TD	Weight Gain	DM Risk	HyperPRL	QTc Prolongation
Chlorpromazine	Sev	Sev	Sev	Mod or sev	Mod	Mod or sev	Mild	Mild	Mod
Perphenazine	Mod	Mod	Mod	Mod	Mod	Mild	Mild	Mild	Mod
Haloperidol	Mild	0	0	Sev	Mod	Mild	0	Mod	Mod
Risperidone	Mild	Mod or sev	0	Mod or sev	Mild	Mod	Mod	Sev	Mod
Ziprasidone	0	Mild	0	Mild[a]	Mild	Mild	Mild	Mild	Sev
Olanzapine	Mod	0	Mild	Mild	Mild	Sev	Sev	Mild	Mod
Aripiprazole	Mild	0	0	Mild[a]	Mild	Mild	Mild	0	0
Quetiapine	Mod	Mod	Mild	0 or mild	0	Mod	Mod	0	Mod
Clozapine	Sev	Mod or sev	Sev	0	0	Sev	Sev	?	?
Iloperidone	Mild	Sev	Mild	Mod	?	Mod or sev	Mod or sev	Mild	Mod or sev
Paliperidone	Mild	Mod or sev	0	Mod	Mild	Mod	Mod	Sev	Mild
Lurasidone	Mild	Mild	0	Mod	?	Mild	Mild	Mod	0
Brexpiprazole	Mild	0	0	Mod	Mild	Mild	Mild	Mild	0
Cariprazine	Mild	Mild	Mild	Mod	Mod	Mild	Mild	Mild	Mild

[a]Moderate frequency and intensity of akathisia.

0, no effect; *?*, insufficient data; *Ach*, anticholinergic effects; *DM*, diabetes mellitus; *EPS*, extrapyramidal symptom; *HyperPRL*, hyperprolactinemia; *Mild*, mild effect; *Mod*, moderate effect; *Sev*, severe effect; *TD*, tardive dyskinesia

BOX 13.6　Extrapyramidal Symptoms

ACUTE DYSTONIA

Signs and Symptoms

- Localized muscular contraction leading to jaw protrusion, torticollis, tongue protrusion, opisthotonos, extremity contraction, or a fixed upward gaze of the eyes (oculogyric crisis) with associated pain

Risk Factors

- Age younger than 30 years, male gender, high-potency typical antipsychotics, IM administration, increased dose, rapid titration of dose

Time Course

- Usually occurs within the first several days of initiation or a dose increase

Treatment

- Moderate to severe reaction: IM diphenhydramine (25–50 mg; repeat as needed) or benztropine (1–2 mg; repeat as needed)
- Mild to moderate reaction: decrease of antipsychotic dose, addition of oral anticholinergic (e.g., benztropine 0.5–1 mg BID–TID, diphenhydramine 25 mg BID)

PARKINSONISM

Signs and Symptoms

- Muscular rigidity, bradykinesia, shuffling gait, masked facies, and resting (usually non–pill-rolling) tremor

Risk Factors

- Female gender, advanced age, high-potency typical antipsychotics, and possibly increased dose

Time Course

- Usually gradual in onset; occurs during first 3 months of treatment

Treatment

- Decrease the dose or switch the agent; if this is ineffective or not feasible, the addition of an anticholinergic (diphenhydramine or benztropine) or amantadine can reduce symptoms; benzodiazepines or beta-blockers may be helpful in refractory cases

AKATHISIA

Signs and Symptoms

- Internal, uncomfortable feeling of restlessness; frequent pacing, inability to remain seated

Risk Factors

- High-potency typical antipsychotics (mid-potency typical agents, risperidone, and aripiprazole to a lesser degree), higher dosage, rapid titration of dose, possibly advanced age, and diabetes mellitus

Time Course

- Usually occurs within the first several days of initiation or a dose increase

Treatment

- Reduction of dose (or change of agent); addition of propranolol (e.g., 10–20 mg BID–TID); benzodiazepines may be effective in refractory cases or when beta-blockers are contraindicated; anticholinergics are occasionally helpful, especially when other EPSs also present

TARDIVE DYSKINESIA

Signs and Symptoms

- Repetitive, involuntary, non-rhythmic movements, most frequently of the tongue and mouth, potentially including facial (e.g., grimacing), extremity (e.g., repetitive hand gestures), truncal (e.g., opisthotonos), and ocular (e.g., oculogyric crisis) movements

Risk Factors

- Typical antipsychotics (risperidone to a lesser degree), time of exposure, advanced age; possibly mood disorders, organic brain disease, and female gender

Time Course

- Approximate incidence of 4% per year for first 5 years of treatment with typical antipsychotics; incidence may somewhat slow thereafter, but the prevalence continues to grow with increased time of exposure

Treatment

- The US FDA has approved valbenazine (Ingrezza) and deutetrabenazine (Austedo) as treatments for tardive dyskinesia.
- Also, change of agent, especially to clozapine, may lead to reduction of symptoms; other treatments (e.g., vitamin E, vitamin B$_6$, benzodiazepines, botulinum toxin, or reserpine) do not appear to be broadly effective

NEUROLEPTIC MALIGNANT SYNDROME (NMS)

Signs and Symptoms

- Confusion, lethargy, rigidity, fever, autonomic instability (with abnormal laboratory values, including significantly increased creatine phosphokinase, elevated hepatic transaminases, and mild leukocytosis)

Risk Factors

- Include dehydration, agitation, use of physical restraint, increased or titration of dose, high-potency typical antipsychotics (though NMS can appear with any antipsychotic), IM administration, and history of catatonia or NMS

Time Course

- Usually occurs within the first several days of treatment

Treatment

- Discontinuation of the offending agent and supportive care to prevent aspiration pneumonia, deep venous thrombosis, renal failure, and other complications in all cases of NMS; dopamine agonists (e.g., bromocriptine), muscle relaxants (e.g., dantrolene), benzodiazepines, and ECT are all options in refractory or severe cases

BID, Twice a day; *ECT*, electroconvulsive therapy; *EPS*, extrapyramidal symptom; *FDA*, Food and Drug Administration; *IM*, intramuscular; *TID*, three times a day.

EPSs than do the typical antipsychotics (i.e., first-generation antipsychotics [FGAs]), and (aside from clozapine) they have relatively negligible anticholinergic effects; overall, they are quite well tolerated. However, several of the atypical antipsychotics have been associated with significant weight gain and with metabolic side effects. These effects appear to be greatest with clozapine and olanzapine; moderate with iloperidone, risperidone, paliperidone, and quetiapine; and

TABLE 13.2 American Diabetes Association Guidelines for Monitoring Patients Taking Antipsychotics

Monitor	Baseline	4 Weeks	8 Weeks	12 Weeks	1 Year	5 Years
Weight	X	X	X	X[a]	X	X
Blood pressure	X			X	X[b]	
Lipid panel	X			X	X	X
Fasting glucose	X			X	X[b]	

[a]Weight should be monitored quarterly after 12 weeks.
[b]Blood pressure and glucose should be monitored yearly after 1 year.
Adapted from American Diabetes Association, American Psychiatric Association, American Association of Clinical Endocrinologists, North American Association for the Study of Obesity. Consensus development conference on antipsychotic drugs and obesity and diabetes. *Diabetes Care.* 2004;27(2):596–601.

low with aripiprazole, brexpiprazole, ziprasidone, cariprazine, and lurasidone (see Tables 13.1 and 13.2 regarding side effects of antipsychotic medications and monitoring guidelines for metabolic side effects).[23,24] In addition, increased rates of cardiovascular events and death have been associated with the use of SGAs among patients with dementia, with a 1.6- to 1.7-fold higher mortality rate in a pooled analysis of more than 5000 patients in 17 clinical trials.[25] These findings have led to a "black box warning" in the package inserts of these agents; of note, a larger analysis found that the rate of stroke with SGAs was not significantly greater than with FGAs among patients with dementia.[26] More information is needed to determine whether there is a differential risk between agents.

Risperidone

Common initial side effects of risperidone include dizziness and OH (caused by alpha$_1$ blockade), headache, and sedation, although sedation is less frequent with this agent than it is with low- and mid-potency FGAs and many of the other SGAs. With respect to longer-term side effects, hyperprolactinemia is greatest with risperidone among all antipsychotics, and weight gain and the risk of diabetes are intermediate. Risperidone also has one of the highest rates of EPS among SGAs. TD has been associated with use of risperidone at lower rates than with FGAs but generally at higher rates than with other SGAs when high doses of risperidone are used. NMS has also been reported in patients taking risperidone.[27] The risk of QTc prolongation appears to be intermediate compared with other SGAs.[24] Overdose with risperidone most commonly results in hypotension and sedation.

Paliperidone

Paliperidone is a metabolite of risperidone, and the side effects of both medications are similar. It is excreted primarily by the kidney and does not undergo hepatic metabolism. Paliperidone's most commonly reported side effects are headache, nausea, dizziness, insomnia, and dyspepsia. Sedation has been noted, although paliperidone appears to be less apt to induce sedation than many other atypicals.[24] Despite early claims that paliperidone was not as likely to cause EPSs as risperidone, several studies have suggested that rates of EPSs are as high as 20%.[28] Paliperidone frequently induces hyperprolactinemia.[24] Paliperidone is thought to have effects on weight gain and metabolic parameters that are comparable to those of risperidone. Paliperidone has been associated with QTc prolongation but less so than most other atypical agents.

Iloperidone

Patients taking iloperidone frequently develop orthostasis, and the dose typically must be titrated very slowly to mitigate this. Common side effects include dizziness, headache, dry mouth, and insomnia. Weight gain with iloperidone is greater than with risperidone, and in a recent meta-analysis, it appears that the frequency of such weight gain may approach rates seen with clozapine in the short-term, though longer-term studies are lacking.[24] EPSs and hyperprolactinemia are less common with iloperidone than with risperidone. Iloperidone has been associated with QTc prolongation of an average of 9.1 milliseconds, which is like that of ziprasidone and greater than with use of oral haloperidol.[29]

Lurasidone

Sedation is the most common side effect of lurasidone. Alpha$_1$-antagonist properties also contribute to a risk of OH and tachycardia. Other common side effects include headache, dry mouth, and constipation. Lurasidone has been linked with higher rates of hyperprolactinemia and EPSs, particularly akathisia and parkinsonism, than with other SGAs. Weight gain and metabolic effects appear to be less frequent than with use of many SGAs. Lurasidone appears to be least likely to cause QTc prolongation.[24]

Ziprasidone

Neurological (e.g., dizziness, sedation, and headache) and GI (e.g., nausea and dyspepsia) side effects are common with use of ziprasidone, but these effects are usually mild. Sedation with ziprasidone is equivalent to that seen with quetiapine. Akathisia is frequently reported, although it may be a result of the activating properties observed at lower doses. TD is less common with ziprasidone than it is with FGAs;[30] however, more long-term data are needed. Orthostasis can occur because of alpha$_1$ blockade. With respect to longer-term side effects, weight gain and the risk for metabolic syndrome appear to be uncommon with this agent. The risk for prolactin elevation is moderate. Ziprasidone has been associated with QTc prolongation—greater than with other SGAs and oral haloperidol[31]—but in the clinical setting, this has not been a major issue. (There has been a single report of TdP associated with ziprasidone monotherapy.) Overdose with ziprasidone alone has been relatively safe; cardiotoxicity has not occurred, and the major symptoms linked with overdose have been sedation and dysarthria.

Aripiprazole

The most common initial side effects of aripiprazole include headache, anxiety, insomnia, akathisia, and GI side effects (nausea, vomiting, and constipation). Sedation may also occur at higher doses, but it is less common than with other SGAs. Akathisia is a common side effect of aripiprazole; other EPSs are rare with its use. As with ziprasidone, significant weight gain and glucose intolerance are less common with aripiprazole; furthermore, this agent appears to have no significant cardiovascular effects (e.g., prolongation of the QTc interval). Additionally, aripiprazole is the only antipsychotic that does not cause hyperprolactinemia, and it may lower prolactin levels.[24] The risk of TD appears to be low. Aripiprazole overdose appears to be relatively safe, with the most common effects being sedation, vomiting, tremor, and OH; however, more clinical experience is needed.

Brexpiprazole

Patients using brexpiprazole can initially experience sedation, anxiety, nausea, insomnia, and akathisia. Akathisia is a common side effect of brexpiprazole, especially at higher doses.[32] However, this occurs less frequently than with aripiprazole. The risk of TD appears to be quite low. Sedation is also a common side effect of brexpiprazole. As with aripiprazole, the risk for cardiometabolic side effects (weight gain, lipid abnormalities, and glucose intolerance) are less common with brexpiprazole than with other atypical antipsychotics (e.g., olanzapine, risperidone, clozapine). However, brexpiprazole has a greater risk of weight gain and hyperprolactinemia than aripiprazole.[32] Brexpiprazole does not seem to have a clinically relevant effect on QTc interval.

Olanzapine

Patients using olanzapine can initially experience sedation, dry mouth, constipation, increased appetite, dizziness (occasionally with OH), and tremor. EPSs occur more frequently with use of olanzapine than with placebo, but they are less frequent than with use of risperidone or high-potency FGAs. The major long-term side effects of olanzapine are metabolic. Weight gain occurs frequently with olanzapine; patients gain, on average, approximately 10 lb in the first 10 weeks of treatment, and they can continue to gain weight with ongoing treatment, with one-third to half of patients gaining more than 7% of their body weight. In one study, the risk of developing diabetes was approximately six times greater than the risk of developing diabetes on a placebo and approximately four times the risk for patients on an FGA.[33] It appears that both insulin resistance and weight gain contribute to this increase in diabetes risk. Hyperlipidemia, likely in the context of increased food intake and weight gain, is also common with long-term olanzapine therapy. The risks of these metabolic side effects are approximately equivalent to those associated with clozapine. Given the risk of these side effects, the American Diabetes Association has developed guidelines for monitoring the metabolic and cardiovascular parameters for patients taking antipsychotics (see Table 13.2).[23] Hyperprolactinemia is uncommon, but it can occur with olanzapine, especially at higher doses. TD can also occur, but it is less common than with use of FGAs. Elevation of hepatic transaminases, without progression to liver failure, occurs in approximately 2% of olanzapine-treated patients; olanzapine has intermediate effects on QTc prolongation. In overdose, olanzapine is relatively safe, with lethargy being the most common effect.

Clozapine

Clozapine has many initial side effects. Anticholinergic side effects, sedation, and OH are common. Sialorrhea occurs frequently, especially at night, and it can be quite upsetting to patients; clonidine, glycopyrrolate, or atropine drops (administered on the tongue) may reduce this symptom. Patients who take clozapine can also have drug-induced fever and tachycardia during the initial days of treatment. Long-term side effects are like those of olanzapine, with weight gain, development of diabetes, and hyperlipidemia all seen commonly; for both clozapine and olanzapine, weight gain is especially common among adolescents. Clozapine appears to be prolactin sparing. Fortunately, TD does not seem to be associated with clozapine (with reports of TD improvement on switching to clozapine).[34]

Several rare but serious adverse effects are associated with use of clozapine. Agranulocytosis is the best-known adverse effect of clozapine; rates of 0.4% have been reported,[35] necessitating the institution of mandatory monitoring of the blood count. Agranulocytosis occurs most often within the first 6 months of treatment, and it appears to be more likely in women and in those of Ashkenazi Jewish ancestry; advanced age may also be a minor risk factor.[36] Specific guidelines (Tables 13.3 and 13.4) serve to guide the clinician regarding when to stop treatment and when to check complete blood counts in both the general population and among patients with benign ethnic neutropenia.[37] Seizures are another risk linked with clozapine treatment, and the risk increases with an increasing dose; 4% to 6% of patients treated with doses of 600 mg/day or greater will have seizures. If clozapine is necessary, patients having seizures on clozapine can be re-started on the agent after adequate anticonvulsant treatment has been initiated. Uncommonly, cardiac complications, such as myocarditis (characterized by chest pain, dyspnea, fatigue, and tachycardia) and cardiomyopathy, arise. In one study, myocarditis was noted in about 5.3% of patients prescribed clozapine, with the

TABLE 13.3 Monitoring Guidelines for Clozapine in the General Population

ANC Level	Treatment Recommendation	ANC Monitoring
ANC ≥1500/μL	Initiate treatment. If treatment interrupted ≥30 days, monitor as if new patient. If treatment interrupted <30 days, continue treatment.	Weekly from initiation to 6 months. Every two weeks from 6 to 12 months. Monthly after 12 months.
Mild neutropenia (1000–1499/μL)	Continue treatment.	Three times weekly until ANC ≥1500/μL. When ANC ≥1500/μL, return to patient's last "normal range" ANC monitoring interval.
Moderate neutropenia (500–999/μL)	Recommend hematology consultation. Interrupt treatment for suspected clozapine-induced neutropenia. Resume treatment after ANC normalizes to ≥1000/μL.	Daily until ANC ≥1000/μL; then three times weekly until ANC ≥1500/μL. When ANC ≥1500/μL, check ANC weekly for 4, then return to patient's last "normal range" ANC monitoring interval.
Severe neutropenia (<500/μL)	Recommend hematology consultation. Interrupt treatment for suspected clozapine-induced neutropenia. Do not re-challenge unless prescriber determines benefits outweigh risks.	Daily until ANC ≥1000/μL. Three times weekly until ANC ≥1500/μL. If patient re-challenged, resume treatment as a new patient under "normal range" monitoring when ANC ≥1500/μL.

ANC, Absolute neutrophil count.

TABLE 13.4 Monitoring Guidelines for Clozapine for Patients with Benign Ethnic Neutropenia

ANC Level	Treatment Recommendation	ANC Monitoring
Normal BEN range (established ANC baseline ≥1000/μL)	Initiate treatment. If treatment interrupted ≥30 days, monitor as if new patient. If treatment interrupted <30 days, continue treatment.	Weekly from initiation to 6 months. Every two weeks from 6 to 12 months. Monthly after 12 months.
BEN neutropenia (500–999/μL)[a]	Recommend hematology consultation. Continue treatment.	Three times weekly until ANC ≥1000/μL or ≥ patient's known baseline. When ANC ≥1000/μL or at patient's known baseline, check ANC weekly for 4 weeks; then return to patient's last "normal BEN range" ANC monitoring interval.[b]
BEN severe neutropenia (<500/μL)[a]	Recommend hematology consultation. Interrupt treatment for suspected clozapine-induced neutropenia. Do not re-challenge unless prescriber determines benefits outweigh risks.	Daily until ANC ≥500/μL. Three times weekly until ANC ≥ patient's baseline. If patient re-challenged, resume treatment as a new patient under "normal range" monitoring when ANC ≥1000/μL or at patient's baseline.

[a]Confirm all initial reports of absolute neutrophil count (ANC) <1500/μL with a repeat ANC measurement within 24 hours.
[b]If clinically appropriate.
BEN, Benign ethnic neutropenia.
Adapted from Clozapine REMS Program. https://newclozapinerems.com/home

highest risk seen in the first 4 weeks of treatment. Although there are no agreed upon guidelines for monitoring to detect myocarditis, there is some suggestion that monitoring weekly troponins for 4 weeks is a sensitive indicator.[38] Hepatotoxicity can occur, although it is exceedingly rare. Clozapine overdose can result in delirium, lethargy, tachycardia, hypotension, and respiratory failure. Cardiac arrhythmias and seizures occur in a minority of cases, and overdose can be fatal. Hemodialysis does not remove clozapine, and management is generally supportive and symptomatic.

Cariprazine

Patients using cariprazine can initially experience dizziness, anxiety, insomnia, headache, and GI side effects (e.g., nausea, constipation, vomiting). EPSs occur more frequently than with use of placebo, including the risk for akathisia, tremors, parkinsonism, and restlessness. Of the SGAs, cariprazine has been associated with a higher risk of akathisia even compared with aripiprazole.[31] With respect to longer-term side effects, cariprazine has favorable metabolic, cardiovascular, and hepatic profiles. No clinically meaningful changes in metabolic variables (hemoglobin A1c, lipids), ECG abnormalities (QTc prolongation), or prolactin levels have been associated with cariprazine treatment. Short-term weight gain has been reported less frequently with cariprazine than with olanzapine. Available data on the safety of cariprazine for patients with severe renal or hepatic impairment are lacking, but the medication appears safe and does not require dosage changes in patients with mild or moderate renal or hepatic disease.[39]

ANTI-ANXIETY AND SLEEP AGENTS

Benzodiazepines

The most common initial side effects of benzodiazepines are sedation and daytime fatigue; these effects are frequently transitory and can be managed by lowering the dose or by moving the dose to before bedtime. Other potential side effects include dizziness, nausea, incoordination, ataxia, anterograde amnesia, and muscle weakness. Uncommon, but possible, psychological effects include increased irritability or hostility and paradoxical disinhibition. Cognitive effects appear to be greatest in older adults, in those with dementia, and in delirious individuals. Long-term side effects are uncommon; a minority of patients report an increase in depressive symptoms while taking benzodiazepines, and memory impairment and motor incoordination may persist. Furthermore, initial side effects can persist and occasionally worsen, especially when longer-acting agents (such as diazepam) are used, or with patients with liver failure or impaired hepatic metabolism. Such effects may be less serious when using benzodiazepines (i.e., lorazepam, oxazepam, temazepam) that do not undergo oxidative metabolism.

Serious adverse events associated with benzodiazepine use include an increased risk of falls and fractures in older adults.[40] Furthermore, patients who take benzodiazepines are at higher risk for motor vehicle accidents and for accidental injuries, the risk of the latter being greatest during the initial period (2 weeks to 1 month) of therapy. Finally, respiratory depression can occur in the context of benzodiazepine use, especially in those with pre-existing respiratory illnesses. Benzodiazepine overdose (when not taken with other sedating agents) is not usually fatal; however, sedation, dysarthria, confusion, ataxia, and incoordination are common.

Benzodiazepines cause physiological dependence and have a characteristic and potentially dangerous withdrawal syndrome. The withdrawal syndrome usually appears within the first 12 to 48 hours after discontinuation (or a drastic decrease in the dose) of short-lasting benzodiazepines (such as lorazepam); it may not appear until 2 to 5 days after discontinuation in patients taking longer-lasting agents (such as clonazepam or diazepam). Given this risk, benzodiazepines should be tapered slowly in all patients. The withdrawal syndrome from benzodiazepines includes anxiety, tremor, diaphoresis, nausea, insomnia, and irritability; vital signs—especially blood pressure and heart rate—are often elevated in untreated benzodiazepine withdrawal. Generalized tonic-clonic seizures may ensue, usually early in the course of the syndrome. As withdrawal continues, delirium may develop, characterized by more intense withdrawal symptoms, and significant autonomic instability and frequently with psychotic symptoms. Delirium from benzodiazepine withdrawal is associated with a significant risk of falls, congestive heart failure, aspiration, deep vein thrombosis, and other serious medical complications.

Short-Acting Sedative-Hypnotic Sleep Agents (Zolpidem, Zaleplon, and Eszopiclone)

The initial side effects of these agents are like those of the benzodiazepines, although they appear to be less frequent. Sedation—their desired effect—is common and may result in daytime somnolence or fatigue. Dry mouth and headache are other common initial effects. Incoordination, memory disturbance, nausea, and dizziness are uncommon when these agents are used at standard doses in patients without impaired metabolism. An unpleasant taste has also been reported by a minority of patients taking eszopiclone. Long-term side effects appear to be uncommon, though these agents have, for the most part, only been studied in short-term use. Tolerance and dose escalation are uncommon. Physiological dependence is also generally uncommon when used as prescribed, but withdrawal syndromes, like those seen with benzodiazepines, can occur when these agents are abruptly discontinued after long-term use; rates of withdrawal are much lower than with the short-lasting benzodiazepines.

One serious adverse effect of zolpidem use involves sleep-associated behavior disorders, including somnambulism and night-eating disorder. These agents are relatively safe in isolated overdose, although respiratory and cardiovascular adverse effects can occur. Treatment of patients with overdose is generally supportive and symptomatic.

Ramelteon

Initial side effects associated with this melatonin receptor agonist are uncommon but can include dizziness, sedation, nausea, and fatigue. Long-term and serious side effects appear to be rare. Overdose has not been reported, but ramelteon was administered in single doses up to 160 mg in an abuse liability trial, and no safety or tolerability concerns were seen. There is no characteristic withdrawal syndrome with discontinuation of ramelteon.

Buspirone

Buspirone is generally well tolerated. Headache, dizziness, and nausea are the most common side effects, and restlessness, insomnia, and increased anxiety may also occur. Sedation, incoordination, and cognitive effects do not appear to be associated with buspirone use. There are no known common long-term side effects, and there is no physiological dependence or withdrawal syndrome. Overdose with buspirone appears to be relatively safe, with dizziness, vomiting, and sedation being the most common effects. However, seizures have been reported in the context of buspirone overdose.[41]

Gabapentin

Gabapentin is frequently used to treat anxiety. Common initial side effects are like those of other anticonvulsants: sedation, dizziness, nausea, ataxia, headache, tremor, and visual changes. In general, these side effects are relatively mild and are often transient. Weight gain can occur as a long-term side effect, but it appears to be less common than with use of valproic acid. Gabapentin undergoes minimal hepatic metabolism and thus is not associated with hepatotoxicity; cardiovascular effects are few as well. In overdose, gabapentin is relatively safe, in part because of dose-limited absorption from the gut, but it is associated with sedation, ataxia, and diplopia; hemodialysis can be used.

OTHER AGENTS USED IN THE TREATMENT OF PSYCHIATRIC CONDITIONS

Beta-Blockers

Initial side effects of the beta-blockers include bradycardia, dizziness or orthostasis, fatigue, nausea, diarrhea, and insomnia. Patients who take beta-blockers for extended periods may develop sexual dysfunction or depressive symptoms. However, a large meta-analysis examining beta-blockers' link with fatigue, sexual dysfunction, and depression found that such associations were quite weak, with no significant associations between depression and the use of beta-blockers;[42] idiosyncratic reactions can occur. Overdose of beta-blockers is serious and can cause bradycardia, hypotension, and more serious cardiac adverse events, up to and including cardiac arrest. Somnolence and lethargy are common in overdose, and propranolol has been associated with seizures in overdose. Abrupt withdrawal after pronged use of beta-blockers has, on occasion, led to angina, MI, and rarely death in patients with (diagnosed or undiagnosed) coronary artery disease (CAD); therefore, these medications should be tapered after long-term use, especially in patients with CAD or with cardiac risk factors.

Clonidine

Dry mouth, sedation, fatigue, and dizziness are the most common side effects of clonidine. Hypotension (and orthostasis) can occur, especially among patients taking other antihypertensive agents. Somewhat less common side effects include nausea, headache, restlessness, and irritability. Vivid dreams, nightmares, and sexual dysfunction are infrequent but have been reported among patients taking clonidine. In overdose, a variety of significant adverse events (including bradycardia, hypotension, respiratory depression, and lethargy) may occur, and in large overdoses, cardiac conduction defects, seizures, and coma can result.[43] Abrupt withdrawal from clonidine has resulted in restlessness, agitation, tremor, and rebound hypertension and has led rarely to hypertensive encephalopathy or cerebrovascular accidents.

Guanfacine

Like clonidine, patients taking guanfacine have reported fatigue, sedation, somnolence, dry mouth, and irritability as initial side effects. Other less common side effects are decreased appetite, abdominal cramps, headaches, and restlessness. Hypotension, bradycardia, and syncope can also occur in both adults and children. Higher doses and concomitant use of blood pressure–lowering medications may elevate the risk of hypotension. Mild prolongation of the QTc interval has been characterized by serious adverse events, including profound sedation, hypotension, bradycardia, syncope, and even death.[43] Abrupt withdrawal from guanfacine can lead to hypertension, irritability, and restlessness.

Stimulants

Frequent side effects of the most commonly used psychostimulants (e.g., methylphenidate, dextroamphetamine, mixed amphetamine salts) include anxiety, insomnia, restlessness, and decreased appetite. Increased blood pressure and heart rate can occur in both children and adults, and these effects are generally dose dependent. Stimulants have been associated with the development of tics; however, meta-analyses of controlled studies have not found elevated rates of tics among children who are taking psychostimulants.[44] In addition, there have been reports of growth retardation among children who receive psychostimulants; however, as with tics, controlled studies have not found a consistent association with growth retardation.[45] More serious adverse effects can include psychosis and disorientation, which are rare except in overdose. Overdose can also be characterized by hyperpyrexia, arrhythmias, seizures, and rhabdomyolysis. There is no characteristic withdrawal syndrome, although abrupt cessation of stimulants after long-term use can be associated with lethargy, dysphoria, irritability, and psychomotor slowing like that seen during withdrawal from illicit amphetamine use.

Modafinil

The most common side effects of modafinil include headache, nausea, anxiety, and insomnia. Hypertension and tachycardia occur infrequently (in <5% of patients) but have occurred more often than with placebo. This agent has not been extensively studied in patients with significant cardiac disease (such as patients with a history of MI). Modafinil has been associated rarely with SJS, angioedema, and multi-organ hypersensitivity. Symptoms most commonly associated with modafinil overdose include restlessness, GI symptoms, disorientation or confusion, and cardiovascular symptoms (tachycardia, hypertension, and chest pain); death has not occurred with modafinil overdose taken in isolation. There is no known withdrawal syndrome.

Atomoxetine

Initial side effects of atomoxetine include GI side effects (e.g., decreased appetite, nausea, constipation, and vomiting), anticholinergic effects (e.g., urinary hesitancy or retention, dry mouth), dizziness, palpitations, and insomnia. Heart rate and blood pressure are elevated in a small percentage of patients. Regarding long-term effects, atomoxetine is associated with sexual dysfunction in both men and women. In addition, growth appears to slow initially in the first 9 months of treatment in pediatric patients, then appears to normalize over the next 36 months of treatment. Rare, but more serious, side effects of atomoxetine include liver dysfunction, which has occurred in at least three patients since its release, all of whom have recovered after discontinuation of atomoxetine; systematic monitoring of liver function tests has not been recommended. In overdose, fatalities have not been reported, and sedation or agitation, GI symptoms, and tachycardia appear commonly. There appear to be no withdrawal symptoms associated with discontinuation of atomoxetine.

Anticholinergics

The most common side effects of anticholinergic medications (such as benztropine and diphenhydramine) include dry mouth, constipation, urinary hesitancy, tachycardia, thickening of secretions, and dry skin (related to effects on muscarinic cholinergic receptors). In addition, sedation is common, especially with diphenhydramine and related compounds, because of their effects on histaminic receptors. Dizziness, tremor, incoordination, dyspepsia, and hypotension can also occur, and these agents should not be used in patients with narrow-angle glaucoma or BPH because of their potential to worsen the effects of these conditions. Long-term effects are generally extensions of their usual initial side effects.

Overdose of anticholinergic medications can lead to a variety of effects (including ataxia, delirium, agitation, tachycardia, prolongation of the QTc interval, hypotension, cardiovascular collapse, seizure, and coma). In most cases, treatment is supportive; vasopressors can be used for hypotension. In patients with refractory symptoms, physostigmine can be used; this agent is often effective, but it can cause bradyarrhythmias, asystole, seizures, and significant GI effects, and it is contraindicated in patients with prolonged PR or QRS intervals. However, it is effective, and one study found that physostigmine was safer and more effective than benzodiazepines in the treatment of patients with delirium with anticholinergic toxicity.[46]

Topiramate

The anticonvulsant topiramate has been used in the treatment of alcohol use disorders (AUDs) and cocaine use disorders. The most prominent initial side effects of topiramate are cognitive and other neurological side effects (including paresthesias, dizziness, sedation, fatigue, anxiety, and impaired taste); insomnia and visual impairment are less common. Cognitive impairment occurs in up to one-third of patients. GI side effects (e.g., nausea, anorexia, dyspepsia, diarrhea) are also common with topiramate. Most of these effects—aside from decreased appetite, paresthesias, and cognitive slowing—tend to improve over time. Longer-term side effects include weight loss (in ~7% of patients who receive 200–400 mg/day).[47] Nephrolithiasis, resulting from inhibition of carbonic anhydrase, occurs in about 1% of patients. One rare but serious adverse effect associated with topiramate is acute myopia with secondary angle-closure glaucoma; this syndrome causes bilateral ocular pain and blurred vision and is a result of increased intraocular pressure. It usually occurs in the first month of treatment and resolves with discontinuation of topiramate. Metabolic acidosis can also occur, and as a result, serum bicarbonate levels should be checked intermittently during topiramate treatment. Topiramate does not have significant cardiac effects, and it has not been associated with liver failure when used alone. Overdose can lead to severe lethargy, confusion, impaired vision, and significant metabolic acidosis, though it is usually not fatal; hemodialysis can be used as needed.

Acamprosate

Acamprosate is used in the treatment of AUDs to reduce the risk of relapse. Diarrhea and GI upset are the most common side effects reported with acamprosate, causing discontinuation rates of up to 2%. Pruritus has also been reported with some frequency. Erythema multiforme has been noted, although it appears to be an extremely rare event. Acamprosate is contraindicated in patients with severe renal impairment, and dose adjustment must be made for patients with moderate renal impairment. Diarrhea is the most common manifestation of overdose; treatment is generally symptomatic and supportive.

Naltrexone

Naltrexone is used in the treatment of substance use disorders to reduce cravings and improve abstinence rates. The most frequent side effects reported with naltrexone include nausea, dizziness, asthenia, and headache. Naltrexone is contraindicated in individuals with acute hepatitis or liver failure. Naltrexone has been associated with elevated liver enzymes, and some clinicians monitor liver function tests before (and periodically after) its initiation. Given its opioid receptor antagonism, it may precipitate acute withdrawal if given to a patient who has used opioids in the past 7 to 10 days, and it should be avoided in such patients. Overdose is generally managed supportively.

Buprenorphine

The partial opioid receptor agonist buprenorphine is used in patients with opioid use disorder both for management of acute withdrawal and as a maintenance treatment for relapse prevention. Side effects of buprenorphine parallel those of other opioids—sedation, nausea, dizziness, constipation, cognitive effects, urinary retention, and respiratory depression, especially at high doses. However, respiratory depression is less likely than with full opioid agonists because of a ceiling effect.

Ketamine

The "s" enantiomer form of the *N*-methyl-D-aspartate (NMDA) antagonist ketamine is used in patients with major depressive disorder for the management of treatment-resistant depression and depressed patients with acute thoughts of suicide. The intranasal form received FDA approval, although its sublingual, oral, and IV forms are also used off-label to treat depression. Common side effects of ketamine include headache, dizziness, euphoria, dissociative phenomena, perceptual disturbances, and blurred vision. Nausea, vomiting, and hypersalivation may also occur. Most of these side effects are transitory, self-limiting, and dose dependent. Agitation and restlessness have been reported with some frequency and may necessitate management with anxiolytics. Ketamine has also been associated with hypertension and with elevations in intracranial and intraocular pressures. It should be used cautiously in patients with co-morbid hypertension, glaucoma, and conditions associated with intracranial hypertension (i.e., head injury, intracranial tumors, and hydrocephalus). Long-term use of ketamine, particularly recreational use, may result in hepatobiliary toxicity, cognitive deficits, and urological complications.[48] Overdose is possible and requires supportive management.

REFERENCES

1. Revet A, Montastruc F, Roussin A, et al. Antidepressants and movement disorders: a postmarketing study in the world pharmacovigilance database. *BMC Psychiatry.* 2020;20(1):1–13.
2. De Picker L, Van Den Eede F, Dumont G, et al. Antidepressants and the risk of hyponatremia: a class-by-class review of literature. *Psychosomatics.* 2014;55:536–547.
3. Weinrieb RM, Auriacombe M, Lynch KG, et al. Selective serotonin re-uptake inhibitors and the risk of bleeding. *Expert Opin Drug Saf.* 2005;4(2):337–344.
4. Beach SR, Celano CM, Noseworthy PA, et al. QTc prolongation, torsades de pointes, and psychotropic medications. *Psychosomatics.* 2013;54(1):1–13.
5. Beach SR, Celano CM, Sugrue AM, et al. QT prolongation, torsades de pointes, and psychotropic medications: a 5-year update. *Psychosomatics.* 2018;59(2):105–122.
6. Thase ME. Effects of venlafaxine on blood pressure: a meta-analysis of original data from 3744 depressed patients. *J Clin Psychiatry.* 1998;59(10):502–508.
7. Whyte IM, Dawson AH, Buckley NA. Relative toxicity of venlafaxine and selective serotonin reuptake inhibitors in overdose compared to tricyclic antidepressants. *QJM.* 2003;96(5):369–374.
8. Delgado PL, Brannan SK, Mallinckrodt CH, et al. Sexual functioning assessed in 4 double-blind placebo- and paroxetine-controlled trials of duloxetine for major depressive disorder. *J Clin Psychiatry.* 2005;66(6):686–692.
9. Maramattom BV. Duloxetine-induced syndrome of inappropriate antidiuretic hormone secretion and seizures. *Neurology.* 2006;66(5):773–774.
10. Asnis GM, Henderson MA. Levomilnacipran for the treatment of major depressive disorder: a review. *Neuropsychiatr. Dis. Treat.* 2015;11:125–135.
11. Roose SP, Laghrissi-Thode F, Kennedy JS, et al. Comparison of paroxetine and nortriptyline in depressed patients with ischemic heart disease. *JAMA.* 1998;279(4):287–291.
12. Rastogi A, Viani-Walsh D, Akbari S, et al. Pathogenesis and management of Brugada syndrome in schizophrenia: a scoping review. *Gen Hosp Psychiatry.* 2020;67:83–91.
13. Cohen HW, Gibson G, Alderman MH. Excess risk of myocardial infarction in patients treated with antidepressant medications: association with use of tricyclic agents. *Am J Med.* 2000;108(1):2–8.
14. Thompson Jr JW, Ware MR, Blashfield RK. Psychotropic medication and priapism: a comprehensive review. *J Clin Psychiatry.* 1990;51(10):430–433.
15. Laughren TP, Gobburu J, Temple RJ, et al. Vilazodone: clinical basis for the US Food and Drug Administration's approval of a new antidepressant. *J Clin Psychiatry.* 2011;72(9):1166–1173.
16. Zhang J, Mathis MV, Sellers JW, et al. The US Food and Drug Administration's perspective on the new antidepressant vortioxetine. *J Clin Psychiatry.* 2014;76:7409.
17. Wisner KL, Stika CS, Ciolino JD. The first Food and Drug Administration-indicated drug for postpartum depression-brexanolone. *JAMA Psychiatry.* 2019;76:1001–1002.
18. Perlis RH, Sachs GS, Lafer B, et al. Effect of abrupt change from standard to low serum levels of lithium: a reanalysis of double-blind lithium maintenance data. *Am J Psychiatry.* 2002;159(7):1155–1159.
19. Restrepo JA, MacLean R, Celano CM, et al. The assessment of cardiac risk in patients taking lamotrigine; a systematic review. *Gen Hosp Psychiatry.* 2022;78:14–27.
20. Joffe H, Hall JE, Cohen LS, et al. A putative relationship between valproic acid and polycystic ovarian syndrome: implications for treatment of women with seizure and bipolar disorders. *Harv Rev Psychiatry.* 2003;11(2):99–108.
21. Latimer PR. Tardive dyskinesia: a review. *Can J Psychiatry.* 1995;40(7 suppl 2):S49–S54.
22. Beach SR, Gross AF, Hartney KE, et al. Intravenous haloperidol: a systematic review of side effects and recommendations for clinical use. *Gen Hosp Psychiatry.* 2020;67:42–50.
23. American Diabetes Association, American Psychiatric Association, American Association of Clinical Endocrinologists, North American Association for the Study of Obesity. Consensus development conference on antipsychotic drugs and obesity and diabetes. *Diabetes Care.* 2004;27(2):596–601.
24. Leucht S, Cipriani A, Spineli L, et al. Comparative efficacy and tolerability of 15 antipsychotic drugs in schizophrenia: a multiple-treatments meta-analysis. *Lancet.* 2013;382(9896):951–962.
25. Schneider LS, Dagerman KS, Insel P. Risk of death with atypical antipsychotic drug treatment for dementia: meta-analysis of randomized placebo-controlled trials. *JAMA.* 2005;294(15):1934–1943.
26. Wang PS, Schneeweiss S, Avorn J, et al. Risk of death in elderly users of conventional vs. atypical antipsychotic medications. *N Engl J Med.* 2005;353(22):2335–2341.
27. Ananth J, Parameswaran S, Gunatilake S, et al. Neuroleptic malignant syndrome and atypical antipsychotic drugs. *J Clin Psychiatry.* 2004;65(4):464–470.
28. Wang SM, Han C, Lee SJ, et al. Paliperidone: a review of clinical trial data and clinical implications. *Clin Drug Investig.* 2012;32(8):497–512.
29. Citrome L. Iloperidone: a clinical overview. *J Clin Psychiatry.* 2011;72(suppl 1):19–23.
30. Huffman JC, Stern TA. QTc prolongation and the use of antipsychotics: a case discussion. *Prim Care Companion J Clin Psychiatry.* 2003;5(6):278–281.
31. Heinrich TW, Biblo LA, Schneider J. Torsades de pointes associated with ziprasidone. *Psychosomatics.* 2006;47(3):264–268.
32. Keks N, Hope J, Schwartz D, et al. Comparative tolerability of dopamine $D_{2/3}$ receptor partial agonists for schizophrenia. *CNS Drugs.* 2020;34:473–507.
33. Koro CE, Fedder DO, L'Italien GJ, et al. Assessment of independent effect of olanzapine and risperidone on risk of diabetes among patients with schizophrenia: population based nested case-control study. *BMJ.* 2002;325(7358):243.
34. Larach VW, Zamboni RT, Mancini HR, et al. New strategies for old problems: tardive dyskinesia (TD). Review and report on severe TD cases treated with clozapine, 12, 8, and 5 years of video follow-up. *Schizophr Res.* 1997;28(2-3):231–246.
35. Li XH, Zhong XM, Lu L, et al. The prevalence of agranulocytosis and related death in clozapine-treated patients: a comprehensive meta-analysis of observational studies. *Psychol Med.* 2020;50:583–594.
36. Alvir JM, Lieberman JA, Safferman AZ, et al. Clozapine-induced agranulocytosis. Incidence and risk factors in the United States. *N Engl J Med.* 1993;329(3):162–167.
37. Clozapine REMS Program. https://newclozapinerems.com/home
38. Sandarsh S, Bishnoi RJ, Shashank RB, et al. Monitoring for myocarditis during treatment initiation with clozapine. *Acta Psychiatr Scand.* 2021;144(2):194–200.
39. Orsolini L, De Berardis D, Volpe U. Up-to-date expert opinion on the safety of recently developed antipsychotics. *Expert Opin Drug Saf.* 2020;19:981–998.
40. Wang PS, Bohn RL, Glynn RJ, et al. Hazardous benzodiazepine regimens in the elderly: effects of half-life, dosage, and duration on risk of hip fracture. *Am J Psychiatry.* 2001;158(6):892–898.

41. Catalano G, Catalano MC, Hanley PF. Seizures associated with buspirone overdose: case report and literature review. *Clin Neuropharmacol*. 1998;21(6):347–350.

42. Ko DT, Hebert PR, Coffey CS, et al. Beta-blocker therapy and symptoms of depression, fatigue, and sexual dysfunction. *JAMA*. 2002;288(3):351–357.

43. Baumgartner K, Mullins M. Pediatric clonidine and guanfacine poisoning: a single-center retrospective review. *Toxicol Commun*. 2021;5:61–65.

44. Cohen SC, Mulqueen JM, Ferracioli-Oda E, et al. Meta-analysis: risk of tics associated with psychostimulant use in randomized, placebo-controlled trials. *J Am Acad Child Adolesc Psychiatry*. 2015;54:728–736.

45. Lahat E, Weiss M, Ben-Shlomo A, et al. Bone mineral density and turnover in children with attention-deficit hyperactivity disorder receiving methylphenidate. *J Child Neurol*. 2000;15(7):436–439.

46. Burns MJ, Linden CH, Graudins A, et al. A comparison of physostigmine and benzodiazepines for the treatment of anticholinergic poisoning. *Ann Emerg Med*. 2000;35(4):374–381.

47. Reife R, Pledger G, Wu SC. Topiramate as add-on therapy: pooled analysis of randomized controlled trials in adults. *Epilepsia*. 2000;41(suppl 1):S66–S71.

48. Zanos P, Moaddel R, Morris PJ, et al. Ketamine and ketamine metabolite pharmacology: insights into therapeutic mechanisms. *Pharmacol Rev*. 2018;70:621–660.

14 Drug–Drug Interactions in Psychopharmacology

Jonathan E. Alpert and David Mischoulon

KEY POINTS

- Drug–drug interactions refer to alterations in drug levels or drug effects (or both) related to the administration of two or more prescribed, recreational, or over-the-counter agents in close temporal proximity.

- Although some drug–drug interactions involving psychotropic medications are life-threatening, most interactions manifest in more subtle ways through increased side effect burden, aberrant drug levels, or diminished efficacy.

- Pharmacokinetic drug–drug interactions involve a change in the plasma level or tissue concentration of one drug following co-administration of one or more other drugs because of an action of the co-administered agents on one of four key pharmacokinetic processes: absorption, distribution, metabolism, or excretion.

- Pharmacodynamic drug–drug interactions involve an effect of one or more drugs on another drug at biological receptor sites of action and do not involve a change in plasma level or tissue concentration.

- The potential for drug–drug interactions should be carefully considered whenever prescribing medications associated with interactions that are uncommon but catastrophic (e.g., hypertensive crises, Stevens-Johnson syndrome, or cardiac arrhythmias) and medications with low therapeutic indices (e.g., warfarin) or narrow therapeutic windows (e.g., cyclosporine) and when prescribing for frail or clinically brittle patients for whom small variations in side effects or efficacy may be particularly troublesome.

OVERVIEW

An understanding of drug–drug interactions is essential to the practice of psychopharmacology.[1,2] As in other areas of medicine, polypharmacy has become an increasingly accepted approach in psychiatry for addressing difficult-to-treat disorders.[3] Moreover, general medical co-morbidity is common among patients with psychiatric disorders, elevating the likelihood of complex medication regimens.[4,5] Similarly, the widespread use of over-the-counter (OTC) supplements by patients receiving treatment for psychiatric disorders may invite additional risk of drug–drug interactions.[6] When they occur, drug–drug interactions may manifest in myriad ways, from perplexing laboratory test results to symptoms that are difficult to distinguish from the underlying psychiatric and physical conditions under treatment. The comprehensive evaluation of patients with psychiatric disorders therefore requires a careful assessment of potential drug–drug interactions.

Drug–drug interactions are alterations in drug levels or drug effects (or both) attributed to the administration of two or more prescribed, illicit, or OTC agents in close temporal proximity. Although many drug–drug interactions involve drugs administered within minutes to hours of each other, some drugs may participate in interactions days or even weeks after their discontinuation because of prolonged elimination half-lives (e.g., fluoxetine) or because of their long-term impact on metabolic enzymes (e.g., carbamazepine). Some drug–drug interactions involving psychotropic medications are life-threatening, such as those involving the co-administration of monoamine oxidase inhibitors (MAOIs) and drugs with potent serotonergic (e.g., meperidine) or sympathomimetic (e.g., phenylpropanolamine) effects.[7–9] These combinations are therefore absolutely contraindicated. However, most drug–drug interactions in psychopharmacology manifest in somewhat more subtle ways, often leading to poor medication tolerability and compliance because of adverse events (e.g., orthostatic hypotension, sedation, or irritability), diminished medication efficacy, or puzzling manifestations (such as altered mental status or unexpectedly high or low drug levels). Drug combinations that can produce these often less than catastrophic drug–drug interactions are usually not absolutely contraindicated. Some of these combinations may, indeed, be valuable in the treatment of some patients while wreaking havoc for other patients. The capacity to anticipate and to recognize both the major, but rare, and the more subtle, but common, potential drug–drug interactions allows the practitioner to minimize the impact of these interactions as an obstacle to patient safety and to therapeutic success. This is both an important goal and a considerable challenge in psychopharmacology.

Although drug–drug interactions are ubiquitous, few studies have systematically assessed in vivo drug–drug interactions of most interest to psychiatrists. Fortunately, well-designed studies of drug–drug interactions are an increasingly integral part of drug development. Beyond these studies, however, the literature on drug–drug interactions remains a patchwork of case reports, post-marketing analyses, extrapolation from animal and in vitro studies, and extrapolation from what is known about other drugs with similar properties. Although these studies often shed some light on the simplest case of a single drug (drug B) exerting an effect on another (drug A), they rarely consider the common clinical scenario in which multiple drugs with numerous potential interactions among them are co-administered. Under these circumstances, the range of possible, if not well-delineated, drug–drug interactions often seems overwhelming.

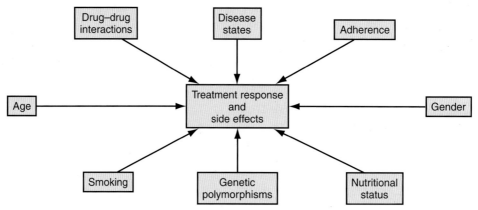

Figure 14.1 Factors contributing to inter-individual variability in drug response.

Fortunately, an increasing range of resources is available (including prescribing software packages and regularly updated websites, such as www.drug-interactions.com) that allow for the prevention and detection of potential interactions. In addition, it is important to recall that numerous factors contribute to inter-individual variability in drug response.[10,11] These factors include treatment adherence, age, gender, nutritional status, disease states, and genetic polymorphisms that may influence risk of adverse events and treatment resistance (Fig. 14.1). Drug–drug interactions can also influence how patients react to drugs, depending on the clinical context. In many cases, the practical impact of drug–drug interactions is likely to be very small compared with other factors that affect treatment response, drug levels, and toxicity. It is reasonable, therefore, to focus special attention on the contexts in which drug–drug interactions are most likely to be clinically problematic.

First, it is crucial to be familiar with the small number of drug–drug interactions in psychopharmacology that, though uncommon, are associated with potentially catastrophic consequences. These include drugs associated with ventricular arrhythmias, hypertensive crisis, serotonin syndrome, Stevens-Johnson syndrome (SJS), seizures, and severe bone marrow suppression. In addition, drug–drug interactions are important to consider when a patient's medications include those with a low therapeutic index (i.e., the closeness between the effective dose and the toxic dose, relevant with lithium, digoxin, or warfarin) or a narrow therapeutic window (i.e., the range of blood levels yielding optimal clinical benefit without toxicity, relevant with indinavir, nortriptyline, or cyclosporine) such that relatively small alterations in pharmacokinetic or pharmacodynamic behavior may jeopardize a patient's well-being. In addition, it is worthwhile to consider potential drug–drug interactions whenever evaluating a patient whose drug levels are unexpectedly variable or extreme and in patients with a confusing clinical picture (such as clinical deterioration) or with unexpected side effects. Finally, drug–drug interactions are likely to be clinically salient for a patient who is medically frail or older, owing to altered pharmacokinetics and vulnerability to side effects, as well as for a patient heavily using alcohol, cigarettes, or illicit drugs or being treated for a drug overdose.

CLASSIFICATION

Drug–drug interactions may be described as pharmacokinetic, pharmacodynamic, mixed, or idiosyncratic, depending on the presumed mechanism underlying the interaction (Box 14.1). *Pharmacokinetic interactions* are those that involve a change in the plasma level or tissue distribution (or both) of one drug by

---

BOX 14.1   Classification of Drug–Drug Interactions

Pharmacokinetic: alteration in blood level or tissue concentration (or both) resulting from interactions involving drug absorption, distribution, metabolism, or excretion

Pharmacodynamic: alteration in pharmacological effect resulting from interactions at the same or inter-related biologically active (receptor) sites

Mixed: alterations in blood levels and pharmacological effects caused by pharmacokinetic and pharmacodynamic interactions

Idiosyncratic: sporadic interactions among drugs not accounted for by their currently known pharmacokinetic or pharmacodynamic properties

---

virtue of co-administration of another drug. These interactions occur because of effects at one or more of the four pharmacokinetic processes by which drugs are acted on by the body: absorption, distribution, metabolism, and excretion. Because of the importance of these factors, particularly metabolism, in drug–drug interactions, a more detailed description of pharmacokinetic processes follows. An example of a pharmacokinetic drug–drug interaction is the inhibition of the metabolism of lamotrigine by valproic acid,[12] thereby raising lamotrigine levels and increasing the risk of potentially serious adverse events, including hypersensitivity reactions (such as SJS). In contrast, *pharmacodynamic interactions* are those that involve a known pharmacological effect at biologically active (receptor) sites. These interactions occur because of effects on the mechanisms through which the body is acted on by drugs and do not involve a change in drug levels. An example of a pharmacodynamic drug–drug interaction is the interference of the antiparkinsonian effects of a dopamine receptor agonist (such as pramipexole) by a dopamine receptor antagonist (such as risperidone). *Mixed interactions* are those that are believed to involve both pharmacological and pharmacodynamic effects. Symptoms of serotonin toxicity, such as agitation and confusion that have been observed in some individuals taking the combination of paroxetine and dextromethorphan, for example, may reflect the shared pharmacodynamic effect of the two agents at serotonin receptor sites as well as the elevation of dextromethorphan levels because of inhibition of its cytochrome (CYP) P450 metabolism by paroxetine. Finally, *idiosyncratic interactions* are those that occur sporadically in a small number of patients in ways that are not yet predicted by the known pharmacokinetic and pharmacodynamic properties of the drugs involved.

PHARMACOKINETICS

As described earlier, pharmacokinetic processes refer to absorption, distribution, metabolism, and excretion, factors that determine plasma levels and tissue concentrations of a drug.[2,11,13] Pharmacokinetics refers to the mathematical analysis of these processes. Advances in analytic chemistry and computer methods of pharmacokinetic modeling and a growing understanding of the molecular pharmacology of the liver enzymes responsible for metabolism of most psychotropic medications have furnished increasingly sophisticated insights into the disposition and interaction of administered drugs. Although pharmacokinetics refers to only one of the two broad mechanisms by which drugs interact, pharmacokinetic interactions involve all classes of psychotropic and nonpsychotropic medications. An overview of pharmacokinetic processes is a helpful prelude to a discussion of drug–drug interactions by psychotropic drug class.

Absorption

Factors that influence drug absorption are generally of less importance to drug–drug interactions involving psychiatric medications than are factors that influence subsequent drug disposition, particularly drug metabolism. Factors relevant to absorption generally pertain to orally rather than parenterally administered drugs, for which alterations in gastrointestinal (GI) drug absorption may affect the rate (time to reach maximum concentration) or the extent of absorption or both. The extent or completeness of absorption, also known as the fractional absorption, is measured as the area under the curve when plasma concentration is plotted against time. The bioavailability of an oral dose of drug refers, in turn, to the fractional absorption for orally compared with intravenously administered drug. If an agent is reported to have a 90% bioavailability (e.g., lorazepam), it would indicate that the extent of absorption of an orally administered dose is nearly that of an intravenously administered dose, although the rate of absorption may well be slower for the oral dose.

Because the upper part of the small intestine is the primary site of drug absorption through passive membrane diffusion and filtration and both passive and active transport processes, factors that speed gastric emptying (e.g., metoclopramide) or diminish intestinal motility (e.g., opiates or marijuana) may facilitate greater contact with, and absorption from, the mucosal surface into the systemic circulation, potentially increasing plasma drug concentrations. Conversely, antacids, charcoal, kaolin-pectin, and cholestyramine may bind to drugs, forming complexes that pass unabsorbed through the GI lumen. Changes in gastric pH associated with food or other drugs alter the non-polar, un-ionized fraction of drug available for absorption. In the case of drugs that are very weak acids or bases, however, the extent of ionization is relatively invariant under physiological conditions. Properties of the preparation administered (e.g., tablet, capsule, or liquid) may also influence the rate or extent of absorption, and for an increasing number of medications (e.g., lithium, bupropion, valproate, and methylphenidate), slow-release preparations are available. Finally, the local action of enzymes in the GI tract (e.g., monoamine oxidase [MAO] and CYP P450 3A4) may be responsible for metabolism of drugs before absorption. As described later, this is of critical relevance to the emergence of hypertensive crises that occur when excessive quantities of the dietary pressor tyramine are systemically absorbed in the setting of irreversible inhibition of the MAO isoenzymes for which tyramine is a substrate.

Distribution

Drugs distribute to tissues through the systemic circulation. The amount of drug ultimately reaching receptor sites in tissues is determined by a variety of factors, including the concentration of free (unbound) drug in plasma, regional blood flow, and physiochemical properties of drug (e.g., lipophilicity or structural characteristics). For entrance into the central nervous system (CNS), penetration across the blood–brain barrier is required. Fat-soluble drugs (such as benzodiazepines, neuroleptics, and cyclic antidepressants) distribute more widely in the body than water-soluble drugs (such as lithium), which disseminate through a smaller volume of distribution. Changes with age, typically including an increase in the ratio of body fat to lean body mass, therefore result in a net greater volume of lipophilic drug distribution and potentially greater accumulation of drug in adipose tissue in older than in younger patients.

In general, psychotropic drugs have relatively high affinities for plasma proteins (some to albumin but others, such as antidepressants, to α_1-acid glycoproteins and lipoproteins). Most psychotropic drugs are more than 80% protein bound. A drug is considered highly protein bound if more than 90% exists in bound form in plasma. Fluoxetine, aripiprazole, and diazepam are examples of the many psychotropic drugs that are highly protein bound. In contrast, venlafaxine, lithium, topiramate, zonisamide, gabapentin, pregabalin, milnacipran, and memantine are examples of drugs with minimal protein binding and therefore minimal risk of participating in drug–drug interactions related to protein binding. A reversible equilibrium exists between bound and unbound drug. Only the unbound fraction exerts pharmacological effects. Competition by two or more drugs for protein-binding sites often results in displacement of a previously bound drug, which in the free state becomes pharmacologically active. Similarly, reduced concentrations of plasma proteins in a severely malnourished patient or a patient with a disease that is associated with severely lowered serum proteins (such as liver disease or nephrotic syndrome) may be associated with an increase in the fraction of unbound drug potentially available for activity at relevant receptor sites. Under most circumstances, the net changes in plasma concentration of active drug are, in fact, quite small because the unbound drug is available for redistribution to other tissues and for metabolism and excretion, thereby off-setting the initial rise in plasma levels. Nevertheless, clinically significant consequences can develop when protein-binding interactions alter the unbound fraction of previously highly protein-bound drugs that have a low therapeutic index (e.g., warfarin). For these drugs, relatively small variations in plasma level may be associated with serious untoward effects.

An emerging understanding of the drug transport proteins, of which P-glycoproteins are the best characterized, indicates a crucial role in regulating permeability of intestinal epithelia, lymphocytes, renal tubules, the biliary tract, and the blood–brain barrier. These transport proteins are thought to account for the development of certain forms of drug resistance and tolerance but are also increasingly seen as likely to mediate clinically important drug interactions.[2] Little is known yet about their relevance to drug interactions involving psychiatric medications; the capacity of St. John's wort to lower blood levels of several critical medications (including cyclosporine and indinavir) is hypothesized to be related, at least in part, to an effect of the botanical agent on this transport system.[14]

Metabolism

Metabolism is the best-characterized pharmacokinetic mechanism implicated in known drug–drug interactions. Metabolism refers to the biotransformation of a drug to another form, a process that is usually enzyme-mediated and that results in a metabolite that may or may not be pharmacologically active and may or may not be subject to further biotransformation before eventual excretion. Most drugs undergo several types of biotransformation, and many psychotropic drug interactions of clinical significance are based on interference with this process. A growing understanding of hepatic enzymes and especially the rapidly emerging characterization of the CYP P450 isoenzymes and other enzyme systems, including the uridine-diphosphate glucuronosyltransferases, flavin-containing monooxygenases, methyltransferases, and sulfotransferases, has significantly advanced a rational understanding and prediction of drug interactions and individual variation in drug responses.[2,15]

Phase I reactions include oxidation, reduction, and hydrolysis, metabolic reactions that typically result in intermediate metabolites, which are then subject to phase II reactions (including conjugation [e.g., glucuronidation and sulfation] and acetylation). Phase II reactions typically yield highly polar, water-soluble metabolites suitable for renal excretion. Most psychotropic drugs undergo both phase I and phase II metabolic reactions. Notable exceptions include valproic acid and a subset of benzodiazepines (i.e., lorazepam, oxazepam, and temazepam), which skip phase I metabolism and undergo only phase II reactions. In addition, certain medications, including lithium and gabapentin, do not undergo any hepatic biotransformation before excretion by the kidneys.

The synthesis or activity of hepatic microsomal enzymes is affected by metabolic inhibitors and inducers, as well as by distinct genetic polymorphisms (stably inherited traits). Table 14.1 lists enzyme inducers and inhibitors common in clinical settings. These should serve as red flags that beckon further scrutiny for potential drug–drug interactions when they are found on a patient's medication list. Imagine two drugs, drug A and drug B, associated with a metabolic enzyme. Drug B may be an inhibitor or an inducer of that enzyme. Drug A may be normally metabolized by this enzyme and would therefore be called a substrate. If drug B is an inhibitor with respect to the metabolic enzyme, it will impede the metabolism of a concurrently administered substrate (drug A), thereby producing a rise in the plasma levels of drug A. If drug B is an inducer of that enzyme, it will enhance the metabolism of the substrate (drug A), resulting in a decline in the plasma levels of drug A (Fig. 14.2). In some circumstances, an inhibitor (such as grapefruit juice) or inducer (e.g., a cruciferous vegetable, such as brussels sprouts) may not be a drug but rather another ingested substance. Moreover, in some circumstances, a drug is not only a substrate of an enzyme, but it can

TABLE 14.1 Commonly Used Drugs and Substances That Inhibit or Induce Hepatic Metabolism of Other Medications

Inhibitors	Inducers
Antifungals (ketoconazole, miconazole, itraconazole)	Barbiturates (e.g., phenobarbital, secobarbital)
Macrolide antibiotics (erythromycin, clarithromycin, triacetyloleandomycin)	Carbamazepine
Fluoroquinolones (e.g., ciprofloxacin)	Oxcarbazepine
Isoniazid	Phenytoin
Antiretrovirals (e.g., ritonavir)	Rifampin
Antimalarials (chloroquine)	Primidone
Selective serotonin reuptake inhibitors (fluoxetine, fluvoxamine, paroxetine, sertraline)	Cigarettes
Duloxetine	Ethanol (chronic)
Bupropion	Cruciferous vegetables
Nefazodone	Charbroiled meats
β-Blockers (lipophilic) (e.g., propranolol, metoprolol, pindolol)	St. John's wort
Quinidine	Oral contraceptives
Valproate	Prednisone
Cimetidine	
Calcium channel blockers (e.g., diltiazem)	
Grapefruit juice	
Ethanol (acute)	

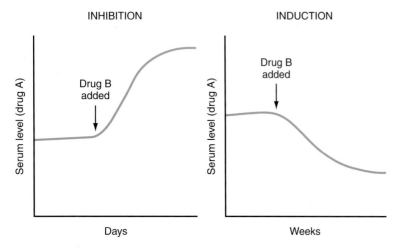

Figure 14.2 Metabolic inhibition and induction. Serum concentrations of drug A rise abruptly if co-administered drug B is an inhibitor of its metabolism, but serum concentrations fall gradually if co-administered drug B is an inducer of its metabolism.

also inhibit the metabolism of other substrates relying on that enzyme, in which case it is considered an inhibitor as well as a substrate. Although inhibition is usually immediate, occurring by one or more of a variety of mechanisms (including competitive inhibition or inactivation of the enzyme), induction, which requires enhanced synthesis of the metabolic enzyme, is typically a more gradual process. A fall in plasma levels of a substrate may not be apparent for days to weeks after introduction of the inducer. This is particularly important when a patient's care is being transferred to another setting where clinical deterioration may be the first sign that drug levels have declined. Reciprocally, an elevation in plasma drug concentrations could reflect the previous discontinuation of an inducing factor (e.g., cigarette smoking or carbamazepine) just as it could reflect the more recent introduction of an inhibitor (e.g., fluoxetine or valproic acid).

Although the CYP P450 isoenzymes represent only one of the many enzyme systems responsible for drug metabolism, they are responsible for metabolizing, at least in part, more than 80% of all prescribed drugs. In addition, growing awareness in the 1990s about the capacity of many of the newer antidepressants to inhibit CYP P450 isoenzymes fueled great interest in the pattern of interaction of psychotropic and other drugs with these enzymes in the understanding and prediction of drug–drug interactions. The CYP P450 isoenzymes represent a family of more than 30 related heme-containing enzymes, largely located in the endoplasmic reticulum of hepatocytes (but also present elsewhere, including the gut and brain), which mediate oxidative metabolism of a wide variety of drugs, as well as endogenous substances (including prostaglandins, fatty acids, and steroids). The majority of

antidepressant and antipsychotic drugs are metabolized by, or inhibit, one or more of these isoenzymes. Table 14.2 summarizes the interactions of psychiatric and non-psychiatric drugs with a subset of isoenzymes that have been increasingly well characterized (1A2, 2C subfamily, 2D6, and 3A4).[16] Further information about the relevance of these and other interactions is highlighted in a later section of this chapter in which clinically important drug–drug interactions are reviewed.

In addition to being influenced by pharmacological inducers or inhibitors, a patient's metabolic status is also under genetic control. Knowledge continues to evolve concerning genetic polymorphisms that affect drug metabolism. Within the group of CYP P450 isoenzymes, there appears to be a polymodal distribution of metabolic activity in the population with respect to certain isoenzymes (including 2C19 and 2D6). Most individuals are normal ("extensive") metabolizers with respect to the activity of these isoenzymes. A smaller number are "poor metabolizers" with deficient activity of the isoenzyme. Probably many fewer individuals are ultra-rapid metabolizers (who have more than normal activity of the enzyme) and intermediate metabolizers (who fall between extensive and poor metabolizers). Individuals who are poor metabolizers with respect to certain CYP P450 isoenzymes are expected to have higher plasma concentrations of a drug that is metabolized by that isoenzyme, thereby potentially being more sensitive, or requiring lower doses of that drug, than a patient with normal activity of that enzyme. They may also have higher-than-usual plasma levels of metabolites of the drug that are produced through other metabolic pathways that are not altered by the polymorphism, thereby potentially incurring pharmacological activity or adverse effects related

TABLE 14.2 Selected Cytochrome P450 Isoenzyme Substrates, Inhibitors, and Inducers

P450 Cytochrome Isoenzymes	Relationship of Medication with Enzyme	Medications
1A2	Substrates	Acetaminophen, aminophylline, asenapine, caffeine, clozapine, cyclobenzaprine, estradiol, fluvoxamine, haloperidol, mirtazapine, ondansetron, olanzapine, phenacetin, procarcinogens, propranolol, ramelteon, riluzole, ropinirole, tacrine, tertiary amine TCAs, theophylline, verapamil, warfarin, zileuton, zolmitriptan
	Inhibitors	Amiodarone, cimetidine, fluoroquinolones, fluvoxamine, grapefruit juice, methoxsalen, ticlopidine
	Inducers	Charbroiled meats, cruciferous vegetables, modafinil, omeprazole, tobacco (cigarette smoking)
2C	Substrates	Barbiturates, cannabidiol, diazepam, fluvastatin, glipizide, glyburide, irbesartan, losartan, mephenytoin, nelfinavir, NSAIDs, phenytoin, primidone, proguanil, propranolol, proton pump inhibitors, rosiglitazone, tamoxifen, tertiary TCAs, THC, tolbutamide, R-warfarin, S-warfarin
	Inhibitors	Armodafinil, fluoxetine, fluvoxamine, ketoconazole, modafinil, omeprazole, oxcarbazepine, ritonavir, sertraline, topiramate
	Inducers	Carbamazepine, norethindrone, prednisone, rifampin, secobarbital
2D6	Substrates	Amphetamines, aripiprazole, atomoxetine, β-blockers (lipophilic), codeine, debrisoquine, deutetrabenazine, dextromethorphan, diltiazem, donepezil, duloxetine, encainide, flecainide, galantamine, haloperidol, hydrocodone, iloperidone, lidocaine, mCPP, metoclopramide, mexiletine, nifedipine, ondansetron, phenothiazines (e.g., perphenazine, thioridazine), promethazine, propafenone, risperidone, SSRIs, tamoxifen, TCAs, tramadol, trazodone, valbenazine, venlafaxine, vortioxetine
	Inhibitors	Amiodarone, antimalarials, bupropion, cimetidine, citalopram, duloxetine, escitalopram, fluoxetine, methadone, metoclopramide, moclobemide, paroxetine, phenothiazines, protease inhibitors (ritonavir), quinidine, sertraline, TCAs, terbinafine, THC, yohimbine
	Inducers	Dexamethasone, rifampin
3A3/4	Substrates	Alfentanil, alprazolam, amiodarone, amprenavir, aripiprazole, armodafinil, brexpiprazole, bromocriptine, buprenorphine, buspirone, Cafergot, caffeine, calcium channel blockers, cannabidiol, carbamazepine, cisapride, clozapine, cyclosporine, dapsone, diazepam, disopyramide, efavirenz, estradiol, fentanyl, HMG-CoA reductase inhibitors (lovastatin, simvastatin), indinavir, lidocaine, loratadine, lurasidone, methadone, midazolam, modafinil, nimodipine, pimozide, prednisone, progesterone, propafenone, quetiapine, quinidine, ritonavir, sildenafil, suvorexant, tacrolimus, testosterone, tertiary amine TCAs, triazolam, valbenazine, vardenafil, vilazodone, vinblastine, warfarin, zaleplon, ziprasidone, zolpidem
	Inhibitors	Antifungals, calcium channel blockers, cimetidine, efavirenz, indinavir, fluoxetine (norfluoxetine), fluvoxamine, grapefruit juice, macrolide antibiotics, mibefradil, nefazodone, nelfinavir, nirmatrelvir, ritonavir, verapamil, voriconazole
	Inducers	Armodafinil, carbamazepine, glucocorticoids, modafinil, oxcarbazepine, phenobarbital, phenytoin, pioglitazone, rifabutin, rifampin, ritonavir, St. John's wort, troglitazone

HMG-CoA, Hydroxymethylglutaryl coenzyme A; *mCPP*, m-chlorophenylpiperazine; *NSAID*, non-steroidal anti-inflammatory drug; *SSRI*, selective serotonin reuptake inhibitor; *TCA*, tricyclic antidepressant; *THC*, tetrahydrocannabinol.

to these alternative metabolites. Poor metabolizers are relatively impervious to drug interactions involving inhibition of the isoenzyme system for which they are already deficient. When the polymorphism is related to an isoenzyme required for conversion of a pro-drug (e.g., tamoxifen, codeine, or tramadol) to its active form, poor metabolizers are also likely to demonstrate a diminished response to those treatments. Studies on genetic polymorphisms affecting the CYP P450 system suggest ethnic differences.[17] Approximately 15% to 20% of Asian Americans and African Americans appear to be poor metabolizers with respect to P450 2C19 compared with 3% to 5% of Whites. Conversely, the proportion of poor metabolizers with respect to P450 2D6 appears to be higher among Whites (~5%–10%) than among Asian Americans and African Americans (~1%–3%). Current understanding of the clinical relevance of genetic polymorphisms in drug therapy in psychiatry remains rudimentary. Commercial genotyping tests for polymorphisms of potential relevance to drug–drug metabolism are increasingly available. Further systematic study of their relevance to the understanding and prediction of drug response is needed before such testing can be meaningfully incorporated into routine psychopharmacological practice.

Excretion

Because most antidepressant, anxiolytic, and antipsychotic medications are largely eliminated by hepatic metabolism, factors that affect renal excretion (glomerular filtration, tubular reabsorption, and active tubular secretion) are generally far less important to the pharmacokinetics of these drugs than to lithium, for which such factors may have clinically significant consequences. Conditions resulting in sodium deficiency (e.g., dehydration, sodium restriction, use of thiazide diuretics) are likely to result in increased proximal tubular reabsorption of lithium, resulting in increased lithium levels and potential toxicity. Lithium levels and clinical status must be monitored especially closely in the setting of vomiting, diarrhea, excessive evaporative losses, or polyuria. Factors, such as aging, that are associated with reduced renal blood flow and glomerular filtration rate (GFR) also reduce lithium excretion. For this reason, as well as for their reduced volume of distribution for lithium because of relative loss of total body water with aging, older adult patients typically require lower lithium doses than younger patients, and a low starting dose (i.e., 150–300 mg/day) is often prudent. Apparently separate from pharmacokinetic effects, however, older adult patients may also be more sensitive to the neurotoxic effects of lithium even at low therapeutic levels. Factors associated with an increased GFR, particularly pregnancy, may produce an increase in lithium clearance and a fall in lithium levels.

For other medications, renal excretion may sometimes be exploited in the treatment of a drug overdose. Acidification of the urine by ascorbic acid, ammonium chloride, or methenamine mandelate increases the rate of excretion of weak bases (such as the amphetamines and phencyclidine [PCP]). Therefore, such measures may be important in the emergency management of a patient with severe PCP or amphetamine intoxication. Conversely, alkalinization of the urine by administration of sodium bicarbonate or acetazolamide may hasten the excretion of weak acids (including long-acting barbiturates, such as phenobarbital).

ANTIPSYCHOTICS

Antipsychotic or neuroleptic drugs include the phenothiazines (e.g., chlorpromazine, fluphenazine, perphenazine, thioridazine, and trifluoperazine), butyrophenones (haloperidol), thioxanthenes (thiothixene), indolones (molindone),

diphenylbutylpiperidines (pimozide), dibenzodiazepines (loxapine), and the newer atypical agents (clozapine, olanzapine, risperidone, quetiapine, ziprasidone, aripiprazole, iloperidone, paliperidone, asenapine, lurasidone, brexpiprazole, cariprazine, lumateperone, and pimavanserin).[18,19] As a class, they are generally rapidly, if erratically, absorbed from the GI tract after oral administration (peak plasma concentrations ranging from 30 minutes to 6 hours). They are highly lipophilic and distribute rapidly to body tissues with a large apparent volume of distribution. Protein binding in the circulation ranges from approximately 90% to 98% except for molindone, paliperidone, and quetiapine, which are only moderately protein bound. The antipsychotics generally undergo substantial first-pass hepatic metabolism (primarily oxidation and conjugation reactions), reducing their systemic bioavailability when given orally compared with intramuscular administration, the fractional absorption of which nearly approximates that of intravenous (IV) administration. Most of the individual antipsychotics have several pharmacologically active and inactive metabolites. Because of their propensity to sequester in body compartments, the elimination half-lives of antipsychotics are quite variable, generally ranging from approximately 20 to 40 hours. For butyrophenones, however, elimination pharmacokinetics appear to be especially complex, and the disappearance of drugs from the systemic circulation, and even more so from brain, may take much longer, as it does for aripiprazole (and its active metabolite, dehydro-aripiprazole), whose half-life may exceed 90 hours.

The lower-potency antipsychotics (including chlorpromazine, mesoridazine, thioridazine, and clozapine) are generally the most sedating and have the greatest anticholinergic, antihistaminic, and α_1-adrenergic antagonistic effects, whereas the higher-potency antipsychotics (including haloperidol, loxapine, molindone, and the piperazine phenothiazines, such as trifluoperazine), are more likely to be associated with an increased incidence of extrapyramidal symptoms (EPSs), including akathisia, dystonia, and parkinsonism. The atypical antipsychotics generally have multiple receptor affinities, including antagonism at dopamine D_{1-4} receptors, serotonin $5-HT_1$, $5-HT_5$, and $5-HT_2$ receptors, α_1- and α_2-adrenergic receptors, histamine-H_1 receptors, and cholinergic muscarinic receptors, with variations across agents; thus, for example, clozapine and olanzapine have notably greater affinity at the muscarinic receptors than the other agents, and aripiprazole is a partial agonist at the D_2 receptor. Although the more complex pharmacological profile of these newer atypical agents, as well as the older low-potency antipsychotics, has generally been associated with a lower risk of EPSs, the same broad range of receptor activity also poses greater risk of pharmacodynamic interactions.

Lower-potency drugs, as well as some atypical antipsychotics, can produce significant hypotension when combined with vasodilator or antihypertensive drugs related to α_1-adrenergic blockade (Table 14.3).[20,21] Hypotension can also occur when low-potency antipsychotics and atypical antidepressants are combined with tricyclic antidepressant (TCA) and MAOI antidepressants. Severe hypotension has been reported when chlorpromazine has been administered with the angiotensin-converting enzyme (ACE) inhibitor captopril. Paradoxical hypotension can develop when epinephrine is administered with low-potency antipsychotics. In this setting, the β-adrenergic stimulant effect of epinephrine, resulting in vasodilation, is thought to be unopposed by its usual pressor effect because α_1-adrenergic receptors are occupied by the antipsychotic. A similar effect may result if a low-potency neuroleptic is administered to a patient with a pheochromocytoma. Finally, hypotension may develop when low-potency antipsychotics are used in combination with a variety of anesthetics (such as halothane, enflurane, and isoflurane).

TABLE 14.3 Selected Drug Interactions with Antipsychotic Medications

Drug	Potential Interaction
Antacids (aluminum-magnesium containing), fruit juice	Interference with absorption of antipsychotic agents
Carbamazepine	Decreased antipsychotic drug plasma levels; additive risk of myelosuppression with clozapine
Cigarettes	Decreased antipsychotic drug plasma levels; reduced EPSs
Rifampin	Decreased antipsychotic drug plasma levels
TCAs	Increased TCA and antipsychotic drug plasma levels; hypotension, depression of cardiac conduction (with low-potency antipsychotics)
SSRIs	Increased SSRI and antipsychotic drug plasma levels; arrhythmia risk with thioridazine and pimozide
Bupropion, duloxetine	Increased antipsychotic drug plasma levels; arrhythmia risk with thioridazine
Fluvoxamine, nefazodone	Increased antipsychotic drug plasma levels; arrhythmia risk with pimozide; seizure risk with clozapine
β-Blockers (lipophilic)	Increased antipsychotic drug plasma levels; improved akathisia
Anticholinergic drugs	Additive anticholinergic toxicity; reduced EPSs
Antihypertensive, vasodilator drugs	Hypotension (with low-potency antipsychotics and risperidone)
Guanethidine, clonidine	Blockade of antihypertensive effect
Epinephrine	Hypotension (with low-potency antipsychotics)
Class I antiarrhythmics	Depression of cardiac conduction; ventricular arrhythmias (with low-potency antipsychotics, ziprasidone)
Calcium channel blockers	Depression of cardiac conduction; ventricular arrhythmias (with pimozide)
Lithium	Idiosyncratic neurotoxicity

EPS, Extrapyramidal symptom; *SSRI,* selective serotonin reuptake inhibitor; *TCA,* tricyclic antidepressant.

In addition, the low-potency antipsychotics have quinidine-like effects on cardiac conduction (and may prolong Q-T and P-R intervals).[22] Ziprasidone may also cause Q-T prolongation, although clinically significant prolongation (QTc >500 ms) appears to be infrequent when administered to otherwise healthy individuals. Significant depression of cardiac conduction, heart block, and life-threatening ventricular dysrhythmias may result from the co-administration of low-potency antipsychotics or ziprasidone with class I antiarrhythmics (e.g., quinidine, procainamide, disopyramide), as well as when administered with high doses of the TCAs or methadone, which also increase the QTc interval, and when administered in the context of other aggravating factors (including hypokalemia, hypomagnesemia, bradycardia, or congenital prolongation of the QTc). Pimozide also can depress cardiac conduction as a result of its calcium channel blocking action, and the combination of pimozide with other calcium channel blockers (e.g., nifedipine, diltiazem, verapamil) is contraindicated.

Another clinically significant pharmacodynamic interaction arises when low-potency antipsychotics, as well as atypical antipsychotics, particularly clozapine or olanzapine, are administered with other drugs that have anticholinergic effects (including TCAs, benztropine, and diphenhydramine). When these drugs are combined, there is greater risk of urinary retention, constipation, blurred vision, impaired memory and concentration, and increased intraocular pressure in the setting of narrow-angle glaucoma. With overdose, a severe anticholinergic syndrome can develop, including delirium, paralytic ileus, tachycardia, and dysrhythmias. Older adult patients are likely to be at increased risk for toxicity because of anticholinergic effects. The high-potency agents and non-anticholinergic atypical agents (e.g., risperidone) are indicated when anticholinergic effects need to be minimized.

The sedative effects of low-potency agents and atypical antidepressants are also often additive to those of the sedative–hypnotic medications and alcohol. In patients for whom sedative effects may be especially dangerous, including older adults, the cautious selection and dosing of antipsychotics should always consider the overall burden of sedation from their concurrent medications. For these patients, starting with a low, divided dose is often an appropriate first step.

Because dopamine receptor blockade is a property common to all antipsychotics, they are all likely to interfere, although to varying degrees, with the efficacy of levodopa and direct dopamine receptor agonists in the treatment of Parkinson disease. When antipsychotic treatment is necessary in this setting, clozapine and the newer atypical agents, or the lower-potency conventional agents, have been preferred. Reciprocally, antipsychotics are likely to be less effective in the treatment of psychosis in the setting of levodopa, stimulants (e.g., dextroamphetamine), and direct agonists (e.g., ropinirole) that facilitate dopamine transmission. Nevertheless, these agents have been combined with antipsychotics in cautious, modestly successful efforts to treat the negative symptoms of schizophrenia (including blunted affect, paucity of thought and speech, and social withdrawal). In addition, elevated prolactin is common on antipsychotics, particularly higher-potency conventional agents and risperidone; it manifests with irregular menses, galactorrhea, diminished libido, or hirsutism. If these agents are necessary and other causes of hyperprolactinemia have been excluded, there is an appropriate role for concurrent, cautious use of dopamine agonists, particularly bromocriptine, to lower prolactin.

The risk of agranulocytosis, which occurs rarely with the low-potency antipsychotics, is much higher with clozapine, with an incidence as high as 1% to 3%. For this reason, the combination of clozapine with other medications associated with a risk of myelosuppression (e.g., carbamazepine) should be avoided. Similarly, because clozapine lowers the seizure threshold to a greater extent than other antipsychotics, co-administration with other medications that significantly lower the seizure threshold (e.g., maprotiline) should be avoided, or combined use with an anticonvulsant should be considered.

The co-administration of lithium with antipsychotic agents (most notably haloperidol) has been associated, very rarely, with potentially irreversible neurotoxicity, characterized by mental status changes; EPSs; and, perhaps in some patients, cerebellar signs and hyperthermia.[23] Related to this concern is the unconfirmed suggestion that lithium co-administration with an antipsychotic may increase the risk of neuroleptic malignant syndrome (NMS). Other clinical variables, including dehydration and poor nutrition, are likely to be of greater significance as putative risk factors for NMS. At present, the evidence is not sufficient to warrant avoidance of the widely used combination of lithium and neuroleptics. Such a possibility, however, should be considered when a patient receiving these medications has neuropsychiatric toxicity of unclear origin.

Pharmacokinetic drug interactions are common among the antipsychotic drugs.[20,21] Plasma levels of the neuroleptics, however, may vary as much as 10-fold to 20-fold among individuals even on monotherapy, and, as a class, antipsychotics fortunately have a relatively wide therapeutic index. Therefore, factors that alter antipsychotic drug metabolism may not have deleterious clinical consequences in many instances. Exceptions include antipsychotic drugs linked to risk of arrhythmia, most notably thioridazine and pimozide. Related to CYP P450 isoenzyme inhibition, agents that interfere with P450 2D6 (such as fluoxetine, paroxetine, duloxetine, or bupropion) can greatly increase levels of low-potency agents, including thioridazine, and thus increase the risk of arrhythmia. Similarly, agents that interfere with P450 3A4 (such as erythromycin, fluvoxamine, or nefazodone) entail similar risk when combined with pimozide. These combinations are contraindicated. The concurrent administration of potent P450 3A4 inhibitors with ziprasidone may increase levels and theoretically increase QTc and risk of arrhythmias. Another exception has to do with patients who are maintained on antipsychotics carefully tapered to the lowest effective dose. In these patients, a small decrease in antipsychotic levels, as may occur with the introduction of a metabolic inducer or an agent that interferes with absorption, may bring them below the threshold for efficacy.

Antipsychotic drug levels may be lowered by aluminum-containing or magnesium-containing antacids, which reduce their absorption and are best given separately. Mixing liquid preparations of phenothiazines with beverages, such as fruit juices, presents the risk of causing insoluble precipitates and inefficient GI absorption. Carbamazepine, known to be a potent inducer of hepatic enzymes, including P450 3A4 and others, has been associated with reduction of steady-state antipsychotic drug plasma levels by as much as 50%. This effect is especially important to bear in mind as a potential explanation when a neuroleptic-treated patient appears to deteriorate in the weeks after the introduction of carbamazepine. Oxcarbazepine may also induce antipsychotic drug metabolism, as can a variety of other anticonvulsants, including phenobarbital and phenytoin. Cigarette smoking may also be associated with a reduction in antipsychotic drug levels through enzyme metabolism. As inpatient units and community residential programs have widely become "smoke-free," there are often substantial differences in smoking frequency between inpatient and outpatient settings. Among patients who smoke heavily, consideration should be given to the impact of these changes in smoking habits on antipsychotic dose requirements.

When an antipsychotic drug is given together with a TCA, the plasma level of each agent may rise, presumably because of mutual inhibition of microsomal enzymes. Reciprocally, when a patient with psychotic depression is tapered off an antipsychotic, it is important to remember that the plasma level of TCAs may also decline. Selective serotonin reuptake inhibitors (SSRIs) and other antidepressants with inhibitory effects on CYP P450 isoenzymes may also produce an increase in the plasma levels of a concurrently administered antipsychotic agent (see Table 14.1). Thus, increases in clozapine, olanzapine, asenapine, and haloperidol plasma levels may occur when co-administered with fluvoxamine. Increases in risperidone, aripiprazole, iloperidone, and typical antipsychotic levels may follow initiation of fluoxetine, paroxetine, bupropion, duloxetine, or sertraline. Quetiapine, lurasidone, and ziprasidone levels may rise following addition of nefazodone, fluvoxamine, or fluoxetine. Phenothiazine drug levels may be increased when co-administered with propranolol, another inhibitor of hepatic microenzymes. Because propranolol is often an effective symptomatic treatment for neuroleptic-associated akathisia, the combined use of the β-blocker with an antipsychotic drug is common. When interactions present a

TABLE 14.4 Selected Drug Interactions with Lithium

Drug	Potential Interaction
Aminophylline, theophylline, acetazolamide, mannitol, sodium bicarbonate, sodium chloride load	Decreased lithium levels
Thiazide diuretics	Increased lithium levels; reduction of lithium-associated polyuria
Non-steroidal anti-inflammatory drugs, COX-2 inhibitors, tetracycline, spectinomycin, metronidazole, angiotensin II receptor antagonists, ACE inhibitors	Increased lithium levels
Neuromuscular blocking drugs (succinylcholine, pancuronium, decamethonium)	Prolonged muscle paralysis
Antithyroid drugs (propylthiouracil, thioamide, methimazole)	Enhanced antithyroid efficacy
Calcium channel blockers (verapamil, diltiazem)	Idiosyncratic neurotoxicity
Antipsychotic drugs	Idiosyncratic neurotoxicity

ACE, Angiotensin-converting enzyme; *COX*, cyclo-oxygenase.

problem, the use of a water-soluble β-blocker, such as atenolol, which is not likely to interfere with hepatic metabolism, provides a reasonable alternative.

MOOD STABILIZERS

Lithium

Lithium is absorbed completely from the GI tract.[18] It distributes throughout total body water and, in contrast to most psychotropic drugs, does not bind to plasma proteins and is not metabolized in the liver. It is filtered and reabsorbed by the kidneys, and 95% of it is excreted in the urine. Lithium elimination is highly dependent on total body sodium and fluid balance; it competes with sodium for reabsorption in the proximal tubules. To a lesser extent, lithium is also reabsorbed in Henle's loop but, in contrast to sodium, it is not reabsorbed in the distal tubules. Its elimination half-life is approximately 24 hours; clearance is generally 20% of creatinine clearance but is diminished in older adults and in patients with renal disease. The risk of toxicity is increased in these patients, as well as in those with cardiovascular disease, dehydration, or hypokalemia. The most common drug–drug interactions involving lithium are pharmacokinetic. Because lithium has a low therapeutic index, such interactions are likely to be clinically significant and potentially serious (Table 14.4).[24]

Several medications are associated with decreased lithium excretion and therefore an increased risk of lithium toxicity. Among the best studied of these interactions are thiazide diuretics. These agents decrease lithium clearance and thereby steeply increase the risk of toxicity. Thiazide diuretics block sodium reabsorption at the distal tubule, producing sodium depletion, which in turn results in increased lithium reabsorption in the proximal tubule. Loop diuretics (e.g., furosemide, bumetanide) appear to interact to a lesser degree with lithium excretion, presumably because they block lithium reabsorption in Henle's loop, potentially off-setting possible compensatory increases in reabsorption more proximally.[25,26] The potassium-sparing diuretics (e.g., amiloride, spironolactone, ethacrynic acid, triamterene) also appear to be somewhat less likely to cause an increase in lithium levels, but close monitoring is indicated when introduced. The potential impact of thiazide diuretics on lithium levels does not contraindicate their combined use, which has been particularly valuable in the treatment of lithium-associated polyuria. Potassium-sparing diuretics have also been used for this purpose.

When a thiazide diuretic is used, a lithium dose reduction and frequent monitoring of lithium levels are required. Monitoring of serum electrolytes, particularly potassium, is also important when thiazides are introduced because hypokalemia enhances the toxicity of lithium. Although not contraindicated with lithium, ACE inhibitors (e.g., captopril) and angiotensin II receptor antagonists (e.g., losartan) can elevate lithium levels, and close monitoring of levels is also required when these agents are introduced. Many of the non-steroidal anti-inflammatory drugs (including ibuprofen, indomethacin, naproxen, ketorolac, meloxicam, and piroxicam) have also been reported to increase serum lithium levels, potentially by as much as 50% to 60% when used at full prescription strength. This may occur by inhibition of renal clearance of lithium by interference with a prostaglandin-dependent mechanism in the renal tubule. The cyclo-oxygenase-2 inhibitors may also raise lithium levels. Limited available data suggest that aspirin is less likely to affect lithium levels.[27,28]

Finally, several antimicrobials are associated with increased lithium levels, including tetracycline, metronidazole, and parenteral spectinomycin. If these agents are required, close monitoring of lithium levels and potential dose adjustment are recommended.

Conversely, a variety of agents can produce decreases in lithium levels, thereby increasing the risk of psychiatric symptom breakthrough and relapse. The methylxanthines (e.g., aminophylline, theophylline) can cause a significant decrease in lithium levels by increasing renal clearance; close blood level monitoring is necessary when co-administration occurs. A reduction in lithium levels can also result from alkalinization of urine (e.g., with acetazolamide or sodium bicarbonate); osmotic diuretics (e.g., urea or mannitol); or ingestion of a sodium chloride load, which also increases lithium excretion.

A probable pharmacodynamic interaction exists between lithium and agents (e.g., succinylcholine, pancuronium, decamethonium) used to produce neuromuscular blockade during anesthesia. Significant prolongation of muscle paralysis can occur when these agents are administered to lithium-treated patients. Although the mechanism is unknown, the possible inhibition by lithium of acetylcholine synthesis and release at the neuromuscular junction is a potential basis for synergism.

Lithium interferes with the production of thyroid hormones through several mechanisms, including interference with iodine uptake, tyrosine iodination, and release of triiodothyronine and thyroxine. Lithium may therefore enhance the efficacy of antithyroid medications (e.g., propylthiouracil, thioamide, methimazole) and has also been used preoperatively to help prevent thyroid storm with the surgical treatment of Graves disease.

There are isolated reports of various forms of neurotoxicity, usually but not always reversible, when lithium has been combined with SSRIs; serotonin–norepinephrine reuptake inhibitors (SNRIs); and other serotonergic agents, calcium channel blockers, antipsychotics, and anticonvulsants (such as carbamazepine). In some cases, features of the serotonin syndrome or NMS have been present. Although it is worthwhile to bear this in mind when evaluating unexplained mental status changes in a lithium-treated patient, the combination of lithium with these classes of medication is neither contraindicated nor unusual.

Valproic Acid

Valproic acid is a simple branched-chain carboxylic acid that, like several other anticonvulsants, has mood-stabilizing properties. Valproic acid is 80% to 95% protein bound and is rapidly metabolized primarily by hepatic microsomal glucuronidation and oxidation. It has a short elimination half-life of about 8 hours. Clearance is essentially unchanged in older adults and in patients with renal disease, but it is significantly reduced in patients with primary liver disease.

TABLE 14.5 Selected Drug Interactions with Valproate and Carbamazepine

Drug	Interaction with Valproate
Carbamazepine	Decreased valproate plasma levels; increased plasma levels of the epoxide metabolite of carbamazepine; variable effects on plasma levels of carbamazepine
Phenytoin	Decreased valproate plasma levels; variable effects on phenytoin plasma levels
Phenobarbital	Decreased valproate plasma levels; increased phenobarbital plasma levels
Oral contraceptives	Decreased valproate plasma levels
Carbapenem antibiotics	Decreased valproate plasma levels
Lamotrigine	Increased lamotrigine levels; hypersensitivity reaction
Aspirin	Increased unbound (active) fraction of valproate
Cimetidine Fluoxetine	Increased valproate plasma levels
Clonazepam	Rare absence seizures
Drug	**Interaction with Carbamazepine**
Phenytoin Phenobarbital Primidone	Decreased carbamazepine plasma levels
Macrolide antibiotics Isoniazid Fluoxetine Verapamil Diltiazem Danazol Propoxyphene	Increased carbamazepine plasma levels
Oral contraceptives Corticosteroids Thyroid hormones Warfarin Cyclosporine Phenytoin Ethosuximide Carbamazepine Valproate Lamotrigine Tetracycline Doxycycline Theophylline Methadone Benzodiazepines TCAs Antipsychotics Methylphenidate Modafinil	Induction of metabolism by carbamazepine
Thiazide diuretics Furosemide	Hyponatremia

TCA, Tricyclic antidepressant.

In contrast to some other major anticonvulsants (such as carbamazepine and phenobarbital), valproate does not induce hepatic microsomes. Rather, it tends to act as an inhibitor of oxidation and glucuronidation reactions, thereby potentially increasing levels of co-administered hepatically metabolized drugs, notably including lamotrigine as well as some TCAs, such as clomipramine, amitriptyline, and nortriptyline (Table 14.5).[29-31] A complex pharmacokinetic interaction occurs when valproic acid and carbamazepine are administered concurrently. Valproic acid not only inhibits the metabolism of carbamazepine and its active metabolite, carbamazepine-10,11-epoxide (CBZ-E), but also displaces both entities from protein-binding sites. Although the effect on plasma carbamazepine levels is variable, the levels of the unbound (active) epoxide metabolite are increased with a concomitant increased risk of carbamazepine neurotoxicity. Conversely, co-administration with carbamazepine results in a decrease in plasma valproic acid levels. Nevertheless, the combination of valproate and carbamazepine has been used successfully in the treatment of patients with bipolar disorder who were only partially responsive to either drug alone. Oral contraceptives as well as carbapenem antibiotics have also been associated with decreases in plasma valproic acid levels; enhanced monitoring of levels and valproate dose adjustments are recommended when these agents are used.

Cimetidine, a potent inhibitor of hepatic microsomal enzymes, is associated with decreased clearance of valproic acid, resulting in increased levels. Dose reductions of valproic acid may be necessary in the patient starting cimetidine but not for other H_2-receptor antagonists. Elevated levels of valproic acid have also been reported sporadically with fluoxetine and other SSRIs. Aspirin and other salicylates may displace protein binding of valproic acid, thereby increasing the unbound (free) fraction, which may increase risk of toxicity from valproate even though total serum levels are unchanged.

Absence seizures have been reported with the combination of clonazepam and valproate, although this is likely to be rare and limited to individuals with neurological disorders.

Lamotrigine

Lamotrigine is a phenyltriazine anticonvulsant that is moderately (50%–60%) protein bound and metabolized primarily by glucuronidation. Its most serious adverse effect is a life-threatening hypersensitivity reaction with rash, typically, but not always, occurring within the first 2 months of use. The incidence among individuals with bipolar disorder is estimated at 0.8 per 1000 among patients on lamotrigine monotherapy and 1.3 per 1000 among patients taking lamotrigine in combination with other agents.

The risk of adverse effects including hypersensitivity reactions and tremor is increased when lamotrigine is combined with valproic acid. As much as a two-fold to three-fold increase in lamotrigine levels occurs when valproic acid is added, related to inhibition of glucuronidation of lamotrigine.[12,30] Accordingly, the *Physicians' Desk Reference* provides guidelines for more gradual dose titration of lamotrigine and lower target doses when introduced in a patient already taking valproate. When valproate is added to lamotrigine, the dose of the latter should typically be reduced by one-half to two-thirds.

Conversely, lamotrigine levels can be decreased by as much as 50% when administered with metabolic inducers, particularly other anticonvulsants (including carbamazepine and phenobarbital). Guidelines have therefore been developed for the dosing of lamotrigine in the presence of these metabolic-inducing anticonvulsants. Of note, similar magnitude reductions in lamotrigine levels have been reported in patients taking oral contraceptives, requiring an increase in the dose of lamotrigine.[32] Lamotrigine levels and symptom status should be monitored closely when oral contraceptives or metabolic-inducing anticonvulsants are started.

Carbamazepine

Carbamazepine is an iminostilbene anticonvulsant structurally related to the TCA imipramine. It is only moderately (60%–85%) protein bound. It is poorly soluble in GI fluids, and as much as 15% to 25% of an oral dose is excreted

unchanged in the feces. Its CBZ-E metabolite is neuroactive. Carbamazepine, a potent inducer of hepatic metabolism, can also induce its own metabolism such that elimination half-life may fall from 18 to 55 hours to 5 to 20 hours over a matter of several weeks, generally reaching a plateau after 3 to 5 weeks.[18]

Most drug–drug interactions with carbamazepine occur by pharmacokinetic mechanisms.[31,33,34] The metabolism of a wide variety of drugs (e.g., valproic acid, phenytoin, ethosuximide, lamotrigine, alprazolam, clonazepam, TCAs, antipsychotics, methylphenidate, doxycycline, tetracycline, thyroid hormone, corticosteroids, oral contraceptives, methadone, theophylline, warfarin, oral hypoglycemics, cyclosporine) is induced by carbamazepine, thereby lowering drug levels and potentially leading to therapeutic failure or symptom relapse (see Table 14.5). Patients of childbearing potential taking oral contraceptives must be advised to use an additional method of birth control.

Several drugs inhibit the metabolism of carbamazepine, including the macrolide antibiotics (e.g., erythromycin, clarithromycin, triacetyloleandomycin), isoniazid, fluoxetine, valproic acid, danazol, and propoxyphene and the calcium channel blockers verapamil and diltiazem. Because of its low therapeutic index, the risk of developing carbamazepine toxicity is significantly increased when these drugs are administered concurrently. Conversely, co-administration of phenytoin or phenobarbital, both microsomal enzyme inducers, can increase the metabolism of carbamazepine, potentially resulting in subtherapeutic plasma levels.

Carbamazepine has been associated with hyponatremia. The combination of carbamazepine with thiazide diuretics or furosemide has been associated with severe, symptomatic hyponatremia, suggesting the need for close monitoring of electrolytes when these medications are used concurrently. Carbamazepine has also been associated with bone marrow suppression, and its combination with other agents that interfere with blood cell production (including clozapine) should generally be avoided.

Oxcarbazepine appears to be a less potent metabolic inducer than carbamazepine, although it still may render certain important agents, particularly P450 3A4 substrates, less effective because of similar pharmacokinetic interactions. Women of childbearing potential should therefore receive guidance about supplementing oral contraceptives with a second non-hormonal form of birth control, as with carbamazepine. Similarly, like carbamazepine, oxcarbazepine is also associated with risk of hyponatremia.

ANTIDEPRESSANTS

The antidepressant drugs include the TCAs, the MAOIs, the SSRIs, the atypical agents (bupropion, trazodone, nefazodone, and mirtazapine), and the SNRIs (duloxetine, venlafaxine, and desvenlafaxine). Although the TCAs and MAOIs are used infrequently, they continue to serve a valuable role in the treatment of more severe, treatment-resistant depressive and anxiety disorders despite the wide range of drug–drug interactions they entail.

Selective Serotonin Reuptake Inhibitors and Other Newer Antidepressants

The SSRIs (fluoxetine, sertraline, paroxetine, fluvoxamine, citalopram, escitalopram, vortioxetine, and vilazodone) share similar pharmacological actions, including minimal anticholinergic, antihistaminic, and α_1-adrenergic blocking effects, and potent pre-synaptic inhibition of serotonin reuptake. Vilazodone is also a partial agonist at the 5-HT$_{1A}$ receptor, and vortioxetine is an antagonist, agonist, or partial agonist at multiple serotonin receptor subtypes. There are important

TABLE 14.6 Potential Drug Interactions with the Selective Serotonin Reuptake Inhibitors and Other Newer Antidepressants

Drug	Potential Interaction
MAOIs	Serotonin syndrome
Secondary amine TCAs	Increased TCA levels when co-administered with fluoxetine, paroxetine, sertraline, bupropion, duloxetine
Tertiary amine TCAs	Increased TCA levels with fluvoxamine, paroxetine, sertraline, bupropion, duloxetine
Antipsychotics (typical) and risperidone, aripiprazole	Increased antipsychotic levels with fluoxetine, sertraline, paroxetine, bupropion, duloxetine
Thioridazine	Arrhythmia risk with P450 2D6 inhibitory antidepressants
Pimozide	Arrhythmia risk with P450 3A4 inhibitory antidepressants (nefazodone, fluvoxamine)
Clozapine and olanzapine	Increased antipsychotic levels with fluvoxamine
Diazepam	Increased benzodiazepine levels with fluoxetine, fluvoxamine, sertraline
Triazolobenzodiazepines (midazolam, alprazolam, triazolam)	Increased levels with fluvoxamine, nefazodone, sertraline
Carbamazepine	Increased carbamazepine levels with fluoxetine, fluvoxamine, nefazodone
Theophylline	Increased theophylline levels with fluvoxamine
Type 1 C antiarrhythmics (encainide, flecainide, propafenone)	Increased antiarrhythmic levels with fluoxetine, paroxetine, sertraline, bupropion, duloxetine
β-Blockers (lipophilic)	Increased β-blocker levels with fluoxetine, paroxetine, sertraline, bupropion, duloxetine
Calcium channel blockers	Increased levels with fluoxetine, fluvoxamine, nefazodone

MAOI, Monoamine oxidase inhibitor; *TCA*, tricyclic antidepressant.

pharmacokinetic differences, which account for distinctions among them with respect to potential drug interactions (Table 14.6).[2,3,16,35] Nefazodone, like trazodone, is distinguished from classic SSRIs by its antagonism of the 5-HT$_2$ receptor (and differs from trazodone in its lesser antagonism of the α_1-adrenergic receptor). Mirtazapine also blocks the 5-HT$_2$ receptor, though it also blocks the 5-HT$_3$ receptor and α_2-adrenergic receptors. Venlafaxine, desvenlafaxine, levomilnacipran, and duloxetine, like TCAs, inhibit serotonin and norepinephrine reuptake but, in contrast to TCAs, are relatively devoid of postsynaptic anticholinergic, antihistaminic, and α_1-adrenergic activity. Milnacipran is also an SNRI, though it is approved by the US Food and Drug Administration only for fibromyalgia. Although venlafaxine is predominantly serotonergic at low to moderate doses, duloxetine is a potent inhibitor of both the norepinephrine and serotonin transporters across its clinical dose range. Although not an approved antidepressant, the norepinephrine reuptake inhibitor atomoxetine, indicated for the treatment of attention-deficit hyperactivity disorder, may have a role in depression pharmacotherapy as a single agent or as adjunctive treatment. It is neither a significant inhibitor nor an inducer of the P450 CYP system, but owing to its adrenergic effects, the risk of palpitations or pressor effects is likely to be greater than with serotonergic agents when combined with prescribed and OTC sympathomimetics, and its use with MAOIs is contraindicated.

All SSRIs, as well as nefazodone, are highly protein bound (95% to 99%), except for fluvoxamine (77%), citalopram (80%), and escitalopram (56%). Mirtazapine and bupropion are moderately protein bound (85%). The SNRI duloxetine is highly protein bound (90%), though venlafaxine, desvenlafaxine, and levomilnacipran are minimally protein bound (15%–30%). All antidepressants are hepatically metabolized, and all of them (except for paroxetine and duloxetine) have active metabolites. The major metabolites of sertraline and citalopram, however, appear to be minimally active. Elimination half-lives range from 5 hours for venlafaxine and 11 hours for its metabolite, O-desmethylvenlafaxine, to 2 to 3 days for fluoxetine and 7 to 14 days for its metabolite, norfluoxetine. Nefazodone, like venlafaxine, has a short half-life (2–5 hours), whereas fluvoxamine, sertraline, paroxetine, citalopram, escitalopram, bupropion, mirtazapine, and duloxetine have half-lives in the intermediate range of 12 to 36 hours. Food may have variable effects on antidepressant bioavailability, including an increase for sertraline and vilazodone but a decrease for nefazodone and no change for escitalopram.

The growing knowledge about the interaction of the newer antidepressants with the CYP P450 isoenzymes has revealed differences among them in their pattern of enzyme inhibition that are likely to be critical to the understanding and prediction of drug–drug interactions.

P450 2D6

Fluoxetine, norfluoxetine, paroxetine, bupropion, duloxetine, sertraline (to a moderate degree), and citalopram and escitalopram (to a minimal extent) inhibit P450 2D6, which accounts for their potential inhibitory effect on TCA clearance and the metabolism of other P450 2D6 substrates. Other drugs metabolized by P450 2D6 whose levels may rise in the setting of P450 2D6 inhibition include the type 1 C antiarrhythmics (e.g., encainide, flecainide, propafenone), as well as lipophilic β-blockers (e.g., propranolol, timolol, metoprolol), antipsychotics (e.g., risperidone, haloperidol, aripiprazole, iloperidone, thioridazine, perphenazine), TCAs, and trazodone. P450 2D6 converts codeine and tramadol into their active form; hence, the efficacy of these analgesics may be diminished when concurrently administered with a P450 2D6 inhibitor. So too, as P450 2D6 converts tamoxifen into its active N-desmethyl tamoxifen form for treatment of neoplasms, the use of inhibitors of 2D6 should be carefully re-evaluated during tamoxifen treatment. These observations underscore the need to exercise care and to closely monitor when prescribing these SSRIs, bupropion, or duloxetine in the setting of complex medical regimens. Plasma TCA levels do not routinely include levels of active or potentially toxic metabolites, which may be altered by virtue of shunting to other metabolic routes when P450 2D6 is inhibited. Therefore, particularly in the case of patients at risk for conduction delay, electrocardiography and blood level monitoring are recommended when combining TCAs with SSRIs, duloxetine, or bupropion.

P450 3A4

Fluoxetine's major metabolite (norfluoxetine), fluvoxamine, nefazodone, and, to a lesser extent, sertraline, desmethylsertraline, citalopram, and escitalopram inhibit P450 3A4. Therefore, all these agents have some potential for elevating levels of pimozide and cisapride (arrhythmia risks), methadone, oxycodone, fentanyl (respiratory depression risks), calcium channel blockers, the "statins," carbamazepine, midazolam, and many other important and commonly prescribed substrates of this widely recruited P450 isoenzyme.

P450 2 C

Serum concentrations of drugs metabolized by this subfamily may be increased by fluoxetine, sertraline, and fluvoxamine.

Reported interactions include decreased clearance of diazepam on all three SSRIs, a small reduction in tolbutamide clearance on sertraline, and increased plasma phenytoin concentrations reflecting decreased clearance on fluoxetine. Warfarin is also metabolized by this subfamily, and levels may be increased by the inhibition of these enzymes. SSRIs may interact with warfarin and potentially increase bleeding diathesis by still other, probably pharmacodynamic, mechanisms (such as depletion of platelet serotonin). Although the combination is common, increased monitoring is recommended when SSRIs are prescribed with warfarin.

P450 1A

Among the SSRIs, only fluvoxamine appears to be a potent inhibitor of P450 1A2. Accordingly, increased serum concentrations of theophylline, haloperidol, clozapine, olanzapine, asenapine, and the tertiary amine TCAs (including clomipramine, amitriptyline, and imipramine) may occur when co-administered with this SSRI. Because theophylline and TCAs have a relatively narrow therapeutic index and because the degree of elevation of antipsychotic blood levels appears to be substantial (e.g., up to four-fold increases in haloperidol concentrations), additional monitoring and consideration of dose reductions of these substrates are necessary when fluvoxamine is co-administered.

Mirtazapine, although neither a potent inhibitor nor inducer of the P450 CYP isoenzymes, has numerous pharmacodynamic effects, including antagonism of the histamine-H_1, α_2-adrenergic, 5-HT_2 and 5-HT_3, and muscarinic receptors, creating the possibility of myriad pharmacodynamic interactions (including blockade of clonidine's antihypertensive activity) but also the possible benefit of attenuated nausea and sexual dysfunction that may occur with SSRIs.

The serotonin syndrome is a potentially life-threatening condition characterized by confusion, diaphoresis, hyperthermia, hyperreflexia, muscle rigidity, tachycardia, hypotension, and coma.[9,36] Although the serotonin syndrome may develop whenever an SSRI is combined with a serotonergic drug (e.g., L-tryptophan, clomipramine, venlafaxine, triptans) and drugs with serotonergic properties (e.g., lithium, mirtazapine, dextromethorphan, tramadol, meperidine, pentazocine), the greatest known risk is associated with the co-administration of an SSRI or SNRI with an MAOI, which constitutes an absolute contraindication. In view of the long elimination half-life of fluoxetine and norfluoxetine, at least 5 weeks must elapse after fluoxetine discontinuation before an MAOI can be safely introduced. With the other SSRIs and SNRIs, an interval of 2 weeks appears to be adequate. Because of the time required for the MAO enzymes to regenerate, at least 2 weeks must elapse after discontinuation of an MAOI before an SSRI or other potent serotonergic drug is introduced. The weak, reversible MAOI antimicrobial linezolid, used for treatment of multi-drug-resistant gram-positive infections, has been implicated in a small number of post-marketing cases of serotonin syndrome in patients on serotonergic antidepressants, typically patients on SSRIs, as well as other medications (including narcotics). Patients on serotonergic antidepressants receiving linezolid should be monitored for the occurrence of symptoms suggesting serotonin syndrome. The co-administration of SSRIs with other serotonergic agents is not contraindicated but should prompt immediate discontinuation in any patient on this combination of drugs who has mental status changes, fever, or hyperreflexia of unknown origin.

Tricyclic Antidepressants

TCAs are thought to exert their pharmacological action by inhibiting the presynaptic neuronal reuptake of norepinephrine and serotonin in the CNS with subsequent modulation of both pre-synaptic and postsynaptic β-adrenergic receptors. TCAs also have significant anticholinergic, antihistaminic, and α-adrenergic activity, as well as quinidine-like effects on cardiac condition, in these respects resembling the low-potency antipsychotic drugs that are structurally similar.

Tricyclic antidepressants are well absorbed from the GI tract and subject to significant first-pass liver metabolism before entry into the systemic circulation, where they are largely protein-bound, ranging from 85% (trimipramine) to 95% (amitriptyline). They are highly lipophilic with a large volume of distribution. TCAs are extensively metabolized by hepatic microsomal enzymes, and most have pharmacologically active metabolites.

With two methyl groups on the terminal nitrogen of the TCA side-chain, imipramine, amitriptyline, trimipramine, doxepin, and clomipramine are called *tertiary amines*. The demethylation of imipramine, amitriptyline, and trimipramine yields the secondary amine TCAs, desipramine, nortriptyline, and protriptyline, which are generally less sedating and have less affinity for anticholinergic receptors. The demethylation of imipramine relies on CYP P450 isoenzymes 1A2 and 3A3/4, whereas that of amitriptyline appears to rely primarily on 1A2. These tertiary amines, as well as their secondary amine offspring, are then hydroxylated via cytochrome P450 2D6, a step sensitive to inhibition by a wide variety of other drugs. The hydroxymetabolites of the most commonly prescribed TCAs can be active. Furthermore, the hydroxymetabolite of nortriptyline may block the antidepressant effect of the parent drug, and some hydroxymetabolites of the TCAs may be cardiotoxic.

Additive anticholinergic effects can occur when the TCAs are co-administered with other drugs possessing anticholinergic properties (e.g., low-potency antipsychotics, antiparkinsonian drugs), potentially resulting in an anticholinergic syndrome. SSRIs, SNRIs, atypical antidepressants, and MAOIs are relatively devoid of anticholinergic activity, although the MAOIs may indirectly potentiate the anticholinergic properties of atropine and scopolamine. Additive sedative effects are common when TCAs are combined with sedative–hypnotics, anxiolytics, narcotics, or alcohol (Table 14.7).

TABLE 14.7 Selected Drug Interactions with Tricyclic Antidepressants

Drug	Potential Interaction
Carbamazepine	Decreased TCA plasma levels
Phenobarbital	
Rifampin	
Isoniazid	
Antipsychotics	Increased TCA plasma levels
Methylphenidate	
SSRIs	
Quinidine	
Propafenone	
Antifungals	
Macrolide antibiotics	
Verapamil	
Diltiazem	
Cimetidine	
Class I antiarrhythmics	Depression of cardiac
Low-potency antipsychotics	conduction; arrhythmias
Guanethidine	Interference with anti-
Clonidine	hypertensive effect
Sympathomimetic amines	Arrhythmias, hypertension
(e.g., isoproterenol, epinephrine)	
Antihypertensives, vasodilator drugs	Hypotension
Anticholinergic drugs	Additive anticholinergic toxicity
MAOIs	Delirium, fever, convulsions
Sulfonylurea hypoglycemics	Hypoglycemia

MAOI, Monoamine oxidase inhibitor; *SSRI*, selective serotonin reuptake inhibitor; *TCA*, tricyclic antidepressant.

Tricyclic antidepressants possess class 1A antiarrhythmic activity and can lead to depression of cardiac conduction, potentially resulting in heart block or ventricular arrhythmias when combined with quinidine-like agents (including quinidine, procainamide, and disopyramide, as well as the low-potency antipsychotics).[37,38] The antiarrhythmics quinidine and propafenone, inhibitors of CYP P450 2D6, may additionally result in clinically significant elevations of the TCAs, thus increasing the risk of cardiotoxicity through both pharmacodynamic and pharmacokinetic mechanisms.

The arrhythmogenic risks of a TCA are enhanced in individuals with underlying coronary or valvular heart disease, recent myocardial infarction, or hypokalemia and in patients receiving sympathomimetic amines, such as dextroamphetamine.

Tricyclic antidepressants also interact with several antihypertensive drugs. TCAs can antagonize the antihypertensive effects of guanethidine, bethanidine, debrisoquine, or clonidine via interference with neuronal reuptake by noradrenergic neurons. Conversely, TCAs can cause or aggravate postural hypotension when co-administered with vasodilator drugs, antihypertensives, and low-potency neuroleptics.

Hypoglycemia has been observed on both secondary and tertiary TCAs, particularly in the presence of sulfonylurea hypoglycemic agents, suggesting the need for close monitoring.

Pharmacokinetic interactions involving the TCAs are often clinically important. The antipsychotic drugs (including haloperidol, chlorpromazine, thioridazine, and perphenazine) are known to increase TCA levels by 30% to 100%. Cimetidine can also raise tertiary TCA levels as predicted by microsomal enzyme inhibition, as can methylphenidate. The antifungals (e.g., ketoconazole), macrolide antibiotics (e.g., erythromycin), and calcium channel blockers (e.g., verapamil and diltiazem) as inhibitors of CYP P450 3A4 may also impair the clearance of tertiary amine TCAs, thereby requiring a TCA dose reduction. SSRIs, particularly fluoxetine, paroxetine, and (to a lesser extent), sertraline, have been associated with clinically significant increases in TCA plasma levels, believed to be the result of inhibition primarily but not exclusively of CYP P450 2D6. Similar elevations in TCA levels are expected with other potent P450 2D6 inhibitor antidepressants (including duloxetine and bupropion).

Inducers of P450 enzymes can increase the metabolism of TCAs. Thus, plasma levels of TCAs may be significantly reduced when carbamazepine, phenobarbital, rifampin, or isoniazid are co-administered or in the setting of chronic alcohol or cigarette use.

Monoamine Oxidase Inhibitors

Monoamine oxidase is an enzyme located primarily on the outer mitochondrial membrane and is responsible for intracellular catabolism of the monoamines. It is found in high concentrations in the brain, liver, intestines, and lungs. In presynaptic nerve terminals, MAO metabolizes cytoplasmic monoamines. In the liver and gut, MAO catabolizes ingested bioactive amines, thus protecting against absorption into the systemic circulation of potentially vasoactive substances, particularly tyramine. Two subtypes of MAO have been distinguished: whereas intestinal MAO is predominantly MAO_A, brain MAO is predominantly MAO_B. MAO_A preferentially metabolizes norepinephrine and serotonin. Both MAO subtypes metabolize dopamine and tyramine. The traditional MAOIs—phenelzine, tranylcypromine, and isocarboxazid—that have been used for the treatment of patients with depression are non-specific inhibitors of both MAO_A and MAO_B. More recently, selegiline, available in transdermal form, has been approved for the treatment of depression. At low doses, selegiline is primarily an inhibitor of MAO_B, though it is a mixed MAO_A and MAO_B inhibitor at higher doses. When patients are using MAOIs, dietary[39,40] and medication restrictions must be closely followed to avoid serious interactions. The MAOIs are therefore generally reserved for use in responsible or supervised patients when adequate trials of other classes of antidepressants have failed.

The two major types of MAOI drug–drug interaction are the serotonin syndrome and the hypertensive (also called hyperadrenergic) crisis.[7,8,35] Hypertensive crisis is an emergency characterized by an abrupt elevation of blood pressure, severe headache, nausea, vomiting, and diaphoresis; intracranial hemorrhage or myocardial infarction can occur. Prompt intervention to reduce blood pressure with the α_1-adrenergic antagonist phentolamine or the calcium channel blocker nifedipine may be life-saving. Potentially catastrophic hypertension appears to be caused by release of bound intraneuronal stores of norepinephrine and dopamine by indirect vasopressor substances. The reaction can therefore be precipitated by the concurrent administration of vasopressor amines, stimulants, anorexiants, and many OTC cough and cold preparations; these include L-dopa, dopamine, amphetamine, methylphenidate, phenylpropanolamine, phentermine, mephentermine, metaraminol, ephedrine, and pseudoephedrine. By contrast, direct sympathomimetic amines (e.g., norepinephrine, isoproterenol, epinephrine), which rely for their cardiovascular effects on direct stimulation of postsynaptic receptors rather than on presynaptic release of stored catecholamines, may be somewhat safer when administered to individuals on MAOIs, although they are also contraindicated.

Hypertensive crises may also be triggered by ingestion of naturally occurring sympathomimetic amines (particularly tyramine), which are present in various food products, including aged cheeses (e.g., stilton, cheddar, blue cheese, or camembert rather than cream cheese, ricotta cheese, or cottage cheese), yeast extracts (e.g., marmite and brewer's yeast tablets), fava (broad) beans, over-ripened fruits (e.g., avocado), pickled herring, aged meats (e.g., salami, bologna, and many kinds of sausage), chicken liver, fermented bean curd, sauerkraut, many types of red wine and beer (particularly imported beer), and some white wines. Although gin, vodka, and whiskey appear to be free of tyramine, their use should be minimized during MAOI treatment, as with other antidepressants, because of the risk of exaggerated side effects and reduced antidepressant efficacy. Other less stringent requirements include moderated intake of caffeine, chocolate, yogurt, and soy sauce. Because MAO activity may remain diminished for nearly 2 to 3 weeks after the discontinuation of MAOIs, a tyramine-free diet and appropriate medication restrictions should be continued for at least 14 days after an MAOI has been discontinued. The lowest dose available of transdermal selegiline has been shown to have minimal risks of hypertensive crisis on a normal diet and therefore does not require the same level of restriction; however, dosages of 9 mg/24 hours and above carry the same dietary recommendations as oral MAOIs.

The serotonin syndrome, the other major drug–drug interaction involving the MAOIs, occurs when MAOIs and serotonergic agents are co-administered. Potentially fatal reactions most closely resembling the serotonin syndrome can also occur with other drugs with less selective serotonergic activity, most notably meperidine, as well as dextromethorphan, a widely available cough suppressant. Both of these medications, similar to the SSRIs, SNRIs, and clomipramine, are absolutely contraindicated when MAOIs are used. The 5-HT$_1$ agonist triptans, used in the treatment of migraine, have been implicated in serotonin syndrome when administered to patients taking MAOIs. This may pose a problem for the triptans that are metabolized in part through the MAO enzymes, including sumatriptan, rizatriptan, and zolmitriptan. Other serotonergic medications (e.g., buspirone and trazodone), although not absolutely contraindicated, should be used with care. Other narcotic analgesics (e.g., propoxyphene, codeine, oxycodone, morphine, alfentanil, or morphine) appear to be somewhat safer alternatives to meperidine, but in conjunction with MAOIs, their analgesic and CNS depressant effects may be potentiated and rare serotonin syndrome–like presentations have been reported.[35,41] If opioid agents are necessary, they should be started at one-fifth to one-half of the standard doses and gradually titrated upward, with monitoring for untoward hemodynamic or mental status changes.

Extremely adverse, although reversible, symptoms of fever, delirium, convulsions, hypotension, and dyspnea were reported on the combination of imipramine and MAOIs. This has contributed to a general avoidance of the once-popular TCA–MAOI combinations. Nevertheless, although incompletely studied, the regimen has been observed in some instances to be successful for exceptionally treatment-refractory patients. When combined, simultaneous initiation of a TCA–MAOI or initiation of the TCA before, but never after, the MAOI has been recommended, although avoidance of the more serotonergic TCAs (including clomipramine, imipramine, and amitriptyline) is prudent.

The sedative effects of CNS depressants (including the benzodiazepines, barbiturates, and chloral hydrate) may be potentiated by MAOIs. MAOIs often cause postural hypotension, and severe additive effects have occurred when co-administered with vasodilator or antihypertensive medications or low-potency antipsychotics.

The MAOIs, like the TCAs, have also been observed to potentiate hypoglycemic agents, including insulin and sulfonylurea drugs, suggesting the need for more frequent glucose monitoring when MAOIs are co-administered with hypoglycemic medications.

Phenelzine has been associated with lowered serum pseudocholinesterase levels and prolonged neuromuscular blockade. The concurrent use of MAOIs is not a contraindication to surgery or electroconvulsive therapy, although it requires a detailed pre-procedure consultation with the anesthesiologist.

St. John's Wort

Although the efficacy of St. John's wort for depression has not been well established in large scale, controlled trials, it has emerged as one of the most carefully studied herbal preparations when it comes to drug–drug interactions. Initial concerns about the generally weak, though potentially variable, MAOI activity of this botanical and the associated risk of serotonin syndrome when combined with serotonergic agents have only been weakly borne out, with few cases of serotonin syndrome reported despite widespread concurrent use of St. John's wort with serotonergic antidepressants. However, both case reports and clinical trials indicate that some critical medications may be rendered less effective in some patients concurrently taking St. John's wort.[14,42] These medications include immunosuppressants (such as cyclosporine and tacrolimus), coumarin anticoagulants, antiretrovirals, theophylline, digoxin, amitriptyline, and oral contraceptives. Although the precise mechanisms and herbal constituents responsible for these effects remain to be elucidated, the primary focus has been on P450 3A4 and P-glycoprotein. A paucity of systematic information exists concerning potential drug interactions and adverse effects of other natural products, including a possible risk of increased bleeding in patients taking gingko biloba and warfarin and of hepatotoxicity in patients on certain kava preparations.[6]

BENZODIAZEPINES

The benzodiazepines are a class of widely prescribed psychotropic drugs that have anxiolytic, sedative, muscle-relaxant, and anticonvulsant properties. Their rate of onset of action, duration of action, presence of active metabolites, and tendency to accumulate in the body vary considerably and can influence both side effects and the success of treatment.[18] Most benzodiazepines are well absorbed on an empty stomach, with peak plasma levels achieved generally between 1 and 3 hours, although with more rapid onset on some (e.g., diazepam, clorazepate) than others (e.g., oxazepam). The duration of action of a single dose of benzodiazepine generally depends more on distribution from systemic circulation to tissue than on subsequent elimination (e.g., more rapid for diazepam than lorazepam). With repeated doses, however, the volume of distribution is saturated, and the elimination half-life becomes the more important parameter in determining duration of action (e.g., more rapid for lorazepam than diazepam). A benzodiazepine that is comparatively short-acting on acute administration may therefore become relatively long-acting on long-term dosing. Benzodiazepines are highly lipophilic and distribute readily to the CNS and to tissues. Plasma protein-binding ranges from approximately 70% (alprazolam) to 99% (diazepam).

Of the benzodiazepines, only lorazepam, oxazepam, and temazepam are not subject to phase I metabolism. Because phase II metabolism (glucuronide conjugation) does not produce active metabolites and is less affected than phase I metabolism by primary liver disease, aging, and concurrently used inducers or inhibitors of hepatic microsomal enzymes, the 3-hydroxy-substituted benzodiazepines are often preferred in older patients and patients with liver disease.

Perhaps the most common and clinically significant interactions involving benzodiazepines are the additive CNS-depressant effects, which can occur when a benzodiazepine is administered concurrently with barbiturates, narcotics, or ethanol. These interactions can be serious because of their potential to cause excessive sedation; cognitive and psychomotor impairment; and at higher doses, potentially fatal respiratory depression. An interesting pharmacodynamic interaction exists between benzodiazepines and physostigmine, which can act as a competitive inhibitor at the benzodiazepine receptor, antagonizing benzodiazepine effects. The specific benzodiazepine antagonist flumazenil, however, is now more commonly the treatment of choice in managing a severe benzodiazepine overdose.

Pharmacokinetic interactions include a decreased rate, but not extent, of absorption of benzodiazepines in the presence of antacids or food. This is more likely to be a factor in determining the subjective effects accompanying the onset of benzodiazepine action for single-dose rather than the overall efficacy of repeated-dose administration. Carbamazepine, phenobarbital, and rifampin may induce metabolism, lowering levels of benzodiazepines that are oxidatively metabolized. In contrast, potential inhibitors of CYP P450 3A4 (including macrolide antibiotics, antifungals [e.g., ketoconazole, itraconazole], nefazodone, fluvoxamine, and cimetidine) may be associated with decreased clearance and therefore increased levels of the triazolobenzodiazepines, as well as the non-benzodiazepine sedative–hypnotics (zolpidem, zaleplon, and eszopiclone), which are metabolized through this pathway.[2] The metabolism of diazepam depends in part on CYP P450 2C19. Decreased diazepam clearance has been reported with concurrent administration of a variety of agents (including fluoxetine, sertraline, propranolol, metoprolol, omeprazole, disulfiram, low-dose estrogen containing oral contraceptives, and isoniazid).

PSYCHOSTIMULANTS AND MODAFINIL

A variety of miscellaneous drug–drug interactions involving the psychostimulants have been reported.[43] These include increased plasma levels of TCAs (and possibly other antidepressants); increased plasma levels of phenobarbital, primidone, and phenytoin; increased prothrombin time on coumarin anticoagulants; attenuation or reversal of the guanethidine antihypertensive effect; and increased pressor responses to vasopressor drugs. The risk of arrhythmias or hypertension should be considered when combining psychostimulants with TCAs. Although methylphenidate has been implicated in putative drug interactions more often than dextroamphetamine or mixed amphetamine salts, drug interactions involving psychostimulants have been insufficiently studied to draw firm conclusions about their comparative suitability for use among patients on complex medical regimens. Although contraindicated because of the risk of hypertensive crisis, the combination of psychostimulants and MAOIs has been cautiously used in patients with exceptionally treatment-refractory depression or in patients with limiting hypotension on MAOIs that proved resistant to other measures.[44,45] Urinary alkalinization (e.g., with sodium bicarbonate) may result in amphetamine toxicity, most likely because of increased tubular reabsorption of un-ionized amphetamine.

Modafinil and armodafinil interact with the P450 CYP isoenzymes as a minimal to moderate inducer of 1A2 and 3A4 and yet as an inhibitor of the 2C isoforms.[2] Modafinil and armodafinil may thereby engage in drug–drug interactions with common substrates, including oral contraceptives (whose levels may decrease) and lipophilic β-blockers, TCAs, clozapine, and warfarin (whose levels may increase), therefore requiring monitoring and patient education. It is important to advise use of a second non-hormonal form of contraception in modafinil and armodafinil-treated patients taking oral contraceptives. Like St. John's wort, modafinil has also been implicated as a factor in lowered cyclosporine levels, presumably through P450 3A4 induction, and should be used with extreme care in patients on immunosuppressants that rely on this enzyme for metabolism. Although modafinil and armodafinil have been widely combined with SSRIs and other first-line antidepressants, its safety in combination with MAOIs is unknown.

Ketamine, Psychedelics, and Cannabinoids

The emergence of exciting new therapies, such as IV and intranasal ketamine and esketamine, the psychedelics, psilocybin and 3,4-methylenedioxymethamphetamine (MDMA), and cannabis-derived products, such as cannabidiol (CBD), also raises concerns about the risk of interactions with standard psychotropics. An exhaustive review is beyond the scope of this chapter, and such data are still in acquisition. Nonetheless, several early reports provide some caveats. A recent review of 40 reports of interactions involving psilocybin and MDMA described interactions between MDMA or psilocybin and various psychotropics, including antipsychotics, anxiolytics, mood stabilizers, N-methyl-D-aspartate antagonists, psychostimulants, and several antidepressants.[46]

A review of 24 studies found no significant interactions between ketamine and lithium but found stronger evidence of attenuation of ketamine's effects when combined with lamotrigine or benzodiazepines. Esketamine had no significant interactions with tranylcypromine. There was mixed evidence for haloperidol and risperidone, and there was some blunting of ketamine-induced positive symptoms in patients with schizophrenia taking clozapine. One report found no interaction with olanzapine. These studies were largely limited by small samples.[47]

Regarding CBD, there have been reports of interactions with several antiepileptic drugs, two of which are often used in psychiatry, carbamazepine and topiramate, both of which result in decreased CBD.[48] Additional investigations suggest potential pharmacokinetic interactions between CBD and gabapentin, oxcarbazepine, phenobarbital, pregabalin, tiagabine, and zonisamide, among others, and pharmacodynamic interactions with valproic acid,[49] as well as some TCAs and benzodiazepines.[50] Further research is needed to better characterize the potential interactions involving standard psychotropics and these newer agents before clear guidelines can be developed.

REFERENCES

1. Ciraulo DA, Shader RI, Greenblatt DJ, et al, eds. *Drug Interactions in Psychiatry*. 3rd ed. Wilkins; 2005.
2. Wynn GH, Cozza KL, Armstrong SC, et al. *Clinical Manual of Drug Interaction Principles for Medical Practice*. American Psychiatric Publishing; 2008.
3. Preskorn SH, Flockhart D. 2010 Guide to psychiatric drug interactions. *Prim Psychiatry*. 2009;16:45–74.
4. Owen JA. Psychopharmacology. In: Levenson JL, ed. *The American Psychiatric Publishing Textbook of Psychosomatic Medicine: Psychiatric Care of the Medically Ill*. 2nd ed. Washington DC, American Psychiatric Publishing; 2011.
5. Alpert JE. Drug-drug interactions in psychopharmacology. 3rd ed. In: Stern TA, Herman JB, Gorrindo T, eds. *Massachusetts General Hospital Psychiatry Update and Board Preparation*. 3rd ed. McGraw-Hill; 2021:401–409.
6. Mills E, Wu P, Johnston B, et al. Natural health product-drug interactions: a systematic review of clinical trials. *Ther Drug Monit*. 2005;27:549–557.
7. Livingston MG, Livingston HM. Monoamine oxidase inhibitors: an update on drug interactions. *Drug Saf*. 1997;14:219–227.
8. Flockhart DA. Dietary restrictions and drug interactions with monoamine oxidase inhibitors: an update. *J Clin Psychiatry*. 2012; 73(suppl 1):17–24.
9. Boyer EW, Shannon M. Current concepts: the serotonin syndrome. *N Engl J Med*. 2005;352:1112–1120.
10. Wilkinson GR. Drug metabolism and variability among patients in drug response. *N Engl J Med*. 2005;352:2211–2221.
11. Buxton ILO. Pharmacokinetics: the dynamics of drug absorption, distribution, metabolism, and elimination. In: Brunton LL, Hilal-Dandan R, Knollman BC, eds. *Goodman and Gilman's the Pharmacological Basis of Therapeutics*. 13th ed. McGraw-Hill; 2017.
12. Patsalos PN, Froscher W, Pisani F, et al. The importance of drug interactions in epilepsy therapy. *Epilepsia*. 2002;43:365–385.
13. Kahn AY, Preskorn SH. Pharmacokinetic principles and drug interactions. In: Soares JC, Gershon S, eds. *Handbook of Medical Psychiatry*. Marcel Dekker; 2003.
14. Zhou S, Chan E, Pan SQ, et al. Pharmacokinetic interactions of drugs with St. John's wort. *J Psychopharmacol*. 2004;18:262–276.
15. Levy R, Thummel K, Trager W, eds. *Metabolic Drug Interactions*. Lippincott Williams & Wilkins; 2000.
16. Daniel WA, Bromek E, Danek PJ, et al. The mechanisms of interactions of psychotropic drugs with liver and brain cytochrome P450 and their significance for drug effect and drug-drug interactions. *Biochem Pharmacol*. 2022;199:115006.
17. Ruiz P, ed. *Ethnicity and Psychopharmacology*. American Psychiatric Press; 2000.
18. Labbate LA, Fava M, Rosenbaum JF, Arana GW. *Handbook of Psychiatric Drug Therapy*. 6th ed. Lippincott Williams & Wilkins; 2009.
19. Pahwa M, Sleem A, Elsayed OH, et al. New antipsychotic medications in the last decade. *Curr Psychiatry Rep*. 2021;23:87.
20. Freudenreich O, Goff DC. Antipsychotics. In: Ciraulo DA, Shader RI, Greenblatt DJ, eds. *Drug Interactions in Psychiatry*. 3rd ed. Williams & Wilkins; 2005.
21. Spina E, de Leon J. Metabolic drug interactions with newer antipsychotics: a comparative review. *Basic Clin Pharmacol Toxicol*. 2007;100:4–22.
22. Taylor DM. Antipsychotics and QT prolongation. *Acta Psychiatr Scand*. 2003;107:85–95.
23. Goldman SA. Lithium and neuroleptics in combination: the spectrum of neurotoxicity. *Psychopharmacol Bull*. 1996;32:299–309.

24. Sarid-Segal O, Creelman WL, Ciraulo DA, et al. Lithium. In: Ciraulo DA, Shader RI, Greenblatt DJ, eds. *Drug Interactions in Psychiatry.* 3rd ed. Williams & Wilkins; 2005.

25. Jefferson JW, Kalin NH. Serum lithium levels and long-term diuretic use. *JAMA.* 1979;241:1134–1136.

26. Saffer D, Coppen A. Furosemide: a safe diuretic during lithium therapy? *J Affect Disord.* 1983;5:289–292.

27. Reinman IG, Diener U, Frolich JC. Indomethacin but not aspirin increases plasma lithium ion levels. *Arch Gen Psychiatry.* 1986;40:283–286.

28. Ragheb MA. Aspirin does not significantly affect patients' serum lithium levels. *J Clin Psychiatry.* 1987;48:425.

29. DeVane CL. Pharmacokinetics, drug interactions, and tolerability of valproate. *Psychopharmacol Bull.* 2003;37(suppl 2):25–42.

30. Fleming J, Chetty M. Psychotropic drug interactions with valproate. *Clin Neuropharmacol.* 2005;28:96–101.

31. Circaulo DA, Pacheco MN, Slattery M. Anticonvulsants. In: Ciraulo DA, Shader RI, Greenblatt DJ, eds. *Drug Interactions in Psychiatry.* 3rd ed. Williams & Wilkins; 2005.

32. Sabers A, Ohman I, Christensen J, et al. Oral contraceptives reduce lamotrigine plasma levels. *Neurology.* 2003;61:570–571.

33. Ketter TA, Post RM, Worthington K. Principles of clinically important drug interactions with carbamazepine: part I. *J Clin Psychopharmacol.* 1991;11:198–203.

34. Ketter TA, Post RM, Worthington K. Principles of clinically important drug interactions with carbamazepine. Part II. *J Clin Psychopharmacol.* 1991;11:306–313.

35. Ciraulo DA, Creelman WL, Shader RI, et al. Antidepressants. In: Ciraulo DA, Shader RI, Greenblatt DJ, eds. *Drug Interactions in Psychiatry.* 3rd ed. Williams & Wilkins; 2005.

36. Keck PE, Arnold LM. The serotonin syndrome. *Psychiatr Ann.* 2000; 30:333–343.

37. Jefferson JW. Cardiovascular effects and toxicity of anxiolytics and antidepressants. *J Clin Psychiatry.* 1989;50:368–378.

38. Witchel HJ, Hancok JC, Nutt DJ. Psychotropic drugs, cardiac arrhythmia and sudden death. *J Clin Psychopharmacol.* 2003;23: 58–77.

39. Van den Eynde V, Gillman PK, Blackwell BB. The prescriber's guide to the MAOI diet-thinking through tyramine troubles. *Psychopharmacol Bull.* 2022;52:73–116.

40. McCabe BJ. Dietary tyramine and other pressor amines in MAOI regimens: a review. *J Am Diet Assoc.* 1986;86:1059–1064.

41. Gratz SS, Simpson GM. MAOI-narcotic interactions. *J Clin Psychiatry.* 1993;54:439.

42. Markowitz JS, DeVane CL. The emerging recognition of herb-drug interactions with a focus on St. John's wort (*Hypericum perforatum*). *Psychopharmacol Bull.* 2001;35:53–64.

43. Markowitz JS, Morrison SD, DeVane CL. Drug interactions with psychostimulants. *Int Clin Psychopharmacol.* 1999;14:1–18.

44. Feighner JP, Herbstein J, Damlouji N. Combined MAOI, TCA, and direct stimulant therapy of treatment-resistant depression. *J Clin Psychiatry.* 1985;46:206–209.

45. Fawcett J, Kravitz HM, Zajecka JM, et al. CNS stimulant potentiation of monoamine oxidase inhibitors in treatment-refractory depression. *J Clin Psychopharmacol.* 1991;11:127–132.

46. Sarparast A, Thomas K, Malcolm B, et al. Drug-drug interactions between psychiatric medications and MDMA or psilocybin: a systematic review. *Psychopharmacology (Berl).* 2022;239:1945–1976.

47. Veraart JKE, Smith-Apeldoorn SY, Bakker IM, et al. Pharmacodynamic interactions between ketamine and psychiatric medications used in the treatment of depression: a systematic review. *Int J Neuropsychopharmacol.* 2021;24:808–831.

48. Karaźniewicz-Łada M, Główka AK, Mikulska AA, et al. Pharmacokinetic drug-drug interactions among antiepileptic drugs, including CBD, drugs used to treat COVID-19 and nutrients. *Int J Mol Sci.* 2021;22:9582.

49. Gilmartin CGS, Dowd Z, Parker APJ, et al. Interaction of cannabidiol with other antiseizure medications: a narrative review. *Seizure.* 2021;86:189–196.

50. Balachandran P, Elsohly M, Hill KP. Cannabidiol interactions with medications, illicit substances, and alcohol: a comprehensive review. *J Gen Intern Med.* 2021;36:2074–2084.

15 Pharmacotherapy of Neurocognitive Disorders and Dementia

Marc S. Weinberg, Sun Young Chung, Nhi-Ha Trinh, Zeina Chemali, and Jennifer R. Gatchel

KEY POINTS

Clinical Findings

- Cognitive disorders are classified in the *Diagnostic and Statistical Manual of Mental Disorders*, Fifth Edition (DSM-5), as "neurocognitive disorders"; they exist on a spectrum of cognitive and functional impairment: delirium, mild neurocognitive disorder, major neurocognitive disorder, and their etiological subtypes.

- The term *dementia* is used to refer to certain etiological subtypes (e.g., Alzheimer disease [AD], frontotemporal dementia [FTD]).

Differential Diagnoses

- An evaluation of a patient with a suspected dementia or major neurocognitive disorder must include a complete history; physical, neurological, and psychiatric examinations; evaluation of cognitive function; and an appropriate laboratory and neuroimaging evaluation.

Epidemiology

- AD accounts for 60% to 80% of all dementias and affects an estimated 6.7 million Americans 65 years of age and older; however, other etiologies, both common (e.g., vascular dementia, Lewy body dementia) and less common (e.g., FTD, progressive supranuclear palsy), must be considered during a comprehensive evaluation.

- Although longevity is the greatest risk factor for AD, as well as for most other dementing disorders, additional factors, such as a genetic propensity (particularly in the rare cases of early-onset AD and in FTD) and vascular pathology, as well as modifiable lifestyle factors contribute to its prevalence.

Pathophysiology

- Animal models, structural and functional imaging studies, and recent advances in molecular imaging and in biofluid biomarkers have provided evidence of neuropathological changes in dementing disorders and AD, even in its pre-clinical or asymptomatic stage.

Treatment Options

- With AD in particular, attention has focused on primary and secondary prevention and on potential curative interventions, including emerging disease-modifying therapies. Neuropsychiatric symptoms (i.e., the behavioral and psychological symptoms of dementia) are among the most disabling and difficult to manage.

OVERVIEW

The *Diagnostic and Statistical Manual of Mental Disorders*, Fifth Edition (DSM-5)[1] places cognitive disorders on a spectrum of cognitive and functional decline: delirium, mild and major neurocognitive disorders, and their etiological subtypes. The term *dementia* is retained for consistency; it was used in the *Diagnostic and Statistical Manual of Mental Disorders*, Fourth Edition (DSM-IV)[2] to describe a syndrome with a decline in memory, as well as an impairment of at least one other domain of higher cognitive function (e.g., aphasia [a difficulty with any aspect of language], apraxia [the impaired ability to perform motor tasks despite intact motor function], agnosia [an impairment in object recognition despite intact sensory function], or executive dysfunction [e.g., difficulty in planning, organizing, sequencing, or abstracting]).

Although dementia is encompassed by the term *major neurocognitive disorder (MNCD)*, for a diagnosis of MNCD to be made, there must be evidence of significant cognitive decline in one or more cognitive domains (e.g., complex attention, executive function, learning and memory, language, perceptual motor, or social cognition) based on concern of the individual, a knowledgeable informant, or the clinician, as well as by objective measures of substantial cognitive impairment on standardized neuropsychological testing or quantified clinical assessments. Several important qualifiers are included in the definition: that is, the condition must represent a change from baseline, social or occupational function must be significantly impaired, and the impairment does not occur exclusively during an episode of delirium or cannot be accounted for by another Axis I disorder, such as major depression.[2]

Many older individuals complain of memory problems (e.g., learning new information, finding words). In most circumstances, such lapses are normal. The term *mild cognitive impairment (MCI)* was coined to recognize an intermediate category between normal cognitive lapses that are associated with aging and with dementia. Although MCI was subsumed under cognitive disorder not otherwise specified in DSM-IV, this less severe level of cognitive impairment most closely corresponds to "mild neurocognitive disorder" in DSM-5.[2] Diagnostic criteria include evidence for a *modest* decline in cognition from a previous level of performance in one or more cognitive domains based on the concern of the individual, a knowledgeable informant, or a clinician and based on objective evidence of cognitive decline. Important qualifiers include a lack of interference with independence in everyday activities (although compensatory strategies may be implemented) and not exclusively occurring during an episode of delirium and not accounted for solely by another Axis I disorder. MCI is common among older adults, although estimates vary widely depending on the diagnostic criteria used (including the criteria of what constitutes a modest decline in cognition) and the assessment methods used; some individuals with MCI progress to dementia. A meta-analysis examining the rate of progression from MCI to AD found that 6.7% progressed to AD each year and overall one-third of those with MCI developed AD during their lifetimes.[3] Risk factors for progression from MCI to AD include carrier status of the E4 allele of the apolipoprotein E *(APOE)* gene, clinical severity, brain atrophy, specific patterns of cerebrospinal fluid (CSF) biomarkers and cerebral glucose metabolism, and amyloid beta (Aβ) deposition. Further work to identify and refine factors that place people at risk for progression of cognitive decline is an area of active research.[4]

EPIDEMIOLOGY OF DEMENTIA

The most common type of dementia (accounting for 60%–80%) is AD.[5] Among the neurodegenerative dementias, Lewy body dementia (LBD) is the next most common followed by frontotemporal dementia (FTD). Vascular dementia (formerly known as multi-infarct dementia) has several etiologies; although it can exist independently from AD, the two frequently co-occur. Indeed, there is increasing awareness that AD is often mixed with other dementia causes. Dementias associated with Parkinson disease (PD) and Creutzfeldt–Jakob disease (CJD) are much less common. Given the challenges of making an accurate diagnosis of dementia subtypes in epidemiological studies and the neuropathological data that suggest that mixed pathologies are more common than discrete subtypes, the proportion of dementias attributed to disparate subtypes must be interpreted with caution.[5]

THE ROLE OF AGE OF ONSET

The onset of dementia is most common in the 70s and 80s; it is rare before the age of 40 years. Both the incidence (i.e., the number of new cases per year in the population) and the prevalence (i.e., the fraction of the population that has the disorder) rise steeply with age. This pattern has been observed both for all dementias and for AD in particular, with the prevalence increasing exponentially with age (i.e., increasing from 3% among those age 65–74 years to nearly 50% in those older than 85 years.[6] Estimates of dementia's prevalence vary depending on which diagnostic criteria are used. The incidence of dementia of almost all types increases with age, such that it affects 15% of all individuals older than 65 years and up to 45% in those older than 80 years. However, the peak age of onset varies somewhat among the dementias, with FTD and vascular dementia typically beginning earlier in life (e.g., in the 60s) and AD developing somewhat later.

Dementia is the main cause of disability among older individuals; not surprisingly, the economic burden is enormous. Moreover, it is expected to rise steeply with anticipated demographic shifts. A substantial fraction of the increased burden will fall on developing countries because a larger fraction of those populations survives to old age. Indeed, by one estimate, although there were 36.5 million people world-wide with dementia in 2010, the number of people living with dementia is expected to double every 20 years, with most of those living in low- and middle-income countries.[6] Because AD and many

other neurodegenerative disorders have an insidious onset, the precise age of onset is indeterminate. However, the approximate age of onset (i.e., within 2–5 years) is critical from both the personal and the public health points of view. Moreover, this knowledge may offer a window into the management of disease risk and morbidity. A sufficient delay in onset can be equivalent to prevention with a late-onset disorder. Later onset can also decrease disease burden by pushing it later into the life span. From a research perspective, age of onset has a robust relationship with genetic risk factors and may have value as an outcome in genetic and other causal models.

EVALUATION OF A PATIENT WITH SUSPECTED COGNITIVE IMPAIRMENT

The diagnostic criteria for dementia require that other disorders (e.g., medical co-morbidities, drug and alcohol use, medication side effects, delirium, and depression) have been ruled out. Of note, an underlying diagnosis of dementia may predispose a patient to delirium; thus, further evaluation of cognitive deficits is required after delirium has been treated successfully. Delirium may be differentiated from dementia in several ways: delirium's onset is typically acute or subacute, the course often has marked fluctuations, and the levels of consciousness and attention are impaired.

At times, depression may be difficult to distinguish from dementia, and the two diagnoses are often co-morbid. Depression in older individuals is associated with cognitive deficits, which may resolve completely after the acute mood episode has been treated. Certain features (such as a more acute onset, poor motivation, prominent negativity, and a strong family history of a mood disorder) favor a diagnosis of depression over dementia. Moreover, depression may represent a risk factor or a prodrome to dementia, in some cases preceding AD by several years. Over time, the definition of depression and other neuropsychiatric symptoms (NPSs) in dementia has become more nuanced because of advancements in the field, including the recognition that NPSs may emerge before cognitive decline. The construct of mild behavioral impairment (MBI), for example, stipulates that symptoms may occur during the preclinical or prodromal stage of a dementia syndrome, with possible symptom domains including decreased motivation, emotional dysregulation, impulse dyscontrol, social inappropriateness, and abnormal perception or thought.

Whenever possible, it is important to establish a precise etiology for dementia (Box 15.1) that can allow for more focused treatments and for an accurate assessment of prognosis. Although reversible causes are found in fewer than 15% of new cases, a diagnosis may help a patient and his or her family understand what the future holds so they can make appropriate personal, medical, and financial plans.

The history is obtained not only from the patient but also from family members or others who have observed the patient and are essential informants. The patient may fail to report deficits, either because of unawareness of cognitive or behavioral symptoms (anosognosia), psychological factors, or both. Loss of insight is characteristic of the behavioral variant of FTD, but it can be present across dementia syndromes. Ideally, family members are interviewed separately from the patient so they can be as candid as possible.

When taking a history, one should obtain the nature of the initial presentation, the course of the illness, and the associated signs and symptoms (including those that are psychiatric or behavioral). These areas are important when determining the disease etiology (e.g., recognizing the characteristic abrupt onset of vascular dementia as opposed to the gradual onset of AD). A valuable scale of independence in functional activities is the Lawton-Brody Instrumental Activities of Daily Living Scale (iADL), available at https://www.alz.org/.[7]

An extensive review of systems must include inquiry about gait and sleep disturbances, falls, sensory deficits, head trauma, and incontinence. Obtaining the full medical history may reveal risk factors for stroke or for other general medical or neurological causes of cognitive difficulties. The psychiatric history may suggest co-morbid illnesses (such as depression or an alcohol use disorder), particularly if prior episodes of psychiatric illness have been elicited.

Up to one-third of cases of cognitive impairment may be at least partially caused by medication effects; common offenders include anticholinergics, antihypertensive agents, various psychotropics, sedative–hypnotics, and narcotics. Any drug should be suspected, especially when it is first prescribed and when the onset of symptoms is temporally related to administration of a medication.

Taking a family history can also help to determine the nature of dementia. A social and occupational history is useful when assessing pre-morbid intelligence and education, changes in the patient's level of function, and environmental risk factors.

A general physical examination is essential, with attention paid to the cardiovascular system. Physical findings can also suggest an endocrine, inflammatory, or infectious etiology. A complete neurological examination (including assessment of cranial nerves, sensory and motor functions, deep tendon reflexes, and cerebellar function) may reveal focal findings that might suggest a vascular dementia or a degenerative disorder, such as PD. Screening for visual acuity and hearing is important because it may reveal sensory losses that can masquerade as, or exacerbate, cognitive decline. A full neurological examination is standard of care.

A psychiatric examination may reveal evidence of delirium, depression, psychosis, or other NPSs. The Neuropsychiatric Inventory (NPI),[8] the Neuropsychiatric Inventory Questionnaire (NPI-Q),[9] and the mild behavioral impairment checklist (MBI-C)[10] are useful scales to assess NPSs in the setting of known or suspected cognitive impairment. The concept of MBI was recently operationalized by Ismail and colleagues[10] to describe emergent NPSs in later life (age 50 years or older) that can create a change in a patient's baseline and persist for more than 6 months. These symptoms may occur in those with or without a psychiatric history and represent early neurobehavioral manifestations in pre-dementia populations. On formal mental status testing, such as with the Folstein Mini-Mental State Examination (MMSE),[11] and other cognitive tests (Table 15.1), documentation of particular findings, in addition to the overall score, allows for cognitive functions to be followed over time.

The laboratory evaluation should include a complete blood count and levels of vitamin B_{12} and folate, sedimentation rate, electrolytes, glucose, homocysteine, blood urea nitrogen, and creatinine, as well as tests of thyroid function and liver function. Screening for cholesterol and triglyceride levels is also useful. Syphilis serology should also be included on an initial panel. Brain magnetic resonance imaging (MRI) is the norm though a computed tomography (CT) scan of the brain without contrast can also identify subdural hematomas, hydrocephalus, stroke, or tumors.

Additional studies are indicated if the initial work-up is uninformative, if a specific diagnosis is suspected, or if the presentation is atypical (Table 15.2). Such investigations are especially important in young patients with a rapidly progressive dementia or an unusual presentation. Neuropsychological testing is essential in cases in which a patient's deficits are mild or difficult to characterize. Briefer screening tools, such as the MMSE, have poor sensitivity and specificity for dementia, particularly in highly educated or intelligent patients. Such tests also generally fail to assess executive function and praxis.

BOX 15.1 Etiologies of Dementia, and of Mild and Major Neurocognitive Disorders

VASCULAR

Stroke, chronic subdural hemorrhages, post-anoxic injury, diffuse white matter disease

INFECTIOUS

Human immunodeficiency virus (HIV) infection, neurosyphilis, progressive multi-focal leukoencephalopathy (PMLE), Creutzfeldt–Jakob disease (CJD), tuberculosis (TB), sarcoidosis, Whipple disease

NEOPLASTIC

Primary versus metastatic carcinoma, paraneoplastic syndrome

DEGENERATIVE

Alzheimer disease (AD), frontotemporal dementia (FTD), dementia with Lewy bodies (DLB), Parkinson disease (PD), progressive supranuclear palsy (PSP), multi-system degeneration, amyotrophic lateral sclerosis (ALS), corticobasal degeneration (CBD), multiple sclerosis (MS)

INFLAMMATORY

Vasculitis

ENDOCRINE

Hypothyroidism, adrenal insufficiency, Cushing syndrome, hypoparathyroidism/hyperparathyroidism, renal failure, liver failure

METABOLIC

Thiamine deficiency (Wernicke encephalopathy), vitamin B_{12} deficiency, inherited enzyme defects

TOXINS

Chronic alcoholism, drugs/medication effects, heavy metals, dialysis dementia (aluminum)

TRAUMA

Dementia pugilistica

OTHER

Normal pressure hydrocephalus (NPH), obstructive hydrocephalus

---

TABLE 15.1 Supplemental Mental State Testing for Patients with Dementia

Area	Test
Memory	Recall name and address: "John Brown, 42 Market Street, Chicago." Recall three unusual words: "tulip, umbrella, fear."
Language	Naming parts: "lab coat: lapel, sleeve, cuff; watch: band, face, crystal" Complex commands: "Before pointing to the door, point to the ceiling." Word list: "In 1 minute, name all the animals you can think of."
Praxis	"Show me how you would slice a loaf of bread." "Show me how you brush your teeth."
Visuospatial	"Draw a clock face with numbers and mark the hands to 10 after 11."
Abstraction	"How is an apple like a banana?" "How is a canal different from a river?" Proverb interpretation

TABLE 15.2 Supplemental Investigations

What	When	Why
Neuropsychological testing	Patient's deficits are mild or difficult to characterize	The sensitivity of the MMSE for dementia is poor, particularly in highly educated or intelligent patients (who can compensate for deficits)
Lumbar puncture (including routine studies and cytology)	Known or suspected cancer, immunosuppression, suspected CNS infection or vasculitis, hydrocephalus by CT, rapid or atypical courses	Look for infection, elevated pressure, and abnormal proteins
MRI with gadolinium; EEG	Any atypical findings on neurological examination; suspected toxic-metabolic encephalopathy, complex partial seizures, CJD	More sensitive than CT for tumor and stroke. Look for diffuse slowing (encephalopathy) vs. focal seizure activity
HIV testing	Risk factors or opportunistic infections	Up to 20% of patients with HIV infection develop dementia, although it is unusual for dementia to be the initial sign
Heavy metal screening, screening for Wilson disease or autoimmune disease	Suggested by history, physical examination, or laboratory findings	May be reversible

CJD, Creutzfeldt–Jakob disease; *CNS*, central nervous system; *CT*, computed tomography; *EEG*, electroencephalogram; *HIV*, human immunodeficiency virus; *MMSE*, Mini-Mental State Examination; *MRI*, magnetic resonance imaging.

Other diagnostic tests can supplement the initial assessment. MRI of the brain is more sensitive for the detection of recent strokes and should be considered when focal findings are found on the neurological examination; in addition, MRI scans can identify lesions that are not apparent on the physical examination, so it should always be considered when the diagnosis is unclear. An electroencephalogram (EEG) may be used to identify a toxic-metabolic encephalopathy, complex partial seizures, or CJD. A lumbar puncture (LP) may be indicated when cancer, infection of the central nervous system (CNS), hydrocephalus, or vasculitis is suspected. Testing of AD biomarkers through CSF (e.g., AD panel) is beneficial for aiding in diagnostic accuracy. Checking for ApoE4 status is becoming routine. Testing for human immunodeficiency virus (HIV) is indicated when a patient has relevant risk factors because up to 20% of patients with HIV infection develop dementia. However, dementia is uncommon as an initial sign. Heavy metal screening, as well as testing for Lyme disease, Wilson disease, and autoimmune diseases, should be reserved for patients in whom these etiologies are suspected.

ALZHEIMER DISEASE

Brief Description

Alzheimer disease (AD) is a progressive, irreversible brain disorder that robs those who have it of memory and overall mental and physical function; it eventually leads to death.

Epidemiology of AD

AD is the most common cause of dementia, affecting one in nine individuals, or more than 6.5 million Americans older than 65 years, possibly increasing to 12.7 million by 2050.[12] Worldwide estimates of dementia (57 million individuals in 2019) may nearly triple to more than 152 million by 2050, which is largely attributable to population growth and population aging.[13]

Currently, AD is the sixth leading cause of death for adults in the United States. In 2022, the direct costs of caring for those with AD in the United States was estimated at $321 billion (in 2021 dollars).[12] Unfortunately, there is significant racial and ethnic disparity in AD burden.[14] The prevalence and incidence of AD and related dementias in Black and Hispanic populations in the United States is approximately 35% higher than that of White or Asian individuals[15] based on meta-analyses from literature and claims data. Interventional AD trials intending to benefit broad swathes of society recruit many fewer individuals from minority backgrounds.[16] Female sex carries an increased risk, even when accounting for differences in longevity, but some of the difference is offset by a greater risk of vascular dementia in men. Many risk factors (except for male sex), such as diabetes, atherosclerosis, hypertension, smoking, atrial fibrillation, and elevated cholesterol, increase the risk of AD, as well as for vascular dementia, although the mechanisms are unclear.[17] Whereas a history of severe head trauma (with loss of consciousness) also increases the risk of AD, education, complexity of occupation, an engaged lifestyle, and exercise have protective effects.[18] Indeed, many modifiable lifestyle factors contribute to the development of AD and other dementias. Barnes and Yaffe,[19] in calculating the population-attributable risk of seven lifestyle factors, found that in the United States, physical inactivity, depression, smoking, and mid-life hypertension were most highly correlated with AD risk. An additional modifiable risk factor is the effect of sleep-disordered breathing; women with sleep-disordered breathing have twice the risk of developing dementia as those without disordered breathing. The effect of diet, meanwhile, is more controversial; there is insufficient evidence to support the association of adherence to a particular diet and development of AD.[18]

Pathophysiology

In his initial 1907 case, Alois Alzheimer identified abnormal nerve cells and fiber clusters in the cerebral cortex at autopsy using what was then a new silver-staining method. These findings, considered to be the hallmark neuropathological lesions of AD, are known as neurofibrillary tangles (NFTs) and neuritic plaques (NPs) (Figure 15.1). Beta-amyloid (Aβ) protein, present in soluble form in the brain but also the primary component of NPs, is thought to play a central pathophysiological role in the disease, perhaps via direct neurotoxicity.[20] NFTs are found in neurons and are primarily composed of anomalous cytoskeletal proteins (such as hyperphosphorylated tau), which may also be toxic to neurons and contribute to AD pathophysiology.[21,22]

However, the mechanisms by which changes in tau and Aβ mediate neuronal death and dysfunction remain important unanswered questions and active areas of research. Two proposed methods of tau-mediated toxicity include NFT toxicity and conformational abnormalities of tangles, including a spreading process through multiple brain regions, in which abnormal tau can catalyze formation of abnormal tau in other cells through a prion-like process.[21,22] Soluble and diffusible Aβ may cause cytotoxicity and synaptotoxicity, with amyloid

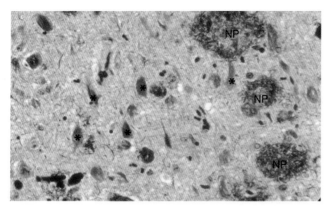

Figure 15.1. Plaques and tangles in Alzheimer disease. *Asterisks* indicate neurofibrillary tangles. *NP*, Neuritic plaque.

plaques serving as reservoirs for sequestration of soluble oligomers.[21,22]

Genetics of AD

Familial heritability of AD is high,[23] leading to the hypothesis that AD risk factors are genetically transmitted. A 2006 study of more than 11,000 Swedish twin pairs 65 years of age and older, including nearly 400 pairs in which at least one twin had AD, estimated a heritability range of 60% to 80%.[24] AD is genetically complex, with fewer than 5% of AD cases caused by single gene mutations and the remainder of inheritance considered as polygenic, involving multiple genomic variants and non-genetic contributions.

Early-onset AD is almost always linked to a family history of dementia. It is highly genetically linked (estimated to have 90%–100% heritability),[25] commonly involving autosomal dominant mutations in the *APP*, *PSEN1*, or *PSEN2* genes.[26] Mutations in these genes account for approximately 10% of early-onset AD but fewer than 1% of all individuals with AD.[27] Amyloid precursor protein (APP) on chromosome 21 was the first identified early-onset AD-linked gene. Presenilin 1 and 2 (*PSEN1* and *PSEN2*) are the other major genes identified as autosomally dominant, also contributing significantly to early-onset AD (as early as in one's 40s).[27] APP, as its name suggests, is a protein precursor to Aβ, the protein aggregate of which is a hallmark pathology of AD. *PSEN1* and *PSEN2* are involved in proteolysis of APP. The discovery and study of these genes and protein interactions has advanced our understanding of the pathophysiology of AD and has led to the ushering of present-day amyloid-based treatment strategies.

Late-onset AD (with no universally appreciated age cutoff but commonly construed as older than 65 years) involves a complex combination of genetic and non-genetic risk factors. The largest genome-wide association study, published in 2022,[28] using genome sequencing from more than 790,000 individuals, identified 75 genomic loci associated with AD. Several gene loci corresponded with other neurodegenerative diseases, such as FTD and PD.[28]

The most well-known AD risk-related gene is *APOE*. Unlike the autosomal dominant genes listed earlier, *APOE* is a *susceptibility* gene that increases the risk for AD without causing the disease and contributes to 40% to 60% of cases. *APOE* has three alleles—2, 3, and 4—which have a complex relationship to risk for both AD and cardiovascular disease, with the 2 allele decreasing the risk of both disorders and increasing longevity and the 4 allele increasing risk and decreasing longevity. The effect of *ApoE4* varies with age; it is most marked in the 60s and decreases substantially beyond the age of 80 or 90 years. Carriers of two *ApoE4* alleles have a markedly higher

risk of AD compared with single allele carriers. *APOE* seems to act principally by modifying the age of onset, which is lowest in those with two copies of the risk allele and intermediate in those with one. The *APOE* effect appears to be stronger in women and in Whites, which may relate to their lower risk of cardiovascular disease.

Aside from those susceptibility-related genes with well-established links to AD pathology (e.g., directly linked to Aβ or tau), other identified genes have known relationships to lipid processing, immunology, and cellular metabolism, activation, and signal transduction pathways.

Patients frequently ask about their risk of AD based on their family history. Those with an autosomal dominant history are best referred for genetic counseling, ideally from an Alzheimer Disease Research Center or a local genetic counselor. Genetic testing is commercially available for *PSEN1*, which is likely to be involved when there is an autosomal dominant family history and the age of onset is 50 years or younger. It can be used both for confirmation of diagnosis and for the prediction of disease onset, but there are complex logistical and ethical issues.[29] Currently, genetic testing is only available for the remaining early-onset genes in research settings. Patients without such a history can be advised that there is an increased risk of AD in first-degree relatives. However, they should be made aware that this increase is modest and that the age of onset tends to be correlated in families. Genetic testing for *APOE* can be used as an adjunct to diagnosis, but it contributes minimally. It is not recommended for the assessment of future risk because it lacks sufficient predictive value at the individual level. Many normal older individuals carry an *ApoE4* allele, and many AD patients do not.

Clinical Features and Diagnosis

The typical clinical profile of AD is one of progressive short-term episodic memory loss. Other common cognitive features include impairment of language, visuospatial ability, and executive function. Patients may be unaware of their cognitive deficits, but this is not uniformly the case. There may be evidence of forgetting conversations, having difficulty with household finances, being disoriented to time and place, and misplacing items frequently. In addition to its cognitive features, several NPSs are common in AD, even in its mildest clinical phases.[30] In particular, irritability, apathy, and depression are frequent early features, with psychosis (delusions and hallucinations) occurring more frequently later in the course of the disease).

According to original diagnostic criteria for AD, a definitive diagnosis required evidence of dementia. Also, it rested on post-mortem findings of a specific distribution and number of its characteristic brain lesions (NFTs and NPs). Detailed clinical assessments (by psychiatry, neurology, and neuropsychology) in combination with structural and functional neuroimaging methods had a high concordance rate with autopsy-proven disease. Structural neuroimaging studies (such as MRI or CT) typically show atrophy in the medial temporal lobes, as well as in the parietal convexities bilaterally (Figure 15.2). Functional imaging studies of resting brain function or blood flow (i.e., positron emission tomography [PET] or single-photon emission computed tomography [SPECT]) display parietotemporal hypoperfusion or hypoactivity (Figure 15.3).

However, recent research advances in the areas of brain imaging and biomarkers have led to the re-conceptualization of AD as existing on a continuum, with a progressive series of biological changes corresponding to pre-clinical and increasingly severe clinical stages of the disorder.[31] These changes, some of which can be measured by AD biomarkers, begin in individuals who are cognitively normal, progress in those with MCI, and accumulate in dementia. Advances in CSF

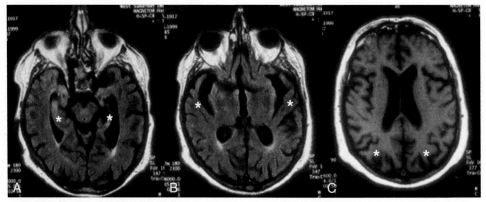

Figure 15.2. A–C, Axial magnetic resonance images of atrophy in Alzheimer disease. *Asterisks* indicate temporal and parietal atrophy.

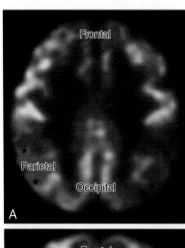

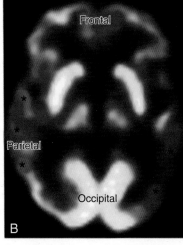

Figure 15.3. A and **B**, Parietotemporal hypoactivity in Alzheimer disease. *Asterisks* indicate regions of hypoactivity.

assays, neuroimaging, and other biomarkers now provide the ability to detect evidence of AD pathophysiology process in vivo.[32] Some promising biomarkers include MRI measurement of atrophy in the hippocampus and other AD-affected brain regions, PET measurements of glucose hypometabolism in AD-affected brain regions, PET measurements of fibrillar Aβ deposition, and CSF measurements of Aβ in combination with total tau and phosphorylated tau,[32] as well as less-invasive and emerging blood-based AD biomarkers. Indeed, increasing evidence from both genetically at-risk cohorts and clinically normal older adults suggests that the pathophysiology of AD

begins years, if not decades, before the diagnosis of dementia is established.[31]

Based on these advances, the National Institute on Aging (NIA) International Working Group and Alzheimer's Association in 2011 and subsequently in 2018 proposed updated criteria for the diagnosis of AD and MCI, in addition to research criteria aimed at clarifying the pre-clinical stages of AD.[31,33] These new criteria reflect increasing knowledge of clinical course and pathophysiology: they take into account that memory impairment may not be a key clinical feature, other potential etiologies (LBD, vascular dementia, and FTD) as well as mixed pathology.[31] New 2018 NIA (in association with the Alzheimer's Association) research criteria focus on defining pre-clinical stages of disease based on biomarkers and genetic testing.[33] The goals of research criteria are to provide insight into factors influencing progression to the clinical stages of AD while evaluating promising AD treatment in pre-clinical stages when they may be most effective. Importantly, these research criteria as well as amyloid imaging and other AD biomarkers are not currently recommended for use in clinical settings;[31,33] this may lie on the horizon because these biomarkers are further evaluated in different populations over time.

Differential Diagnosis

For AD, like other dementias, it is important to exclude reversible or partially reversible causes of cognitive dysfunction or of other brain diseases that could manifest as a dementia (see Box 15.1). Beyond this, the key features are insidious onset, gradual progression, and a characteristic pattern of deficits, particularly early prominent deficits in short-term memory.

Treatments

Behavioral strategies, including environmental cues, such as re-orientation to the environment with the addition of a clock and a calendar, can be reassuring to patients. In addition, clear communication should be emphasized in this population, including keeping the content of communication simple and to the point and speaking clearly and loudly enough, given that decreased hearing acuity is common in older adults. For patients who are easily distressed or are psychotic, reassurance and distraction are strategies that can be calming.

The re-conceptualization of AD on a continuum of neuropathological and clinical impairment and identification of pre-clinical AD through biomarker studies has led to a shift in focus toward intervention with potential disease-modifying treatments in the early stages of AD.[21] Such early intervention among asymptomatic individuals before clinical or biomarker changes develop is termed *primary prevention* and has been

TABLE 15.3 Food and Drug Administration–Approved Pharmacotherapy for Alzheimer Disease

Mechanism of action	Drug name
Acetylcholinesterase inhibitors	Donepezil (Aricept)
	Rivastigmine (Exelon)
	Galantamine (Razadyne), formerly Reminyl
Normalizes glutamate	Memantine (Namenda)
Anti-amyloid monoclonal antibodies	Aducanumab (Aduhelm)
	lecanemab (Leqembi)

effective for other chronic diseases.[34] Along these lines, general interventions include risk reduction for the general public, prevention in those with mutations or pre-clinical disease, and treatment aimed at delaying the progression of clinical signs and symptoms.[34] Possible preventive measures include weight control and exercise, as well as normalizing blood pressure, blood sugar, and cholesterol, which have been associated with the risk for AD and other major neurocognitive disorders. Thus far, AD trials based on lowering specific risk factors, such as cholesterol levels, did not slow progression in the symptomatic stage of disease. However, this remains an active area of investigation.

Current pharmacotherapy in AD (Table 15.3) addresses both the cognitive symptoms and the pathogenesis of AD and involves primarily cholinesterase inhibitors and *N*-methyl-D-aspartate receptor antagonists. More recently, several anti-amyloid monoclonal antibody (mAb) therapies have received US Food and Drug Administration (FDA) accelerated pathway approval, conferring the first new disease-modifying therapies for AD in decades.

Conventional AD Treatments

AD has been linked to a deficiency of acetylcholine (ACh). Three of the four medications approved by the FDA now in use for treatment of AD are designed to prevent the breakdown of ACh, thereby increasing concentrations of ACh in the hippocampus and neocortex, areas of the brain important for memory and for other cognitive symptoms. These cholinesterase inhibitors include donepezil (Aricept), rivastigmine (Exelon), and galantamine (Razadyne). All have been shown to slow AD symptoms by stabilizing cognition and behavior, participation in activities of daily living, and global function in mild to moderate AD, improving cognition and behavior in moderate to severely affected patients with AD, delaying nursing home placement, and reducing both health care expenditures and caregiver burden for patients with AD.[35] However, the effects are modest, and they are not apparent in some individuals.

Certain pharmacokinetic properties should be kept in mind while prescribing these medications: whereas donepezil and extended-release galantamine are given once daily, both galantamine and rivastigmine are given twice daily; rivastigmine should be administered with meals to reduce gastrointestinal (GI) side effects. Common side effects include nausea, vomiting, diarrhea, insomnia or vivid dreams, fatigue, muscle cramps, incontinence, bradycardia, and syncope. A daily transdermal patch form of rivastigmine (Exelon) reduces GI side effects, which often limit adoption of this class of medications by patients. Data also suggest that a cholinesterase inhibitor should be initiated as soon as a diagnosis of AD becomes apparent. Treatment should be continued into the severe stages of the disease, provided that the medication is well tolerated.[35,36] Increasing numbers of studies are investigating the potential efficacy of introducing treatment at the stage of MCI; although studies have not been positive, interventions with these and other agents in pre-clinical AD and MCI remain active areas of investigation.

Another medication, memantine (Namenda), has proven effective in patients with more severe forms of AD. Memantine normalizes levels of glutamate, a neurotransmitter involved in learning and memory, which in excessive quantities, is thought to contribute to neurodegeneration. Memantine has been used in combination with cholinesterase inhibitors for greater efficacy in slowing the progression of AD. Common side effects include dizziness, agitation, headache, and confusion. In patients with moderate to severe AD receiving donepezil, those assigned to continue donepezil had less cognitive decline than those assigned to discontinue the medication, and the combination of donepezil and memantine did not confer additional benefits above those of donepezil alone.[37]

Anti-amyloid Monoclonal Antibodies

Brain Aβ deposition is a hallmark pathological finding in AD pathology,[38] and clearance of this peptide has been shown in preclinical and several recent clinical trials to slow AD progression. There are currently two FDA-approved mAb-based therapies aimed at targeting Aβ deposits in the brains with MCI or early AD. Aducanumab (Aduhelm), is a human immunoglobulin that targets aggregated Aβ in the brain. Aduhelm was approved by the FDA in June 2021 through their accelerated approval pathway.[39] Accelerated approval uses surrogate endpoint effects (cerebral amyloid deposit as a surrogate for cognitive decline) in treatments thought to have a high likelihood of clinical benefit. Full approvals are conditioned on finding clinical benefit. Aduhelm's approval was controversial because of mixed clinical efficacy findings.[40] A decision by the US Centers for Medicare and Medicaid Services (CMS) to restrict coverage of Aduhelm to clinical trials has restricted the commercialization of this first-in-class FDA-approved mAb treatment for AD.

The other mAb with current FDA approval is lecanemab (Leqembi), an mAb that binds to soluble Aβ protofibril forms. In an 18-month, double-blinded phase III trial among patients with MCI (with evidence of cerebral amyloid accumulation) or early AD, lecanemab treatment resulted in lower levels of amyloid in the brain and a 27% reduction in the rate of cognitive decline compared with those in the placebo group.[39] Subgroup analyses of cognitive endpoints found that men benefited from the treatment more than women. Leqembi was approved by the FDA in January 2023, through its accelerated approval pathway (like Aduhelm). Prescribing information for Leqembi includes indications for initiating treatment for individuals with MCI and early AD. A subcutaneous form of lecanemab is under investigation, with preliminary evidence supporting its efficacy shared at the 2023 Clinical Trials in Alzheimer's Disease conference (Boston, MA).

Safety of Anti-amyloid Monoclonal Antibodies

Using anti-amyloid mAbs can result in vasogenic cerebral edema and cerebral microhemorrhage. This phenomenon, coined amyloid-related imaging abnormalities (ARIAs), was first identified through brain MRIs of subjects receiving bapineuzumab, one of the first studied amyloid-targeting mAbs for AD.[41] ARIA subtypes include ARIA-E (vasogenic edema) and ARIA-H (microhemorrhage). Interestingly, MRI scan abnormalities do not necessarily correlate with symptoms. In clinical trials, the propensity for ARIAs has been higher in participants with homozygous *ApoE ε4* genotype. (Individuals with the *ApoE ε4* genotype show higher rates of AD and amyloid accumulation, including in cerebral vessels, predisposing them to cerebral amyloid angiopathy, a likely partial link between anti-amyloid mAb treatment and ARIA phenomenology.) Risk reduction through patient selection and safety monitoring will be essential as this new class of medications enters widespread use.

Treatment of Neuropsychiatric Symptoms of AD and Related Dementias

NPSs are among the most distressing and disabling symptoms for patients and their care partners with AD and the related dementia discussed later. They occur across the clinical spectrum (from preclinical stages, to MCI, to dementia) and span multiple affective and behavioral domains (e.g., apathy, depression, irritability, anxiety, aggression or agitation, psychosis, sleep disturbance, disinhibition or perseveration, and loss of empathy) and are among the most challenging symptoms to manage. The profile of NPSs may differ among dementia subtypes, (i.e., depression, apathy, psychosis, and agitation are more common in AD than disinhibition or perseveration and loss of empathy early in the course of FTD). Despite the prevalence and clinical relevance of NPSs, they are associated with disease progression, mortality, decreased patient functional ability and quality of life, as well as care-partner stress and health care system burden; their neurobiology is incompletely understood. As a result, there are few effective treatments, and these symptoms often go unrecognized or mistreated or under-treated.

The FDA has not yet approved any drugs to treat NPSs in dementia syndromes. Very recently, pimavanserin, a 5-HT$_{2A}$ receptor selective inverse agonist, was approved to treat PD psychosis.[42] Thus far pimavanserin and dextromethorphan/quinidine (Nuedexta)—approved for treatment of pseudobulbar affect across a range of conditions including amyotrophic lateral sclerosis (ALS)—are the only FDA-approved medications to treat NPSs in neurodegenerative disease.

Before the initiation of pharmacotherapy for NPSs in Alzheimer's disease and related dementias (ADRDs), possible exacerbating medical (e.g., urinary infection, delirium) or environmental triggers should be carefully investigated and resolved. In addition, non-pharmacological approaches should be considered as an initial strategy because they have fewer adverse events and are generally viewed more favorable by patients and care partners than are medications. Principles of non-pharmacological management of NPSs conceptualize NPSs as originating from unmet needs, overstimulation in the environment, and interaction between patient-care partners and environmental factors. Thus, examples of such approaches include using anti-inflammatory agents to manage minor pain that a patient may be unable to describe, avoiding confrontation, redirecting to pleasurable activities, minimizing stimulating activities in the evening, and implementing massage and aromatherapy. Other treatment considerations include removing deleterious medications, reducing excessive alcohol intake, and promoting restorative sleep by diagnosing and treating underlying sleep apnea. The DICE (describe, investigate, create, and evaluate) approach is an example of a framework that was developed to provide a structured strategy for implementing both non-pharmacological as well as pharmacological approaches to treatment of NPSs.[43] In this patient–care-partner–clinician collaborative approach, the care-partner describes the patient's behavior(s) to the clinician or clinical team. This is followed by investigation of contributing etiologies and creation of a management plan that addresses the observations and findings during the investigation. This plan is then implemented and evaluated, with adjustments made as needed.

In cases when pharmacologic approaches are used to treat NPSs in combination with non-pharmacological approaches, different classes of psychotropics (including antidepressants, antipsychotics, anticonvulsants, and mood stabilizers) are used off-label. Such medications have variable efficacy and can be associated with significant side effects. For example, when antipsychotics are used to manage NPSs in ADRD (often for psychosis, agitation, disinhibition, or anxiety), clinical experience suggests that second-generation antipsychotics (SGAs) (such as olanzapine, quetiapine, risperidone, and aripiprazole) are preferred over the older conventional antipsychotics that are more likely to produce extrapyramidal symptoms (such as parkinsonism and dystonia). One recent review compared trials of atypical antipsychotics used for the treatment of NPSs in dementia and concluded that olanzapine and risperidone had the best evidence for efficacy, although their effects were modest.[44] On the other hand, a recent clinical trial suggested that these and other SGAs may be little better than placebo.[45]

Although these agents may work well when used judiciously, reports of a small but statistically significant increase in risk of cerebrovascular adverse events and death have led to an FDA warning for use of SGAs in older individuals with dementia. The potential for an increased risk of serious adverse events is of concern, and the risk-to-benefit ratio of antipsychotic medication use remains controversial; clinicians must weigh the risks against the potential benefits of these medications with patients and their families.

In general, such agents should be used only when necessary, at the lowest efficacious dose, and for as limited a time as possible and while continuing non-pharmacologic strategies. Psychosis does not require treatment unless it leads to dangerous behavior, causes distress to the patient, or is disruptive to the family or other caregivers. When such agents are used, choosing lower doses and titrating upward slowly is advised for this population. When the target symptoms are controlled, it is prudent to consider tapering the medications after 2 to 3 months to determine whether longer-term treatment is necessary. Indeed, with longer-term treatment, the benefits are less clear, and risks of severe adverse outcomes increase.

Other agents that have shown promise for management of NPSs in ADRD include pimavanserin and muscarinic receptor agonists for psychosis in AD; citalopram, prazosin, and cannabinoid agonists for agitation; methylphenidate for apathy in AD; and trazodone, melatonin, and orexin antagonists for sleep disturbances. This is an evolving area in which more research is needed to develop effective and safe treatments that target NPS neurobiology and reduce patient and care-partner burden.

Supportive and Long-Term Care for Patients with AD and Related Dementias

Because AD and the related dementias are chronic, progressive illnesses with limited available disease-modifying therapy or cures, they are associated with significant burdens for patients, their families, and the health care system. Identifying resources for families and care partners, including resources for caregiving at home, can provide essential support to patients and care partners and is the foundation of patient-care and partner– and family-centered care. This may include a home health aide, Meals on Wheels, or a visiting nurse. Structured activities outside of the home, such as adult day care or exercise programs, are also important. Moreover, it is critical that such support be provided in a culturally sensitive manner, given varying attitudes and understanding of ADRD across cultures and ethnic groups. In addition, although difficult for the patient and family, it is crucial to think through the future care requirements as well as legal and financial planning while the patient is in the early stages of the disease and can communicate her or his wishes for their own care and estate. This includes consideration of in-home and external care arrangements (e.g., assisted living, a skilled nursing facility) and consultation with an elder affairs lawyer or other legal representative.

Prognosis

Patients who live through the full course of the disease may survive for 10 to 20 years. However, many patients die in the early or middle stages of the illness. The landscape of AD treatments is rapidly shifting, although no treatments have yet been found that increase survival or halt disease progression definitively.

LEWY BODY DEMENTIA

Definition

Lewy body dementia is a progressive brain disease that involves cognitive, behavioral, and motor system deterioration like that seen in PD. LBD broadly refers to two disorders—dementia with Lewy bodies (DLB) and Parkinson disease dementia (PDD). Whereas in DLB, cognitive symptoms precede motor symptoms, in PDD, cognitive symptoms do not begin until 1 year or more after onset of movement symptoms. Cytoplasmic Lewy bodies are the common pathological substrate. In DLB, these develop in the cytoplasm of cortical neurons; in PDD, Lewy bodies are found in the substantia nigra.

Epidemiology and Risk Factors

Lewy body dementia is arguably the second-leading cause of dementia in older adults. Some researchers estimate that it accounts for up to 20% of dementia in the United States, affecting 800,000 individuals.[12] Slightly more men than women are affected. As with most dementias of adult onset, advanced age is a main risk factor for LBD. Disease onset is usually in the seventh decade of life or later. LBD may cluster in families.

Pathophysiology

The main pathological features of LBD are proteinaceous deposits called Lewy bodies (Figure 15.4), named for Frederic H. Lewy, who first described them in the early 1900s. Among other proteins, Lewy bodies are composed of alpha-synuclein in the cortex and brainstem.[46] In PD, Lewy bodies are primarily restricted to the brainstem and dopaminergic cells of the substantia nigra. In LBD, Lewy bodies are found in the cortex and amygdala, as well as in the brainstem. Triplication or mutations of the alpha-synuclein gene are rare causes of LBD. The mechanisms by which Lewy bodies cause neuronal dysfunction and eventual death are uncertain, but both the cholinergic and dopaminergic neurotransmitter systems are severely disrupted. Of note, Lewy body and AD pathology frequently co-occur.[47]

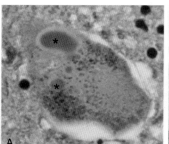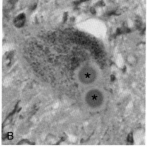

Figure 15.4. Lewy body pathology. *Asterisks* indicate Lewy bodies.

Clinical Features and Diagnosis

Lewy body dementia typically presents with cortical and subcortical cognitive impairments and with visuospatial and executive dysfunction that is worse than that found in AD, with relatively spared language and memory function. A recent international consortium on LBD resulted in revised criteria for the clinical and pathological diagnosis of LBD.[48] Core clinical features include fluctuating attention, recurrent visual hallucinations, and parkinsonism. Parkinsonian symptoms are also necessary for the diagnosis of LBD, with the motor symptoms occurring in most cases within about 1 year of the cognitive problems. Suggestive clinical features include rapid eye movement (REM) behavior disorder, extreme sensitivity to neuroleptics, disorientation, and low dopamine transporter uptake on neuroimaging.[48] Other manifestations (such as apathy, irritability, depression, and agitation), repeated falls and syncope, autonomic dysfunction, delusions, hallucinations in other modalities, prominent slowing on the EEG, and low uptake on MIBG (iodine-123 meta-iodobenzylguanidine) myocardial scintography are considered supportive of the diagnosis but not as specific. Although clinical features of the disease (e.g., hallucinations, fluctuations, visuospatial deficits, and REM behavior disorder) are helpful in the identification of possible cases of this disease, clinical–pathological concordance has not been great, and post-mortem pathological findings of Lewy bodies in the cerebral cortex, amygdala, and brainstem are necessary to confirm the diagnosis.[48]

Structural imaging is not usually helpful because atrophy may not be apparent early on in patients with LBD (Figure 15.5A). Sometimes pallor of the substantia nigra can be identified on MRI; as the disease progresses, there may be atrophy with a frontotemporal, insular, and visual cortex predominance. PET and SPECT may show evidence of decreased activity or perfusion in the occipitotemporal cortices (Figure 15.5B) in early clinical disease stages. In later stages, only the primary sensorimotor cortex may be spared.

Differential Diagnosis

As with AD, metabolic, inflammatory, infectious, vascular, medication-related, and structural causes of cognitive decline in the setting of parkinsonism should be excluded with testing. If the clinical picture is not highly consistent with LBD, other dementias with parkinsonism should be considered, including corticobasal degeneration (CBD), progressive supranuclear palsy (PSP), the "Parkinson-plus" syndromes (e.g., multiple-system atrophy), and vascular parkinsonism with dementia. It is also sometimes difficult to distinguish between PD with dementia and LBD depending on the characteristics, severity, and presentation sequence of the cognitive and motor symptoms. This distinction is primarily based on whether parkinsonism precedes dementia for more than 1 year, as occurs in PD with dementia. Furthermore, the motor symptoms of PD tend to respond better to dopaminergic therapies than they do in LBD.

Treatment

There are currently no FDA-approved treatments specific for LBD. Given the severe cholinergic losses that occur in LBD, the frequent co-occurrence of AD pathology, and several small trials that suggest their effectiveness, cholinesterase inhibitors have been the off-label treatment of choice. Rivastigmine has been effective for cognitive deficits and behavioral problems in LBD compared with placebo.[48] However, in a recent Cochrane review summarizing the evidence from six trials investigating cholinesterase inhibitors in PD dementia, LBD,

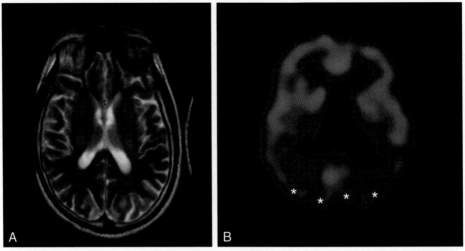

Figure 15.5. Lewy body dementia neuroimaging. **A**, Magnetic resonance imaging. **B**, Single-photon emission computed tomography.

and MCI associated with PD, the authors concluded that efficacy of cholinesterase inhibitors in LBD remained unclear in contrast to their use in PDD.[49] Although memantine may also be a logical choice because it enhances cognition in disorders with cholinergic deficits and it has dopaminergic effects that could benefit the parkinsonism in LBD, its efficacy has thus far been modest in two recent controlled trials.[50,51] Low dosages of levodopa and carbidopa (dopamine replacement) are sometimes helpful for the motor symptoms of LBD, although higher dosages of dopamine replacement therapy and direct dopamine agonists may exacerbate NPSs (e.g., hallucinations). Given that patients with LBD are sensitive to neuroleptics, typical antipsychotics and risperidone should be strictly avoided in patients with LBD because even a single dose can lead to prolonged drug-induced akinesia and rigidity. Other atypical antipsychotics (such as quetiapine) may be very useful for management of LBD's behavioral symptoms, with fewer untoward motor side effects than typical antipsychotics. However, these agents pose other potential side effects (e.g., metabolic syndrome, weight gain, increased mortality risk). Tricyclic antidepressants (TCAs) or benzodiazepines may help with REM behavior disorder in LBD, but given their anticholinergic and sedative properties, they should be used with caution in older individuals with dementia.

Supportive Care and Long-Term Management

These issues are similar to those for AD except that the neuropsychiatric features of LBD may be more severe than in AD, requiring additional supportive care. Greater levels of depression may occur in caregivers of patients with LBD than in caregivers of patients with AD; thus, early support for patients and their families is important.

Prognosis

The average duration of the disease is 5 to 7 years, although there may be substantial variability in the outcome of LBD.

The frequency of co-occurring AD and LBD pathologies in the same individual is greater than is anticipated by chance. Clinical syndromes with overlapping AD and LBD symptoms and the pathological findings have led to several diagnostic categories, such as AD with Lewy bodies or the Lewy body variant of AD. Future research in this area may elucidate the relationship and pathophysiology of both AD and LBD.

FRONTOTEMPORAL DEMENTIAS
Definition

Definitions of FTDs are currently in flux. FTDs may be understood as a genetically and pathologically heterogenous group of neurodegenerative disorders that involve degeneration of different regions of the frontal and temporal lobes to differing extents. The clinical pictures and underlying pathologies are also heterogeneous.[52] Currently subsumed under the term FTDs are Pick disease, frontotemporal lobar degeneration, primary progressive aphasia, and semantic dementia.[53] Additionally, there can be significant overlap between FTD and motor ALS (FTD-ALS) as well as the atypical parkinsonian syndromes, PSP, and corticobasal syndrome (CBS).[48]

Epidemiology and Genetic Risk Factors

Frontotemporal dementia tends to manifest at younger ages than typical AD, with most cases occurring in people younger than 65 years old, and it is the most common form of dementia with an onset before age 60 years, with most cases presenting between 45 and 64 years of age.[54] In contrast, FTD diagnoses account for only 2.7% of dementia diagnoses for patients older than 65 years old. FTD sometimes runs in families. In fact, 25% to 50% of patients with FTD have a first-degree relative with the disease, and autosomal dominant inheritance is frequently observed. Many of these families are found to harbor a mutation in *MATP*, the gene encoding the tau protein, which is found in NFTs. Patients with *MATP* mutations often have a motor syndrome, such as PD or PSP, along with their FTD. A total of 40 tau mutations have been reported across 113 families. In addition, FTD can sometimes be associated with mutations in *GRN*, *VCP*, *TARDBP*, *PSEN1*, and *CHMP2B*,[52,54] along with a recently identified C9ORF72 hexanucleotide repeat expansion.[53]

Pathophysiology

The pathophysiology of FTD is poorly understood, and it likely represents a constellation of syndromes with different underlying causes. This notion is reflected in the variable pathologies that underlie the disease and somehow all lead to neuronal dysfunction and to death. Individuals with clinically defined FTD may exhibit variable combinations of abnormal

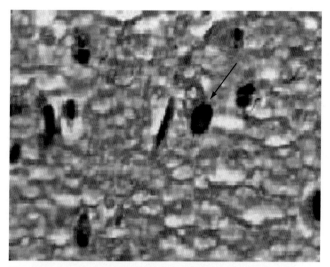

Figure 15.6. Neuropathology of frontotemporal disease: Pick bodies *(arrow).*

tau protein deposits, including tangles and Pick bodies (as in Pick disease; see Figure 15.6); ubiquitin-positive inclusions; gliosis; non-specific spongiform degeneration; and prion-related spongiform changes. In some cases, AD pathology distributed in the frontotemporal cortex can cause an FTD-like syndrome. Furthermore, transactive response DNA-binding protein 43 (TDP-43) was identified in 2006 as the major inclusion protein in most patients with ALS and in the most common subtype of FTD, frontotemporal lobar degeneration with TDP-43 pathology (FTLD-TDP).[52,54] Indeed, FTLD can be classified into three general categories based on the predominant neuropathological protein: microtubule-associated tau (FTLD-TAU), TAR DNA-binding protein 43 (FTLD-TDP), and fused in sarcoma protein (FTLD-FUS). Recently, the clinicopathologic overlap between ALS and FTD was supported by discovery of C9ORF72 repeat expansions, a GGGGCC hexanucleotide repeat in a non-coding region of C9ORF72 (chromosome 9 open reading frame 72), encoding an unknown C9ORF72 protein.[53] Although genetic causes of FTD include tau mutations on chromosome 17 (FTD-17) (these cases often have associated symptoms of parkinsonism), repeat expansions in C9ORF72 are currently the most important genetic cause of familial ALS and FTD.[53]

Clinical Features, Diagnosis, and Differential Diagnosis

The classic hallmarks of FTD are behavioral features out of proportion to amnesia. Behavioral variant FTD (bvFTD) refers to a gradual, progressive loss of judgment; disinhibition; impulsivity; social misconduct; loss of awareness; and withdrawal. Other typical symptoms are stereotypies, excessive oral or manual exploration, hyperphagia, wanderlust, excessive joviality, sexually provocative behaviors, and inappropriate words or actions. Given the overlaps between behavioral syndromes associated with an FTD diagnosis, distinction of this neurodegenerative disease from primary psychiatric illness can be challenging. This may, in part, account for underreporting of incidence and delayed diagnosis.

In some cases, language is initially or primarily affected and can remain as the relatively isolated deficit for years. In these cases, there is often primarily left hemisphere pathology selectively involving the frontal or temporal lobes, or the peri-Sylvian cortex. Primary progressive aphasia (PPA) refers to symptomatic involvement of the frontal (or other peri-Sylvian) language areas leading to changes in both expressive and receptive language function.[55] Depending on the localization of left hemisphere pathology, patients may exhibit different degrees of impairment of word-finding, object-naming, syntax, or word-comprehension abilities. Semantic variant PPA is characterized by significant loss of word meaning (i.e., semantic losses) with relatively preserved fluency, which results from left anterior temporal lobe involvement. In contrast, progressive non-fluent aphasia (PFNA) results in difficulty in the production of language. This can manifest as changes in the manner of speech, for example, speaking more slowly, with grammatical errors or with omitted or improperly ordered words. The definitions of these syndromes have been in flux, and in more recent years, PPA syndromes have been further divided into three patterns: semantic variant PPA and PNFA (as earlier) and logopenic progressive aphasia (LPA), also referred to as the logopenic or phonological variant of PPA. LPA is characterized by impaired naming and single word retrieval in the absence of motor speech abnormalities and generally preserved object knowledge and comprehension of single words and simple sentences. The clinicopathological correlates of these syndromes are not uniform.[56,57] They can range from tauopathy to AD pathology, which can often make the distinction between FTD and AD more complex. Although beyond the scope of this chapter, this is an area of active research.

Clinical presentations of FTD vary based on the relative involvement of the hemisphere (right or left) or lobe (frontal or temporal) involved. Patients may initially have right greater than left temporal lobe involvement and exhibit primarily a behavioral syndrome with emotional distance; irritability; and disruption of sleep, appetite, and libido. With greater initial left than right temporal lobe involvement, patients exhibit more language-related problems, including anomia, word-finding difficulties, repetitive speech, and loss of semantic information (e.g., semantic dementia).[55] In some cases of FTD, the frontal lobes may be involved to a greater extent than the temporal lobes. In these instances, patients exhibit symptoms of elation, disinhibition, apathy, and aberrant motor behavior. Depending on the combination of regions involved, patients with FTD exhibit specific cognitive and NPSs. As the disease progresses to involve greater expanses of the frontotemporal cortex, the clinical features become similar. The presumption is that the atrophy and underlying pathology that accompanies FTD is regionally specific, but it becomes more generalized as the disease progresses.

The evaluation and diagnosis of FTD is like that of the other dementias and includes clinical evaluation, laboratory studies, neuropsychological testing (often including tests of social cognition), and brain imaging (structural and functional imaging). The work-up supports the exclusion of other medical and primary psychiatric disorders and reflects diagnostic confidence: As defined by the latest FTD Criteria Consortium guidelines,[58] whereas *possible* bvFTD is based solely on clinical syndrome, *probable* bvFTD incorporates clinical features including functional decline, and neuroimaging, such as fluorodeoxyglucose-PET and MRI, with evidence of hypoperfusion, hypometabolism, or focal atrophy. Findings on CT or MRI scans may show frontotemporal atrophy (Figure 15.7A), which can be quite striking at autopsy (Figure 15.7B). Clinical findings of motor system or brainstem abnormalities should be investigated when considering the various diagnoses. For example, some cases of FTD are associated with parkinsonism (FTD-17) or motor neuron disease (e.g., ALS), with increasing evidence that ALS and FTD may be on a disease continuum with shared underlying pathogenesis. Other clinically defined

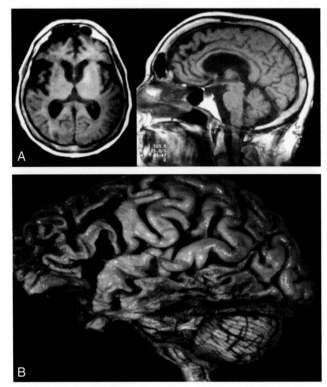

Figure 15.7. Frontotemporal atrophy on magnetic resonance imaging (**A**) and at autopsy (**B**).

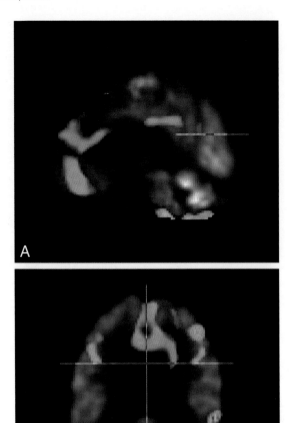

Figure 15.8. Regional hypoactivity in frontotemporal disease. Colored areas in sagittal (**A**) and horizontal (**B**) brain sections indicate activity 2 standard deviations below the population mean. (Courtesy of Keith Johnson.)

disorders may have features of FTD but are distinguished by eye movement, sensory, or gait abnormalities (e.g., PSP, CBD, and NPH). Brain imaging studies of FTD may show focal atrophy in the frontotemporal cortices along with frontotemporal hypoperfusion or hypoactivity (Figure 15.8).

Behavioral variant FTD, characterized by changes in behavior and social comportment, may clinically resemble many primary psychiatric disorders, ranging from bipolar disorder to personality and autism spectrum disorders. NPSs may represent a prodromal stage of FTD, a co-morbid psychiatric disorder, or both. A recent International Consortium put forth a set of consensus guidelines to aide in distinguishing bvFTD from a psychiatric disorder.[59]

Treatment

There are no specific treatments or cures for FTD. The behavioral features are sometimes helped by use of selective serotonin reuptake inhibitors, and these are probably the best-studied treatments for these disorders. Cholinesterase inhibitors and memantine may exacerbate the NPSs. Antipsychotics (preferably atypical ones), mood stabilizers, and benzodiazepines are sometimes necessary to treat aggression and agitation, but they should be used sparingly.

Supportive Care and Long-Term Management

As in the other dementias, supportive, long-term care is crucial for FTD because it is often accompanied by loss of insight, lack of judgment, and severe behavioral symptoms.

Prognosis

There are no specific medical treatments for FTD. Across the disorders, the time between illness and death is typically about 7 years.

Although not all cases of FTD have the same underlying pathology, there is a developing notion that there is a group of associated dementias (including some instances clinically consistent with FTD) based on the presence of abnormal forms of the tau protein and TDP-43. These disorders cut across the regional neuroanatomic boundaries that typically characterize FTD and may exhibit features atypical for frontotemporal lobar degeneration. Not only do some cases of clinically defined FTD have tau pathology, but they also have certain characteristic motor, sensory, and brainstem-related clinical features, as found in PSP, CBD, and FTD with parkinsonism or motor neuron disease. Other focal atrophies outside of the frontotemporal lobes may also reflect underlying tau pathology (such as progressive visuospatial and language dysfunction) that can occur in posterior (parietal) cortical atrophy.

VASCULAR DEMENTIA

Definition

Vascular dementia has become an overarching term that encompasses a variety of vascular-related causes of dementia, including multi-infarct dementia (MID) and small vessel disease. More recently, the term *vascular cognitive impairment* has been used to account for all forms of cognitive dysfunction caused by vascular disease, ranging from prodromal stages and mild

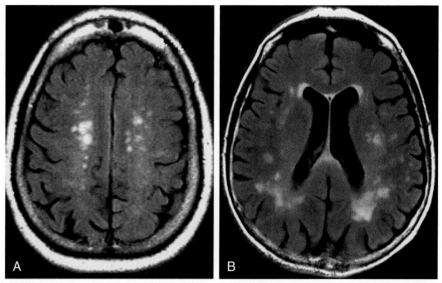

Figure 15.9. Magnetic resonance imaging (MRI) of vascular dementia: small-vessel disease. **A**, Coronal fluid attenuation inversion recovery (FLAIR) MRI showing centrum semiovale ischemic white matter disease. **B**, Coronal FLAIR MRI showing periventricular ischemic white matter disease.

cognitive dysfunction to dementia, or major neurocognitive impairment.

Epidemiology and Risk Factors

Various types of vascular dementia account for approximately 20% of all dementia cases, making it the second or third most common form of dementia. It is equally prevalent in women and men, but the frequency may be higher in men and in African Americans. Risk factors are like those for cardiovascular illness (including diabetes, hypercholesterolemia, hyperhomocysteinemia, hypertension, cigarette smoking, and physical inactivity). To the extent that these factors have familial or genetic bases, so does vascular dementia. Not all genetic risk factors have the same relevance for the different forms of vascular dementia. For example, it is uncertain whether an elevated cholesterol level is as crucial a risk factor as is hypertension for microvascular ischemic white matter disease; several large studies have failed to show a clinical benefit of decreased cholesterol for cognitive impairments even when rates of stroke and transient ischemic attacks are reduced.

Pathophysiology

There are several underlying causes of vascular dementia. Recurrent or specifically localized embolic strokes (from sources such as the heart or carotid arteries or local thromboses of larger-caliber intracranial vessels) can lead to vascular dementia. These causes are most closely associated with the clinical entity of MID. Smaller subcortical strokes (e.g., lacunar infarctions) in gray and white matter structures may also lead to a form of vascular dementia.

White matter disease without clearly symptomatic strokes or gross tissue damage may cause an insidiously progressive cognitive decline (Figure 15.9). It is important to keep in mind that cerebral hemorrhages caused by hypertension or amyloid angiopathy are possible mechanisms of vascular-induced cognitive impairment, but they require a different type of clinical management than does typical vascular occlusive disease. There are specific gene mutations (e.g., *notch 3*) that cause certain forms of vascular dementia (e.g., cerebral autosomal dominant arteriopathy with subcortical infarcts and leukoencephalopathy [CADASIL]), but these are extremely rare.

Clinical Features and Diagnosis

Vascular dementia has variable clinical features that depend on the localization of the vascular lesions. Overall, left hemisphere lesions tend to cause language problems, and right hemisphere lesions tend to cause visuospatial problems. Both the type of cognitive deficits and the time course of the cognitive changes are variable. Embolic or large-vessel stroke-related dementia may progress in a characteristic step-wise pattern, with intervening periods of stability punctuated by abrupt declines in cognitive function; the type of cognitive symptoms is affected by the brain areas affected over time. This might be considered the classic presentation for vascular dementia associated with multiple infarcts; however, it may not be the most common presentation of vascular dementia.[60,61]

Multiple small subcortical infarcts may cause a more insidious decline even in the absence of recognized stroke symptoms. However, small cortical infarcts at specific locations (e.g., the thalamus or caudate) can cause significant cognitive and motor symptoms. So-called small-vessel or microvascular ischemic disease preferentially involves the white matter, particularly in the centrum semiovale and periventricular regions (see Figure 15.9), and is also a common cause of vascular dementia. This has been called *leukoaraiosis*. Symptoms in this case tend to develop in a gradual and insidious fashion and can be difficult to distinguish from AD. Memory or mood complaints are usually a presenting feature. Sometimes the memory disorder can be distinguished from that in AD. Spontaneous recall is affected in both disorders, but recognition memory is often preserved in vascular dementia, which is not the case for AD. Presentations involving relatively isolated psychotic symptoms in the setting of preserved memory should also raise the possibility of vascular dementia. Likewise, apathy, executive dysfunction, and a relatively intact memory are suggestive of a small-vessel ischemic process. Vascular dementia is also often referable to altered frontal systems dysfunction by which there is disconnection or damage to white matter tracts that relay information to and from the region.

Differential Diagnosis

The main difficulty in diagnosing vascular dementia is distinguishing it from AD. Classically, vascular dementia is distinguished from AD based on an abrupt onset and a step-wise course. In addition, prominent executive dysfunction and preserved recognition memory are also suggestive of vascular dementia. However, in many cases, the symptoms of vascular dementia overlap with those of AD. Furthermore, autopsy studies show that the co-occurrence of AD and CNS vascular pathology is frequent; the interaction may cause cognitive impairment that might not otherwise occur if the same level of AD or vascular dementia pathology was present alone.

In addition, because the clinical features of vascular cognitive impairment may be variable, specific vascular lesions can mimic a variety of different dementias and even PD. The finding of focal features on examination or CNS vascular disease on structural imaging studies helps to determine the correct diagnosis.

Treatment

Treatment for vascular dementia involves control of vascular risk factors (e.g., hypercholesterolemia, hypertension, inactivity, diabetes, excess alcohol use, cigarette smoking, hyperhomocysteinemia). If strokes are found on brain imaging studies, a stroke work-up should be initiated to determine if surgery (e.g., for carotid stenosis), anticoagulation (for atrial fibrillation), or antiplatelet agents (e.g., for small-vessel strokes) are indicated. Such an evaluation may show hemorrhages from amyloid angiopathy or hypertension, in which case avoidance of anticoagulant or antiplatelet therapies may be prudent. In addition to treating these causes of CNS vascular disease, some literature indicates that symptomatic treatments (such as cholinesterase inhibitors or memantine) may be helpful for cognition.[62] However, there are no FDA-approved treatments for vascular dementia. Neuropsychiatric features (e.g., depression or psychosis) are common in vascular dementia and should be treated accordingly.

Recent work has highlighted a significant incidence of vascular-related cognitive impairment that does not reach clinical criteria for dementia. This is akin to the notion of MCI or prodromal AD. Although definitions for vascular-related cognitive impairment are currently under development, the idea highlights the importance of recognizing cognitive difficulties caused by CNS vascular disease in their earliest stages so vascular risk factors can be identified and treated.[61]

CORTICOBASAL DEGENERATION

CBD is a rare form of dementia that is related to FTD and typically involves specific motor and cognitive deficits. It usually occurs between the ages of 45 and 70 years and may have a slight female predominance. It rarely runs in families; however, it may be associated with a specific tau gene haplotype. Pathologically, there are abnormal neuronal and glial tau accumulations in the cortex and basal ganglia, including the substantia nigra. Swollen, achromatic neurons are typical. The pathophysiology is unknown, and although thought to primarily relate to the toxic effects of the tau protein, it has been increasingly recognized to involve Tar-DNA binding protein-43 (TDP-43)–positive inclusions as well as AD pathology.[63] Clinically, CBD is typically characterized by asymmetric sensorimotor symptoms involving one hemi-body to a greater degree than the other, with features of cortical and basal ganglionic dysfunction. Patients tend to have problems performing complex sequenced movements and movements on command (i.e., apraxia). Dystonia and action- or stimulus-induced myoclonus are also common. One classic sensorimotor feature of CBD is the alien hand or limb phenomenon, in which a part of the body feels as if it is not one's own or like it is being moved by an external or alien force. Parkinsonian

rigidity and walking problems may also develop in addition to these sensorimotor problems, as well as problems with language and memory, personality changes, and inappropriate behavior.

Structural imaging studies may show frontotemporal atrophy, asymmetric parietal atrophy, or both. Functional imaging studies may demonstrate asymmetric hypometabolism and hypoperfusion in the parietal cortex and basal ganglia with or without frontotemporal hypometabolism and hypoperfusion. In the setting of mild motor symptoms with more prominent cognitive or behavioral manifestations, CBD can be confused for AD or FTD or vascular dementia with vascular parkinsonism. Some studies indicate that up to 20% of clinically diagnosed FTDs turn out to have the pathology of CBD. Because of the significant clinicopathologic heterogeneity, the term *CBS* is sometimes used for patients with characteristic clinical features, and *CBD* is reserved for diagnosis based on neuropathological analysis.

There are no FDA-approved or other treatments specific for CBD. Treatment is therefore supportive or symptomatic based on the individual patient's specific disease manifestations.

PROGRESSIVE SUPRANUCLEAR PALSY

PSP is another dementia characterized by the presence of cognitive and behavioral features along with specific motor abnormalities. PSP tends to occur in middle age and is slightly more common in men than in women. It is a rare and sporadic disease, but, like CBD, it has been associated with specific tau gene haplotypes. The pathology of PSP involves (usually) abnormal tau-reactive deposits in neurons and glia that are typically concentrated in various brainstem nuclei (including the substantia nigra) but sometimes also in the cortex. In addition to involvement of systems that coordinate somatic movement, the supranuclear systems that govern the cranial nerves are also affected.

The classic clinical features of the disease are progressive difficulties with balance and gait, resulting in frequent falls early in the disease, progressive loss of voluntary control of eye movements, and progressive cognitive and behavioral difficulties. Patients with PSP often have difficulties with the coordination of eyelid opening and closing, dysarthria, dysphagia, and fixed facial expression akin to surprise. Symptoms like those of PD are also present, particularly akinesia and axial rigidity. The cognitive and behavioral features are usually referable to frontal lobe dysfunction and may closely resemble those of FTD (such as executive dysfunction, apathy, and reduced processing speed). CT or MRI scans may show an atrophic brainstem with frontotemporal atrophy as the disease progresses.

There are no approved therapies or cures for PSP, and management is supportive or symptomatic. It is important to assess safety issues to reduce the risk of falls and injury. Swallowing evaluations help to determine diet modifications that delay aspiration from dysphagia.

NORMAL-PRESSURE HYDROCEPHALUS

Normal-pressure hydrocephalus is a condition that involves enlargement of the ventricles leading to cognitive and motor difficulties. About 250,000 people in the United States have this disease; it usually occurs in adults 55 years of age or older. Intermittent pressure increases are thought to cause ventricular expansion over time, with damage to the adjacent white matter tracts that connect the frontal lobes. The main clinical features are gait disturbance, frontal systems dysfunction, and urinary incontinence.[64] Patients need not have all three symptoms to have NPH. There are no clear genetic causes. The main risk factors relate to conditions that adversely affect the function of the ventricular system for CSF egress, which include history of head trauma, intracranial hemorrhage, meningitis, or any inflammatory or structural process that might damage the meninges.

Evaluation usually includes structural brain imaging (MRI or CT) demonstrating the presence of ventricular enlargement out of proportion to atrophy. Reversal of CSF flow in the cerebral aqueduct or the presence of transependymal fluid on MRI may suggest NPH.

If NPH is suspected, it is prudent to remove CSF and to measure the CSF pressure, which can be done by a variety of techniques. It is most important to perform cognitive and motor testing before and after the removal of a large volume of CSF. LP, lumbar catheter insertion, or CSF pressure and outflow-resistance monitoring in combination with pre-procedure and post-procedure neuropsychological and motor testing can be very helpful in making a diagnosis and in estimating the likelihood of treatment success.[65] Placement of a CSF shunt is the treatment of choice and can arrest or even significantly improve a patient's condition.[66]

RAPIDLY PROGRESSING DEMENTIAS: PRION DISEASES WITH CREUTZFELDT–JAKOB DISEASE AS AN EXAMPLE

Creutzfeldt–Jakob disease is a rare disorder that causes a characteristic triad of progressive dementia, myoclonus, and distinctive periodic EEG complexes; cerebellar, pyramidal and extrapyramidal findings are also characteristic, as are psychiatric symptoms, which may be among the first signs of the disease. The typical age of onset is around 60 years. CJD is caused by prions, novel proteinaceous infective agents. Prion protein (PrP), an amyloid protein encoded on chromosome 20, is the major constituent of prions. PrP normally exists in a PrPc isoform; in a pathological state, it is transformed to the PrPSc isoform, which condenses in neurons and causes their death. As prion-induced changes accumulate, the cerebral cortex takes on the distinctive microscopic, vacuolar appearance of spongiform encephalopathy. The CSF in almost 90% of patients with CJD contains traces of prion proteins detected by a routine LP. CJD is transmissible and can occur as three general forms: sporadic, familial, or acquired, including a variant form of CJD. Treatment in these cases is supportive because it follows a characteristically rapid and fatal course over an average of 6 months.[67]

Anti-sense oligonucleotide-based treatments targeting PrP have shown promise in preclinical models of CJD.[68] Several longitudinal studies of familial prion diseases have been established, and a clinical trial is expected to begin within the next several years, sponsored by Ionis Pharmaceuticals.

CONCLUSIONS

As the population ages, the number of people with dementing disorders is increasing dramatically; most have AD, vascular dementia, LBD, or a combination of these disorders. Although none is curable, all have treatable components—whether they are reversible, static, or progressive. Furthermore, the increasing recognition of the spectrum of cognitive impairment in mild and major neurocognitive disorders and in pre-clinical stages of AD has the potential for identifying people at earlier stages of impairment and preventing progression. The role of a psychiatrist in the diagnosis and treatment of dementing disorders is extremely important, particularly in the identification of treatable psychiatric and behavioral symptoms, which are common sources of care partner distress and institutionalization.

Family members and care partners are also significantly impacted and at risk in cases of all progressive dementias. Caregiving is mentally and physically challenging. Spousal and other family caregivers are often on duty 24 hours a day and are at increased risk of loneliness, depression, and medical problems. This makes it important that the psychiatrist communicates with them about the diagnosis and the expected course of the disease and provides psychoeducation on the risk of caregiver burnout and sources of support. They can benefit from advice on how best to relate to the patient, how to restructure the home environment for safety and comfort, and how to seek out legal and financial guidance when appropriate. Most hospitals and health care systems have social workers who can assist with providing support on the caregiving journey and navigating health care systems, as well as programs akin to the Dementia Care Collaborative at Massachusetts General Hospital (www.dementiacarecollaborative.org). Family members should also be made aware of the potential assistance available to them through support networks, such as nonprofit organizations (e.g., Alzheimer's Association, Alzheimer's Foundation, The Association for Frontotemporal Degeneration, Lewy Body Dementia Association) as well as other community or religious organizations.

Overall, great advances have been made in our understanding of the pathophysiology, epidemiology, and genetics of various dementing disorders. The likelihood of having measures for early detection, prevention, and intervention in the future is very promising.

REFERENCES

1. American Psychiatric Association. *Diagnostic and Statistical Manual of Mental Disorders.* American Psychiatric Association; 2013. 5th ed.
2. American Psychiatric Association. *Diagnostic and Statistical Manual of Mental Disorders.* American Psychiatric Association; 1994. 4th ed.
3. Mitchell AJ, Shiri-Feshki M. Rate of progression of mild cognitive impairment to dementia—meta-analysis of 41 robust inception cohort studies. *Acta Psychiatr Scand.* 2009;119(4):252–265.
4. Petersen RC, Roberts RO, Knopman DS, et al. Mild cognitive impairment ten years later. *Arch Neurol.* 2009;66:1447–1455.
5. Mayeux R, Stern Y. Epidemiology of Alzheimer disease. *Cold Spring Harbor Perspect Med.* 2012;2(8):a006239.
6. Sosa-Ortiz AL, Acosta-Castillo I, Prince MJ. Epidemiology of Alzheimer's disease. *Arch Med Res.* 2012;43:600–608.
7. The Hartford Institute for Geriatric Nursing, New York University, College of Nursing. *Try This: Best Practices in Nursing Care to Older Adults.* 2007;23.
8. Cummings JL, Mega M, Gray K, et al. The Neuropsychiatric Inventory: comprehensive assessment of psychopathology in dementia. *Neurology.* 1994;44(12):2308–2314.
9. Kaufer DI, Cummings JL, Ketchel P, et al. Validation of the NPI-Q, a brief clinical form of the Neuropsychiatric Inventory. *J Neuropsychiatry Clin Neurosci.* 2000;12(2):233–239.
10. Ismail Z, Agüera-Ortiz L, Brodaty H, et al. The Mild Behavioral Impairment Checklist (MBI-C): a rating scale for neuropsychiatric symptoms in pre-dementia populations. *J Alzheimers Dis.* 2017;56(3):929–938.
11. Folstein MF, Folstein SE, McHugh PR. Mini-mental state exam: a practical method for grading the cognitive state of patients for the clinician. *J Psychiatr Res.* 1975;12:189–198.
12. 2022 Alzheimer's disease facts and figures. *Alzheimers Dement.* 2022;18(4):700–789.
13. GBD 2019 Dementia Forecasting Collaborators. Estimation of the global prevalence of dementia in 2019 and forecasted prevalence in 2050: an analysis for the Global Burden of Disease Study 2019. *Lancet Public Heal.* 2022;7(2):e105–e125.
14. Matthews KA, Xu W, Gaglioti AH, et al. Racial and ethnic estimates of Alzheimer's disease and related dementias in the United States (2015-2060) in adults aged ≥65 years. *Alzheimers Dement.* 2019;15(1):17–24.
15. Akushevich I, Kravchenko J, Yashkin A, et al. Expanding the scope of health disparities research in Alzheimer's disease and related

dementias: recommendations from the "Leveraging Existing Data and Analytic Methods for Health Disparities Research Related to Aging and Alzheimer's Disease and Related Dementias" Workshop Series. *Alzheimers Dement (Amst).* 2023;15(1):e12415.

16. Canevelli M, Bruno G, Grande G, et al. Race reporting and disparities in clinical trials on Alzheimer's disease: a systematic review. *Neurosci Biobehav Rev.* 2019;101:122–128.

17. Reitz C, Brayne C, Mayeux R. Epidemiology of Alzheimer disease. *Nat Rev Neurol.* 2011;7:137–152.

18. Carillo MC, Brashear HR, Logovinsky V, et al. Can we prevent Alzheimer's disease? Secondary "prevention" trials in Alzheimer's disease. *Alzheimers Dement.* 2013;9:123–131.e1.

19. Barnes DE, Yaffe K, Byers AL, et al. Midlife vs late-life depressive symptoms and risk of dementia: differential effects for Alzheimer disease and vascular dementia. *Arch Gen Psychiatry.* 2012;69(5):493–498.

20. Selkoe DJ. Aging, amyloid, and Alzheimer's disease: a perspective in honor of Carl Cotman. *Neurochem Res.* 2003;28:1705–1713.

21. Iqbal K, Alonso Adel C, Chen S, et al. Tau pathology in Alzheimer disease and other tauopathies. *Biochim Biophys Acta.* 2005;1739:198–210.

22. Hyman BT. The neuropathological diagnosis of Alzheimer's disease: clinical-pathological studies. *Neurobiol Aging.* 1997;18:S27–S32.

23. Heston LL, Mastri AR, Anderson VE, et al. Dementia of the Alzheimer type: clinical genetics, natural history, and associated conditions. *Arch Gen Psychiatry.* 1981;38(10):1085–1090.

24. Gatz M, Reynolds CA, Fratiglioni L, et al. Role of genes and environments for explaining Alzheimer disease. *Arch Gen Psychiatry.* 2006;63:168–174.

25. Wingo TS, Lah JJ, Levey AI, et al. Autosomal recessive causes likely in early-onset Alzheimer disease. *Arch Neurol.* 2012;69:59–64.

26. Karch CM, Goate AM. Alzheimer's disease risk genes and mechanisms of disease pathogenesis. *Biol Psychiatry.* 2015;77(1):43–51.

27. Sirkis DW, Bonham LW, Johnson TP, et al. Dissecting the clinical heterogeneity of early-onset Alzheimer's disease. *Mol Psychiatry.* 2022;27:2674–2688.

28. Bellenguez C, Kucukali F, Jansen IE, et al. New insights into the genetic etiology of Alzheimer's disease and related dementias. *Nat Genet.* 2022;54:412–436.

29. Bird TD. Risks and benefits of DNA testing for neurogenetic disorders. *Semin Neurol.* 1999;19:253–259.

30. Kawas CH. Clinical practice. Early Alzheimer's disease. *N Engl J Med.* 2003;349:1056–1063.

31. Sperling RA, Aisen PS, Beckett LA, et al. Toward defining the preclinical stages of Alzheimer's disease: recommendations from the National Institute on Aging-Alzheimer's Association workgroups on diagnostic guidelines for Alzheimer's disease. *Alzheimers Dement.* 2011;7:280–292.

32. Reiman EM, McKhann GM, Albert MS, et al. Alzheimer's disease: implications of the updated diagnostic and research criteria. *J Clin Psychiatry.* 2011;72(9):1190–1196.

33. Jack Jr CR, Bennett DA, Blennow K, et al. NIA-AA Research framework: toward a biological definition of Alzheimer's disease. *Alzheimers Dement.* 2018;14(4):535–562.

34. Pillai JA, Cummings JL. Clinical trials in predementia stages of Alzheimer disease. *Med Clin North Am.* 2013;97(3):439–457.

35. Trinh N, Hoblyn J, Mohanty S, et al. Efficacy of cholinesterase inhibitors in the treatment of neuropsychiatric symptoms and functional impairment in Alzheimer disease. *JAMA.* 2003;289:210–216.

36. Lyketsos CG, Colenda C, Beck C, et al. Position statement of the American Association for Geriatric Psychiatry regarding principles of care for patients with dementia resulting from Alzheimer disease. *Am J Geriatr Psychiatry.* 2006;14(7):561–572.

37. Howard R, McShane R, Lindesay J, et al. Donepezil and memantine for moderate-to-severe Alzheimer's disease. *N Engl J Med.* 2012;366(10):893–903.

38. Murphy MP, LeVine III H. Alzheimer's disease and the amyloid-β peptide. *J Alzheimers Dis.* 2010;19(1):311–323.

39. Shi M, Chu F, Zhu F, et al. Impact of anti-amyloid-β monoclonal antibodies on the pathology and clinical profile of Alzheimer's disease: a focus on aducanumab and lecanemab. *Front Aging Neurosci.* 2022;14:870517.

40. Caleb AG, Knopman DS, Emerson SS, et al. Revisiting FDA approval of aducanumab. *N Engl J Med.* 2021;5(9):769–771.

41. Lacorte E, Ancidoni A, Zaccaria V, et al. Safety and efficacy of monoclonal antibodies for Alzheimer's disease: a systematic review and meta-analysis of published and unpublished clinical trials. *J Alzheimers Dis.* 2022;87(1):101–129.

42. Cummings J, Isaacson S, Mills R, et al. Pimavanserin for patients with Parkinson's disease psychosis: a randomised, placebo-controlled phase 3 trial. *Lancet.* 2014;383(9916):533–540. Erratum in: *Lancet.* 2014;384(9937):28.

43. Kales HC, Gitlin LN, Lyketsos CG. Detroit Expert Panel on Assessment and Management of Neuropsychiatric Symptoms of Dementia. Management of neuropsychiatric symptoms of dementia in clinical settings: recommendations from a multidisciplinary expert panel. *J Am Geriatr Soc.* 2014;62(4):762–769.

44. Carson S, McDonagh MS, Peterson K. A systematic review of the efficacy and safety of atypical antipsychotics in patients with psychological and behavioral symptoms of dementia. *J Am Geriatr Soc.* 2006;54:354–361.

45. Schneider LS, Tariot PN, Dagerman KM, et al. Effectiveness of atypical antipsychotic drugs in patients with Alzheimer's disease. *N Engl J Med.* 2006;355:1525–1538.

46. Weisman D, McKeith I. Dementia with Lewy bodies. *Semin Neurol.* 2007;27(1):42–47.

47. Jellinger KA. Alpha-synuclein pathology in Parkinson's and Alzheimer's disease brain: incidence and topographic distribution—a pilot study. *Acta Neuropathol (Berl).* 2003;106:191–201.

48. McKeith IG, Dickson DW, Lowe J, et al. Diagnosis and management of dementia with Lewy bodies: third report of the DLB Consortium. *Neurology.* 2005;65:1863–1872.

49. Rolinski M, Fox C, Maidment I, et al. Cholinesterase inhibitors for dementia with Lewy bodies, Parkinson's disease dementia and cognitive impairment in Parkinson's disease. *Cochrane Database Syst Rev.* 2012;14(3).

50. Aarsland D, Ballard C, Walker Z, et al. Memantine in patients with Parkinson's disease dementia or dementia with Lewy bodies: a double-blind, placebo-controlled, multicentre trial. *Lancet Neurol.* 2009;8(7):613–618.

51. Johansson C, Ballard C, Hansson O, et al. Efficacy of memantine in PDD and DLB: an extension study including washout and open-label treatment. *Int J Geriatr Psychiatry.* 2011;26(2):206–213.

52. Forman MS, Farmer J, Johnson JK, et al. Frontotemporal dementia: clinicopathological correlations. *Ann Neurol.* 2006;59:952–962.

53. Van Blitterswijk M, DeJesus-Hernandez M, Rademakers R. How do C9ORF72 repeat expansions cause amyotrophic lateral sclerosis and frontotemporal dementia: can we learn from other noncoding repeat expansions disorders? *Curr Opin Neurol.* 2012;25(6):689–700.

54. Seltman RE, Matthews BR. Frontotemporal lobar degeneration: epidemiology, pathology, diagnosis and management. *CNS Drugs.* 2012;26(10):841–870.

55. Mesulam MM. Primary progressive aphasia—a language-based dementia. *N Engl J Med.* 2003;349:1535–1542.

56. Kertesz A, McMonagle P, Blair M, et al. The evolution and pathology of frontotemporal dementia. *Brain.* 2005;128:1996–2005.

57. Seeley WW, Bauer AM, Miller BL, et al. The natural history of temporal variant frontotemporal dementia. *Neurology.* 2005;64:1384–1390.

58. Rascovsky K, Hodges JR, Knopman D, et al. Sensitivity of revised diagnostic criteria for the behavioural variant of frontotemporal dementia. *Brain.* 2011;134(Pt 9):2456–2477.

59. Ducharme S, Dols A, Laforce R, et al. Recommendations to distinguish behavioural variant frontotemporal dementia from psychiatric disorders. *Brain.* 2020;143(6):1632–1650.

60. Hachinski VC, Bowler JV. Vascular dementia. *Neurology.* 1993;43:2159–2160. Author reply 2160-2161.

61. Bowler JV. Vascular cognitive impairment. *J Neurol Neurosurg Psychiatry.* 2005;76(suppl 5):v35–v44.

62. Bowler JV. Acetylcholinesterase inhibitors for vascular dementia and Alzheimer's disease combined with cerebrovascular disease. *Stroke.* 2003;34:584–586.

63. Shelley BP, Hodges JR, Kipps CM, et al. Is the pathology of corticobasal syndrome predictable in life? *Mov Disord.* 2009;24(11):1593–1599.

64. Nowak DA, Topka HR. Broadening a classic clinical triad: the hypokinetic motor disorder of normal pressure hydrocephalus also affects the hand. *Exp Neurol.* 2006;198:81–87.

65. Relkin N, Marmarou A, Klinge P, et al. Diagnosing idiopathic normal-pressure hydrocephalus. *Neurosurgery.* 2005;57(suppl): S4–S16. Discussion ii-v.

66. Aygok G, Marmarou A, Young HF. Three-year outcome of shunted idiopathic NPH patients. *Acta Neurochir Suppl.* 2005;95: 241–245.

67. Gencer AG, Pelin Z, Kucukali C, et al. Creutzfeldt-Jakob disease. *Psychogeriatrics.* 2011;11(2):119–124.

68. Vallabh SM, Minikel EV, Schreiber SL, et al. Towards a treatment for genetic prion disease: trials and biomarkers. *Lancet Neurol.* 2020;19(4):361–368.

15

16 Pharmacotherapy of Substance Use Disorders

Mladen Nisavic

KEY POINTS

Incidence

- Problematic use of alcohol, opioids, and other substances is one of the leading causes of morbidity and mortality in the United States.

Epidemiology

- The highest rates of alcohol use, heavy binge use, and alcohol use disorders occur between the ages of 18 and 29 years and in men. Opioid use disorder (OUD) remains a public health crisis with more patients affected, as well as the higher rates of OUD-associated complications, overdoses, and deaths.

Prognosis

- Integrated treatment that is delivered in settings where both mental health and substance use disorders (SUDs) are treated will significantly improve outcomes.

Treatment Options

- Several effective pharmacological and psychosocial treatments exist for disorders related to the use of alcohol, opioids, and other substances that produce outcomes similar to or better than outcomes for other chronic illnesses.

Complications

- Unrecognized and untreated SUDs are associated with poor outcomes and treatment failure for co-occurring mental health disorders. Likewise, they contribute significantly to accidents, violence, medical morbidity, and mortality (primarily from drug overdoses).

OVERVIEW

The chronic, relapsing nature of substance use is erroneously thought to imply that treatment for patients with these disorders is futile or even unhelpful and commonly results in clinicians ignoring opportunities to intervene in the disease process. Most clinicians fail to appreciate that the relapse rate of other common chronic medical disorders (e.g., diabetes, hypertension, asthma) exceeds that for SUDs and that compared with other chronic conditions, response rates with treatment are comparable to if not superior to those of chronic medical conditions.[1]

Substance use is highly co-morbid with other psychiatric conditions, with nearly half of those with SUDs having a co-occurring psychiatric disorder.[2] Accordingly, it is essential for psychiatrists to be knowledgeable about safe and evidence-driven treatment strategies for SUDs.

Substance use is common across the United States. In 2020, the National Survey on Drug Use and Health found that 162.5 million Americans aged 12 years or older (accounting for 58.7% of the population) used tobacco, alcohol, or an illicit drug in the past month. This number included 50% (138.5 million individuals) who drank alcohol and 13.5% (37.3 million) who used illicit drugs.[2] Of the 138.5 million active alcohol users, 61.6 million engaged in binge drinking, and 17.7 million were heavy drinkers. Cannabis was the most commonly used illicit substance (with 49.6 million people reporting use in the past year). Past-year stimulant use was endorsed by 10.3 million individuals, and roughly 33% of this cohort used only cocaine, another 33% reported misusing prescription stimulant medications, and 15% endorsed using methamphetamine. Opioid (e.g., heroin, prescription pain medications) use was reported by 3.4% (9.5 million people), with most admitting to prescription pain reliever misuse (9.3 million people).[2]

During the past decade, the number of patients treated for substance–related problems in the United States has grown steadily. The top five drugs involved in drug-related emergency department (ED) visits in 2021 were alcohol (41.7%), opioids (14.8%), methamphetamine (11.3%), marijuana (11.12%), and cocaine (4.8%).[3] Fentanyl-related ED visits rose throughout 2021, peaking in the fourth quarter, which reflected the increasing availability of fentanyl in the communities at risk.

Disruption of the endogenous reward systems in the brain is a common feature of SUDs; in fact, most addictive drugs act as functional dopamine analogues in the nucleus accumbens–ventral tegmental area (NAcc–VTA) reward circuit. Whether through the direct effect of the drug (e.g., cocaine, amphetamines), or indirectly (opioids, alcohol), a common sequela of acute intoxication is an increase in synaptic availability of dopamine within circuits that mediate motivation and drive, conditioned learning, and inhibitory control participants (Figure 16.1). With chronic drug use comes long-lasting compensatory changes in the reward circuits (e.g., reduced dopamine availability and receptor density) and in the orbitofrontal cortex (salience attribution), the cingulate gyrus (inhibitory control and mood regulation), the amygdala (fear processing), and the hippocampus (memory). As a result, with chronic use, addiction becomes less about "seeking a high" and more about attempting to retrieve a state of relative normalcy. Those with SUDs require higher drug doses to obtain the same response (because of tolerance) and exhibit physiologically unpleasant reactions on drug discontinuation (because of dependence and withdrawal). Furthermore, patients with SUDs may exhibit a diminished response to other previously rewarding cues (e.g., food, sex, physical exercise) due to compensatory changes in the NAcc–VTA circuit. Chronic changes in the prefrontal cortex result in diminished ability to prioritize rational and safe behaviors, and context-based priming of the hippocampus and the amygdala may

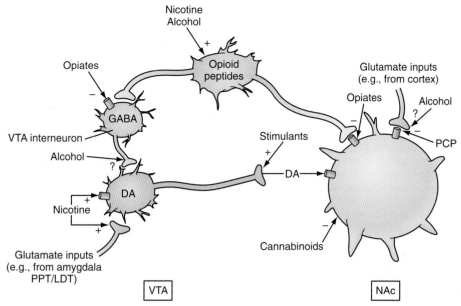

Figure 16.1 Converging acute actions of addictive drugs on the ventral tegmental area and nucleus accumbens. *DA*, Dopamine; *GABA*, gamma aminobutyric acid; *LDT*, laterodorsal tegmentum; *NAc*, nucleus accumbens; *PCP*, phencyclidine; *PPT*, pedunculopontine tegmentum; *VTA*, ventral tegmental area. (Redrawn from Nestler EJ. Is there a common molecular pathway for addiction? *Nat Neurosci*. 2005;8(11):1445–1449.)

contribute to the emergence of cravings when the individual is exposed to heightened emotional states, locations, or sensory cues that were previously associated with drug use.

ALCOHOL USE DISORDER AND RELATED CONDITIONS

Overview

Ethanol, often referred to as "man's oldest friend and oldest enemy," possesses a simple chemical structure (C_2H_5OH) that belies the complexities of its medical, psychological, and social impact. Recreational alcohol use is characterized by euphoria, disinhibition, anxiety reduction, and mild sedation. These effects commonly contribute to culturally sanctioned perceptions of alcohol as a means to relax and facilitate social endeavors. With increased use, however, acute alcohol intoxication develops and leads to behavioral disinhibition, impairments in memory and executive function, and motor and coordination deficits. With severe use, alcohol-induced amnesia ("blackouts"), coma, and even death can occur.[4]

Beyond the effects of acute intoxication, alcohol can result in direct toxicity of multiple organ systems, including the central nervous system (CNS), heart, kidneys, and liver.[5] Although these complications are commonly associated with heavy or chronic use, individuals who infrequently binge drink can develop life-threatening alcoholic hepatitis as a result of acute toxicity or present with an alcohol-associated cancer diagnosis[6] (Figure 16.2). Alcohol use is an important risk factor for development of cancers of the esophagus and liver, heart disease, cirrhosis, and end-stage liver disease. Alcohol is also strongly associated with violent behavior and aggression, homicide, falls and trauma, and motor vehicle accidents (MVAs).[7] Not surprisingly, alcohol consumption is a significant cause of death in the United States, accounting for approximately 100,000 deaths annually, and it is a source of considerable financial burden, estimated at $224 billion annually in United States alone.[8–10]

Effects of high-risk drinking

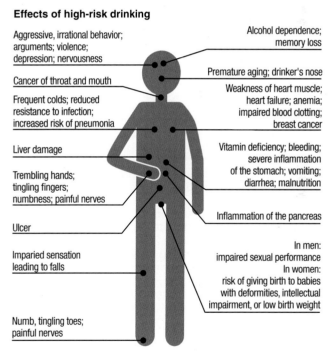

Aggressive, irrational behavior; arguments; violence; depression; nervousness

Cancer of throat and mouth

Frequent colds; reduced resistance to infection; increased risk of pneumonia

Liver damage

Trembling hands; tingling fingers; numbness; painful nerves

Ulcer

Imparied sensation leading to falls

Numb, tingling toes; painful nerves

Alcohol dependence; memory loss

Premature aging; drinker's nose

Weakness of heart muscle; heart failure; anemia; impaired blood clotting; breast cancer

Vitamin deficiency; bleeding; severe inflammation of the stomach; vomiting; diarrhea; malnutrition

Inflammation of the pancreas

In men: impaired sexual performance
In women: risk of giving birth to babies with deformities, intellectual impairment, or low birth weight

Figure 16.2 Alcohol-related disorders associated with high-risk drinking. (From Rehm J, Room R, Monteiro M, et al. Alcohol use. In: Ezzati M, Lopez AD, Rodgers A, Murray CJL, eds. Comparative Quantification of Health Risks: Global and Regional Burden of Disease Attributable to Selected Major Risk Factors. World Health Organization; 2004.)

Finally, with persisting heavy alcohol use, individuals are at risk for developing alcohol use disorder (AUD), in which continued drinking despite growing medical and social consequences can exact a considerable toll on patients' lives (including financial problems, family disintegration, loss of employment, and an increased risk of medical complications). In the United States, an estimated 18 million individuals meet criteria for an active AUD. Not surprisingly, these individuals have a considerably higher risk of developing alcohol-related complications, including neurocognitive sequelae secondary to alcohol toxicity. It is estimated that some degree of impairment in cognitive or motor processes is observed in half of all patients who meet criteria for an AUD, and up to 2 million US adults will require lifelong supportive care because of alcohol-induced CNS damage.[11,12]

Integral to all these pathways to harm is the volume and frequency of alcohol consumption. Low-risk consumption is defined as 14 drinks or fewer per week and 1 to 2 drinks or fewer per day for men aged 21 to 65 years. For men older than 65 years of age and for women (regardless of their age) low-risk consumption is defined as 7 drinks or fewer in any given week and 1 drink or fewer per day.[13]

Pathophysiology of Alcohol Use

Understanding the complexity of the CNS regions adversely impacted by alcohol use is central to the understanding of the pathophysiologic effects of ethanol. The cerebral cortex (including the dorsolateral and orbitofrontal cortex) and subcortical areas, including the limbic system (e.g., amygdala), thalamus, hypothalamus, and hippocampus (that are involved with learning and memory), are the key brain regions susceptible to alcohol-related damage. Areas that influence posture and movement, such as the cerebellum, are likewise affected frequently.[14–18] Loss of prefrontal cortex volume, an area that is normally necessary for planning, problem-solving, and behavioral regulation, is associated with increased rates of impulsivity and susceptibility to alcohol relapse.[19–21] Hippocampal toxicity may have a direct impact on memory storage and retrieval and may augment the damage caused by deficiencies of vitamins and other micronutrients associated with chronic use. Furthermore, the neurotoxic effects of alcohol may be exacerbated by an individual's poor cardiovascular care and by a higher incidence of head trauma (including falls, being a victim of violence, and MVAs).

Most symptoms of acute alcohol intoxication—increased euphoria, disinhibition, anxiety reduction, and sedation—reflect the effects of alcohol on the gamma aminobutyric acid (GABA) and glutamate neurotransmitter systems. GABA is the major inhibitory neurotransmitter, and acute alcohol ingestion has direct pro-GABAergic, CNS-depressant effects that result in the signs and symptoms of intoxication. With chronic use, the CNS attempts to down-regulate endogenous GABA activity (e.g., through reduction in GABA receptors) to balance the exogenous pro-GABA effects of alcohol, thus contributing to the emergence of tolerance. Chronic alcohol consumption likewise impacts glutamate receptor availability and leads to an increase in glutaminergic CNS activity, again an attempt to counter-balance increased exogenous GABAergic input. Alcohol withdrawal is a syndrome of CNS hyperexcitation that occurs when sudden cessation or dose reduction of alcohol use results in decreased inhibitory exogenous GABAergic tone and increased endogenous glutaminergic tone caused by a relative glutamate–GABA imbalance associated with chronic use.[22] Given the degree of impact on the two most common CNS neurotransmitters, it is not surprising that the effects of alcohol will (directly or indirectly) impact other neurotransmitter systems, including serotonin, endorphins, and dopamine.[23–26] The extent to which these monoamine neurotransmitter systems become implicated may contribute toward the heterogeneity of alcohol withdrawal syndrome. Furthermore, alcohol-related dopamine increases in the NAcc–VTA circuit have been linked with euphoric and rewarding effects associated with alcohol use.[27]

Alcohol Use Disorder

AUD has been re-classified in the *Diagnostic and Statistical Manual of Mental Disorders*, Fifth Edition (DSM-5), into an 11-item category that was constructed by combining three of the four former "abuse" criteria (repeated legal consequences was dropped) with the seven "alcohol dependence" criteria specified in the Fourth Edition (DSM-IV) and by adding a new "craving" criterion.[28] Only 2 of the 11 symptoms are required to meet a diagnostic threshold in the DSM-5; this highlights a degree of heterogeneity within the syndrome that has both typological and clinical implications for diagnosis and treatment. The DSM-5 criteria include a problematic pattern of alcohol use leading to significant impairment or distress; with alcohol often taken in larger amounts or over a longer period than was intended; with a persistent desire or unsuccessful efforts to cut down or to control alcohol use; with a great amount of time spent on activities necessary to obtain or use alcohol or recovery from its effects; with craving to use alcohol; with recurrent alcohol use resulting in a failure to fulfill major role obligations at work, school, or home; with continued alcohol use despite having persistent or recurrent social or interpersonal problems caused or exacerbated by the effects of alcohol; with important social, occupational, or recreational activities given up or reduced because of alcohol use; with recurrent alcohol use in situations in which it is physically hazardous; with ongoing alcohol use despite knowledge of having a persistent or recurrent physical or psychological problem that is likely to have been caused or exacerbated by alcohol; with tolerance, as defined by a need for increased amounts of alcohol to achieve intoxication or its desired effect, or by a markedly diminished effect with continued use of the same amount of alcohol; and with withdrawal.

First described in the 1970s as alcohol dependence syndrome, AUD is conceptualized as an integration of physiological and psychological processes that leads to a pattern of heavy alcohol use that is increasingly unresponsive to external circumstances or to adverse consequences.[29] The syndrome is characterized by neuroadaptation to chronic alcohol use (tolerance and withdrawal) and by an impaired ability to alter or to stop alcohol consumption despite the personal suffering it causes (impaired control over use). The syndrome is not an all-or-nothing phenomenon; instead, it occurs with graded intensity, and its presentation is often influenced by personality, as well as by social and cultural contexts.

The term *alcoholism* was originally coined to describe alcohol addiction and continues to have considerable colloquial use. As with terms *abuse* and *dependence*, this terminology is antiquated and largely stigmatizing; therefore, we encourage using the term AUD in all clinical settings.

Etiology and Epidemiology of Alcohol Use Disorder

Understanding epidemiology and etiology of AUD can help us better understand the heterogeneity of patient experiences and thus inform clinical assessment, prevention, and treatment strategies. Genetic and other biological factors, along with cognitive, behavioral, and sociocultural factors, are all involved in the emergence of AUD.[30] Genes confer at least four separate domains of risk: alcohol metabolizing enzymes (e.g., the functional genetic variants of alcohol dehydrogenase that demonstrate high alcohol-oxidizing activity and the genetic variant of aldehyde dehydrogenase that has low acetaldehyde-oxidizing activity, protect against heavy drinking and alcoholism), impulsivity and disinhibition (e.g., dopaminergic *DRD2* genes), psychiatric disorders (e.g., the miRNA biogenesis pathway), and individual level of response to alcohol.[31-34] Genetic heritability for alcohol dependence is commonly estimated at approximately 50%, with the other 50% attributable to environmental causes.

Factors that influence the initiation of alcohol consumption should be distinguished from those that affect patterns of consumption once drinking has been initiated. Studies of adolescent twins have demonstrated that initiation of drinking is primarily influenced by cultural factors, including the drinking status of parents, siblings, and peers, as well as by environmental variation across geographical regions.[35-37] Conversely, after being initiated, progression to AUD is strongly influenced by genetic factors, although these influences continue to be modulated by family- and peer-context effects and by environmental variation.[38] Pedigree, twin, and adoption studies all point to an increased risk for AUD in offspring when there is a history of alcohol and substance use in the family.[39] For example, a positive family history of AUD may result in a four-fold increased risk for developing the disorder, especially in individuals with multiple close relatives with AUD.[40]

Rates of alcohol use and AUD vary along several dimensions, including gender, life stage, ethnicity, geographic location, social context (e.g., college setting), and presence of psychiatric co-morbidity. Men have higher rates of AUD (12.4%) than women (4.9%). Likewise, AUD rates are higher among 18- to 29-year-olds (16.2%) and lowest among individuals 65 years and older (1.5%).[3] Under-age drinking is a major public health problem in its own right, with about 11 million (28.7%) individuals aged 12 to 20 years reporting past-month alcohol use and 10 million disclosing heavy or binge use.[2] Heavy drinking in this age group is a significant risk factor for unwanted complications, including MVAs, trauma, violence, and unwanted pregnancies; therefore, screening for alcohol use in adolescents and teenagers should be routine. Early exposure to alcohol is a significant independent risk factor for developing AUD. The National Epidemiologic Survey on Alcohol and Related Conditions (NESARC) showed that individuals who began drinking before age 14 years had a significantly increased chance of developing AUD at some point in their life (47% vs 9%) as compared with individuals who began drinking after age 20 years.[41] In the United States, Whites and persons reporting two or more races are more likely to report current alcohol use compared with other ethnic groups.[2] An estimated 55% of Whites and 52% of persons reporting two or more races used alcohol in the past month, compared with 40% of Hispanics, 37% of Asians, 37% of African Americans, and 36% of American Indians or Alaska Natives. Problem drinking and AUD rates likewise vary with ethnicity with the highest 12-month prevalence noted among Native Americans and Alaska Natives (12.1%) followed by Whites (8.9%), Hispanics (7.9%), African Americans (6.9%), and Asian and Pacific Islanders (4.5%).

Alcohol Use Disorder and Co-occurring Psychiatric Illness

The co-morbidity of AUD with other psychiatric disorders has been widely recognized.[42] The most common life-time occurrences of psychiatric disorders for individuals with AUD are anxiety disorders (47%), other SUDs (43%), and affective disorders (41%); these are followed by conduct (32%) and antisocial personality disorder (13%). There is a moderately strong correlation between the severity of mental illness and the prevalence of AUD.[42] There are several possible explanations for these co-occurrences: both conditions may be caused by a common pathway (e.g., a genetic predisposition), one

disorder may substantially influence the onset of the other (e.g., an individual uses alcohol to cope with psychiatric distress), or there are methodological determinants (e.g., unmeasured common causes or selection biases in clinical studies).

The interplay of alcohol use and behavioral determinants is often observed in clinical settings and can result in diagnostic challenges and have an impact on treatment considerations and the overall prognosis. Because acute intoxication or withdrawal can closely resemble symptoms of a primary mood or anxiety disorder, it is the prerogative of the evaluating clinician to screen for, diagnose, and offer treatment for any co-morbid non–substance-related mental health syndromes. Historically labeled "dual diagnosis," patients with co-occurring addictions and behavioral health conditions may not respond as readily to standard addiction care, leading to greater rates of relapse, attrition, and re-admissions. Teachings have encouraged a sequential approach to treatment, commencing with addiction, which practically resulted in "dual diagnosis" patients being allocated to treatment through specialized addiction programs, often with minimal attention paid to their other mental health needs. This approach has since been shown to be ineffective. Instead, we recommend attending to both disorders simultaneously; whether it is medication-based therapy, counseling, or peer support, there is now robust evidence that concurrent management of addiction and primary mood and anxiety disorders is associated with optimal outcomes.[43,44]

It is important to note that any generalizations about "dual diagnosis" patients should be made with caution. The term obviously covers an immense amount of clinical territory because it covers the presence of an alcohol or other SUD, which are heterogeneous and vary greatly in severity but also covers a vast array of psychopathological disturbances, each with its own sub-variations and degrees of severity. Thus, the specific type, severity, and relative clinical significance of the co-morbid psychiatric disorder on the patient's presentation and future function should always be considered when approaching these dual problems.[45,46]

Typologies and Classifications of Alcohol Use Disorder

Various typologies have been proposed over the past 50 years to better classify the heterogeneous syndrome of AUD. Early typologies relied largely on theoretically framed clinical observations. More recently, data-driven, multi-variate sub-classifications have been derived that have etiological significance, predictive validity, and potential clinical utility.

One of the first and most well-known was Jellinek's typology of five subspecies of "alcoholism" labeled using the letters of the Greek alphabet: alpha, beta, delta, gamma, epsilon.[47] This typology was not successfully validated, but it highlighted the importance of heterogeneity of the syndrome and sparked further interest in the topic. Cloninger's type I/type II and Babor's type A/B typologies followed. Cloninger and colleagues[48] described two forms of alcohol use based on differences in alcohol-related symptoms, patterns of transmission, and personality characteristics using data derived from a cross-fostering study of Swedish adoptees. Type I was characterized by either mild or severe alcohol use in the probands and no criminality in the fathers. These individuals came from relatively high socioeconomic backgrounds; showed higher rates of maternal alcohol use; and were thought to be more responsive to environmental influence, to have milder alcohol-related problems, and to show a later age of onset (older than 25 years) of drinking. On the other hand, Cloninger's type II was characterized as being associated with a family history of alcohol use, more severe alcohol-related problems, other drug use, and an early onset (before age 25 years). Although multi-variate statistical methods were used to identify subtypes, Cloninger's classification has since been criticized because of its small sample sizes (<200), selection methods, and indirect assessment of family variables.[49]

A second typology was proposed by Babor and colleagues[50] based on a sample of 321 inpatients with AUD. Type A resembled Cloninger's type I and was characterized by a later age of onset, fewer childhood behavior problems, and less psychopathology. Type B resembled Cloninger's type II and was defined by a high prevalence of childhood behavior or conduct problems, a family history of alcohol use, early onset of alcohol use, more severe psychopathology, and higher rates of treatment resistance. Across these classifications, a broad distinction of early- versus late-onset alcohol use emerges, which may have some clinical utility, although its overall evidence remains limited.

More recent multi-variate, multi-dimensional analyses have revealed that there may be as many as four general, homogeneous subtypes of AUD: chronic or severe, depressed or anxious, mildly affected, and antisocial.[51,52] These four subtypes are found within both genders and across different ethnic subgroups, but more prospective research is needed to examine their relative clinical course and responsiveness to various pharmacological and psychosocial interventions. Using data from the NESARC, Moss and colleagues[53] described five subtypes of alcohol use, distinguished by family history, age of dependence onset, endorsement of DSM-IV AUD criteria, and the presence of co-morbid psychiatric and SUDs. These general population-derived subtypes await further study, but they may enhance our understanding of the etiology and natural history of AUD and lead to improved and more targeted treatment interventions.

Screening for Problem Drinking and Alcohol Use Disorder

Given the extent of alcohol use in the United States, routine screening for problematic alcohol use and AUD should be a standard practice in all clinical settings. There are brief and effective screening measures that can yield high rates of detection, and importantly, even a brief, compassionate discussion by a clinician can yield a measurable impact on the extent and severity of a patient's alcohol use (Figure 16.3).[54,55]

The National Institute on Alcohol Abuse and Alcoholism has recommended either the use of a single alcohol screening question (SASQ) or administration of the Alcohol Use Disorders Identification Test (AUDIT) self-report questionnaire as standard screening procedures for the detection of alcohol-related problems. The AUDIT (Table 16.1) screen is readily available and has been validated across a variety of cultural and ethnic groups. When using the SASQ, clinicians are advised to ask if an individual has consumed a threshold number of standard drinks on any one occasion during the past year (four for women, five for men). A positive response may signal the presence of an alcohol-related problem and requires further assessment. When even more brevity is required because of time constraints, a shorter three-item version of the AUDIT called the AUDIT-C can be used. It includes only the first three AUDIT items (i.e., the three "Consumption" items; hence the "C"), and has comparable sensitivity and specificity as the full 10-item AUDIT with a cut-off score of 4 or more for a man and 3 or more for a woman.[55] Compared with the SASQ, AUDIT, or AUDIT-C, the often-used cutting down, annoyance by criticism, feeling guilty, and eye-opener (CAGE) questionnaire may lack sensitivity to detect hazardous or problem drinking, though its simplicity has potential benefits in busy clinical settings.

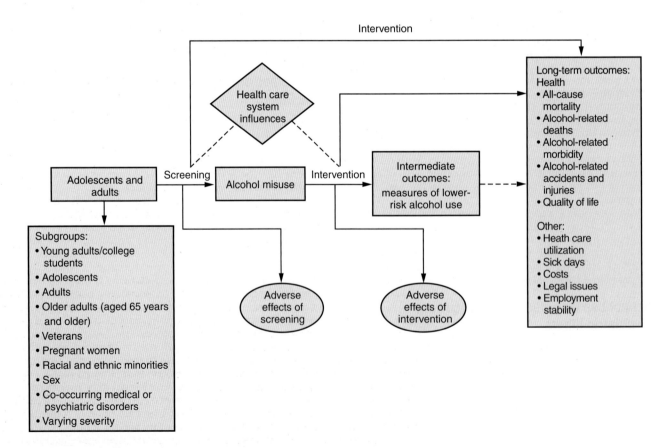

Figure 16.3 Screening and assessment process. (From Jonas DE, Garbutt JC, Brown JM, et al. *Screening, Behavioral Counseling, and Referral in Primary Care to Reduce Alcohol Use.* Agency for Health Research and Quality; 2012.)

TABLE 16.1 The AUDIT/AUDIT-C (IN BOX) for Alcohol Screening[a]

Patient: Because alcohol use can affect your health and can interfere with certain medications and treatments, it is important that we ask some questions about your use of alcohol. Your answers will remain confidential so please be honest. Place an X in one box that best describes your answer to each question.

Questions	0	1	2	3	4	Score
How often do you have a drink containing alcohol?	Never	Monthly or less	2 to 4 times a month	2 to 3 times a week	4 or more times a week	
How many drinks containing alcohol do you have on a typical day when you are drinking?	1 or 2	3 or 4	5 or 6	7 to 9	10 or more	
How often do you have five or more drinks on one occasion?	Never	Less than monthly	Monthly	Weekly	Daily or almost daily	
How often during the past year have you found that you were not able to stop drinking after you had started?	Never	Less than monthly	Monthly	Weekly	Daily or almost daily	
How often during the past year have you failed to do what was normally expected of you because of drinking?	Never	Less than monthly	Monthly	Weekly	Daily or almost daily	
How often during the past year have you needed a first drink in the morning to get yourself going after a heavy drinking session?	Never	Less than monthly	Monthly	Weekly	Daily or almost daily	
How often during the past year have you had a feeling of guilt or remorse after drinking?	Never	Less than monthly	Monthly	Weekly	Daily or almost daily	
How often during the past year have you been unable to remember what happened the night before because of your drinking?	Never	Less than monthly	Monthly	Weekly	Daily or almost daily	
Have you or someone else been injured because of your drinking?	No		Yes, but not in the past year		Yes, during the past year	
Has a relative, friend, doctor, or other health care worker been concerned about your drinking or suggested you cut down?	No		Yes, but not in the past year		Yes, during the past year	
Total:						

[a]This self-report questionnaire (the Alcohol Use Disorders Identification Test [AUDIT]) is from the World Health Organization. To reflect standard drink sizes in the United States, the number of drinks in question 3 was changed from 6 to 5. A free AUDIT manual with guidelines for use in primary care is available online at http://www.who.org.
Information from Reinert DF, Allen JP. The alcohol use disorders identification test: an update of research findings. *Alcohol Clin Exp Res.* 2007;31(2):185–199 and Bradley KA, DeBenedetti AF, Volk RJ, et al. AUDIT-C as a brief screen for alcohol misuse in primary care. *Alcohol Clin Exp Res.* 2007;31(7):1208–1217.

For adolescents, the CRAFFT screen is recommended. As with other screening tools, the title is an acronym for having ever ridden in a *car* driven by someone who had been using alcohol or drugs; ever used alcohol or drugs to *relax*, feel better about oneself, or fit in; ever used alcohol or drugs *alone*; ever *forgot* things because of using alcohol or drugs; ever had *family* or *friends* recommend cutting down on drinking or drug use; and ever gotten into *trouble* while using alcohol or drugs. These questions have excellent sensitivity and specificity.[56] One point is given for each endorsed item, and a score of 2 or more is indicative of a potential AUD that requires further assessment.

Medical biomarker screens may also prove useful, especially if there is concern that the patient may be deliberately minimizing the extent of alcohol use. Active or recent use can be detected with a Breathalyzer or by testing a sample of patient's urine or saliva for alcohol. To assess for chronic use, other laboratory markers can be used, including serum γ-glutamyl transpeptidase, mean corpuscular volume, and percent carbohydrate-deficient transferrin.[57–59] Although often non-specific, elevation in these markers may be indicative of consistent heavy use over time. Ethyl glucuronide is a direct metabolite of alcohol that can be detected in the urine up to 7 days after alcohol consumption.[57–59] Although excellent in detecting chronic use, this screen may yield false-positive results from incidental exposures (including mouthwash, foods prepared with alcohol, hand sanitizers, and over-the-counter medications). Phosphatidyl ethanol can be detected for up to 12 days after a single drinking event and can be an excellent tool to monitor abstinence.

Treatment for Alcohol Use Disorders

Given the significant variability in the extent of alcohol use across the population, as well as different ways in which alcohol can impact patients' lives, it should be no surprise that several treatment options exist for managing AUD.[2,60–63] As with other SUDs, the heterogeneity of AUD implies that there is no "one size fits all" treatment; instead, a wide array of empirically based, effective treatments should be considered when approaching patients with AUD who are in need of assistance. These interventions can range from brief supportive counseling by the patient's primary care provider (PCP) to more extensive individual and group-based psychosocial interventions to peer support (e.g., recovery coaching, Alcoholics Anonymous [AA], self-management and recovery training [SMART] recovery) or pharmacological interventions to minimize cravings and relapse risk.[60–63]

Brief Counseling Interventions for Alcohol Use

A concerned and focused assessment with brief advice by a health care provider can make a meaningful difference on a patient's drinking habits. Generally recommended for patients who drink problematically but who may not meet other criteria for AUD, these interventions often aim to reduce or moderate drinking rather than result in total abstinence.[63-65] Brief interventions are generally limited to four or fewer sessions, can last from a few minutes to 1 hour each, and are designed to be conducted by all clinicians (not necessarily specialized in addiction).[66] Research indicates that brief interventions for AUD are more effective than no intervention and, in some cases, can be as effective as more extensive intervention.[67-70]

Capitalizing on these findings and to expand access to treatment for alcohol-related problems, the Center for Substance Abuse Treatment has devised an initiative known as "Screening, Brief Intervention, Referral, and Treatment" (SBIRT). Rejecting the notion that only people meeting criteria for AUD need targeted interventions, SBIRT assumes that everyone, regardless of their current level of alcohol consumption, can benefit from learning the facts about safe alcohol consumption and knowing how their own usage compares to accepted limits. Using the AUDIT or AUDIT-C as a screening device, front-line clinicians in any setting can assess for alcohol-related problems quickly and easily. SBIRT triage guidelines provide recommendations along the lines of an individual's alcohol involvement. Simple clinical advice to cut down or stop is recommended if someone scores between 7 and 16 on the AUDIT; multiple sessions of brief treatment and monitoring are recommended if an individual scores between 16 and 19 (or has consumed alcohol to intoxication five or more days per month, as disclosed on a screening interview); and last if an individual scores 20 or more on the AUDIT, a referral for more intensive assessment and treatment is recommended.[71]

What is it about brief interventions that make them effective? After reviewing the key ingredients in a variety of brief intervention protocols, Miller and Sanchez[69] proposed six critical elements that they summarized with the acronym FRAMES: feedback, responsibility, advice, menu, empathy, and self-efficacy. The clinician completes assessment and provides *feedback* on the patient's alcohol-related problems ("Your results show"), stresses the patient's *responsibility* to address the problem ("It's your choice"); gives clear *advice* to change drinking behavior ("I would recommend that you cut down or stop"), provides a *menu* of treatment strategies ("There a several things you might do"), expresses *empathy* for the patient's problem ("This can be difficult to hear, and making changes is not always easy"), and stresses *self-efficacy* ("However, it is quite possible for you to achieve this"). The expectation is that the patient may already have some of the skills needed to successfully resolve their drinking problem. Additional components of goal-setting, follow-up, and timing have also been identified as important to the efficacy of brief interventions.[70] Although non-specialist clinicians, such as PCPs, can have an impact on patients who show at-risk drinking through brief intervention, patients may experience better outcomes when seen by clinicians specifically trained in addiction,[72-74] perhaps because of their more specific education and training. Given the relative paucity of addiction-trained specialists nationwide, especially when considering the sheer numbers of US adults with problematic drinking, we recommend that all providers learn some of these strategies; the impact on their patients' well-being may be considerable.

Intensive Interventions for Alcohol Use

Three broad elements are important for prolonged recovery from AUD or other SUDs: de-conditioning, skills training, and cognitive re-structuring.[75] There is a broad array of evidence-based interventions that address these critical elements. Some of these include Twelve-Step Facilitation (TSF), a professional therapy designed to engage patients and support long-term involvement in the fellowship of AA; motivational enhancement therapy, an intervention based on the principles

of motivational interviewing; a variety of cognitive-behavioral approaches, such as the Community Reinforcement Approach, designed to engage multiple therapeutic elements in the community; interpersonal system-based interventions, such as behavioral marital therapy and family therapies; and pharmacotherapies (e.g., naltrexone, acamprosate) targeting the reinforcing effects of alcohol use.[76-85]

Despite vastly differing theoretical assumptions regarding the specifics of treatment content and for how long, at what intensity, and by whom the treatment should be delivered, comparisons of the relative efficacy of active treatments reveal surprisingly similar effects, suggesting that they may all mobilize common change processes in patients. However, it seems clear that the *duration* and *continuity* of care are linked to treatment outcome rather than amount or intensity.[82] Consequently, there have been recent shifts from intensive short-term inpatient service models toward longitudinal outpatient models of addiction recovery management that more closely reflect the chronic relapse–remission nature of SUDs.[86,87] Furthermore, in recent years, there has been an increasing recognition of the importance of a non-stigmatizing, patient-centered, and empathic approach to delivering addiction care, which is a shift from a moralistic and often prejudiced approach used throughout the 1990s. In fact, there is now a growing recognition that the traditional confrontational engagement may only increase the patient's resistance to seeking treatment.[87]

Emanating from the brief intervention literature and humanistic psychology, motivational interviewing (MI) has been shown to be an important and effective way to interact with patients with a range of alcohol problems. It has been defined as a patient-centered, yet directive, method for enhancing intrinsic motivation to change by exploring and resolving patient ambivalence.[70] This approach has been shown to be helpful for many patients and can be used as a stand-alone approach, as well as in-tandem with other interventions[83] (Table 16.2). MI reinforces the importance of avoiding arguments with the patient, teaches us to "roll with resistance" (e.g., trying to understand the patient's frame of reference), helps the provider develop discrepancies between the patient's values and behaviors observed, supports the patient's self-efficacy and confidence to achieve the desired outcome, and helps the provider to deliver empathic care to the patient. There are four main processes of MI: engaging (establishing a helpful connection and working relationship), focusing (developing and maintaining specific direction in the conversation about change), evoking (eliciting the patients' own motives about change), and planning (developing commitment to change and forming a specific action plan to change).[73]

Although addiction is traditionally perceived as "impossible to fix," which leads to provider and patient burnout and frustration, this could not be further from the truth. Multiple studies show that the clinical outcomes of patients with addiction are similar to those with other chronic diseases.[87] For example, 40% to 60% of patients treated for an AUD remain

TABLE 16.2 Motivational Interviewing Processes	
Engaging	Establishing a helpful connection and working relationship
Focusing	Developing and maintaining specific direction in the conversation about change
Evoking	Eliciting the patient's own motives about change
Planning	Developing commitment to change and forming a specific action plan to change

From Miller WR, Rollnick S. *Motivational Interviewing: Helping People Change.* 3rd ed. Guilford Press; 2012.

in remission after 1 year, and another 15% maintain clinically meaningful improvement in their alcohol use problems; remission rates are comparable to those seen with asthma, high blood pressure, or diabetes.[88] Although full remission and recovery can take years to achieve and patients may require more than one attempt at stopping,[89] full sustained remission is the likely final outcome for most of patients with AUD.[90] Consequently, we believe that AUD can be a good prognosis disorder as long as adequate monitoring, patient-centered management, and access to appropriate resources and re-intervention, whenever necessary, are in place.

Pharmacological Interventions for Alcohol Use Disorder

Three medications have been approved by the Food and Drug Administration (FDA) for the treatment of AUD: disulfiram (approved in 1947), naltrexone (approved as an oral formulation in 1994 with the long-acting injectable formulation approved in 2006), and acamprosate (approved in 2004) (Table 16.3). Although without formal FDA approval, other medications (gabapentin and topiramate) have likewise been used in clinical settings for longitudinal management of AUD.

Disulfiram inhibits acetaldehyde dehydrogenase, leading to a build-up of the ethanol metabolite acetaldehyde and associated symptoms of flushing, hypotension, headache, nausea, and vomiting. These symptoms are uncomfortable; thus, through negative reinforcement, the patient is discouraged from drinking while taking the medication. Although theoretically promising, the practical effectiveness of disulfiram is compromised by poor compliance and considerable side effects (including cardiovascular complications and rare hepatotoxicity). Accordingly, unless the patient is strongly and specifically motivated to take this medication or their compliance is externally monitored or enforced, we recommend *against* use of disulfiram because considerably safer alternatives exist.

The opioid antagonist naltrexone has helped to reduce the number of drinking days presumably through its inhibitory effect on the CNS reward pathways.[91,92] The medication is generally safe with minimal drug–drug interactions or significant side effects, and it can be administered orally as well as intramuscularly. Patients should be followed for a change in liver enzymes (reversible with naltrexone discontinuation) and advised against taking opioid agonists while taking this agent. Naltrexone may be more effective in those with a strong family history of AUD and in individuals with the *OPRM1* genotype.[93]

Acamprosate is thought to act primarily at glutamate *N*-methyl-d-aspartate (NMDA) receptors by moderating symptoms related to prolonged alcohol withdrawal and mitigating cravings and intent to use. It may be preferred for those with significant liver damage given its predominantly renal metabolism, and it is generally well-tolerated with few drug interactions or side effects. The primary challenge with acamprosate administration comes from its dosing (three times per day).

Other agents, including the anticonvulsants topiramate and gabapentin, have been used off-label for mitigating the cravings and relapse to drinking with some success. They appear to have similar efficacy to the FDA-approved agents already discussed, and they may be of benefit in specific clinical settings (e.g., because patients with concurrent cocaine and alcohol use can derive benefit for both conditions from taking topiramate).[94,95]

Long-Term Supports for Alcohol Use Disorder

As with other chronic illnesses, relapses can occur during or after successful treatment episodes. Hence, patients may require prolonged treatment and multiple episodes of care to achieve long-term abstinence and fully restored function. Participation in mutual-help organizations, such as AA, SMART Recovery, Secular Organization for Sobriety, and Women for Sobriety, is often helpful to many patients and can be an inexpensive adjunct to conventional addiction care.[96-104]

Compared with conventional interventions, AA and SMART recovery are often more accessible and flexible, with meetings held several times a day in many communities, allowing for more choices for the patient. AA members always make themselves available to their peers, providing a degree of flexibility not seen in professional settings. This degree of availability means that peer support is self-adaptive: patients can access resources at times of high relapse risk (e.g., unstructured time, evenings, and weekends) or whenever they feel they need it. Furthermore, it provides recovery-specific experience and support, with members serving as role models. AA meeting formats also provide continuing reminders of past negative experiences and the positive benefits of staying sober that help maintain and enhance recovery momentum.[105] AA also possesses a low threshold for entry, with no paperwork or third-party insurance approval, and AA can be attended free of charge for as long as individuals desire, making it a highly cost-effective public health resource. Studies with adults and adolescents reveal that participation in AA can enhance recovery outcomes and remission rates while simultaneously and substantially reducing health care costs.[105,106]

Figure 16.4 illustrates the relationship between common high-risk precursors to relapse and how mutual-help organizations (MHOs), such as AA, might attenuate this risk through facilitating changes in social networks, psychological factors (e.g., enhancing coping, abstinence self-efficacy, motivation for abstinence), and bio- and neurobiological factors.[107]

Empirically, there have now been rigorous scientific studies conducted on how exactly MHOs, like AA, confer recovery benefits. These studies suggest that the main ways that AA aids remission and recovery is through facilitating changes in the social networks of attendees and by boosting abstinence self-efficacy and coping and by maintaining abstinence motivation.[108,109]

TABLE 16.3 Pharmacological Treatments for Alcohol Use Disorder

Drug (Trade Name)	Pharmacokinetics and Pharmacodynamics	Effects
Disulfiram (Antabuse)	Inhibits acetaldehyde dehydrogenase, leading to a build-up of acetaldehyde	Produces undesirable consequences when alcohol is consumed, including flushing, palpitations, nausea, vomiting, and headache
Naltrexone (ReVia, Long acting = Vivitrol)	μ-Opioid receptor antagonist	Reduces the reinforcement and euphoria produced by alcohol
Acamprosate	Antagonist at glutamatergic NMDA receptors and agonist at GABA type A receptors	Reduces alcohol cravings

GABA, Gamma aminobutyric acid; *NMDA*, N-methyl-D-aspartate.

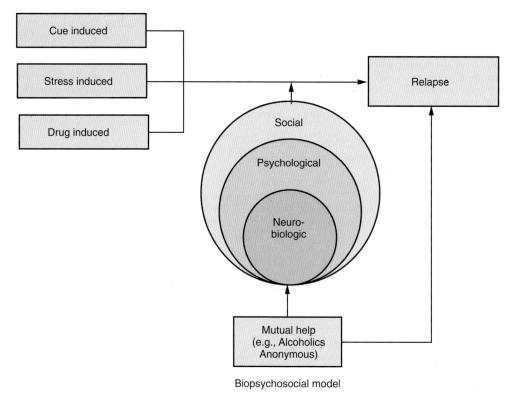

Biopsychosocial model

Figure 16.4 Biopsychosocial model of how mutual help organizations, such as Alcoholics Anonymous, may attenuate relapse risk over time. (From Kelly JF, Yeterian JD. Mutual-help groups for alcohol and other substance use disorders. In: McCrady BS, Epstein EE, eds. *Addictions: A Comprehensive Guidebook*. 2nd ed. Oxford University Press; 2013.)

Acute Alcohol Intoxication

Even though the effect of alcohol on the brain is complex, in the absence of significant tolerance, there is generally a predictable correlation between the blood alcohol level (BAL) and the behavior observed. Whereas lower BALs are usually associated with euphoria, mild disinhibition, and inattentiveness, argumentativeness and assaultive behavior develop at 0.1% to 0.19% BAL and growing sedation and impairment in memory (blackouts) at 0.2% to 0.3% BAL. Severe complications of acute intoxication, including over-sedation, coma, or death are usually noted at 0.40% to 0.50% BAL. In the absence of significant hepatic impairment, resolution of intoxication follows steady-state kinetics: a 70-kg man tends to metabolize 10 mL of ethanol per hour (10 mL = 1.5–2 drink equivalents; 1 standard drink = 0.5 oz of whiskey, 4 oz of wine, or 12 oz of beer) (Figure 16.5).

For most individuals, treatment of acute intoxication is largely supportive and focused on providing a safe and comfortable environment for patients to recover and minimizing risk for unintended harm. In a medically hospitalized patient, the latter should include aspiration and fall precautions, minimization of non-essential interventions, and even one-on-one observation if the patient requires frequent re-direction. If agitation is unresponsive to supportive measures or redirection, different medications can be used to prevent unintended self-harm or harm to others. Oral medications should be always offered first, with intravenous (IV) or intramuscular (IM) options reserved for cases of severe agitation. We recommend against use of benzodiazepines or barbiturates to manage agitation in a patient with acute alcohol intoxication; these agents may increase the risk of over-sedation and aspiration, as well as potentiate intoxication and thus contribute to worsening delirium and disinhibition. Neuroleptics can be administered orally (e.g., quetiapine or olanzapine), intramuscularly (e.g.,

olanzapine), or intravenously (e.g., haloperidol) and present a safe and versatile choice in an acutely intoxicated patient who presents with significant agitation.

Alcohol Withdrawal Syndrome

Alcohol withdrawal syndrome (AWS) can vary from mild discomfort that requires no treatment to a potentially life-threatening condition involving seizures, delirium, and multi-organ failure requiring intensive care. Reassuringly, uncomplicated withdrawal is common, with more than 90% of patients with AUD requiring nothing more than supportive treatment on cessation of use.[110] Unsurprisingly, the rates of AWS and associated complications are considerably higher in medically hospitalized patients.

In most cases, symptoms of alcohol withdrawal emerge within hours and resolve after 3 to 5 days. A hallmark symptom is generalized tremor (fast in frequency and more pronounced when the patient is under stress), and patients may otherwise complain of irritability and insomnia. Alcohol withdrawal seizures occur in roughly 1% of patients in alcohol withdrawal, although the prevalence is increased in individuals with inadequately treated prior episodes of withdrawal, a history of withdrawal seizures, a co-morbid seizure disorder, or a prior brain injury. Withdrawal seizures can occur 6 to 24 hours after cessation of alcohol or with a significant reduction in alcohol intake. Multiple prior detoxification attempts may predispose patients to withdrawal seizures more than the quantity or duration of drinking, implying a kindling cause.[111] Whereas a generalized single tonic-clonic ictal episode is most commonly observed (i.e., in 75% of cases), status epilepticus is rare (occurring in <10% of cases). Multiple seizures in the setting of alcohol withdrawal should prompt consideration for potential additional contributors (e.g., a primary seizure

As BAC increases, so does impairment

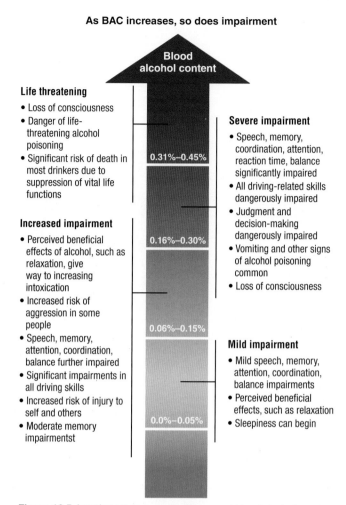

Figure 16.5 Impairment as a result of increased blood alcohol content (BAC). (From National Institute on Alcohol Abuse and Alcoholism. Alcohol Overdose: the Dangers of Drinking Too Much. NIAAA Brochures and Fact Sheets. 2013. http://pubs.niaaa.nih.gov/publications/AlcoholOverdoseFactsheet/Overdosefact.htm)

disorder; another substance, such as cocaine; or a CNS lesion). Although brain imaging may not be necessary in all cases of withdrawal-related seizure episodes, it is an important consideration given the high co-morbidity of head injuries with AUD and frequent challenges in obtaining a consistent medical history or a reliable neurological examination from a patient in acute alcohol withdrawal.[112]

Prompt treatment of early withdrawal symptoms with benzodiazepines or barbiturates, as described later, is the most effective measure to prevent the development of seizures. There is little evidence to support preferential treatment with alternative anticonvulsant agents, as benzodiazepines have generally been shown to be superior for both prevention and treatment of withdrawal seizures.

Alcohol Withdrawal Delirium

Alcohol withdrawal delirium (AWD), historically known as delirium tremens, is the major acute complication of alcohol withdrawal. First described in the medical literature more than 150 years ago, AWD was historically associated with mortality rates of 10% to 25%, although reassuringly, these statistics have improved with earlier recognition and a focus on the prevention and treatment of symptoms. Nonetheless, it remains imperative to be on the alert for this life-threatening condition.

The incidence of AWD is now approximately 5% among hospitalized patients with AUD and about 33% in patients with alcohol withdrawal seizures, with symptoms commonly observed 2 to 3 days after a significant reduction or cessation of alcohol use. The principal features are inattentiveness; tremor; hyperactivity and wakefulness; hallucinations; and autonomic imbalance, including fever, increased tone, and prominent hypertension and tachycardia. Hallucinations, when present, are most commonly visual and perceived as frightening by the patient. Untreated, AWD symptoms will persist for 2 to 3 days, although complications including unintentional trauma or injury, aspiration (e.g., pneumonia, acute respiratory distress syndrome), and cardiovascular events may further prolong a patient's recovery and cause significant morbidity and mortality (estimated at <5%).

Treatment of AWS relies on the early recognition of patients at risk for developing the syndrome and prompt treatment of withdrawal after initial symptoms have been observed. Although it can be challenging to predict which patients may develop AWS, a history of withdrawal or associated complications (e.g., seizures, AWD) is most strongly associated with risk for recurrent AWS.

Given the heterogeneity of the syndrome, rigid adherence to a single protocol for all cases of alcohol withdrawal is unrealistic. This noted, most patients with AWS should respond well to symptom-triggered benzodiazepine-based withdrawal protocol, in which benzodiazepine dosage and timing is individualized based on symptom severity and clinical need and only administered after the withdrawal symptoms are observed. Assessment of the severity of withdrawal is best accomplished with the use of standardized scales, such as the Clinical Institute Withdrawal Assessment Alcohol Scale Revised (CIWA-Ar).[113] Although it is more involved than standard taper protocols and often may require education of clinical staff (physicians and nurses), the benefits of symptom-triggered treatment are considerable because it ensures the patients are receiving treatment only when they need *and* as much as they need. This has significant clinical implications and has been shown to reduce the overall use of benzodiazepines by a factor of 4, shorten the length of treatment, and reduce symptom duration by a factor of 6.[114-116] Chlordiazepoxide, diazepam, and lorazepam are the three most commonly used benzodiazepines for the management of alcohol withdrawal, with the first two often used in outpatient detoxification or psychiatric hospital settings; lorazepam is a preferred agent in medically hospitalized patients. Lorazepam, temazepam, and oxazepam all have low rates of hepatic metabolism and thus may be preferred agents in patients with significant liver disease. In patients unable or unwilling to take medications orally, lorazepam can be administered intravenously or intramuscularly (which further adds to its versatility in hospital settings).

As previously reviewed, we generally recommend against using standing benzodiazepine tapers or continuous infusions, given higher risk for complications and overall inferior treatment outcomes compared with symptom-triggered treatment. This noted, in a small subset of patients, symptom-triggered treatment may prove challenging (e.g., medical confounders that resemble signs of withdrawal, deception by the patient). In these cases, considering alternatives to benzodiazepines or a structure taper may prove beneficial.

The α2-agonist dexmedetomidine is commonly used in cases of alcohol withdrawal in the intensive care setting, especially when a patient requires escalating doses of benzodiazepines that result in intubation and mechanical ventilation to protect the airway.[117] Propofol may also be used in cases of severe AWS that are unresponsive to other medications.[118]

Over the past decade, phenobarbital (a long-acting barbiturate) has been increasingly recognized as a viable and safe alternative to conventional benzodiazepine treatment. A prospective, randomized, double-blind, placebo-controlled study with 102 patients, half of whom received either a single dose of IV phenobarbital (10 mg/kg in 100 mL of normal saline) or placebo (100 mL of normal saline) in addition to a symptom-guided lorazepam-based alcohol withdrawal protocol, found that patients who received phenobarbital had fewer intensive care unit (ICU) admissions (8% vs 25%), and there were no differences in adverse events.[119]

Similarly, recent large retrospective work from our institution showed that a phenobarbital-driven protocol was comparable in efficacy and safety to conventional benzodiazepine treatment and was a potentially superior choice in patients with benzodiazepine tolerance and in surgical trauma patients in whom symptom-triggered treatment may be difficult to institute because of substrate limitations.[120,121]

Though antiepileptic agents have generally shown to be inferior to benzodiazepines for AWS management, there is growing interest in benzodiazepine-sparing protocols, especially for cases of mild alcohol withdrawal. Accordingly, there is some evidence that gabapentin co-administered with clonidine may prove effective in managing most symptoms of mild to moderate AWS.[122]

In addition to active pharmacologic management of alcohol withdrawal, supportive care is key to minimizing the risk of potential complications. In hospitalized patients, this includes consideration of fall and aspiration precautions and frequent re-direction or re-orientation if the patient is delirious. As noted, benzodiazepines/barbiturates are essential in treatment of alcohol withdrawal, yet these agents should not be used solely for agitation management because there is a risk for over-medicating the patient, and through this potentiating acute intoxication, disinhibition, agitation, and impulsivity. Neuroleptics, including quetiapine or olanzapine, are commonly used in conjunction with GABAergic agents in hospital settings, (when a patient can take medications orally) and haloperidol (when IV medications are required).

Although rare, Wernicke–Korsakoff syndrome is markedly challenging to diagnose in patients in active withdrawal. We recommend proactive use of B vitamins in all patients deemed at risk of developing the syndrome given minimal risks and considerable potential benefits. Thiamine (we usually recommend 200–500 mg IV two to three times per day) should be given for at least 3 days until a normal diet is resumed, at which point the dosing can be changed to oral. Repletion of other vitamins, including folate, with concurrent proper nutrition and hydration, is likewise important for most patients in active withdrawal.

Wernicke–Korsakoff Syndrome

Observed in a small subset (5%) of patients with chronic alcohol use, this syndrome is commonly missed in clinical setting, including upward of 80% of cases.[123] Wernicke's encephalopathy is characterized by the triad of ophthalmoplegia, ataxia, and mental disturbance, although the presence of all three is not necessary to make the diagnosis, and the findings may prove non-specific (e.g., in a patient in acute alcohol withdrawal). The ocular findings are observed in 17% of cases and consist of paresis or paralysis of the external recti, nystagmus, and a disturbance in conjugate gaze. Cognitive findings include inattentiveness, amnesia, apathy or amotivation, and impaired arousal, leading to lethargy and unresponsiveness. After treatment with thiamine is initiated, improvement in ocular findings may occur within hours, with full recovery over days to weeks. Cognitive findings may begin to improve within 1 week (in 30% of cases), although most patients will require more than 1 to 2 months to recover fully.[124] Functional magnetic resonance imaging (MRI) studies show substantially

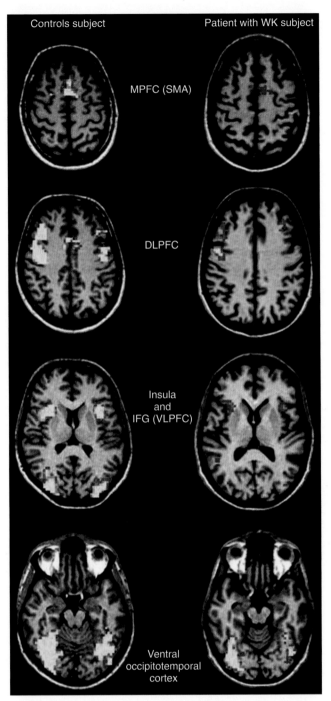

Figure 16.6 Brain activation in patients with Wernicke–Korsakoff *(WK)* compared with control participants. *DLPFC,* Dorsolateral prefrontal cortex; *IFG,* inferior frontal gyrus; *MPFC,* medial prefrontal cortex; *SMA,* supplementary motor area; *VLPFC,* ventrolateral prefrontal cortex. (From Caulo M, Van Hecke J, Toma L, et al. Functional MRI study of diencephalic amnesia in Wernicke–Korsakoff syndrome. *Brain.* 2005;128(pt 7):1584–1594.)

diminished global activation in the brain among patients with Wernicke–Korsakoff's syndrome compared with normal control participants (Figure 16.6).

Korsakoff's psychosis, also referred to as confabulatory psychosis and alcohol-induced persisting amnestic disorder, is characterized by impaired memory in an otherwise alert and responsive individual. Curiously, confabulation, long regarded as the hallmark of the syndrome, is only seen in a subset of patients.[123,124] Most of these patients have diminished spontaneous verbal output, have a limited understanding of the extent of their memory loss, and lack insight into the nature of their illness. The memory loss is commonly bipartite, including both a retrograde (inability to recall the past) and an anterograde component (lack of capacity for retention of new information). At times, the patient may not be able to recall simple items (such as the examiner's name, the day, or the time) even when provided with the information repeatedly. Patients with the syndrome tend to improve over time, although 25% to 30% of patients never regain premorbid function, and some degree of chronic impairment persists in 50% of cases.[125] The electroencephalogram may be unremarkable or show diffuse slowing, and the MRI scan may reveal changes in the periaqueductal area and medial thalamus.[123–125] The specific memory structures affected in Korsakoff's psychosis are the medial dorsal nucleus of the thalamus and the hippocampal formations.

Administration of the B vitamin thiamine (IM or IV) should be routine for *all* suspected cases of alcohol intoxication and AUD given difficulties in diagnosing the syndrome in acute settings. Because subclinical cognitive impairments can occur even in apparently well-nourished patients, routine management should include not only administration of thiamine but also of other micronutrients, including folic acid, and multi-vitamins.

Fetal Alcohol Spectrum Disorder

Fetal alcohol spectrum disorder (FASD) is an umbrella term that describes the range of effects that can occur in an individual whose mother drank alcohol during pregnancy. These effects may include physical, mental, behavioral, or learning disabilities with possible lifelong implications.[126] Formerly known as "fetal alcohol syndrome," these disorders can include a set of birth defects caused by alcohol during pregnancy.[127] Children with this condition may have facial deformities, mis-proportioned heads, intellectual disability, and behavioral problems (Figure 16.7).

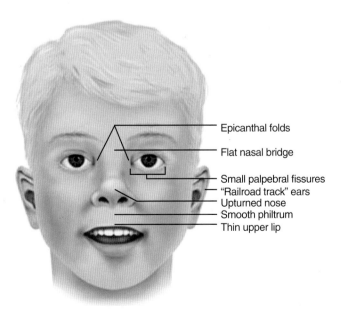

Figure 16.7 Characteristics of fetal alcohol spectrum disorder. (From Wattendorf DJ, Muenke M. Fetal alcohol spectrum disorders. *Am Fam Physician.* 2005;72(2):279–282, 285.)

However, even when these abnormalities are not evident, brain damage may still have occurred. Approximately 30% to 40% of all women who drink heavily during pregnancy will have a baby with some degree of FASD. It is the leading cause of preventable intellectual disability in the Western Hemisphere. MRI studies show that the areas that regulate movement and cognitive processes related to attention, perception, thinking, and memory are particularly sensitive to pre-natal alcohol exposure and that brain size is reduced.[128]

The minimum amount of alcohol needed to produce harmful effects in exposed children is not known. Thus, the safest approach is to completely avoid alcohol during pregnancy. People with pre-natal alcohol exposure have a high risk of developing learning and mental disabilities, school dropout, delinquency, alcohol and other SUDs, mental illness, and poor psychosocial function. Education, screening, and early intervention are critical.

COCAINE USE DISORDER AND ASSOCIATED CONDITIONS

The National Survey on Drug Use and Health (NSDUH) has estimated that 3.1 million people in the United States aged 12 years and older primarily used cocaine, with another 500,000 adults using cocaine in conjunction with other stimulants.[2] Despite the overall downward trend in usage, cocaine, after alcohol, remains a significant contributor to drug-related ED visits, general hospital admissions, family violence, and other social problems. In 2011, cocaine use resulted in 40% of all illicit drug-related ED visits.[3]

Use of cocaine leads to intense euphoria, increased energy, a reduced need for sleep, an increased sense of productivity and well-being, and increased sexual function. On cessation of use, individuals may experience a "crash," marked by hypersomnia, irritability, withdrawal, and even depression, each of which provides a strong incentive for further cocaine use. Pharmacologically, these responses are primarily mediated by the effects of cocaine on the dopamine reuptake transporter (DAT), where cocaine inhibits the reuptake of synaptic dopamine, thus resulting in increased dopamine bioavailability. With chronic use, downregulation of dopamine receptors and ultimately depletion of synaptic dopamine is observed; this contributes to the emergence of tolerance and may be the physiologic mechanism behind postuse depression observed in many individuals (Figure 16.8). Like other stimulants, cocaine also disrupts the synthesis and reuptake of serotonin, and it has been implicated in other neurotransmitter systems, including norepinephrine, NMDA, and GABA. Plasma cholinesterases rapidly convert cocaine into benzoylecgonine, an inactive metabolite that can be detected in the urine for 3 days after cocaine use. When alcohol is taken in conjunction with cocaine, liver esterases produce cocaethylene, an active metabolite that has a longer half-life (2–4-hours) and is more cardiotoxic than cocaine.

Patients who experience uncomfortable acute effects of cocaine ingestion often complain of anorexia, insomnia, increased anxiety, hyperactivity, or rapid speech or thinking ("speeding"). Their physical examination may reveal signs of adrenergic hyperactivity, including hyperreflexia, tachycardia, diaphoresis, and dilated pupils that are responsive to light. More severe sequelae of acute intoxication include hyperpyrexia, hypertension, cocaine-induced vasospastic events (e.g., stroke, myocardial infarction), or seizures. Although uncommon in the general population, these complications account for most cocaine-associated ED visits. Insufflating the drug may produce rhinitis or sinusitis and, rarely, perforations of the nasal septum, and free-basing (inhalation of cocaine alkaloid vapors) may produce bronchitis.

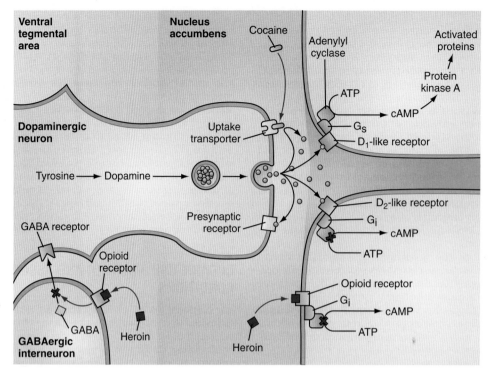

Figure 16.8 Schematic of the effects of cocaine and heroin on a synapse. *ATP*, Adenosine triphosphate; *cAMP*, cyclic adenosine monophosphate; *GABA*, gamma aminobutyric acid. (Redrawn and adapted from Leshner A and the US National Institute on Drug Abuse. *New Understandings of Drug Addiction, Hospital Practice Special Report*. McGraw-Hill; 1997.)

The most notable psychiatric problems associated with acute cocaine use are the emergence of heightened or severe anxiety, mania, or psychosis. The presence of visual or tactile hallucinations (e.g., "coke bugs," a perception of something crawling under the skin) and symptom onset during periods of active drug use help differentiate these episodes from a primary mood or thought disorder. With discontinuation of use, those who have used cocaine may note apathy, anhedonia, and even depression; rarely, the symptoms may be so severe that thoughts of suicide emerge. Psychiatric sequelae of acute cocaine intoxication and withdrawal tend to improve relatively quickly with drug discontinuation and supportive care, especially compared with the primary mood and thought disorders these syndromes otherwise resemble closely.

Management of Cocaine Intoxication and Acute Withdrawal

Most individuals who use cocaine do not require any specific treatment after the drug's use; when patients present with active psychiatric symptoms after cocaine ingestion, the primary intervention involves ensuring a safe and supportive recovery environment. However, benzodiazepines, neuroleptics, or both can be helpful for those who have more severe anxiety or for those with acute mania or psychosis. Appropriate screening and medical support should be offered for patients who present with potential CNS (e.g., stroke) or cardiovascular complications related to acute use of cocaine.

As with other SUDs, cocaine use disorder is marked by the emergence of tolerance, dependence, and an inability to stop using the drug despite significant psychosocial complications related to the drug use. Compared with patients who present with recreational cocaine use, patients with cocaine use disorder may be at higher risk for the emergence of withdrawal

after the drug is discontinued. As with acute intoxication, the care of patients who present with cocaine discontinuation is largely supportive; this syndrome, although unpleasant, is self-limited and non–life-threatening. There are no specific pharmacologic interventions that shorten the duration or extent of cocaine withdrawal, although benzodiazepines and neuroleptics are commonly used to mitigate emergent anxiety or irritability. A rare but major complication of cocaine discontinuation is the onset of severe depression with thoughts of suicide.[129] If this occurs, close monitoring (e.g., one-on-one observation) is required, and unless symptoms resolve rapidly, psychiatric hospitalization for further stabilization and safety may be necessary. A less severe anhedonic state may persist for 2 to 3 months after cocaine use, and it is thought to reflect a more persistent state of dopamine depletion.

Treatment of Cocaine Use Disorder

Manual-guided cognitive-behavioral therapy (CBT) has been efficacious in the treatment of patients with cocaine use.[130] Twelve-step facilitation and CBT appear to be helpful, especially in individuals with more severe cocaine use and in those with other co-morbid SUDs.[131]

There is no FDA-approved pharmacotherapy for cocaine use disorder. Trials with desipramine, fluoxetine, bupropion, amantadine, and carbamazepine have found inconsistent results, as have trials using both short- and long-acting stimulants. Positive responses have been reported in some trials with baclofen and modafinil, but these drugs require further investigation. Topiramate has shown most consistent benefit in reducing cocaine use, cravings, and risk for relapse; thus, it remains a potential treatment strategy, whether alone or in conjunction with individual or group counseling or peer support (e.g., AA, Narcotics Anonymous, recovery coaching).

AMPHETAMINE USE DISORDER

In 2020, roughly 5.1 million individuals 12 years of age and older were active non-medical users of prescription stimulants, and 2.5 million (0.9%) adults used methamphetamine.[2]

Like cocaine, the primary CNS effect of amphetamines is an increase in synaptic dopamine availability. Unlike cocaine, which exerts its effect through blocking of DAT, most amphetamines have a dual effect through direct potentiation of dopamine release into the synapse and by blocking of dopamine reuptake through DAT inhibition. Thus, compared with cocaine, most amphetamines produce a "high" that is both more intense and longer lasting. Methamphetamine, invented for military use by the Japanese in World War I, is the most commonly used street amphetamine; it is commonly known as "speed" (when taken orally) or "crystal meth" (when smoked).

The signs and symptoms of acute amphetamine intoxication are like those of cocaine. Given the increased potency of amphetamines, patients may be more likely to present with significant anxiety, mood lability, and even mania or psychosis. Supportive care helps to diminish distressing sensory cues (and in some cases, it may be the only intervention necessary). For patients with significant behavioral distress or agitation, atypical antipsychotics (e.g., oral olanzapine or quetiapine, or IV haloperidol) may mitigate the patient's distress. Benzodiazepines can likewise be of use and may be useful in those with an increased risk for seizures. If these agents are used, monitoring for the emergence of benzodiazepine-associated disinhibition or delirium is required.

With chronic amphetamine use, dental problems (e.g., caries, missing teeth, bleeding and infected gums) may arise, as can muscle cramps (related to dehydration and low levels of magnesium and potassium), constipation (caused by dehydration), weight loss, and excoriated skin lesions ("speed bumps"). Chronic amphetamine use is associated with significant changes within the reward circuits, including loss of DAT in the caudate and putamen, and decreased perfusion in the putamen. Furthermore, loss of perfusion has been noted within the frontal cortex, and loss of volume of both the amygdala and the hippocampus can be seen on MRI scans of those with chronic amphetamine use.

Treatment of Amphetamine Intoxication and Withdrawal

Amphetamines can be withdrawn abruptly; like with cocaine, the acute withdrawal is unpleasant but not associated with significant medical or psychiatric complications in most individuals. Patients may describe irritability, an increased appetite, and an increased need for sleep, especially if they are recovering from a prolonged binge during which they were unable to access food or consistent sleep for days or weeks. As with cocaine, the major behavioral complication is the emergence of severe depression with suicidal ideation. Some patients may note the persistence of psychosis for days or weeks after discontinuation of amphetamine use. If significant anxiety or agitation develops that warrants medication, benzodiazepines, neuroleptics, or both are the most commonly used treatment options.

Most signs of acute amphetamine intoxication and withdrawal resolve in 2 to 4 days after the last drug exposure. However, clinicians should monitor patients for symptoms of a chronic mood or thought disorder, which may take 3 to 6 months to resolve.

As with cocaine, there is currently no FDA-approved treatment for patients with amphetamine use disorder. Long-acting stimulants have not been shown to be of benefit, and there is a risk for drug diversion.

CLUB DRUGS

During the 1990s, the use of "club drugs," primarily 3,4-methylenedioxy-methamphetamine (MDMA), also called "Molly" or "Ecstasy", γ-hydroxybutyrate (GHB), and ketamine steadily increased. This trend was reversed in the early 2000s when the Monitoring the Future Survey reported a steep decline in the use of club drugs.[132] Use of many of these substances has diminished since, and only a brief overview of key "club drugs" is presented here.

MDMA has both amphetamine-like and hallucinogenic effects. Its primary mechanism of action is via indirect serotonin agonism, but it also affects dopamine and other neurotransmitter systems. MDMA was initially used experimentally to facilitate psychotherapy, but its use was banned after it was found to be neurotoxic to animals. With ingestion, most users describe a stimulant-like experience (reflective of drug's pro-dopaminergic effects), in addition to an increased sense of connection to others and empathy (reflection of strong serotonergic function of MDMA). In toxic amounts, MDMA can result in distorted perceptions, confusion, hypertension, hyperactivity, and potentially fatal hyperthermia. Concurrent use of MDMA and other serotonergic agents (e.g., selective serotonin reuptake inhibitors) has been associated with the development of a potentially life-threatening serotonin syndrome. With chronic MDMA use, serotonin stores become depleted, leading to tolerance and unpleasant side effects (e.g., teeth gnashing, restlessness). Frequent users learn to anticipate these effects, and they limit their long-term consumption of the drug.

GHB (sodium oxybate) is structurally like GABA, and it acts as a CNS depressant. It has been approved by the FDA as a Schedule III controlled substance for the treatment of patients with narcolepsy. GHB has a relatively low therapeutic index; as little as twice the dose that produces euphoria can cause CNS depression. In overdose, it can cause coma; it has also been identified as a "date rape" drug.

Ketamine ("Special K," "Super K," or "K") is a non-competitive NMDA antagonist that is classified as a dissociative anesthetic. In addition to causing a dissociative high, this drug can cause delirium, amnesia, and respiratory depression. More recently, studies suggest that ketamine can treat those with severe depression and suicidal ideation.

"Bath salts" is the street name used to describe a heterogeneous drug group including various synthetic derivatives of methcathinone, either mephedrone or methylenedioxypyrovalerone (MDPV).[133] These compounds are Drug Enforcement Administration (DEA) schedule I substances that are considered illegal only if intended for human consumption. Accordingly, they were sold legally and labeled "plant food or bath salts, not for human consumption" (thus the name). In 2011, the DEA, using its emergency scheduling authority, made sale and possession of these substances illegal in the United States. Methcathinone is derived from compounds found in Khat (or qat; *Catha edulis*), a flowering plant from East Africa.[134] Existing as a white or tan crystalline powder, the compound can be ingested orally or administered nasally, rectally, IM, or IV. The average dose is 5 to 20 mg; psychoactive effects begin at 3 to 5 mg. The typical package contains 500 mg, thus creating a high risk for overdose. Consumption increases intracellular dopamine and serotonin levels by their effects on dopamine and serotonin reuptake transporters. Subjective effects observed with use include euphoria, an emphatic mood, sexual stimulation, a greater mental focus, and enhanced energy (feelings like those produced by MDMA). The peak "rush" occurs at 90 minutes, with effects lasting for 3 to 4 hours. The total experience lasts for 6 to 8 hours, and it is often followed by a crash. More intense psychic effects can include panic attacks; agitation; paranoia; hallucinations; psychosis; and aggressive, violent, or bizarre self-destructive behavior. Use may also lead to anorexia, delirium, and depression. Physical effects included tachycardia, hypertension, mydriasis, arrhythmias, hyperthermia, sweating, rhabdomyolysis, seizures, stroke, cerebral edema, myocardial infarction, cardiovascular collapse, and death. Bath salts are commonly not detected by routine toxicology screens. Clinical management usually involves the use of benzodiazepines for acute agitation. Cardiac monitoring and IV fluids are recommended; autonomic instability may require monitoring in an ICU.

OPIOID USE DISORDER AND ASSOCIATED CONDITIONS

Over the past 3 decades, there has been a persistent and dramatic increase in opioid use in the United States, with an estimated 9.5 million people reporting past-year misuse of heroin or prescription pain relievers in 2020. The vast majority of those who have used opioids (9.3 million) used prescription opioids (e.g., fentanyl, oxycodone), reflecting an increased availability and distribution of these drugs.[2] This is more than twice the number of people who used opioids just a decade ago and starkly emphasizes the ongoing impact of the opioid epidemic in our country. Nearly one-third (31%) of individuals with acquired immunodeficiency syndrome in the United States are related to injection drug use.[135] An estimated 70% to 80% of the new hepatitis C virus (HCV) infections occurring in the United States each year are among IV drug users. Other public health problems that have emerged over the past decade include increased ED visits and deaths caused by opioid overdoses. Specifically, prescription methadone-, oxycodone-, and hydrocodone-related ED visits quadrupled between 2004 and 2008.[136]

Opioids act by binding to the opioid receptors, with most of the clinically relevant effects attributed to opioid effect on the mu receptors (Figure 16.9). As with other addictive substances, opioids impact CNS reward circuits; opioid binding to mu receptors in the VTA indirectly stimulates dopamine release and thus contributes to reinforcing the effects of the drug (Figure 16.10). Beyond the reward circuits, opioid receptors exist throughout both central and peripheral nervous system, thus accounting for the wide range of effects attributed to this drug class, including analgesia, reduced secretions, antinausea and antiemetic effects, constipation, miosis, urinary hesitation, and hypotension (Table 16.4). Given their significant role in pain control, reduction of secretions, and nausea, opioids remain an important drug class in a wide variety of medical and surgical conditions.

Acute opioid intoxication is marked by a subjective perception of euphoria and slight sedation.[137] The physical examination after use of opioids is notable for miosis. With significant use, the patient may exhibit more pronounced sedation and reduced respiratory rate; this condition may be rapidly fatal (overdose) if left untreated. The classic signs of opioid withdrawal usually begin 8 to 12 hours after the last dose of a short-acting agent or more than 24 to 48 hours after using a long-acting agent, such as methadone (Box 16.1). These include the emergence of sweating, yawning, lacrimation, rhinorrhea, marked irritability, dilated pupils, and piloerection ("gooseflesh"). Rare tremor, or even myoclonus, may occur. More severe signs of opioid withdrawal include insomnia, nausea or vomiting, and abdominal cramps. Untreated, the

syndrome usually subsides in 3 to 7 days, though it may persist for weeks if the patient is withdrawing from a long-acting agent (e.g., methadone, buprenorphine). Although non–life-threatening, opioid withdrawal is described as markedly distressing by most patients. Appropriate treatment should be offered in a timely fashion to avoid the risk of premature discharge and relapse.

Overdose Prevention and Reversal

Opioid overdoses are medical emergencies and they require immediate attention to the maintenance of airway, breathing, and circulation (i.e., ABCs of resuscitation). Opioid-induced respiratory depression can be treated with 0.4 mg/mL of IV or IM naloxone. This medication can be repeated every 2 minutes as needed (up to a total dose of 2 mg). If the patient does not respond after 20 minutes, he or she should be treated for a combined drug overdose. Because of methadone's long duration of action, overdoses of this drug often require multiple boluses or even an IV naloxone drip.

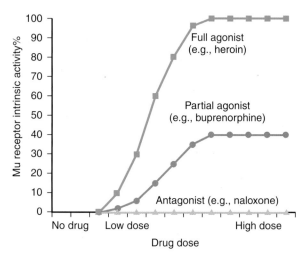

Figure 16.9 Comparison of activity levels of opiates at the mu receptor.

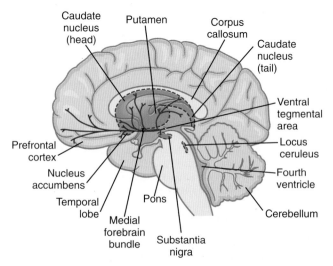

Figure 16.10 Schematic of reward pathways in the brain. (Redrawn and adapted from Leshner A, US National Institute on Drug Abuse. *New Understandings of Drug Addiction, Hospital Practice Special Report*, McGraw-Hill; 1997.)

TABLE 16.4 Opioid Agonist Drug Effects

Acute-use effects	Euphoria
	Vomiting
	Constricted pupils
	Depressed respiration
	Drowsiness
	Decreased pain sensation
	Decreased awareness
	Decreased consciousness
Large-dose acute-use effects	Non-responsiveness
	Pin-point pupils
	If severe anoxia, pupils may dilate
	Bradycardia and hypotension
	Skin cyanotic
	Skeletal muscle flaccid
	Pulmonary edema in ~50%
	Slow or absent respiration
Chronic-use effects	Physical dependence
	Psychological dependence
	Lethargy and indifference
	Reduction in bowel movement

BOX 16.1 Signs and Symptoms of Opiate Withdrawal

- Dysphoric mood
- Nausea with or without vomiting
- Body aches
- Lacrimation
- Rhinorrhea
- Pupillary dilation
- Sweating
- Piloerection
- Diarrhea
- Yawning
- Mild fever
- Insomnia
- Irritability
- Opioid craving

As a response to the prescription pain-reliever epidemic, many states have implemented intranasal Narcan *overdose-prevention programs*. Intranasal Narcan can be provided at no cost by state public health agencies or prescribed to high-risk individuals and to members of their households. Between 2007 and 2011, intranasal Narcan reversed more than 1000 opiate overdoses in Massachusetts.[138]

Opioid Use Disorder Treatment

Food and Drug Administration regulations define opiate substitution therapy (with either methadone or buprenorphine) as treatment with an approved opiate that extends beyond 30 days. There are currently three agents carrying FDA approval for treatment of opioid use disorder (OUD), methadone (a full agonist), buprenorphine (a partial agonist), and IM naltrexone (a full antagonist).

Methadone, a long-acting opioid agonist, has been available for many decades and has been extensively studied for treatment of patients with OUD. Compared with conventional detoxification, treatment with methadone carries favorable data on helping patients maintain sobriety from opioids, helps increase engagement in treatment, and reduces rates of overdose and opioid-related death. Furthermore, treatment with methadone has been shown to result in reduced rates of infections associated with IV drug use (IVDU) (e.g., human immunodeficiency virus [HIV], HCV). Although methadone can be prescribed for pain by all appropriately licensed physicians, special designation is required for dispensing methadone for OUD. Accordingly, methadone can often be initiated only in specially designated facilities (so-called "methadone clinics"). However, hospitals and other treatment facilities can continue methadone for a patient already in treatment or initiate methadone for management of withdrawal without concerns.

A common starting dose of methadone for a patient beginning treatment is 30 to 40 mg/day. Although this dose may mitigate signs of major withdrawal, it is rarely sufficient in managing cravings, and patients commonly require a gradual dose increase toward 80 to 120 mg/day on average, at which point most withdrawal symptoms and cravings abate. As the methadone dose increases, patients should be monitored for sedation (that may be delayed by 24–48 hours after a dose adjustment) and prolongation of the QTc interval. Polypharmacy is likewise a potential concern because patients may use other opioids or sedatives (e.g., "the cocktail," a combination of clonidine, clonazepam, gabapentin, and tizanidine) to potentiate the sedating effect of methadone. Success in methadone treatment has been associated with higher doses (with a range from 60–120 mg/day), length of treatment, and the provision of comprehensive counseling and rehabilitation services, although counseling should never be forced on the patient and only offered if the patient expresses a willingness to engage in this treatment modality.

Buprenorphine, a partial opioid agonist, has a high affinity for the mu receptors, a long half-life, and a slow dissociation constant. Accordingly, it tends to out-compete most other opioids at the receptor, which helps it mitigate cravings and block potential agonist effects of any other opioids co-ingested with buprenorphine. The tendency of buprenorphine to out-compete or displace other opioids at the mu receptor likewise contributes to precipitated withdrawal if the patient is given buprenorphine while still acutely intoxicated on a full agonist agent. To avoid this problem, buprenorphine should not be started until the patient demonstrates mild to moderate symptoms of withdrawal.

Buprenorphine, with its partial agonist effect and thus reduced risk for potential complications, including overdose, is an excellent agent for the treatment of patients with OUD.[28] Unlike methadone, treatment with buprenorphine does not require significant oversight, and it can be initiated in office-based treatment setting, thus providing an alternative for patients who struggle with rigid guidelines in place at most methadone clinics. Office-based treatment also helps reduce the potential stigma associated with OUD and helps increase overall buprenorphine availability. When sublingual (SL) buprenorphine is dispensed in a combination tablet with naloxone, it has minimal potential for IV misuse (because of the immediate opioid antagonist effects of IV naloxone).[139] Similar to methadone, buprenorphine has been highly effective in the treatment of OUD, including positive effects on overall patient sobriety; treatment retention; reduction in IVDU-associated infections; and most important, reduction in opioid-related overdose and mortality rates.

To initiate buprenorphine, the patient should be instructed to refrain from use of opioids for at least 24 hours. Treatment can be initiated as early as 12 hours after the last use of a short-acting agent, when the patient is showing signs of moderate to severe opioid withdrawal. When the presence of withdrawal is observed, buprenorphine induction can begin with 4 mg/1 mg of SL buprenorphine–naloxone (which can be given as two 2-mg doses separated 1 hour apart). If no concerns for worsened withdrawal emerge 1 to 4 hours after the initial dose is given, an additional 4 mg/1 mg can be given every 4 to 6 hours as needed to stabilize the patient, with most patients needing 8 to 12 mg of buprenorphine on the first day. Traditionally done in hospital or clinic settings, there is now increased recognition that most patients can safely start buprenorphine while at home. After induction, most patients can be maintained on buprenorphine 16 to 24 mg/day (either as a single daily dose or divided twice or thrice daily). Because of the ceiling effect seen with partial opiate agonists, there is no clear pharmacological benefit from buprenorphine doses higher than 32 mg/day; even at 24 mg/day, buprenorphine has greater than 90% mu receptor occupancy. If precipitated withdrawal occurs, more aggressive buprenorphine dosing is recommended to manage the withdrawal symptoms in addition to liberal use of other supportive medications (e.g., clonidine, benzodiazepines) to manage discomfort.

If a patient taking methadone was to be transitioned to buprenorphine, traditionally, methadone would be gradually tapered to 30 mg/day and then discontinued. Some 2 to 4 days later, the patient would customarily note the onset of significant withdrawal, and at this point, buprenorphine would be initiated. Not only was this approach time-consuming, but it also carried a significant risk of precipitating withdrawal (because of the long half-life and variable metabolism of methadone), thus resulting in significant patient discomfort and anxiety. More recently, there has been a general recognition of potential benefits of buprenorphine micro-dosing in this clinical scenario. Specifically, progressively increasing doses of buprenorphine are offered over 7 days, while the patient continues to take the full dose of opioid agonist (e.g., methadone). Patients are usually started on 0.5 mg of buprenorphine per day, and the dose is doubled every 24 hours until the patient reaches a therapeutic dose of 16 mg/day. At this point, patients can be safely tapered off methadone or any other opioid agonist without significant withdrawal or discomfort.

Extensive research has shown that OUD treatment with methadone or Suboxone is highly effective. It reduces illicit drug use, the mortality rate, criminal behavior, and transmission of hepatitis and HIV infection, and it permits many of those with addictions to attain normal levels of social function.[140]

Naltrexone is an opioid receptor antagonist that fully occupies the opioid receptor and prevents the euphoric effects of opioids, thus blocking the reinforcing "high" and resulting in reduced opioid use in patients taking this medication. In a patient with opioid dependence, naltrexone can precipitate withdrawal if it is given too soon after an agonist; therefore, it is best to wait 7 to 10 days after last opioid use to prevent patient discomfort. In clinical practice, this waiting period can prove to be challenging, especially for those in the community or outside a controlled treatment setting. In fact, many patients return to drug use because of acute withdrawal or cravings before being able to initiate the medication. Oral naltrexone has been of some benefit for highly motivated patients and within the criminal justice system population (where administration can be closely monitored). In the general population, it fares poorly because of a lack of adherence. In 2010, an injectable form of naltrexone (Vivitrol) was approved by the FDA, which is now the recommended standard for all patients who request naltrexone for OUD treatment. When taken consistently, Vivitrol can reduce relapse rates and help mitigate cravings, although effectiveness remains limited by poor compliance. Therefore, we recommend IM naltrexone only if it is specifically requested by the patient or if there are significant barriers to other treatment options.[141]

Managing the Patients with Opioid Use Disorder in Hospital Settings

If a patient has been receiving OUD treatment before admission to a hospital, the dose of methadone or buprenorphine should be confirmed by the inpatient staff and should not be changed without consultation with the patient and the physician responsible for the patient's outpatient treatment. Under current FDA regulations, hospital-based physicians may prescribe methadone or buprenorphine to any hospitalized person without a specialized treatment waiver or an opioid treatment program registration. The patient should not be withdrawn from their outpatient opioid therapy unless there is full agreement between the patient, the hospital-based physician, and the outpatient treatment staff on this course of action.

Patients receiving long-term methadone therapy should continue to receive daily methadone treatment while hospitalized. If a switch to a parenteral medication is necessary, methadone can be given as an IV formulation, although clinicians should note that the dose given as the IV methadone is twice as potent as the oral formulation. As soon as oral medication can be tolerated, the oral methadone dose should be re-instated.[142] The patient's methadone dose should not be assumed to be sufficient for pain control, and we advise against dose fractionation of the home dose even though it may provide some benefit for pain control; fractionation may generate logistical challenges if the patient leaves prematurely, and it may prove inferior regarding craving control. If additional methadone is required for pain control, we recommend increasing by 5 to 10 mg every 24 to 48 hours while closely monitoring for sedation or QTc prolongation (Table 16.5). Methadone has significant drug–drug interactions, and patients should be monitored for these as well. These interactions include QTc prolongation, with concurrent use of antifungals or neuroleptics, or the risk for methadone induction with concurrent rifampin administration.

Inpatient Withdrawal Management ("Detoxification") for Patients with Opioid Use Disorder

Although techniques that permit a safe, rapid, and medically effective detoxification from opioids seem highly attractive in an era of managed care, clinicians must recognize that detoxification alone is rarely successful as a treatment for any addiction. Unless the patient is highly motivated or transitions to a long-term structured residential treatment program where access to drug is minimal, relapse rates after detoxification are extremely high. The resulting costs to the patient, to society, and to the health care system far outweigh any savings realized from a rapid "cost-effective" detoxification protocol.

TABLE 16.5 Equivalent Doses of Narcotic Pain Medications

Drug	Parenteral Dose (mg)
Morphine	10
Oxycodone (Percocet, OxyContin)	5–10
Hydrocodone (Vicodin, Lortab)	10
Hydromorphone (Dilaudid)	2.5
Methadone*	5

*There is considerable variability across patients as regards to methadone bioavailability, storage and metabolism so that exact equivalency dosage may be challenging to reliably determine

Accordingly, patients should be counseled about these risks and encouraged to consider long-term treatment options, given their superior safety and efficacy record. In most optimal scenarios, the choice to initiate methadone or Suboxone to help mitigate withdrawal should be based on the patient's choice of which medication they prefer for longitudinal treatment of their OUD.

If, however, the patient demands to be withdrawn from opioids ("detox"), controlled withdrawal can be best achieved with methadone. Commonly, the patient is initiated on methadone, and the dose is titrated to a point where acute withdrawal is stabilized (usually 40–60 mg/day). At this point, methadone can be reduced by 20% each day until it is discontinued. In addition, the patients may benefit from Bentyl (for gastrointestinal distress) and clonidine (for anxiety and insomnia). Patients taking clonidine should be monitored closely for side effects (particularly hypotension and sedation), and the medication can be tapered off over 3 to 4 days.[143,144]

Discharge planning should be initiated as quickly as possible after admission. For patients who are not already in treatment, days to weeks may be required to arrange for access to an appropriate treatment setting. Physicians who are able to provide office-based buprenorphine treatment can be identified via the "physician locator" at Substance Abuse and Mental Health Services Administration's website (http://www.buprenorphine.samhsa.gov) or at the website maintained by the National Alliance of Advocates for Buprenorphine Treatment (http://www.naabt.com). Methadone clinics can likewise be readily identified, and patients should be involved in the conversation regarding local politics of methadone dosing on discharge, namely, whether the patient is expected to fully taper off methadone before discharge or whether they can transition to the methadone clinic on a stable dose initiated during the hospitalization.

Regardless of the form of medication treatment, many patients benefit from counseling and rehabilitation services; these should include educational and vocational services as needed. CBT has been more effective than drug counseling alone. Contingency management has also helped to reduce illicit drug use in patients on maintenance therapy.

Pain Management for Patients Receiving Opioid Use Disorder Treatment

Determining the appropriate dosage of pain medications for a patient receiving chronic OUD therapy is a common clinical problem, one further complicated by the diverse binding profiles of various medications used to manage OUD and the potential effects they may have on conventional pain management. Furthermore, patients on chronic methadone or Suboxone may present with tolerance that may greatly increase the doses required for adequate pain control. Hyperalgesia has likewise been described with chronic opioid treatment and may result in heightened pain perception and difficulties in pain control. Finally, patient factors (e.g., limited distress tolerance, fear of stigma or discrimination, anxiety about potential unsolicited changes to outpatient OUD treatment) and provider factors (e.g., prejudice, fear of patient deception, concern about inadvertently inducing overdose) can provide additional challenges to safe and adequate pain control in this population.

The analgesic effect of methadone is minimal in those receiving maintenance therapy, and if pain control is required, the clinician should anticipate the need to gradually increase the maintenance methadone dose (for baseline pain control) and consider use of short-acting opioid agents for acute pain control. Patients on Suboxone may need a dose reduction if significant pain control needs are estimated; at dosages of 8 mg/

day, patients have sufficient Suboxone to prevent buprenorphine withdrawal yet not so much to fully block conventional agonists from acting on the mu receptor. Accordingly, patients should be counseled about reducing buprenorphine toward this dose, and then when acute pain needs subside, they can be quickly returned to their home dosing before discharge. Patients on naltrexone should be tapered off this medication before potential surgery if at all possible; if more pain control is warranted, the clinician should consider using non-opioid alternatives (e.g., regional nerve block).

BENZODIAZEPINES AND BARBITURATES

The use of CNS depressants accounts for a significant component of ED visits related to both suicide attempts and accidental overdoses. Although benzodiazepines have become the most commonly misused sedative–hypnotics in the United States, there are still areas where the non-medical use of barbiturates (such as butalbital [Fiorinal and Esgic]), carisoprodol (Soma), or other sedative–hypnotics (such as methaqualone, glutethimide) leads to serious clinical problems (Table 16.6). More recently, a significant increase with zolpidem-related ED visits has been noted.[145]

A person intoxicated on a CNS depressant typically has many of the same diagnostic features as occurs with alcohol intoxication. Slurred speech, unsteady gait, and sustained vertical or horizontal nystagmus in a patient without objective evidence of recent alcohol use may support the diagnosis of acute benzodiazepine or barbiturate intoxication. Symptom progression and variability resemble alcohol intoxication, including the risk for disinhibition or assaultive behavior, over-sedation, and coma at high doses. As tolerance to barbiturates develops, there is no concomitant increase in the lethal dose, so that as little as a 10% to 25% increase over the usual daily dosage may be fatal to a patient using barbiturates. Thus, a barbiturate overdose should always be considered potentially life-threatening. Supportive measures with suspected overdose include maintenance of adequate airway, mechanical ventilation, alkalinization of the urine, correction of acid–base disorders, and diuresis with furosemide or mannitol. Severe overdoses may require dialysis or charcoal resin hemoperfusion.[146]

Withdrawal from sedative–hypnotics can be accompanied by a wide variety of signs and symptoms, like those seen with AWS, including anxiety, insomnia, hyperreflexia, diaphoresis, nausea or vomiting, or sometimes delirium and convulsions. Pulse and respiration rates are usually elevated, pupil size is normal, there may be significant tachycardia and hypertension, and fever is generally rare without associated complications (e.g., aspiration).

Several techniques are available for the management of patients with suspected benzodiazepine or barbiturate withdrawal. The basic principle is usually to withdraw the suspected agent slowly to avoid convulsions. The long-acting

TABLE 16.6 Neurobiology of Drug Reinforcement

Drug Type	Mechanism of Reinforcement
Cocaine Amphetamines Nicotine	Mesolimbic dopamine system
Opioids Alcohol	Mesolimbic dopamine system GABA and glutamate Dopamine and serotonin Opioid peptide systems
Cannabinoids	Dopamine in the nucleus accumbens

GABA, Gamma aminobutyric acid.

TABLE 16.7 Equivalent Doses of Common Sedative–Hypnotics

Generic Name	Dose (mg)
Phenobarbital	30
Secobarbital	100
Pentobarbital	100
BENZODIAZEPINES	
Alprazolam	1
Diazepam	10
Chlordiazepoxide	25
Lorazepam	2
Clonazepam	0.5–1
OTHER	
Meprobamate	400

barbiturate phenobarbital may be a superior drug of choice for the management of detoxification for drugs in this class (Table 16.7).

REFERENCES

1. O'Brien CP, McLellan AT. Myths about the treatment of addiction. *Lancet.* 1996;347:237–240.
2. Substance Abuse and Mental Health Services Administration. (2021). Key substance use and mental health indicators in the United States: results from the 2020 National Survey on Drug Use and Health (HHS Publication No. PEP21-07-01-003, NSDUH Series H-56). Center for Behavioral Health Statistics and Quality, Substance Abuse and Mental Health Services Administration. Accessed January 15, 2023. https://www.samhsa.gov/data
3. Substance Abuse and Mental Health Services Administration. Drug Abuse Warning Network: Findings from Drug-Related Emergency Department Visits, 2021 (HHS Publication No. PEP22-07-03-002). 2022. Accessed January 15, 2023. Center for Behavioral Health Statistics and Quality, Substance Abuse and Mental Health Services Administration. Retrieved from https://www.samhsa.gov/data
4. Goodwin DW, Crane JB, Guze SB. Alcoholic "blackouts": a review and clinical study of 100 alcoholics. *Am J Psychiatry.* 1969;126(2):191–198.
5. Yao H, Takashima Y, Hashimoto M, et al. Subclinical cerebral abnormalities in chronic kidney disease. *Contrib Nephrol.* 2013;179:24–34.
6. Bagnardi V, Rota M, Botteri E, et al. Light alcohol drinking and cancer: a meta-analysis. *Ann Oncol.* 2013;24(2):301–308.
7. World Health Organization. *Global Status Report on Alcohol and Health.* World Health Organization; 2011.
8. Mokdad AH, Marks JS, Stroup DF, et al. Actual causes of death in the United States, 2000. *JAMA.* 2004;291(10):1238–1245.
9. Bouchery EE, Harwood HJ, Sacks JJ, et al. Economic costs of excessive alcohol consumption in the U.S. 2006. *Am J Prev Med.* 2011;41(5):516–524.
10. Harwood H. *Updating Estimates of the Economic Costs of Alcohol abuse In the United States: estimate, Update Methods and Data.* National Institute on Alcohol Abuse and Alcoholism, National Institutes of Health, Department of Health and Human Services; 2000.
11. Rourke S, Loberg T. *Neurobehavioral Correlates of Addiction.* Oxford University Press; 1996.
12. Bates ME, Bowden SC, Barry D. Neurocognitive impairment associated with alcohol use disorders: implications for treatment. *Exp Clin Psychopharmacol.* 2002;10(3):193–212.
13. U.S. Department of Health and Human Services, U.S. Department of Agriculture. *Dietary Guidelines for Americans* 2005.
14. Sullivan EV, Deshmukh A, Desmond JE, et al. Cerebellar volume decline in normal aging, alcoholism, and Korsakoff's syndrome: relation to ataxia. *Neuropsychology.* 2000;14(3):341–352.
15. Oscar-Berman M, Marinkovic K. Alcohol: effects on neurobehavioral functions and the brain. *Neuropsychol Rev.* 2007; 17(3):239–257.
16. Zahr NM, Sullivan EV. Translational studies of alcoholism: bridging the gap. *Alcohol Res Health.* 2008;31(3):215–230.
17. Oscar-Berman M. *Neuropsychological Vulnerabilities in Chronic Alcoholism.* National Institute on Alcohol Abuse and Alcoholism; 2000.
18. Moselhy HF, Georgiou G, Kahn A. Frontal lobe changes in alcoholism: a review of the literature. *Alcohol Alcohol.* 2001; 36(5):357–368.
19. Everitt BJ, Robbins TW. Neural systems of reinforcement for drug addiction: from actions to habits to compulsion. *Nature Neurosci.* 2005;8(11):1481–1489.
20. Kalivas PW. The glutamate homeostasis hypothesis of addiction. *Nat Rev Neurosci.* 2009;10(8):561–572.
21. Kalivas PW, Volkow ND. The neural basis of addiction: a pathology of motivation and choice. *Am J Psychiatry.* 2005;162 (8):1403–1413.
22. Valenzuela CF. Alcohol and neurotransmitter interactions. *Alcohol Health Res World.* 1997;21(2):144–148.
23. Enoch MA, Gorodetsky E, Hodgkinson C, et al. Functional genetic variants that increase synaptic serotonin and 5-HT3 receptor sensitivity predict alcohol and drug dependence. *Mol Psychiatry.* 2011;16(11):1139–1146.
24. Sari Y, Johnson VR, Weedman JM. Role of the serotonergic system in alcohol dependence: from animal models to clinics. *Prog Mol Biol Transl Sci.* 2011;98:401–443.
25. Gianoulakis C. Influence of the endogenous opioid system on high alcohol consumption and genetic predisposition to alcoholism. *J Psychiatry Neurosci.* 2001;26(4):304–318.
16. Ramchandani VA, Umhau J, Pavon FJ, et al. A genetic determinant of the striatal dopamine response to alcohol in men. *Mol Psychiatry.* 2011;16(8):809–817.
27. Weiss F, Porrino LJ. Behavioral neurobiology of alcohol addiction: recent advances and challenges. *J Neurosci.* 2002; 22(9):3332–3337.
28. American Psychiatric Association. *Diagnostic and Statistical Manual of Mental Disorders.* 5th ed. American Psychiatric Publishing; 2013.
29. Edwards G, Gross MM. Alcohol dependence: provisional description of a clinical syndrome. *BMJ.* 1976;1(6017):1058–1061.
30. Schuckit MA. An overview of genetic influences in alcoholism. *J Subst Abuse Treat.* 2009;36(suppl 1):S5–S14.
31. Li TK. Pharmacogenetics of responses to alcohol and genes that influence alcohol drinking. *J Stud Alcohol.* 2000;61(1):5–12.
32. Filbey FM, Claus ED, Morgan M, et al. Dopaminergic genes modulate response inhibition in alcohol abusing adults. *Addict Biol.* 2012;17(6):1046–1056.
33. Mulligan MK, Dubose C, Yue J, et al. Expression, covariation, and genetic regulation of miRNA biogenesis genes in brain supports their role in addiction, psychiatric disorders, and disease. *Front Genet.* 2013;4:126.
34. Schuckit MA, Tapert S, Matthews SC, et al. fMRI differences between subjects with low and high responses to alcohol during a stop signal task. *Alcohol Clin Exp Res.* 2012;36(1):130–140.
35. Heath AC, Madden PA, Martin NG. Assessing the effects of cooperation bias and attrition in behavioral genetic research using data-weighting. *Behav Genet.* 1998;28(6):415–427.
36. Koopmans JR, Boomsma DI. Familial resemblances in alcohol use: genetic or cultural transmission? *J Stud Alcohol.* 1996; 57(1):19–28.
37. Prescott CA, Hewitt JK, Heath AC, et al. Environmental and genetic influences on alcohol use in a volunteer sample of older twins. *J Stud Alcohol.* 1994;55(1):18–33.
38. Rose MK. Genetics and alcoholism: implications for advanced practice psychiatric/mental health nursing. *Arch Psychiatr Nurs.* 1998;12(3):154–161.
39. Urbanoski KA, Kelly JF. Understanding genetic risk for substance use and addiction: a guide for non-geneticists. *Clin Psychol Rev.* 2012;32(1):60–70.
40. Schuckit MA. *Vulnerability Factors for Alcoholism.* Lippincott Williams & Wilkins; 2002.
41. Hingson RW, Heeren T, Winter MR. Age at drinking onset and alcohol dependence: age at onset, duration, and severity. *Arch Pediatr Adolesc Med.* 2006;160(7):739–746.
42. Kessler RC, Crum RM, Warner LA, et al. Lifetime co-occurrence of DSM-III-R alcohol abuse and dependence with other psychiatric disorders in the National Comorbidity Survey. *Arch Gen Psychiatry.* 1997;54(4):313–321.

43. Kelly TM, Daley DC, Douaihy AB. Treatment of substance abusing patients with comorbid psychiatric disorders. *Addict Behav.* 2012;37(1):11–24.

44. Ray GT, Weisner CM, Mertens JR. Relationship between use of psychiatric services and five-year alcohol and drug treatment outcomes. *Psychiatr Serv.* 2005;56(2):164–171.

45. Brown SA, Inaba RK, Gillin JC, et al. Alcoholism and affective disorder: clinical course of depressive symptoms. *Am J Psychiatry.* 1995;152(1):45–52.

46. Brown SA, Irwin M, Schuckit MA. Changes in anxiety among abstinent male alcoholics. *J Stud Alcohol.* 1991;52(1):55–61.

47. Jellinek EM. *The Disease Concept of Alcoholism.* College & University Press; 1960.

48. Cloninger CR, Bohman M, Sigvardsson S. Inheritance of alcohol abuse. Cross-fostering analysis of adopted men. *Arch Gen Psychiatry.* 1981;38(8):861–868.

49. Hesselbrock M. *Genetic Determinants of Alcoholic Subtypes.* Oxford University Press; 1995.

50. Babor TF, Dolinsky ZS, Meyer RE, et al. Types of alcoholics: concurrent and predictive validity of some common classification schemes. *Br J Addict.* 1992;87(10):1415–1431.

51. Del Boca FK, Hesselbrock M. Gender and alcoholic subtypes. *Alcohol Health Res World.* 1996;20(1):56–62.

52. Hesselbrock VM, Hesselbrock MN. Are there empirically supported and clinically useful subtypes of alcohol dependence? *Addiction.* 2006;101(suppl 1):97–103.

53. Moss HB, Chen CM, Yi HY. DSM-IV criteria endorsement patterns in alcohol dependence: relationship to severity. *Alcohol Clin Exp Res.* 2008;32(2):306–313.

54. Reinert DF, Allen JP. The alcohol use disorders identification test: an update of research findings. *Alcohol Clin Exp Res.* 2007;31(2):185–199.

55. Bradley KA, DeBenedetti AF, Volk RJ, et al. AUDIT-C as a brief screen for alcohol misuse in primary care. *Alcohol Clin Exp Res.* 2007;31(7):1208–1217.

56. Knight JR, Sherritt L, Shrier LA, et al. Validity of the CRAFFT substance abuse screening test among adolescent clinic patients. *Arch Pediatr Adolesc Med.* 2002;156(6):607–614.

57. Anton RF. Carbohydrate-deficient transferrin for detection and monitoring of sustained heavy drinking. What have we learned? Where do we go from here? *Alcohol.* 2001;25(3):185–188.

58. Miller PM, Anton RF. Biochemical alcohol screening in primary health care. *Addict Behav.* 2004;29(7):1427–1437.

59. Thon N, Weinmann W, Yegles M, et al. Direct metabolites of ethanol as biological markers of alcohol use: basic aspects and applications. *Fortschr Neurol Psychiatr.* 2013;81(9):493–502.

60. Bien TH, Miller WR, Tonigan JS. Brief interventions for alcohol problems: a review. *Addiction.* 1993;88(3):315–335.

61. Graham A. *Brief Interventions.* American Society of Addiction Medicine; 1998.

62. O'Connor PG, Schottenfeld RS. Patients with alcohol problems. *N Eng J Med.* 1998;338(9):592–602.

63. Madras BK, Compton WM, Avula D, et al. Screening, brief interventions, referral to treatment (SBIRT) for illicit drug and alcohol use at multiple healthcare sites: comparison at intake and 6 months later. *Drug Alcohol Depend.* 2009;99(1–3):280–295.

64. Fleming MF, Barry KL, Manwell LB, et al. Brief physician advice for problem alcohol drinkers. A randomized controlled trial in community-based primary care practices. *JAMA.* 1997;277(13):1039–1045.

65. Kristenson H, Ohlin H, Hulten-Nosslin MB, et al. Identification and intervention of heavy drinking in middle-aged men: results and follow-up of 24–60 months of long-term study with randomized controls. *Alcohol Clin Exp Res.* 1983;7(2):203–209.

66. Wallace P, Cutler S, Haines A. Randomised controlled trial of general practitioner intervention in patients with excessive alcohol consumption. *BMJ.* 1988;297(6649):663–668.

67. A cross-national trial of brief interventions with heavy drinkers. WHO Brief Intervention Study Group. *Am J Public Health.* 1996;86(7):948–955.

68. Edwards G, Orford J, Egert S, et al. Alcoholism: a controlled trial of "treatment" and "advice." *J Stud Alcohol.* 1977;38(5):1004–1031.

69. Miller WR, Sanchez V. *Motivating Young Adults for Treatment and Lifestyle Change.* Notre Dame Press; 1994.

70. Miller WR, Rollnick S. *Motivational Interviewing: Helping People Change.* 3rd ed. Guilford Press; 2012.

71. Alaja R, Seppa K. Six-month outcomes of hospital-based psychiatric substance use consultations. *Gen Hosp Psychiatry.* 2003;25(2):103–107.

72. Ettner SL, Hermann RC, Tang H. Differences between generalists and mental health specialists in the psychiatric treatment of Medicare beneficiaries. *Health Serv Res.* 1999;34(3):737–760.

73. Moos RH, Finney JW, Federman EB, et al. Specialty mental health care improves patients' outcomes: findings from a nationwide program to monitor the quality of care for patients with substance use disorders. *J Stud Alcohol.* 2000;61(5):704–713.

74. Hillman A, McCann B, Walker NP. Specialist alcohol liaison services in general hospitals improve engagement in alcohol rehabilitation and treatment outcome. *Health Bull.* 2001;59(6):420–423.

75. Marlatt GA, Gordon JR, eds. *Relapse Prevention: Maintenance Strategies in the Treatment of Addictive Behaviors.* Guilford Press; 1985.

76. Swearingen CE, Moyer A, Finney JW. Alcoholism treatment outcome studies, 1970–1998. An expanded look at the nature of the research. *Addict Behav.* 2003;28(3):415–436.

77. Miller WR, Rollnick S. *Motivational Interviewing: Preparing People to Change Addictive Behaviour.* Guilford Press; 1991.

78. Meyers RJ, Smith JE, Lash DN. The community reinforcement approach. *Rec Dev Alcohol.* 2003;16:183–195.

79. Moos RH. Addictive disorders in context: principles and puzzles of effective treatment and recovery. *Psychol Addict Behav.* 2003;17(1):3–12.

80. Humphreys K, Tucker JA. Romance, realism and the future of alcohol intervention systems. *Addiction.* 2002;97(2):138–140.

81. White W.L. *Recovery Management and Recovery-Oriented Systems of Care: Scientific Rationale and Promising Practices.* Northeast Addiction Technology Transfer Center, Great Lakes Addiction Technology Transfer Center, Philadelphia Department of Behavioral Health/Mental Retardation Services; 2008.

82. Dennis ML, Scott CK. Four-year outcomes from the Early Re-Intervention (ERI) experiment using Recovery Management Checkups (RMCs). *Drug Alcohol Depend.* 2012;121(1–2):10–17.

83. McKay J, Lynch K, Shepard D. Do patient characteristics and initial progress in treatment moderate the effectiveness of telephone-based continuing care for substance use disorders? *Addiction.* 2005;100(2):216–226.

84. Stout RL, Rubin A, Zwick W, et al. Optimizing the cost-effectiveness of alcohol treatment: a rationale for extended case monitoring. *Addict Behav.* 1999;24(1):17–35.

85. Miller WR, Benefield RG, Tonigan JS. Enhancing motivation for change in problem drinking: a controlled comparison of two therapist styles. *J Consult Clin Psychol.* 1993;61(3):455–461.

86. Stephens RS, Roffman RA, Curtin L. Comparison of extended versus brief treatments for marijuana use. *J Consult Clin Psychol.* 2000;68(5):898–908.

87. McClellan A, Lewis D, O'Brien C, et al. Drug dependence, a chronic medical illness: implications for treatment, insurance, and outcomes evaluation. *JAMA.* 2000;284(13):1689–1695.

88. Fuller RK, Hiller-Sturmhofel S. Alcoholism treatment in the United States. An overview. *Alcohol Res Health.* 1999;23(2):69–77.

89. Dennis ML, Scott CK, Funk R, et al. The duration and correlates of addiction and treatment careers. *J Subst Abuse Treat.* 2005;28(suppl 1):S51–S62.

90. White WL. *Recovery/Remission from Substance Use Disorders: Analysis of Reported Outcomes in 415 Scientific Reports, 1868–2011.* Philadelphia: Department of Behavioral Health and Intellectual Disability Services, Great Lakes Addiction Technology Transfer Center; 2012.

91. Froehlich J, O'Malley S, Hyytia P, et al. Preclinical and clinical studies on naltrexone: what have they taught each other? *Alcohol Clin Exp Res.* 2003;27(3):533–539.

92. Volpicelli JR, Alterman AI, Hayashida M, et al. Naltrexone in the treatment of alcohol dependence. *Arch Gen Psychiatry.* 1992;49(11):876–880.

93. Chamorro AJ, Marcos M, Miron-Canelo JA, et al. Association of micro-opioid receptor (OPRM1) gene polymorphism with response to naltrexone in alcohol dependence: a systematic review and meta-analysis. *Addict Biol.* 2012;17(3):505–512.

94. Arbaizar B, Diersen-Sotos T, Gomez-Acebo I, et al. Topiramate in the treatment of alcohol dependence: a meta-analysis. *Actas Esp Psiquiatr.* 2010;38(1):8–12.

95. Paparrigopoulos T, Tzavellas E, Karaiskos D, et al. Treatment of alcohol dependence with low-dose topiramate: an open-label controlled study. *BMC Psychiatry.* 2011;11:41.

96. Emrick C, Tonigan J, Montgomery H, et al. *Alcoholics Anonymous: What is Currently Known.* Rutgers Center of Alcohol Studies; 1993.

97. Humphreys K. *Circles of Recovery: Self-Help Organizations for Addictions.* Cambridge University Press; 2004.

98. Humphreys K, Moos R. Can encouraging substance abuse patients to participate in self-help groups reduce demand for health care? A quasi-experimental study. *Alcohol Clin Exp Res.* 2001;25(5):711–716.

99. Humphreys K, Moos RH. Encouraging posttreatment self-help group involvement to reduce demand for continuing care services: two-year clinical and utilization outcomes. *Alcohol Clin Exp Res.* 2007;31(1):64–68.

100. Kelly JF. Self-help for substance use disorders: history, effectiveness, knowledge gaps, and research opportunities. *Clin Psychol Rev.* 2003;23(5):639–663.

101. Kelly JF, Stout R, Zywiak W, et al. A 3-year study of addiction mutual-help group participation following intensive outpatient treatment. *Alcohol Clin Exp Res.* 2006;30(8):1381–1392.

102. Moos RH, Moos BS. The interplay between help-seeking and alcohol-related outcomes: divergent processes for professional treatment and self-help groups. *Drug Alcohol Depend.* 2004;75(2):155–164.

103. Kelly JF, White W. Broadening the base of addiction recovery mutual aid. *J Groups Addict Recover.* 2012;7(2–4):82–101.

104. Hester RK, Lenberg KL, Campbell W, et al. Overcoming addictions, a web-based application, and SMART recovery, an online and in-person mutual help group for problem drinkers, Part 1: three-month outcomes of a randomized controlled trial. *J Med Internet Res.* 2013;15(7):e134.

105. Kelly JF, Humphreys K, Youngson H. Mutual aid groups. In: Harrison S, Carver V, eds. *Alcohol and Drug Problems: A Practical Guide for Counselors.* 4th ed. Centre for Addiction and Mental Health; 2012:169–197.

106. Mundt MP, Parthasarathy S, Chi FW, et al. 12-Step participation reduces medical use costs among adolescents with a history of alcohol and other drug treatment. *Drug Alcohol Depend.* 2012;126(1–2):124–130.

107. Kelly JF, Hoeppner B, Stout RL, et al. Determining the relative importance of the mechanisms of behavior change within Alcoholics Anonymous: a multiple mediator analysis. *Addiction.* 2012;107(2):289–299.

108. Kelly JF, Magill M, Stout RL. How do people recover from alcohol dependence? A systematic review of the research on mechanisms of behavior change in Alcoholics Anonymous. *Addict Res Theory.* 2009;17(3):236–259.

109. Kelly JF, Stout RL, Magill M, et al. Mechanisms of behavior change in Alcoholics Anonymous: does Alcoholics Anonymous lead to better alcohol use outcomes by reducing depression symptoms? *Addiction.* 2010;105(4):626–636.

110. Sullivan JT, Sykora K, Schneiderman J, et al. Assessment of alcohol withdrawal: the revised Clinical Institute Withdrawal Assessment for Alcohol Scale (CIWA-Ar). *Br J Addict.* 1989;84(11):1353–1357.

111. Alldredge BK, Lowenstein DH, Simon RP. Placebo-controlled trial of intravenous diphenylhydantoin for short-term treatment of alcohol withdrawal seizures. *Am J Med.* 1989;87(6):645–648.

112. Schoenenberger RA, Heim SM. Indication for computed tomography of the brain in patients with first uncomplicated generalized seizure. *BMJ.* 1994;309(6960):986–989.

113. Sullivan JT, Sykora K, Schneiderman J, et al. Assessment of alcohol withdrawal: the revised Clinical Institute Withdrawal Assessment for Alcohol Scale (CIWA-Ar). *Br J Addict.* 1989;84(11):1353–1357.

114. Daeppen JB, Gache P, Landry U, et al. Symptom-triggered vs fixed-schedule doses of benzodiazepine for alcohol withdrawal: a randomized treatment trial. *Arch Intern Med.* 2002;162(10):1117–1121.

115. Jaeger TM, Lohr RH, Pankratz VS. Symptom-triggered therapy for alcohol withdrawal syndrome in medical inpatients. *Mayo Clinic Proc.* 2001;76(7):695–701.

116. Sellers EM, Naranjo CA, Harrison M, et al. Diazepam loading: simplified treatment of alcohol withdrawal. *Clin Pharmacol Ther.* 1983;34(6):822–826.

117. Rayner SG, Weinert CR, Peng H, et al. Dexmedetomidine as adjunct treatment for severe alcohol withdrawal in the ICU. *Ann Intensive Care.* 2012;2(1):12.

118. Coomes TR, Smith SW. Successful use of propofol in refractory delirium tremens. *Ann Emerg Med.* 1997;30(6):825–828.

119. Rosenson J, Clements C, Simon B, et al. Phenobarbital for acute alcohol withdrawal: a prospective randomized double-blind placebo-controlled study. *J Emerg Med.* 2013;44(3):592–598. e592.

120. Nejad S, Nisavic MD, Larentzakis A, et al. Phenobarbital for acute alcohol withdrawal management in surgical trauma patients—a retrospective comparison study. *Psychosomatics.* 2020;61(4):327–335.

121. Nisavic M, Nejad S, Isenberg B, et al. Use of phenobarbital in alcohol withdrawal management - a retrospective comparison study of phenobarbital and benzodiazepines for acute alcohol withdrawal management in general medical patients. *Psychosomatics.* 2019;60(5):458–467.

122. Levine AR, Carrasquillo L, Mueller J, et al. High-dose gabapentin for the treatment of severe alcohol withdrawal syndrome: a retrospective cohort analysis. *Pharmacotherapy.* 2019;39(9):881–888.

123. Isenberg-Grzeda E, Kutner HE, Nicolson SE. Wernicke-Korsakoff-syndrome: under-recognized and under-treated. *Psychosomatics.* 2012;53(6):507–516.

124. Victor M, Adams RD, Collins GH. The Wernicke-Korsakoff syndrome. A clinical and pathological study of 245 patients, 82 with post-mortem examinations. *Contemp Neurol Ser.* 1971;7:1–206.

125. Thomson AD, Marshall EJ. The natural history and pathophysiology of Wernicke's encephalopathy and Korsakoff's psychosis. *Alcohol Alcohol.* 2006;41(2):151–158.

126. de Sanctis L, Memo L, Pichini S, et al. Fetal alcohol syndrome: new perspectives for an ancient and underestimated problem. *J Matern Fetal Neonatal Med.* 2011;24(1):34–37.

127. Lipinski RJ, Hammond P, O'Leary-Moore SK, et al. Ethanol-induced face-brain dysmorphology patterns are correlative and exposure-stage dependent. *PLoS One.* 2012;7(8):e43067.

128. National Institute on Alcohol Abuse and Alcoholism. *10th Special Report to the U.S. Congress on Alcohol and Health: Highlights from Current Research from the Secretary of Health and Human Services.* US Department of Health and Human Services; 2000.

129. Gawin F, Kleber H. Abstinence symptomatology and psychiatric diagnosis in cocaine abusers. *Arch Gen Psychiatry.* 1986;43:107–113.

130. Carroll KM. Relapse prevention as a psychosocial treatment approach: a review of controlled clinical trials. *Exp Clin Psychopharmacol.* 1996;4:46–54.

131. American Psychiatric Association. Practice guidelines: treatment of patients with substance use disorders. *Am J Psychiatry.* 2006;163(suppl):8.

132. Johnston LD, O'Malley PM, Bachman JG, et al. *Monitoring the Future National Results on Drug Use: 2012 Overview, Key Findings on Adolescent Drug Use.* Institute for Social Research, The University of Michigan; 2013.

133. Ross EA, Watson M, Goldberger B. "Bath salts" intoxication. *N Engl J Med.* 2011;365(10):967–968.

134. Coppola M, Mondola R. Synthetic cathinones: chemistry, pharmacology and toxicology of a new class of designer drugs of abuse marketed as "bath salts" or "plant food". *Toxicol Lett.* 2012;211(2):144–149.

135. Centers for Disease Control and Prevention. Reported US AIDS cases by HIV-exposure category—1994. *MMWR Morb Mortal Wkly Rep.* 1995;44:4.

136. Substance Abuse and Mental Health Services Administration, Center for Behavioral Health Statistics and Quality. Drug Abuse Warning Network. *National Estimates of Drug-Related Emergency Department Visits,* HHS Publication No. SMA 11-4618 Department of Health and Human Services; 2011.

137. Centers for Disease Control and Prevention. Vital signs: over-doses of prescription opioid pain relievers —United States, 1999–2008. *MMWR Morb Mortal Wkly Rep.* 2011;60:1–6.

138. Massachusetts Department of Public Health. Overdose Education and Naloxone Distribution (OEND) Program Data. Author; 2011.

139. Ling W, Charuvastra C, Collins JF, et al. Buprenorphine mainte-nance treatment of opiate dependence: a multicenter, random-ized clinical trial. *Addiction.* 1998;93:475–486.

140. Ball JC, Ross A. *The Effectiveness of Methadone Maintenance Treatment.* Springer-Verlag; 1991.

141. Syed YY, Keating GM. Extended-release intramuscular nal-trexone (VIVITROL®): a review of its use in the prevention of relapse to opioid dependence in detoxified patients. *CNS Drugs.* 2013;27(10):851–861.

142. Fultz JM, Senay EC. Guidelines for the management of hospital-ized narcotics addicts. *Ann Intern Med.* 1975;82:815–818.

143. Charney DS, Sternberg DE, Kleber HD, et al. The clinical use of clonidine in abrupt withdrawal from methadone. *Arch Gen Psychiatry.* 1981;38:1273–1277.

144. Jaffe JH, Kleber HD. Opioids: general issues and detoxification. In: American Medical Association., ed. *Treatment of Psychiatric Disorders: A Task force Report of the American Psychiatric Association.* Vol 2. American Psychiatric Association; 1989.

145. Substance Abuse and Mental Health Services Administration, Center for Behavioral Health Statistics and Quality. *The Dawn Report. Emergency Department Visits for Adverse Reactions Involving the Insomnia Medication Zolpidem.* 2013.

146. Wiviott SD, Wiviott-Tishler L, Hyman SE. Sedative-hypnotics and anxiolytics. In: Friedman L, Fleming NF, Roberts DH, eds. *Source Book of Substance Abuse and Addiction.* Williams & Wilkins; 1996.

17 Pharmacotherapy of Sexual Disorders and Sexual Dysfunction

Linda Carol Shafer

KEY POINTS

Incidence

- Sexual disorders are common, occurring in 43% of women and 31% of men in the United States.

Epidemiology

- Advanced age and co-morbid medical (particularly cardiovascular) and psychiatric conditions are associated with higher rates of sexual dysfunction in both genders. Paraphilic disorders are associated with attention-deficit hyperactivity disorder.

Pathophysiology

- Sexual function depends on a complex interplay of biological, social, cultural, and psychological factors, many of which are poorly understood. The human sexual response cycle is a useful framework for understanding sexual problems.

Clinical Findings

- The *Diagnostic and Statistical Manual of Mental Disorders*, Fifth Edition, is the reference standard for the classification of sexual disorders. A careful sexual history remains the most important tool for facilitating diagnosis.

Differential Diagnoses

- These include many medical and surgical conditions, adverse effects of medications, and other psychiatric disorders.

Treatment Options

- Phosphodiesterase type 5 (PDE-5) inhibitors have revolutionized the treatment of erectile dysfunction and may benefit some women with selective serotonin reuptake inhibitor–induced sexual dysfunction. Flibanserin, a centrally acting serotonin mixed agonist and antagonist, and bremelanotide, a subcutaneous-injectable melanocortin receptor agonist, are newer US Food and Drug Administration–approved medications for low sexual desire in premenopausal women. Otherwise, pharmacological options for patients with sexual disorders remain limited, although many are under study, complemented by therapy.

Complications

- PDE-5 inhibitors are well-tolerated, although adverse effects, such as headache and low blood pressure, may occur. Flibanserin is associated with fatigue, hypotension, and syncope and contraindicated with recent alcohol use. Bremelanotide is linked to nausea, headache, injection site pain, and local hyperpigmentation. Hormonal agents used in women are linked to potential risks of cardiovascular disease and breast cancer.

Prognosis

- Sexual disorders are often multifaceted and require a multidisciplinary approach to achieve clinically significant improvement.

OVERVIEW

Sexual disorders are extremely common. It has been estimated that 43% of women and 31% of men in the United States have sexual dysfunction.[1] Lack of sexual satisfaction is associated with significant emotional distress (e.g., depression, marital conflict) and physical problems (e.g., cardiovascular disease, diabetes mellitus). Individuals with sexual problems are often reluctant to seek assistance from a physician and may first experiment with any number of self-help methods. With the introduction of phosphodiesterase type 5 (PDE-5) inhibitors, such as sildenafil (Viagra), for the treatment of erectile dysfunction (ED) and the increased interest in pharmacological therapy for female sexual disorders, the frequency of complaints related to sexual dysfunction in primary care practices has increased. Nevertheless, the incidence of sexual problems is related to the frequency with which providers take a sexual history, many of whom remain reluctant to broach the topic despite strong patient interest.[2]

The *Diagnostic and Statistical Manual of Mental Disorders*, Fifth Edition (DSM-5) is the reference standard for the classification of sexual disorders.[3] Sexual disorders are separated into three chapters: sexual dysfunctions, paraphilic disorders, and gender dysphoria.

Sexual dysfunction is characterized by a clinically significant disturbance in the ability to respond sexually or to experience sexual pleasure, lasting at least 6 months. Some disorders are gender-specific (e.g., male hypoactive sexual desire disorder). The sexual dysfunctions are further assigned a severity rating and classified as lifelong or acquired and situational or generalized. In addition, the DSM-5 includes "associated features," such as relationship and medical factors, which support some selected diagnoses.

The DSM-5 distinguishes between paraphilias and paraphilic disorders.[4] Paraphilias are defined as persistent and intense sexual interests that are atypical but not harmful to oneself or others and thus are considered normal. Paraphilic disorders are paraphilias, which, in contrast, cause distress or

TABLE 17.1 Classification of Sexual Dysfunctions

Impaired Sexual Response Phase	Female	Male
Desire	Female sexual interest/ arousal disorder Other specified sexual dysfunction: sexual aversion	Male hypoactive sexual desire disorder Other specified sexual dysfunction: sexual aversion
Excitement (arousal, vascular)	Female sexual interest/ arousal disorder	Erectile disorder
Orgasm (muscular)	Female orgasmic disorder	Delayed ejaculation Premature ejaculation
Sexual pain	Genito-pelvic pain/ penetration disorder	Other specified or unspecified sexual dysfunction

TABLE 17.2 Medical and Surgical Conditions Causing Sexual Dysfunctions

Organic Disorders	Sexual Impairment
ENDOCRINE Hypothyroidism, adrenal dysfunction, hypogonadism, diabetes mellitus	Low libido, (early) erectile dysfunction, decreased vaginal lubrication
VASCULAR Hypertension, atherosclerosis, stroke, venous insufficiency, sickle cell disorder	Erectile dysfunction, but ejaculation and libido intact
NEUROLOGICAL Spinal cord damage, diabetic neuropathy, herniated lumbar disk, alcoholic neuropathy, multiple sclerosis, temporal lobe epilepsy	Sexual disorder—early sign, low libido (or high libido), erectile dysfunction, impaired orgasm
LOCAL GENITAL DISEASE *Male*: priapism, Peyronie disease, urethritis, prostatitis, hydrocele *Female*: imperforate hymen, vaginitis, pelvic inflammatory disease, endometriosis	Low libido, erectile dysfunction Genito-pelvic pain, low libido, decreased arousal
SYSTEMIC DEBILITATING DISEASE Renal, pulmonary, or hepatic diseases, advanced malignancies, infections	Low libido, erectile dysfunction, decreased arousal
SURGICAL-POSTOPERATIVE STATES *Male*: prostatectomy (radical perineal), abdominal-perineal bowel resection *Female*: episiotomy, vaginal repair of prolapse, oophorectomy *Male and female*: amputation (leg), colostomy, and ileostomy	Erectile dysfunction, no loss of libido, ejaculatory impairment Genito-pelvic pain, decreased lubrication Mechanical difficulties in sex, low self-image, fear of odor

impairment to the individual or that result in personal harm or risk of harm to others.

Finally, gender dysphoria describes dissatisfaction with one's assigned birth sex, causing clinically significant distress or an impairment of social function. Notably, the term allows for the possibility of an alternative or undefined gender rather than simply male or female gender roles.[3]

EPIDEMIOLOGY AND RISK FACTORS

Sexual disorders affect individuals across the epidemiological spectrum. They occur more often in women than in men and are more frequent with advanced age, lower socioeconomic status, obesity, sedentary lifestyle, co-existing medical (e.g., cardiovascular) and psychiatric conditions, and a history of sexual trauma.[5] The prototypical paraphilic is young, White, and male and more likely to have attention-deficit hyperactivity disorder (ADHD), substance abuse, major depression or dysthymia, or a phobic disorder.[6] More broadly, the coronavirus disease 2019 (COVID-19) pandemic, although waning in global impact, is likely to have profound persistent effects on sexual health. Potential consequences include short- and long-term complications of virus infection; delayed medical and psychiatric care, in turn worsening sexual function; heightened vigilance toward hygienic and quarantining protocols, potentially inhibiting sexual relationships; increased social isolation and reliance on virtual intimacy; exacerbation of mental health and psychosocial stressors; and potential for greater partner conflict or compulsive sexual behaviors (e.g., internet pornography) with work-from-home arrangements, among other factors.[7]

PATHOPHYSIOLOGY

Sexual function depends on complex interactions among the brain, hormones, and the vascular system. Neural modulators of sexual desire, arousal, and orgasm include dopamine, oxytocin, melanocortin, estrogen, and testosterone. At the vascular level, nitric oxide (NO) plays a critical role in regulating vaginal smooth muscle tone and intrapenile blood flow.[8] In fact, PDE-5 inhibitors act by prolonging the effects of NO.

The sexual response cycle concept is useful in understanding sexual problems. The stages vary with age and physical status and are affected by medications, diseases, injuries, and psychological conditions (Table 17.1). Three major models have been proposed.

Masters and Johnson developed the first model of the human sexual response, consisting of a linear progression through four distinct phases: (1) excitement (arousal), (2) plateau (maximal arousal before orgasm), (3) orgasm (rhythmic muscular contractions), and (4) resolution (return to baseline). After resolution, a refractory period exists in men.[9]

Kaplan modified the Masters and Johnson[10] model by introducing a desire stage (neuropsychological input). The Kaplan model consists of three stages: (1) desire, (2) excitement or arousal, and (3) orgasm (muscular contraction).

Most recently, Basson,[11] recognizing the complexity of the female sexual response, proposed a biopsychosocial model of female sexuality that consists of four overlapping components: (1) biology, (2) psychology, (3) sociocultural factors, and (4) interpersonal relationships. The model acknowledges that many factors may stimulate a woman's receptivity for sex. Indeed, sexual satisfaction may be prompted by such factors as emotional closeness and may still be achieved without direct desire. Additionally, it is known that physical measurements of female arousal (such as increased vaginal secretions) are poorly correlated with sexual satisfaction.

Aging is associated with changes in the normal human sexual response. Men are slower to achieve erections and require more direct genital stimulation. Women have decreased levels of estrogen, leading to decreased vaginal lubrication and narrowing of the vagina. Testosterone levels in both sexes decline with age, which may result in decreased libido.[12]

CLINICAL FEATURES AND DIAGNOSIS

The diagnosis of a sexual problem relies on a thorough medical and sexual history, supplemented by physical examination and laboratory testing. A mixed organic–psychological basis is often present. Physical disorders, surgical conditions (Table 17.2), medications, and use or abuse of drugs (Table 17.3) can affect sexual function directly or cause

TABLE 17.3 Drugs and Medicines That Cause Sexual Dysfunction

Drug	Sexual Side Effect
CARDIOVASCULAR	
Methyldopa	Low libido, erectile dysfunction, anorgasmia
Thiazide diuretics	Low libido, erectile dysfunction, decreased lubrication
Clonidine	Erectile dysfunction, anorgasmia
Propranolol	Low libido
Digoxin	Gynecomastia, low libido, erectile dysfunction
Clofibrate	Low libido, erectile dysfunction
PSYCHOTROPICS	
Sedatives	
Alcohol	Higher doses cause sexual problems
Barbiturates	Erectile dysfunction
Anxiolytic	
Alprazolam; diazepam	Low libido, delayed ejaculation
Antipsychotics	
Thioridazine	Delayed or retrograde ejaculation
Haloperidol	Low libido, erectile dysfunction, anorgasmia
Antidepressants	
MAOIs (phenelzine)	Erectile dysfunction, delayed ejaculation, anorgasmia
Tricyclics (imipramine)	Low libido, erectile dysfunction, delayed ejaculation
SSRIs (fluoxetine, sertraline)	Low libido, erectile dysfunction, delayed ejaculation
Atypical (trazodone)	Priapism, delayed or retrograde ejaculation
Lithium	Low libido, erectile dysfunction
HORMONES	
Estrogen	Low libido in men
Progesterone	Low libido, erectile dysfunction
GASTROINTESTINAL	
Cimetidine	Low libido, erectile dysfunction
Methantheline bromide	Erectile dysfunction
Opiates	Orgasmic dysfunction
Anticonvulsants	Low libido, erectile dysfunction, priapism

MAOIs, Monoamine oxidase inhibitors; *SSRIs*, selective serotonin reuptake inhibitors.

BOX 17.1 Psychological Causes of Sexual Dysfunction

PREDISPOSING FACTORS
Lack of information or experience
Unrealistic expectations
Negative family attitudes to sex
Sexual trauma: rape, incest

PRECIPITATING FACTORS
Childbirth
Infidelity
Dysfunction in the partner

MAINTAINING FACTORS
Interpersonal issues
Family stress
Work stress
Financial problems
Depression
Performance anxiety
Gender dysphoria

Clinicians should be aware of the growing numbers of patients with concerns about "hypersexuality" and "sexual addiction," in part spurred by ease of access to internet pornography and "cybersex" activities.[15,16] In fact, a "hypersexual disorder," conceptualized as a non-paraphilic sexual desire disorder with an impulsivity component, was proposed for the DSM-5, although ultimately rejected.[17] Nevertheless, the sexual history-taker should actively explore the role of the internet in the patient's sexual and non-sexual functioning and the potential for excessive or compulsive sexual activities, which may only be exacerbated in the aftermath of the COVID-19 pandemic.

Physical Examination and Laboratory Investigation

Although history-taking is often the most important tool in the diagnosis of sexual disorders, the physical examination and pertinent laboratory testing are useful in excluding an organic cause. There is no "routine" work-up. However, special attention should be paid to the endocrine, neurological, vascular, urological, and gynecological systems.[18]

Tests for systemic illness include complete blood count, urinalysis, creatinine, lipid profile, thyroid function studies, and fasting blood sugar. Endocrine studies (including testosterone, prolactin, luteinizing hormone, and follicle-stimulating hormone) can be performed to assess low libido and ED. An estrogen level and microscopic examination of a vaginal smear can be used to assess vaginal dryness. Cervical culture and a Papanicolaou (Pap) smear can be performed to investigate genital pain. The nocturnal penile tumescence (NPT) test is valuable in the assessment of ED. If NPT occurs regularly (as measured by a Rigi-Scan monitor), problems with erection are unlikely to be organic. Penile plethysmography is used to assess paraphilic disorders by measurement of an individual's sexual arousal in response to visual and auditory stimuli.

Diagnostic Features of Specific Sexual Dysfunctions

Male Disorders of Sexual Function

Erectile Disorder. Erectile dysfunction ("impotence") is characterized by marked difficulty obtaining or maintaining an erection during sexual activity or by a marked decrease in

secondary psychological reactions that lead to a sexual problem.[13] Psychological factors may predispose to, precipitate, or maintain a sexual disorder (Box 17.1).

Approach to Sexual History-Taking

The sexual history provides an invaluable opportunity to uncover sexual problems. Patients and physicians alike may be reluctant to discuss sexual problems. Thus, the need to make sexual history-taking a routine part of practice is paramount. Physicians should always attempt to be sensitive and non-judgmental in their interviewing technique, moving from general topics to more specific ones. Questions about sexual function may follow naturally from aspects of the medical history (such as introduction of a new medication or investigation of a chief complaint that involves a gynecological or urological problem).

Screening questions include: Are you sexually active? With men, women, or both? Is there anything you would like to change about your sex life? Have there been any changes in your sex life? Are you satisfied with your present sex life? To maximize its effectiveness, the sexual history may be tailored to the patient's needs and goals.[14] Physicians should recognize that patients with paraphilic disorders are often secretive about their activities, in part because of legal and societal implications. Patients should be reassured about the confidentiality of their interaction (except in cases where their behavior requires mandatory legal reporting, e.g., as with child abuse).

BOX 17.2 Risk Factors Associated with Erectile Disorder

- Hypertension
- Diabetes mellitus
- Smoking
- Coronary artery disease
- Peripheral vascular disorders
- Blood lipid abnormalities
- Peyronie disease
- Priapism
- Pelvic trauma or surgery
- Renal failure and dialysis
- Hypogonadism
- Alcoholism
- Depression
- Lack of sexual knowledge
- Poor sexual technique
- Interpersonal problems

erectile rigidity. Symptoms should be present during 75% to 100% of sexual encounters.[3] More than 18 million American men older than aged 20 years and more than 50% of men aged 40 to 70 have ED.[19,20] Up to 86% of cases of ED have an organic basis.[21] Numerous risk factors for ED have been identified (Box 17.2). ED itself may be a symptom of a generalized vascular disease and should prompt further investigation. Depression is a common co-morbidity.

Delayed Ejaculation. Also known as "retarded ejaculation," this uncommon disorder is characterized by a marked delay, infrequency, or absence of ejaculation after normal sexual excitement that is not desired by the individual, occurring in 75% to 100% of partnered sexual activity.[3] It is among the least common and least well-studied male sexual dysfunctions, with an overall estimated prevalence of 1% to 4%. However, ejaculatory difficulties are known to increase with increasing age and co-morbid medical conditions, affecting up to 43% of men in their 70s.[22] Symptoms of delayed ejaculation are classically restricted to failure to reach orgasm in the vagina during intercourse. The disorder ejaculation must be differentiated from retrograde ejaculation, in which the bladder neck does not close off properly during orgasm, causing semen to spurt backward into the bladder. Delayed ejaculation should also be excluded in couples with infertility of unknown cause; the man may not have admitted his lack of ejaculation to his partner. Men with delayed ejaculation report lower levels of sexual arousal and satisfaction despite strong penile response during psychophysiological testing.

Premature (Early) Ejaculation. This disorder is defined as recurrent ejaculation with minimal sexual stimulation before, on, or shortly after penetration (within ~1 minute) and before the person wishes it. Rapid ejaculation is a common complaint reported in 20% to 30% of men aged 18 to 70 years internationally. However, only 1% to 3% of men meet the strict DSM-5 criteria for the disorder.[3] Prolonged periods of no sexual activity make premature ejaculation worse. If the problem is chronic and untreated, secondary ED often occurs.

Male Hypoactive Sexual Desire Disorder. This disorder is characterized by persistently or recurrently deficient or absent sexual or erotic thoughts or fantasies and desire for sexual activity. The prevalence of problems with sexual desire increases from 6% of men aged 18 to 24 years to 41% of men aged 66 to 74 years. However, only 1.8% of men aged 16 to 44 years meet the strict DSM-5 definition of the disorder requiring symptoms to last at least 6 months.[3]

Female Disorders of Sexual Function

Female Sexual Interest/Arousal Disorder. Female sexual interest/arousal disorder (FSIAD) is characterized by absent or reduced interest in sexual activity, erotic thoughts, sexual excitement, arousal, or genital sensation and lack of initiation of sexual activity. Low sexual interest is reported in 20% to 40% of women.[23] However, the prevalence of FSIAD as defined by DSM-5 criteria has yet to be precisely defined.

Female Orgasmic Disorder. This disorder is defined as a marked delay in, or infrequency or lack of intensity of, orgasm occurring in 75% to 100% of occasions of sexual activity. Some women who can have orgasm with direct clitoral stimulation find it impossible to reach orgasm during intercourse. The estimated prevalence of female orgasmic problems ranges from 10% to 42%, but only a fraction of women report associated distress.[3] The ability to reach orgasm increases with sexual experience. Claims that stimulation of the Gräfenberg spot, or G-spot, in a region in the anterior wall of the vagina will cause orgasm and female ejaculation have never been substantiated.[24] Premature ejaculation in the male may contribute to female orgasmic dysfunction.

Genito-Pelvic Pain/Penetration Disorder. This disorder is characterized by persistent or recurrent difficulties with vulvo-vaginal pain or fear of pain during intercourse or penetration. There may be associated marked tensing of the pelvic floor muscles during attempted vaginal penetration. The prevalence is unknown; however, approximately 15% of North American women report recurrent pain during intercourse.[3]

Sexual Dysfunctions Affecting Both Genders

Substance-/Medication-Induced Sexual Dysfunction. This disorder is characterized by a clinically significant disturbance in sexual function with objective evidence that the symptoms occurred soon after ingestion of a substance and could have been caused by the substance. It should cause clinically significant distress and not occur during an episode of delirium.[3]

Other Specified and Unspecified Sexual Dysfunction. These diagnoses are used to describe entities that are not diagnostic of the aforementioned sexual dysfunctions. If the clinician wishes to explain why the symptoms do not meet full criteria for another disorder, the "other specified" diagnosis should be used. Otherwise, the "unspecified" diagnosis should be used. Of note, the uncommonly encountered "sexual aversion" (persistent extreme aversion to genital sexual contact with a partner) is not designated as a discrete disorder in DSM-5. However, a clinician could elect to use the "other specified" designation followed by "sexual aversion" as the specific reason to indicate this diagnosis if clinically most appropriate.[3]

Diagnostic Features of Specific Paraphilic Disorders

Most paraphilic disorders are thought to have a psychological basis. Individuals with paraphilic disorders have difficulty forming more socialized sexual relationships. Paraphilic disorders may involve a conditioned response in which non-sexual objects become sexually arousing when paired with a pleasurable activity (masturbation).[3] The diagnostic criteria and clinical features of the major paraphilic disorders are summarized in Table 17.4.

Diagnostic Features of Gender Dysphoria

Gender dysphoria is subcategorized into disorders that affect children and disorders that affect adolescents and adults.

Gender Dysphoria in Children. Children with this disorder express a strong desire to be of the opposite gender and

TABLE 17.4 Features of Specific Paraphilic Disorders

Disorder	Definition	Features
Exhibitionistic disorder	Exposure of genitals to unsuspecting strangers in public	Primary intent is to evoke shock or fear in victims; offenders are usually male
Fetishistic disorder	Sexual arousal using non-living objects (e.g., female lingerie) or intense focus on a non-genital body part	Masturbation occurs while holding the fetish object; the sexual partner may wear the object
Frotteuristic disorder	Sexual arousal by touching and rubbing against a non-consenting person	The behavior occurs in a crowded public place from which the offender can escape arrest
Pedophilic disorder	Sexual activity with a prepubescent child; the patient must be at least 16 years of age and be at least 5 years older than the victim	Pedophilia is the most common paraphilic disorder; most of the victims are girls, often relatives with the perpetrator; most pedophiles are heterosexual
Sexual masochism disorder	Sexual pleasure comes from physical or mental abuse or humiliation	A dangerous form involves hypoxyphilia, in which oxygen deprivation enhances arousal and accidental deaths can occur
Sexual sadism disorder	Sexual arousal is derived from causing mental or physical suffering to another person	Sexual sadism is mostly seen in men; it can progress to rape; 50% of those afflicted have alcoholism
Transvestic disorder	Cross-dressing in heterosexual males for sexual arousal	The wife (partner) may be aware of the activity and help in the selection of clothes or insist on treatment
Voyeuristic disorder	Sexual arousal by watching an unsuspecting person who is naked, disrobing, or engaging in sexual activity	Most commonly occurs in men, but it can occur in women; masturbation commonly occurs
Other specified paraphilic disorder	Paraphilic disorders that do not meet criteria for any of the above categories	Categories include necrophilia (corpses), zoophilia (animals), urophilia (urine), and coprophilia (feces)
Unspecified paraphilic disorder	Paraphilic disorders that do not meet criteria for any of the above categories	Clinician chooses not to specify the reason that criteria are not met; insufficient diagnostic information

TABLE 17.5 Psychiatric Differential Diagnosis of Sexual Dysfunction

Psychiatric Disorder	Sexual Complaint
Depression (major depression or dysthymic disorder)	Low libido, erectile dysfunction
Bipolar disorder (manic phase)	Increased libido
Generalized anxiety disorder, panic disorder, post-traumatic stress disorder	Low libido, erectile dysfunction, lack of vaginal lubrication, anorgasmia
Obsessive-compulsive disorder	Low libido, erectile dysfunction, lack of vaginal lubrication, anorgasmia, "anti-fantasies" focusing on the negative aspects of a partner
Schizophrenia	Low desire, bizarre sexual desires
Paraphilic disorder	Deviant sexual arousal causing distress, harm, or both
Gender dysphoria	Dissatisfaction with one's own sexual preference or phenotype
Personality disorder (passive-aggressive, obsessive-compulsive, histrionic)	Low libido, erectile dysfunction, premature ejaculation, anorgasmia
Marital dysfunction or interpersonal problems	Varied
Fears of intimacy or commitment	Varied, deep intrapsychic issues

exhibit behaviors stereotypical of the other sex. They may participate in such activities as cross-dressing and cross-gender roles in fantasy play and prefer toys and sex characteristics of the opposite gender. Identification with a non-stereotypical or non-binary gender is also possible. Children with gender dysphoria may have co-existing separation anxiety, generalized anxiety, and depression and are 2 to 4.5 times more likely to be birth-assigned males.[3] Although of late the diagnosis of gender dysphoria in children has been mired in sociopolitical controversy, recent research suggests that in fact the disorder generally manifests in early childhood, usually by age 7 years.[25]

Gender Dysphoria in Adolescents and Adults. This disorder is similar to the childhood form, but there is emphasis on incongruent sexual identity rather than participation in gender-atypical behaviors. Patients reject their own gender and secondary sex characteristics and desire those of the opposite (or an alternative) gender. The disorder is equally likely in adolescent birth-assigned males and females but is more common in birth-assigned males as adults. The overall prevalence in adult birth-assigned males and females ranges from 0.005% to 0.014% and 0.002% to 0.003%, respectively. These statistics are based on patients seeking gender reassignment and therefore are likely underestimates.[3] Associations include homosexual or bisexual orientation, anxiety, depression, suicidal ideation or attempts, and paraphilias.

DIFFERENTIAL DIAGNOSIS OF SEXUAL DISORDERS

The differential diagnosis of sexual disorders includes medical and surgical conditions (see Table 17.2), adverse effects of medications (see Table 17.3), and other psychiatric disorders (Table 17.5).[13,26,27] Before a primary sexual disorder is diagnosed, it is important to identify potentially treatable conditions (both organic and psychiatric) that manifest as sexual problems. For example, treatment of depression may improve erectile function. Although paraphilic disorders often have a psychological basis, an organic cause should be considered if the behavior begins at a late age, there is regression from previously normal sexuality, or there are abnormal physical findings. Box 17.3 lists the psychiatric differential diagnosis of paraphilic disorders. Patients with gender dysphoria generally have normal physical and laboratory findings. The differential diagnosis includes non-conformity to stereotypical sex role behaviors, transvestic fetishism (cross-dressing), and schizophrenia (e.g., with the delusion that one belongs to the other sex).

TREATMENT

Organically Based Treatment

The essence of treatment for sexual disorders involves treatment of pre-existing illnesses, stoppage of or substitution for

BOX 17.3 Psychiatric Differential Diagnosis of Paraphilic Disorders

- Intellectual disability
- Dementia
- Substance intoxication
- Manic episode (bipolar disorder)
- Schizophrenia
- Obsessive-compulsive disorder
- Gender dysphoria
- Personality disorder
- Sexual dysfunction
- Non-paraphilic compulsive sexual behaviors:
  - Compulsive use of erotic videos, magazines, or cybersex
  - Uncontrolled masturbation
  - Unrestrained use of prostitutes
  - Numerous brief, superficial, sexual affairs
  - Hypersexuality/sexual addiction

offending medications, lifestyle modification (e.g., reduction in alcohol and smoking, improvement in diet and exercise), and addition of medications for psychiatric conditions (e.g., depression). Although many medications for the treatment of hypertension inhibit sexual function, the angiotensin II receptor blockers (e.g., losartan) may ameliorate sexual problems.[28] Any hormone deficiency should be corrected (e.g., addition of testosterone for hypogonadism, thyroid hormone for hypothyroidism, estrogen/testosterone [Estratest] for post-menopausal females, or bromocriptine for elevated prolactin).[13]

Selective serotonin reuptake inhibitor (SSRI)–induced sexual dysfunction is a frequent complaint that has received significant attention. Treatment strategies include awaiting spontaneous remission, decreasing the dose of the SSRI, taking a drug holiday, switching SSRIs, switching to a non-SSRI, and adding an "antidote" drug, the last two options being the most efficacious. Non-SSRI antidepressants less likely to cause sexual dysfunction include bupropion (Wellbutrin), mirtazapine (Remeron), vortioxetine (Trintellix), possibly duloxetine (Cymbalta), trazodone (Desyrel), vilazodone (Viibryd), nefazodone (brand name Serzone withdrawn in the United States), and transdermal selegiline (EMSAM).[29,30] Non-approved antidepressants with fewer sexual side effects include: tianeptine (Stablon), reboxetine (Edronax, Vestra), moclobemide (Aurorix, Manerix), agomelatine (Valdoxan, Melitor, Thymanax), and gepirone (Ariza, Variza).[31,32] PDE-5 inhibitors are the "antidotes" of choice followed by bupropion and high-dose buspirone (Buspar). Additional possible antidotes include herbal agents, such as maca root and *Gingko biloba*, and a variety of medications including amantadine (Symmetrel), dextroamphetamine (Dexedrine), methylphenidate (Ritalin), granisetron (Kytril), cyproheptadine (Periactin), yohimbine (Yocon), and atomoxetine (Strattera).[33,34]

Premature Ejaculation

There is no Food and Drug Administration (FDA)–approved treatment for premature ejaculation. However, the SSRIs (e.g., fluoxetine [Prozac], sertraline [Zoloft], and paroxetine [Paxil]), used continuously or intermittently (2–12 hours before sex), can cause delayed ejaculation, which can treat premature ejaculation. The tricyclic clomipramine (Anafranil) is also efficacious. Dapoxetine (Priligy), an SSRI with a rapid onset and short half-life, was developed specifically to treat premature ejaculation but is not approved. Tramadol taken on-demand (in re-development for premature ejaculation

under the brand name Zertane) appears promising, but as a weak opioid, it is limited by potential dependency. Topical anesthetic agents under investigation include the lidocaine/prilocaine eutectic mixture (EMLA cream) and topical eutectic-like mixture for premature ejaculation (TEMPE or PSD 502/Fortacin).[35] However, these can cause skin irritation and penile numbing. Co-existing ED if present should be treated first with PDE-5 inhibitors.

Erectile Disorder

The mainstay of treatment for ED is the use of oral PDE-5 inhibitors, which can help men with a wide range of conditions; they are easy to use and have few adverse effects (Table 17.6). Available agents are sildenafil (Viagra), vardenafil (Levitra; Staxyn orally disintegrating tablet [ODT]), tadalafil (Cialis), and avanafil (Stendra) (see Table 17.6). PDE-5 inhibitors in development include mirodenafil (Mvix), udenafil (Zydena), and lodenafil (Helleva).[36,37] Of note, the PDE-5 inhibitors are metabolized by P450 3A4 and 2C9 isoenzyme systems. Patients who take potent inhibitors (including grapefruit juice, cimetidine, ketoconazole, erythromycin, and ritonavir) of these P450 isoenzyme systems should have a lower starting dose of a PDE-5 inhibitor.[38] Statins may also help improve the efficacy of PDE-5 inhibitors.

The only other oral pharmacological agent approved by the FDA for the treatment of ED is yohimbine (Yocon), an α_2-adrenergic inhibitor, although its efficacy is uncertain. Other (non-approved) agents include α-receptor blocker phentolamine (Vasomax), dopamine agonist apomorphine (Uprima), melanocortin agonist bremelanotide (Vyleesi; only approved for low sexual desire in women), amino acid L-arginine (ArginMax), opioid antagonist naltrexone (Depade, Revia) and serotonin/dopamine modulator, clavulanic acid (Zoraxel).[39] 5-HT$_{2C}$ serotonin receptor agonists including trazodone appear to stimulate erections in some studies. Topical agents include alprostadil cream (Topiglan), minoxidil solution, and nitroglycerine ointment. Herbal agents are of uncertain benefit with *Panax ginseng*, *Butea superba*, and *Lepidium meyenii* (maca root) appearing more promising; some herbals may contain traces of PDE-5 inhibitors.[40] Transdermal testosterone and/or clomiphene citrate (Clomid) may be considered for hypogonadal men with ED.

Second-line treatments for ED include use of intrapenile injection therapy, intraurethral suppository therapy, and vacuum-assisted devices (Table 17.7). Injectable gene therapies for ED, such as hMaxi-K, are promising, but clinical trials are in the early stages.[41] The third-line treatment for ED is surgical implantation of an inflatable or malleable rod or penile prosthesis. Endarterectomy may correct ED in certain patients with underlying vascular disease. Pelvic drug-eluting vascular stents (e.g., zotarolimus) are in investigational stages.[42]

Female Sexual Dysfunction

Medical options for treating female sexual dysfunction are increasing but remain sparse. EROS-CTD, an approved (non-pharmacologic) clitoral suction device, can be used to increase vasocongestion and engorge the clitoris for better sexual arousal and orgasm. Two agents are now available for treating premenopausal women with generalized, acquired hypoactive sexual desire disorder (according to *Diagnostic and Statistical Manual of Mental Disorders*, Fourth Edition [DSM-IV] criteria, most similar but not equivalent to FSIAD in DSM-5): flibanserin (Addyi), an oral centrally acting serotonin receptor agonist/antagonist, and bremelanotide (Vyleesi), a subcutaneous-injectable melanocortin 4 receptor agonist. The most

TABLE 17.6 First-line Treatment for Erectile Dysfunction: Comparison of Phosphodiesterase Type 5 Inhibitors

Medication	Dose	Onset	Duration	Food Interaction	Advantages	Side Effects	Contraindications
Sildenafil (Viagra)	25–100 mg (maximum)	30–60 min	≤12 h	Delayed absorption with high-fat foods	>65% efficacy Longest track record	Headache, low BP, flushing, dyspepsia, vasodilation, diarrhea, visual changes (blue tinge to vision), hearing loss (rare) NAION (not proven)	Active CAD, hypotension No nitrates for 24 h after dose Caution with α-blockers
Vardenafil (Levitra)	2.5–20 mg (maximum)	30–60 min	≤10 h	Delayed absorption with high-fat foods	>65% efficacy Available as ODT preparation (Staxyn)	Headache, low BP, flushing, dyspepsia, vasodilation, diarrhea, visual changes, hearing loss (rare) NAION (not proven)	Active CAD, hypotension May prolong QTc May increase LFT No nitrates for 24 h after dose Avoid α-blockers Hytrin and Cardura Cautious use with Flomax or Uroxotra
Tadalafil (Cialis)	2.5–20 mg (maximum) Only PDE-5 inhibitor approved for daily use (5 mg)	60–120 min	Up to 36 h	None	>65% efficacy No visual side effects Can be taken with food	Headache, low BP, flushing, dyspepsia, vasodilation, diarrhea, back pain, myalgias, hearing loss (rare) NAION (not proven)	Active CAD, hypotension No nitrates for 48 h after dose Avoid α-blockers Hytrin and Cardura Cautious use with Flomax or Uroxotra
Avanafil (Stendra)	50–200 mg (maximum)	15–30 min	≤6 h	None	Similar efficacy to other PDE-5 inhibitors Can be taken with food Shortest onset of action Shortest duration of action and interaction with nitrates	Headache, low BP, flushing, dyspepsia, nasal congestion, dizziness, hearing loss (rare) NAION (not proven)	No nitrates for 12 h after dose Start at lower dose (50 mg instead of 100 mg) if taking (stable) α-blocker

BP, Blood pressure; *CAD*, coronary artery disease; *LFT*, liver function test; *NAION*, non-arteritic anterior ischemic optic neuropathy; *ODT*, orally disintegrating tablet; *PDE-5*, phosphodiesterase type 5.

TABLE 17.7 Second-Line Treatments for Erectile Dysfunction

Treatment	Effects	Advantages	Disadvantages
Intraurethral suppository: alprostadil (MUSE)	Prostaglandin E₁ gel delivered by applicator into meatus of penis Induces vasodilation to cause erection	60% efficacy Less penile fibrosis and priapism than with penile injections Can be used twice daily	Not recommended with pregnant partners Mild penile or urethral pain
Penile self-injection: alprostadil (Caverject and Edex)	Prostaglandin E₁ injected into base of penis Induces vasodilation to cause erection	50%–87% efficacy Few systemic side effects	Can cause penile pain, priapism, fibrosis Not recommended for daily use
Intracavernosal injection: VIP + phentolamine: aviptadil (Senatek)	VIP causes veno-occlusion while phentolamine increases arterial flow	Associated with less pain than alprostadil and therefore preferred by patients	Less effective than alprostadil
Vacuum constriction device (pump)	Creates vacuum to draw blood into penile cavernosa Elastic band holds blood in penis	67% efficacy No systemic side effects Safe if erection not maintained more than 1 h	May not be acceptable to partner Erection hinged at base; does not allow for external ejaculation

VIP, Vasoactive intestinal polypeptide.

common adverse effects of flibanserin include nausea, fatigue, dizziness, and dry mouth. Hypotension and syncope have also been reported and may be potentiated with alcohol consumption, which is therefore contraindicated within 2 hours of flibanserin use. Bremelanotide is associated with nausea, headache, flushing, injection site pain or reaction, and local hyperpigmentation of the face, breasts, and gingiva.[43]

Ospemifene (Osphena), an oral selective estrogen receptor modulator, is another approved agent used to treat postmenopausal dyspareunia (genital pain associated with sex) or vaginal dryness caused by vulvar and vaginal atrophy. Otherwise, most agents used to treat sexual dysfunction in men have been tried in women with limited success. Studies have demonstrated a reduction in SSRI-induced adverse sexual effects in women receiving sildenafil.[44] Bupropion may be helpful for female sexual dysfunction with or without concomitant depression.[45] Hormonal agents have been studied extensively, although enthusiasm has been tempered by links with cardiovascular disease and breast cancer; they should not be prescribed in premenopausal women in whom there is no clear benefit and only potential risk.[46] Transdermal/topical preparations include estrogen/testosterone (Estratest), testosterone (LibiGel—Phase III trials; Intrinsa—rejected by the FDA), and prostaglandin E₁ (alprostadil). Oral hormonal therapies include estrogen for vasomotor symptoms, novel steroid tibolone (Livial—rejected), and dehydroepiandrosterone (DHEA) for women with adrenal insufficiency.

Paraphilic Disorders

Pharmacological therapy for patients with paraphilic disorders is aimed at suppression of compulsive sexual behavior. The anti-androgen drugs, cyproterone acetate (CPA—not FDA-approved) and medroxyprogesterone acetate (MPA, Depo-Provera), are used to reduce aberrant sexual tendencies. Treatment with synthetic gonadotropin-releasing hormone (GnRH) analogues (approved for prostate cancer), including leuprorelin (Prostap), triptorelin (Trelstar), and goserelin (Zoladex), is also effective; oral estrogen (ethinyl estradiol) is less so. The SSRIs and clomipramine (Anafranil) reduce aberrant sexual urges by decreasing the compulsivity or impulsivity of the act.[47] Paraphilic disorders commonly co-exist with ADHD, and the addition of psychostimulants, such as methylphenidate sustained-release (Ritalin-SR), to SSRIs appears beneficial in controlling paraphilic behaviors.[48]

Gender Dysphoria

The major treatment for gender dysphoria is gender-affirming (reassignment) hormonal or surgical therapy or both. Hormones may be used to suppress original sex characteristics, for example, with GnRH agonists, CPA, estrogens, or testosterone.[49]

Psychologically Based Treatments

Sexual Dysfunction

General principles of treatment include improving communication (verbally and physically) between partners, encouraging experimentation, decreasing the pressure of performance by changing the goal of sexual activity away from erection or orgasm to feeling good about oneself, and relieving the pressure of the moment. The PLISSIT model provides a useful framework for approaching treatment of sexual problems and can be tailored to the desired level of intervention. The stages are (1) P, permission; (2) LI, limited information; (3) SS, specific suggestions; and (4) IT, intensive therapy. Permission-giving involves reassuring the patient about sexual activity, alleviating guilt about activities the patient feels are "bad" or "dirty," and reinforcing the normal range of sexual activities. Limited information includes providing basic knowledge about anatomy and physiology and correcting myths and misconceptions. Specific suggestions include techniques of behavioral sex therapy (Table 17.8). Intensive therapy may be useful for patients with chronic sexual problems or complex psychological issues.[50] Although the first three stages (P, LI, SS) may be implemented by any health care provider, the last stage (IT) usually requires an expert with special training in sex therapy.

Paraphilic Disorders

Paraphilic disorders are often refractory to treatment, and recidivism is high, but several non-pharmacological modalities have been used with varying success. Insight-oriented or supportive psychotherapy is relatively ineffective. Cognitive-behavioral therapy can be used to help patients identify aberrant sexual tendencies, alter their behavior, and avoid sexual triggers to prevent relapse.[4] Aversive therapy, via conditioning with ammonia, is used to reduce paraphilic behavior. Orgasmic reconditioning is used to teach the paraphilic

TABLE 17.8 Specific Behavioral Techniques of Sex Therapy

Sexual Disorder	Suggestions
Male hypoactive sexual desire disorder	Sensate focus exercises (non-demand pleasuring techniques) to enhance enjoyment without pressure Erotic material and masturbation training
Female sexual interest/arousal disorder	Sensate focus exercises Lubrication: saliva, KY Jelly for vaginal dryness
Other specified sexual dysfunction: sexual aversion	Sensate focus exercises For phobic or panic symptoms, use antianxiety or antidepressant medications
Erectile disorder	Sensate focus exercises (non-demand pleasuring techniques) Use female superior position (heterosexual couple) for non-demanding intercourse Female manually stimulates penis, and if erection is obtained, she inserts the penis into the vagina and begins movement Learn ways to satisfy partner without penile–vaginal intercourse
Female orgasmic disorder	Self-stimulation Use of fantasy materials Kegel vaginal exercises (contraction of pubococcygeus muscles) Use of controlled intercourse in female superior position "Bridge technique": male stimulates female's clitoris manually after insertion of the penis into the vagina
Delayed ejaculation (during intercourse)	Female stimulates male manually until orgasm becomes inevitable Insert penis into vagina and begin thrusting
Premature ejaculation	Increased frequency of sex "Squeeze technique": female manually stimulates penis until ejaculation is approaching, then squeezes the penis with her thumb on the frenulum; pressure is applied until male no longer feels the urge to ejaculate (15–60 seconds); use the female superior position with gradual thrusting and the "squeeze" technique as excitement intensifies "Stop–start technique": female stimulates the male to the point of ejaculation, then stops the stimulation; she resumes the stimulation for several stop–start procedures until ejaculation is allowed to occur
Genito-pelvic pain/penetration disorder	Treat any underlying gynecological problem first Treat insufficient lubrication using, e.g., KY Jelly Female is encouraged to accept larger and larger objects into her vagina (e.g., her fingers, her partner's fingers, Hegar graduated vaginal dilators, syringe containers of different sizes) Recommend use of the female superior position, allowing female to gradually insert erect penis into the vagina Practice Kegel vaginal exercises to develop a sense of control

patient how to become aroused by more acceptable mental images. Social skills training (individual or group) is used to help the paraphilic form better interpersonal relationships. Surveillance systems (using family members to help monitor patient behavior) may be helpful. Lifelong maintenance is required.

Gender Dysphoria

Individual psychotherapy is useful both in helping patients understand their gender dysphoria and in addressing other psychiatric issues. A thorough psychological evaluation and appropriate informed consent are generally required before initiating gender-affirming medical treatment, particularly if irreversible (e.g., with surgery) or in minors.[49] Marital and family therapy can help with adjustment to a new gender.

OUTLOOK

Sexual disorders remain common and are associated with significant long-term emotional, physical, and psychosocial stress, likely only exacerbated in the post COVID-19 era. However, decreasing societal stigma, combined with increasing understanding of the medical basis of sexual disorders, has enabled more patients to feel comfortable seeking treatment. The DSM-5 is the current reference standard for the classification of sexual disorders. However, research is ongoing to clarify the nuances of these conditions, many of which have been substantively redefined or newly described compared with previous DSM editions.

Phosphodiesterase type 5 inhibitors remain among the most effective agents for the treatment of patients with sexual

dysfunction and have revolutionized the treatment of ED in men. Interest in developing effective therapies for female sexual dysfunction is on the rise, with the notable FDA approval of flibanserin and bremelanotide for premenopausal women with low sexual desire. Nonetheless, pharmacological options remain limited, although investigation continues. Further elucidation of the brain mechanisms behind sexual desire and arousal should allow for new therapeutic targets. Genetic research also heralds a new era in drug development aimed at personalized medicine through application of pharmacogenetic principles.

Although sex is increasingly "medicalized," the role of psychological interventions in the treatment of patients with sexual problems should not be overlooked. Evidence-based clinical guidelines for the treatment of those with sexual disorders may help in optimizing short- and long-term management strategies. Overall, a multidisciplinary approach appears to be advantageous and will continue to evolve with time.

REFERENCES

1. Laumann EO, Paik A, Rosen RC. Sexual dysfunction in the United States: prevalence and predictors. *JAMA*. 1999;281:537–544.
2. Clark RD, Williams AA. Patient preferences in discussing sexual dysfunctions in primary care. *Fam Med*. 2014;46:124–128.
3. American Psychiatric Association. *Diagnostic and Statistical Manual of Mental Disorders*. 6th ed. American Psychiatric Press; 2013: 423–459, 685–705.
4. Yakeley J, Wood H. Paraphilias and paraphilic disorders: diagnosis, assessment and management. *Adv Psychiatr Treat*. 2014;20: 202–213.
5. McCabe MP, Sharlip ID, Lewis R, et al. Risk factors for sexual dysfunction among women and men: a consensus statement from the Fourth International Consultation on Sexual Medicine 2015. *J Sex Med*. 2016;13:153–167.

6. Korchia T, Boyer L, Deneuville M, et al. ADHD prevalence in patients with hypersexuality and paraphilic disorders: a systematic review and meta-analysis. *Eur Arch Psychiatry Clin Neurosci.* 2022;272(8):1413–1420.

7. Pennanen-Iire C, Prereira-Lourenço M, Padoa A, et al. Sexual health implications of COVID-19 pandemic. *Sex Med Rev.* 2021;9:3–14.

8. Melis MR, Argiolas A. Erectile function and sexual behavior: a review of the role of nitric oxide in the central nervous system. *Biomolecules.* 2021;11:1866.

9. Masters WH, Johnson VE. *Human Sexual Response.* Little, Brown and Company; 1966. 1st ed.

10. Kaplan HS. *The Sexual Desire Disorders: Dysfunctional Regulation of Sexual Motivation.* Brunner-Routledge; 1995. 1st ed.

11. Basson R. The female sexual response: a different model. *J Sex Marital Ther.* 2000;26:51–65.

12. Curley CM, Johnson BT. Sexuality and aging: is it time for a new sexual revolution? *Soc Sci Med.* 2022;301:114865.

13. Basson R, Schultz WW. Sexual sequelae of general medical disorders. *Lancet.* 2007;369:409–424.

14. Savoy M, O'Gurek D, Brown-James A. Sexual health history: techniques and tips. *Am Fam Physician.* 2020;101:286–293.

15. Asiff M, Sidi H, Masiran R, et al. Hypersexuality as a neuropsychiatric disorder: the neurobiology and treatment options. *Curr Drug Targets.* 2018;19:1391–1401.

16. de Alarcón R, de la Iglesia JI, Casado NM, et al. Online porn addiction: what we know and what we don't-a systematic review. *J Clin Med.* 2019;8:9.

17. Montgomery-Graham S. Conceptualization and assessment of hypersexual disorder: a systematic review of the literature. *Sex Med Rev.* 2017;5:146–162.

18. Bhugra D, Colombini G. Sexual dysfunction: classification and assessment. *Adv Psychiatr Treat.* 2013;19:48–55.

19. Selvin E, Burnett AL, Platz EA. Prevalence and risk factors for erectile dysfunction in the US. *Am J Med.* 2007;120:151–157.

20. Feldman HA, Goldstein I, Hatzichristou DG, et al. Impotence and its medical and psychosocial correlates: results of the Massachusetts Male Aging Study. *J Urol.* 1994;151:54–61.

21. Pozzi E, Fallara G, Capogrosso P, et al. Primary organic versus primary psychogenic erectile dysfunction: findings from a real-life cross-sectional study. *Andrology.* 2022;10:1302–1309.

22. Chen J. The pathophysiology of delayed ejaculation. *Transl Androl Urol.* 2016;5:549–562.

23. Laumann EO, Nicolosi A, Glasser DB, et al. Sexual problems among women and men aged 40-80 y: prevalence and correlates identified in the Global Study of Sexual Attitudes and Behaviors. *Int J Impot Res.* 2005;17:39–57.

24. Hoag N, Keast JR, O'Connell HE. The "G-spot" is not a structure evident on macroscopic anatomic dissection of the vaginal wall. *J Sex Med.* 2017;14:1524–1532.

25. Zaliznyak M, Bresee C, Garcia MM. Age at first experience of gender dysphoria among transgender adults seeking gender-affirming surgery. *JAMA Netw Open.* 2020;3:e201236.

26. Basson R. Clinical practice. Sexual desire and arousal disorders in women. *N Engl J Med.* 2006;354:1497–1506.

27. Bhasin S, Enzlin P, Coviello A, et al. Sexual dysfunction in men and women with endocrine disorders. *Lancet.* 2007;369:597–611.

28. Ismail SB, Noor NM, Hussain NHN, et al. Angiotensin receptor blockers for erectile dysfunction in hypertensive men: a brief meta-analysis of randomized control trials. *Am J Mens Health.* 2019; 131557988319892735.

29. Schweitzer I, Maguire K, Ng C. Sexual side-effects of contemporary antidepressants: review. *Aust N Z J Psychiatry.* 2009;43:795–808.

30. Jacobsen PL, Nomikos GG, Zhong W, et al. Clinical implications of directly switching antidepressants in well-treated depressed patients with treatment-emergent sexual dysfunction: a comparison between vortioxetine and escitalopram. *CNS Spectr.* 2020;25:50–63.

31. La Torre A, Giupponi G, Duffy D, et al. Sexual dysfunction related to psychotropic drugs: a critical review—part I: antidepressants. *Pharmacopsychiatry.* 2013;46:191–199.

32. Wagstaff AJ, Ormrod D, Spencer CM. Tianeptine: a review of its use in depressive disorders. *CNS Drugs.* 2001;15:231–259.

33. Montejo AL, Prieto N, de Alarcón R, et al. Management strategies for antidepressant-related sexual dysfunction: a clinical approach. *J Clin Med.* 2019;8:1640.

34. da Silva Leitão Peres N, Cabrera Parra Bortoluzzi L, Medeiros Marques LL, et al. Medicinal effects of Peruvian maca (Lepidium meyenii): a review. *Food Funct.* 2020;11:83–92.

35. Hisasue S. The drug treatment of premature ejaculation. *Transl Androl Urol.* 2016;5:482–486.

36. Jiann B-P. Evolution of phosphodiesterase type 5 inhibitors in treatment of erectile dysfunction in Taiwan. *Urol Sci.* 2016;27:66–70.

37. Alshehri YM, Al-Majed AA, Attwa MW, et al. Lodenafil. *Profiles Drug Subst Excip Relat Methodol.* 2022;47:113–147.

38. Huang SA, Lie JD. Phosphodiesterase-5 (PDE5) inhibitors in the management of erectile dysfunction. *P T.* 2013;38:407–419.

39. Albersen M, Shindel AW, Mwamukonda KB, et al. The future is today: emerging drugs for the treatment of erectile dysfunction. *Expert Opin Emerg Drugs.* 2010;15:467–480.

40. Ho CC, Tan HM. Rise of herbal and traditional medicine in erectile dysfunction management. *Curr Urol Rep.* 2011;12:470–478.

41. Yoshimura N, Kato R, Chancellor MB, et al. Gene therapy as future treatment of erectile dysfunction. *Expert Opin Biol Ther.* 2010;10: 1305–1314.

42. Kim ED, Owen RC, White GS, et al. Endovascular treatment of vasculogenic erectile dysfunction. *Asian J Androl.* 2015;17:40–43.

43. Pachano Pesantez GS, Clayton AH. Treatment of hypoactive sexual desire disorder among women: general considerations and pharmacological options. *Focus (Am Psychiatr Publ).* 2021;19:39–45.

44. Nurnberg HG, Hensley PL, Heiman JR, et al. Sildenafil treatment of women with antidepressant-associated sexual dysfunction: a randomized controlled trial. *JAMA.* 2008;300:395–404.

45. Segraves RT, Clayton A, Croft H, et al. Bupropion sustained release for the treatment of hypoactive sexual desire disorder in premenopausal women. *J Clin Psychopharmacol.* 2004;24:339–342.

46. Davis SR, Baber R, Panay N, et al. Global consensus position statement on the use of testosterone therapy for women. *J Clin Endocrinol Metab.* 2019;104:4660–4666.

47. Thibaut F, Cosyns P, Fedoroff JP, et al. The World Federation of Societies of Biological Psychiatry (WFSBP) 2020 guidelines for the pharmacological treatment of paraphilic disorders. *World J Biol Psychiatry.* 2020;21:412–490.

48. Kafka MP, Hennen J. Psychostimulant augmentation during treatment with selective serotonin reuptake inhibitors in men with paraphilias and paraphilia-related disorders: a case series. *J Clin Psychiatry.* 2000;61:664–667.

49. Meyer G, Boczek U, Bojunga J. Hormonal gender reassignment treatment for gender dysphoria. *Dtsch Arztebl Int.* 2020;117:725–732.

50. Keshavarz Z, Karimi E, Golezar S, et al. The effect of PLISSIT based counseling model on sexual function, quality of life, and sexual distress in women surviving breast cancer: a single-group pretest-posttest trial. *BMC Womens Health.* 2021;21:417.

18 Device Neuromodulation and Brain Stimulation Therapies

James Luccarelli, Michael E. Henry, Carlos G. Fernandez Robles, Cristina Cusin, Joan A. Camprodon, and Darin D. Dougherty

KEY POINTS

- Somatic therapies are a group of device-based techniques that modulate disease-relevant structures of the nervous system via surgical ablation or electrical stimulation with the goal of therapeutically modifying pathological patterns of brain activity and circuit connectivity.

- Repetitive transcranial magnetic stimulation uses an external magnetic field to electrically stimulate the cortical surface. It received US Food and Drug Administration (FDA) approval for the treatment of major depressive disorder (MDD) in 2008, with further approvals in 2018 for the treatment of obsessive-compulsive disorder (OCD), in 2020 for smoking cessation, and in 2021 for co-morbid anxiety symptoms in patients with depression.

- Electroconvulsive therapy (ECT) uses an electrical stimulus applied to the scalp to induce a generalized seizure. In clinical use since 1938, ECT devices received FDA approval for the treatment of depression (unipolar or bipolar) and catatonia in 2018.

- Vagus nerve stimulation, approved by the FDA in 2005 for treatment-resistant depression, involves intermittent stimulation of the left vagus nerve that results in electrical stimulation to brain regions involved in mood regulation.

- Deep brain stimulation involves placement of electrodes at target regions within the brain. It received FDA approval for the treatment of refractory OCD in 2009.

- Ablative limbic system surgical procedures (such as anterior cingulotomy, sub-caudate tractotomy, limbic leucotomy, and anterior capsulotomy) are viable treatment options for patients with treatment-refractory MDD or OCD.

OVERVIEW

Therapeutic options for patients with affective, behavioral, or cognitive disorders include psychotherapy, pharmacotherapy, and somatic therapies. This chapter focuses on the latter.

Somatic therapies, also known as *brain stimulation* or *neuromodulation*, are a group of device-based techniques that target specific structures of the nervous system via surgical ablation or electrical modulation with the goal of therapeutically modifying pathological patterns of brain activity and circuit connectivity. Somatic therapies can be divided into two general groups: invasive and non-invasive modalities. Invasive treatments require the surgical implantation of stimulating electrodes (or surgical ablative disconnection of aberrant pathways) and include ablative limbic system surgeries, deep brain stimulation (DBS), and vagus nerve stimulation (VNS). Non-invasive techniques can modulate brain activity trans-cranially without surgical intervention and include transcranial magnetic stimulation (TMS) as its most paradigmatic modality. Electroconvulsive therapy (ECT), the oldest of all somatic therapies, occupies a space in between the two categories because it does not require surgical intervention but does require general anesthesia; it is generally considered minimally invasive.

Studies have demonstrated that only 30% to 40% of patients with major depressive disorder (MDD) treated with pharmacotherapy achieve full remission, and 10% to 15% experience no symptom improvement.[1] Thus, somatic therapies provide an important therapeutic option for patients who do not respond to initial pharmacotherapy. Although invasive neuromodulation should be reserved for the most refractory patients, non-invasive techniques (including ECT) can be considered in earlier phases of the therapeutic process, given their efficacy and relatively benign safety profile (which can be significantly better than certain pharmacological options).

TRANSCRANIAL MAGNETIC STIMULATION

Transcranial magnetic stimulation (TMS) is a non-invasive neuromodulation modality that uses powerful and rapidly changing magnetic fields applied over the surface of the skull to generate targeted electrical currents in the brain, painlessly and without the need for surgery, anesthesia, or the induction of seizures. In 2008, the FDA approved the use of high-frequency repetitive TMS (rTMS) over the left dorsolateral prefrontal cortex (DLPFC) for the treatment of MDD. Deep TMS H-coils were approved for MDD in 2013, with further approvals in 2018 for the treatment of OCD, in 2020 for smoking cessation, and in 2021 for co-morbid anxiety symptoms in patients with depression.

One of the primary advantages of TMS is its non-invasive nature, which is made possible by the application of Faraday's principle of electromagnetic induction. Briefly (and overly simplified), this principle states that a changing electrical current flowing through a circular coil generates a magnetic field tangential to the plane of the coil. If this magnetic field contacts another conductive material (e.g., a pick-up coil) it will generate a secondary electrical current (Figure 18.1). TMS systems use an electrical capacitor to generate a brief powerful current that flows through the TMS coil, which is a circular loop of wire connected to the capacitor and embedded in a protective plastic case. According to Faraday's principle, when the electrical current flows through the circular coil, a rapidly changing magnetic field is generated. If the TMS coil is placed on the surface of the skull, this magnetic field will travel towards the intra-cranial space unaltered by the structures it

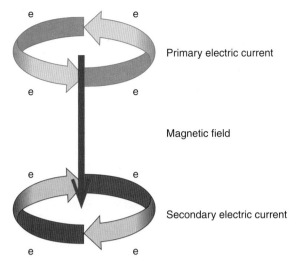

Primary electric current

Magnetic field

Secondary electric current

Figure 18.1 The principle of electromagnetic induction, by which a primary electrical current (e, yellow) generates a perpendicular magnetic field that, when in contact with a conductive material, leads to a secondary electrical current in the same plane, but opposite sense than the primary (e, red). How this principle of physics is applied in transcranial magnetic stimulation: a coil is placed on the scalp surface, leading to electrical stimulation of the cortex. (Redrawn from Jalinous R. *A Guide to Magnetic Stimulation.* Magstim Company; 1998.)

will cross (e.g., soft tissue, bone, cerebrospinal fluid), until it reaches the electrically conductive neurons of the cortex. These neurons will then act as an organic pick-up coil, and a secondary electrical current will be generated that is able to trigger action potentials and force brain cells to fire (Figure 18.1). As a result, the stimulation of neurons in TMS is really electrical, not magnetic, and the term "magnetic stimulation" is a misnomer: the magnetic pulses are used only as a vehicle for the non-invasive transfer of electrical currents from the coil to the cortex.

Although the magnetic field is essentially unaltered by the various structures it encounters on its path to the cortex, the strength of the field weakens as it moves from its source in the TMS coil. As a result, the 1- to 2-Tesla magnetic pulse originated in the TMS coil becomes too weak to generate neuronal action potentials 2 to 4 cm away from its origin on the skull's surface. This sets a practical limitation to this technique because only superficial cortical structures can be directly stimulated by TMS. Nevertheless, the effects of TMS are not only local but circuit-wide; after an action potential is generated in a cortical neuron, the volley of activation travels through its axon and stimulates the post-synaptic neuron, leading to a cascade of events through the entire neural circuit (including deep cortical, sub-cortical, and contralateral regions). This cascade of electrical events is specific to the brain circuit that the target region is connected with and not generalized like the effects of ECT. Therefore, although it is true that TMS only directly modulates superficial cortical nodes, these nodes act as windows that provide modulatory access to an entire functional network of cortical and sub-cortical neurons.[2]

The effects of TMS are not only specific to the target of stimulation but also to the parameters used. This is important as we consider statements such as "TMS is (or is not) effective for a given condition," which lack meaning and are not informative. Alternatively, "TMS applied over a determined anatomical target at a specific frequency and dose for a particular condition" is more clinically and scientifically meaningful. Because the effects of TMS are specific to the stimulated region and the parameters used, we should expect that stimulating prefrontal

cortical areas that process working memory or spatial attention will have little effect on mood, anhedonia, or neurovegetative symptoms of depression. Similarly, inhibiting a pathologically hypoactive region will most likely worsen a patient's condition, though its activation may prove therapeutic. Last, applying 2 weeks of stimulation when 4 to 6 or more weeks are needed should have minimal or no therapeutic impact. This highlights the need to have a basic understanding of the TMS parameters that clinicians and scientists can manipulate: the location or target of stimulation, the focality and depth, the frequency, and the dose of stimulation (which is a composite measure of stimulation intensity and duration) (Box 18.1).

As already mentioned, the choice of the anatomical site of stimulation is crucial because it grants us access to modulate a specific functional network of interest. Similarly, the focality of stimulation is of relevance because the clinical impact and specificity are not the same if one modulates a cortical area of 0.25 or 1 cm². Although the intensity of stimulation has an influence on the focality of its effects (the stronger the magnetic field, the deeper and less focal its effects),[3] focality is primarily controlled by the choice of TMS coil. Various types of coils are manufactured with differences in their internal architecture that allow varying degrees of focality and depth. The most common types are the circular coils (less focal), the figure-of-eight or butterfly coils (more focal), and the H-coils (deep).

Transcranial magnetic stimulation can either inhibit (downregulate) or activate (up-regulate) populations of neurons depending on the frequency of stimulation. With parameters similar to the ones leading to long-term depression or long-term potentiation, low frequencies of 1 Hz are known to be inhibitory,[4] and high frequencies greater than 5 Hz (typically 10 or 20 Hz) are activating.[5] Newer TMS protocols with more complex patterns of stimulation (such as theta burst stimulation [TBS]) have been developed more recently and allow for longer-lasting behavioral effects despite a significantly shorter stimulation time. (Whereas a traditional therapeutic protocol for MDD lasts 37.5 minutes, TBS can be performed in 3 minutes.) After the target of stimulation and direction of modulation are set, the dose is determined by deciding the strength of the magnetic field (pulse intensity) and the total number of pulses (duration). Duration also relates to the total number of sessions, typically daily sessions over the course of weeks. Other more complex variables, such as the waveform of the electromagnetic current, are also relevant to define the dose.[6] As we improve our understanding of the mechanism of action of TMS, the parameter space available becomes more complex, granting greater control and specificity to clinicians and scientists.[7]

The safety profile of TMS is notoriously benign, given its non-invasive nature. The only contraindication considered to be absolute is the presence of metallic hardware in the area of stimulation, such as cochlear implants, brain stimulators, or medication pumps.[7] Still, the use of TMS on patients with DBS has been tested and considered relatively safe when the DBS system is off, although data are still very limited and extreme caution (in addition to an accurate risk/benefit analysis) should be used in these cases.[8] The primary safety concern with TMS remains the induction of seizures with repetitive trains, even if this is a very rare phenomenon; approximately 20 seizures have been reported out of the estimated 300,000 sessions (clinical or research) since its development in the early 1980s.[7] Since the 2008 FDA approval of the NeuroStar TMS Therapy system (Neuronetics), seven seizures have been reported in the United States from 250,000 treatment sessions in 8000 patients.[9] This represents 1 case in 35,000 patients, which is similar or fewer than the seizure risk of most antidepressant medications. It should be noted that TMS may trigger a seizure but not cause epilepsy; seizures are always during (not after) rTMS and do not lead to spontaneous events afterward. Nevertheless, one should screen patients for a personal history of epilepsy and possible risk factors that increase their seizure risk (such as brain lesions or medications that lower the seizure threshold). Other less severe but more common side effects include headaches, local discomfort in the area of stimulation, facial twitching, tinnitus, anxiety, and vasovagal syncope.[7]

The evidence for the use of high-frequency rTMS to the left DLPFC, low-frequency rTMS to the right DLPFC, a combination of the two techniques (termed bilateral treatments), deep TMS over the left DLPFC, and TBS in the treatment of depression is supported by multiple clinical studies including more than 4000 patients, demonstrating robust odds ratios of 2.54 to 4.66 for response relative to sham TMS.[10] Recent developments in image-guided TMS using neuro-navigation have proved to increase the anatomical specificity and clinical efficacy of TMS. One protocol involved functional magnetic resonance imaging (MRI) to locate the region of the left DLPFC most functionally anticorrelated with the subgenual anterior cingulate cortex, which is then targeted with 10 TMS sessions per day over a 5-day period. This accelerated protocol resulted in a 69% reduction in depression scores in 5 days compared with 14% in those receiving sham treatment.[11] A device using this protocol received FDA approval for the treatment of depression in 2022.

As TMS has entered clinical practice with more homogeneous protocols leading to greater effects sizes and decreased variability, researchers have explored what variables may predict the antidepressant response of TMS. Fregni and colleagues[12] analyzed the pooled data for 195 patients from six independent studies. They reported that age and the number of previously failed medication trials were negative predictors of response (i.e., younger and less treatment-refractory patients had better outcomes). As the field moves toward identifying not only clinical or demographic variables but also biological markers that predict response to treatment, the hope is that the biomarkers linked to the therapeutic targets specifically modulated by the different treatment modalities will help stratify patients and individually select the most effective treatments.[13]

ELECTROCONVULSIVE THERAPY

Electroconvulsive therapy involves delivery of an electrical current to the brain through the scalp and skull to induce a generalized seizure. ECT has been in use since 1938; it received FDA clearance in 2018 for the treatment of severe unipolar depression, bipolar depression, and catatonia in patients aged 13 years and older. There is additional evidence for ECT as an effective treatment for both mania and schizophrenia, with recent treatment guidelines recommending ECT in patients with treatment-resistant disease refractory to clozapine. Compared with other antipsychotic augmentation strategies, it is evident that the effectiveness of ECT exceeds any other option and can accelerate the initial response by a few weeks. Furthermore, augmenting clozapine with ECT yields a response rate of 76% in patients with severe disease. In current practice, it remains a critical treatment for patients whose symptoms are unresponsive to drugs or who are intolerant of their side effects.[14] The neurobiological mechanism of ECT remains unknown and likely involves both neurohormonal effects resulting from the clinical seizure and changes in brain structure after treatment.[15]

Although most patients initially receive a medication trial regardless of their diagnosis, several groups of patients are appropriate for ECT as a primary treatment. These include patients who are severely malnourished, dehydrated, and exhausted because of protracted depressive or catatonic illnesses (however, they should be treated promptly after careful re-hydration); patients who have been unresponsive to medications during previous episodes (because they are often better served by proceeding directly to ECT); and patients with catatonia who are showing signs of metabolic failure (as they respond promptly to ECT). In addition, because of its life-threatening nature, patients with significant suicidal ideation or a recent suicide attempt, especially in the context of psychotic illness, may be appropriate candidates for initial ECT treatment because of the speed of response.

To minimize the risks of injury from a generalized seizure, general anesthesia and muscle relaxant are given before ECT. Because of the numerous physical effects of ECT, careful patient selection and collaboration with an experienced anesthesia team are essential for the safe delivery of ECT. The routine pre-ECT work-up usually includes a thorough medical history and physical examination, along with an electrocardiogram, urinalysis, complete blood count, and serum electrolytes. Additional studies may be necessary at the clinician's discretion, particularly in the presence of baseline medical illness. As the technique for ECT delivery has improved, factors that were formerly considered near-absolute contraindications to ECT have become relative risk factors. The patient is best served by weighing the risk of treatment against the morbidity or lethality of remaining depressed. The prevailing view is that there are no longer any absolute contraindications to ECT, but several conditions (e.g., space-occupying lesions with increased intracranial pressure [ICP], recent cerebral infarction, cardiac conditions) warrant careful work-up and management.

The brain is physiologically stressed during ECT, with cerebral oxygen consumption doubling during treatment and cerebral blood flow increasing several-fold. Increases in ICP and the permeability of the blood–brain barrier also develop. These acute changes may increase the risk of ECT in patients with a variety of neurological conditions.[16] Space-occupying brain lesions with associated increased ICP were previously considered essentially an absolute contraindication to ECT; however, more recent reports indicate that with careful management, patients with a brain tumor or a chronic subdural hematoma may be safely treated. Recent cerebral infarction probably represents the most common intracranial risk factor. Case reports of ECT after recent cerebral infarction indicate that the complication rate is low,[16] and consequently, ECT can be used for post-stroke depression, although clinical trials in this setting are lacking. Although 1 month is considered a standard amount of time for healing, the interval between infarction and time of ECT should be determined by the urgency of treatment for depression. ECT is instrumental in treating severe depression during pregnancy, and its safety has been documented extensively. The most common risks to the mother are premature contractions and pre-term labor, which occur infrequently and are not clearly caused by ECT; nonetheless, fetal monitoring is recommended before and after each ECT treatment.[17]

In addition to therapeutic brain effects, the electrical stimulus administered during ECT causes cardiac stimulation.[18] Cardiac work increases abruptly at the onset of the seizure initially because of sympathetic outflow from the diencephalon, through the spinal sympathetic tract, to the heart (Figure 18.2). This outflow persists for the duration of the seizure and is augmented by a rise in circulating catecholamine levels that peak about 3 minutes after the onset of seizure activity (Figure 18.3A).[19] After the seizure ends, parasympathetic tone remains strong, often causing transient bradycardia and hypotension, with a return to baseline function in 5 to 10 minutes (see Figure 18.3B). The cardiac conditions that most often worsen under this autonomic stimulus are ischemic heart disease, hypertension, congestive heart failure (CHF), and cardiac arrhythmias. These conditions, if properly managed, have proved to be surprisingly tolerant to ECT. Vascular aneurysms should be repaired before ECT if possible, but in practice, they have proved surprisingly durable during treatment.[20] Critical aortic stenosis should be surgically corrected before ECT to avoid ventricular overload during the seizure. Patients with cardiac pacemakers generally tolerate ECT uneventfully, although proper pacer function should be ascertained before treatment. The 2020 American Society of Anesthesiologists Practice Advisory recommends "suspending the implantable cardioverter defibrillator anti-tachycardia

therapy with either a magnet or a programmer" before ECT.[21] Patients with compensated CHF generally tolerate ECT well, although a transient decompensation into pulmonary edema for 5 to 10 minutes may occur in patients with a baseline ejection fraction below 20%. It is unclear whether the underlying cause is a neurogenic stimulus to the lung parenchyma or a reduction in cardiac output because of increased heart rate and blood pressure.

Antidepressants are generally continued during ECT treatment. However, if the current antidepressant trial has been of adequate dose and duration, it is a good time to consider changing medications. As tolerated, anticonvulsants are prescribed because mood stabilizers may be tapered before ECT to enhance seizure quality. Likewise, benzodiazepines should be reduced if possible and withheld the night before treatment and the morning of ECT. When tapering, the anticonvulsant load, including benzodiazepines, should be reduced carefully because too aggressive a taper can increase the risk of severe post-treatment agitation. In patients with a preexisting seizure disorder, the anticonvulsant regimen should be continued for patient safety. The elevated seizure threshold can almost always be over-ridden with an ECT stimulus, and patients managed in this manner usually have the same clinical response as patients not taking anticonvulsants.[22]

The typical course of ECT treatment includes two phases: acute treatment, with the goal of rapidly improving symptoms, followed by continuation and maintenance treatment with the goal of prolonging the time to symptom relapse. In the acute phase, treatments are generally given two to three times per week and continued until symptom remission or a plateau in treatment response. In prospective trials, the median number of treatments required to reach remission is 7.3,[23,24] but in ordinary clinical practice, longer courses are often required,[25] and for patients who continue to demonstrate clinical benefit, there is no absolute number of acute course treatments that may be administered.

Electroconvulsive therapy is not a single technique but rather a range of stimulation types. The ECT electrodes can be placed to stimulate both sides of the brain (bilateral) or just one hemisphere (typically the right) (Figure 18.4). Present evidence suggests equal efficacy of the two electrode placements in depression, with fewer cognitive effects of right unilateral treatment,[24] but optimal electrode placement for particular patients and disorders remains an active area of research. Additionally, the width of the electrical stimulus is variable, with modern brief pulse and ultra-brief pulse retaining treatment efficacy while reducing cognitive side effects relative to earlier sine wave stimuli (Figure 18.5). The efficacy of acute course ECT in the treatment of depression is established by numerous clinical trials and meta-analyses, with demonstrated response rates of around 75% for both unipolar and bipolar depression.[26] The efficacy of ECT is higher than that of TMS and other non-surgical brain stimulation techniques, with similar tolerability.[27,28] Older age is associated with greater benefit from ECT treatment,[29] although efficacy remains high even in children and adolescents.[30]

After successful treatment with ECT, without any continuation therapy, the risk of depressive relapse is greater than 80% at 6 months.[31] As a result, ongoing treatment with pharmacotherapy, additional ECT, or both is necessary. Ongoing treatment with ECT following symptom improvement is termed continuation or maintenance ECT. In a recent comparison of pharmacotherapy alone versus ECT plus pharmacotherapy, relapse rates at 1 year were 61% with pharmacotherapy alone and 32% with pharmacotherapy plus maintenance ECT.[32] Continuation ECT alone (weekly for 4 weeks, biweekly for 8 weeks, and monthly for 3 months) lowers the relapse rate at 6 months to below 40%.[23] Large controlled trials of other antidepressant

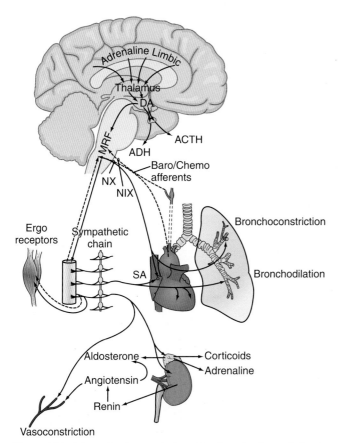

Figure 18.2 Schematic of sympathetic outflow from the diencephalon to the heart and other organs. *ACTH*; adrenocorticotropic hormone, *ADH*; antidiuretic hormone, *DA*; dopamine, *MRF*; medial reticular formation, *NIX*; cranial nerve 9, *NX*; cranial nerve 10, *SA*; sinoatrial node

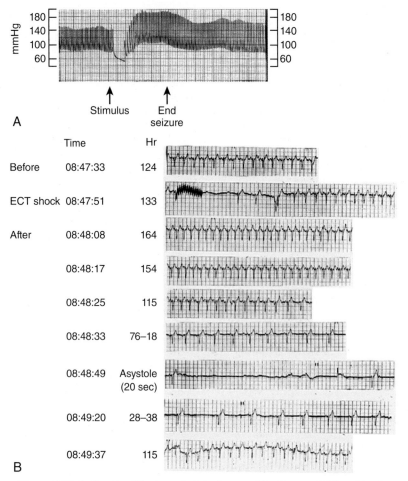

Figure 18.3 A, Graphic of the impact of electroconvulsive therapy (ECT) on blood pressure and **B**, on cardiac rhythm.

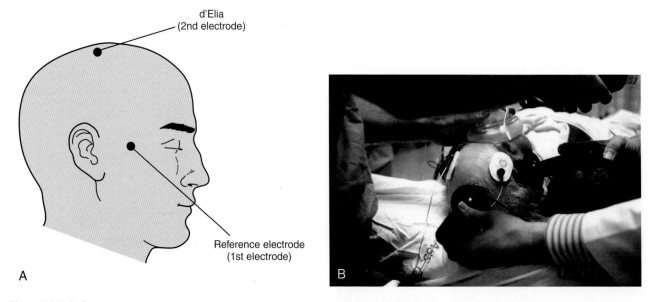

Figure 18.4 A, Schematic of electrode placements during electroconvulsive therapy (ECT). **B**, Photograph of electrodes being placed during ECT.

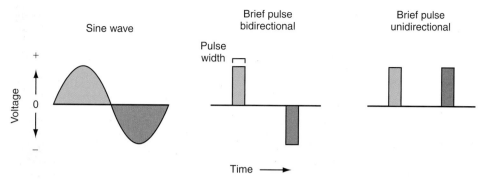

Figure 18.5 Schematic of sine wave and brief pulse stimuli for electroconvulsive therapy.

drugs after ECT have not yet been conducted. Although questions remain about the relative effectiveness of continuation ECT and continuation pharmacotherapy, the cumulative evidence over the past decade indicates that continuation ECT is a valuable and effective strategy for most patients, with a cohort of 100 maintenance ECT patients maintaining benefit from 50 or more treatments over a median of 22 months.[33]

Pooled data indicate a mortality rate of ECT of 2.1 per 100,000 treatments, which is lower than the general anesthesia mortality rate of 3.4 per 100,000 in surgical procedures.[34] Although there is no evidence for structural brain damage as a result of ECT, there are important effects on cognition. Memory impairment varies greatly in severity and is associated with bilateral electrode placement, high stimulus intensity, inadequate oxygenation, prolonged seizure activity, advanced age, alcohol abuse, and lower pre-morbid cognitive function. Difficulty recalling new information (anterograde amnesia) is usually experienced during the ECT series, but it normally resolves within 1 month after the last treatment. Difficulty remembering events before ECT (retrograde amnesia) is usually more severe for events closer to the time of treatment. A meta-analysis of cognitive function testing in 2981 patients in 84 studies found significant decreases in cognitive performance scores 0 to 3 days after completion of a series of ECT.[35] However, within 15 days of the last ECT treatment, almost all mean test scores were at or above pre-ECT levels. After 15 days, improvements compared to baseline were observed in processing speed, working memory, anterograde memory, and aspects of executive function.

VAGUS NERVE STIMULATION

Vagus nerve stimulation was approved for treatment-refractory MDD and bipolar disorder in 2005. The FDA-approval language states that VNS is an adjunctive treatment for treatment-resistant depression (TRD) and that it should be used in patients with severe, chronic, recurrent TRD who have failed at least four adequate antidepressant trials. Implantation of the VNS device involves surgical placement of electrodes around the left vagus nerve via an incision in the neck (only the left vagus nerve is used for VNS because the right vagus has a much higher percentage of parasympathetic branches to the heart) (Figure 18.6). A second incision is used to place an internal pulse generator (IPG) sub-cutaneously in the left sub-clavicular region, and the wire between the electrodes on the vagus nerve and the IPG is connected by means of sub-cutaneous tunneling between the two incision sites.

The interest in studying the efficacy of VNS for MDD arose from the clinical experience of treating more than 40,000 patients with treatment-resistant epilepsy with VNS. Depression is more prevalent in patients with epilepsy than it is in the general population, and it was noted that many

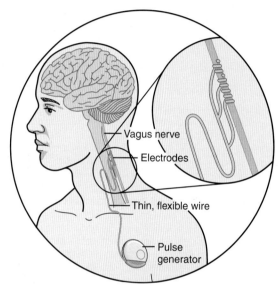

Figure 18.6 A schematic demonstrating the locations of the electrode lead on the left vagus nerve and the internal pulse generator after vagus nerve stimulation device implantation. (Redrawn from Cyberonics, Inc. *Physician's Manual for the VNS Therapy™ Pulse Model 102 Generator and VNS Therapy™ Pulse Duo Model 102R generator. Cyberonics; 2003.*)

patients with treatment-resistant epilepsy being treated with VNS experienced improvement in symptoms of MDD.[36] The left vagus nerve enters the brain and first innervates the nucleus tractus solitarius (NTS). Although the mechanism of action of VNS is not completely understood, the NTS communicates with the parabrachial nucleus (PBN); the cerebellum; the dorsal raphe; the periaqueductal gray; the locus coeruleus; and ascending projections to limbic, paralimbic, and cortical regions.[37] Functional neuroimaging studies of participants receiving VNS show increased cerebral blood flow in many of these brain regions that are implicated in the pathophysiology of MDD.[38] For instance, the locus coeruleus and dorsal raphe nuclei contain the cell bodies of noradrenergic and serotonergic neurons that then project throughout the central nervous system. Last, the PBN communicates with other brain regions (including the hypothalamus, thalamus, amygdala, and nucleus of the stria terminalis) implicated in the pathophysiology of MDD.[37]

Vagus nerve stimulation is an adjunctive treatment for depression; therefore, all patients who receive VNS should continue to receive pharmacotherapy, psychotherapy, or both (and even ECT, if necessary), referred to as *treatment as usual*. In an 8-week clinical trial of 112 patients in the active VNS treatment group and 110 patients in the sham VNS treatment group, active VNS failed to demonstrate statistically significant efficacy on the primary outcome measure, the Hamilton Depression Rating Scale (a clinician-administered scale), at 8 weeks.[39] However, step-wise increases in response and remission at 3, 6, 9, and 12 months were demonstrated during the subsequent open-label phase of the study and the FDA approved VNS for TRD in 2005 based on these data. Greater results have been demonstrated in longer-term studies. In a 5-year open label study of 795 patients, 494 receiving VNS and 301 receiving treatment as usual, 5-year cumulative remission rates were 43.3% in the VNS arm compared with 25.7% in the treatment as usual arm.[40] Moreover, the rate of suicide deaths and all-cause mortality in the VNS arm was less than half of that in the treatment-as-usual group.

Adjustment of the VNS stimulation parameters is performed by using a device that communicates trans-cutaneously with the IPG. The dose parameters used by the clinician for VNS therapy include the magnitude of the electrical charge delivered to the left vagus nerve, the stimulation frequency, the stimulation pulse width, and the duration of stimulation. Finally, decreasing the stimulation pulse width or stimulation frequency is often helpful for addressing potential side effects associated with VNS therapy.

Potential risks associated with VNS include standard risks associated with the surgical procedure itself. Most common side effects associated with active VNS therapy are likely caused by stimulation of the laryngeal and pharyngeal branches of the left vagus nerve. The most common side effect is voice alteration during the active phase (seen in 54%–60% of patients). Other relatively common side effects include cough, neck pain, paresthesia, and dyspnea.[41] These side effects typically decrease or dissipate over time. Despite these side effects, the device is well tolerated, and patients also can turn off the device at any time by placing a magnet provided by the manufacturer over the IPG. The IPG will remain off (i.e., no stimulation will occur) as long as the magnet is in place. When the magnet is removed, the IPG returns to its previously set stimulation parameters.

DEEP BRAIN STIMULATION

Deep brain stimulation grew from the therapeutic tradition of ablative stereotaxic surgery and the technical developments that led to cardiac pacemakers.[42] It requires the surgical placement of stimulating electrodes in disease-specific deep brain structures via craniotomy and stereotaxic surgery. The intracranial electrodes are connected to an IPG, which consists of a battery and mini-processor that can generate electrical currents according to clinician-determined parameters. The IPG is surgically implanted in the pectoral region (although other sites are also possible) and connects to the intra-cranial electrodes via a wire that travels through the head and neck's subcutaneous tissue. Clinicians who employ DBS use devices that communicate trans-cutaneously with the IPG to control and interrogate the system. Clinicians can change the voltage, frequency, and pulse width of the electrical pulses according to safety and efficacy criteria. Most commercially available DBS systems have four contact positions in each stimulating electrode, which can be independently activated to provide positive or negative electrical charges, therefore changing the size and shape of the electric field. This flexibility allows clinicians a significant range of electrode combinations that increase the anatomical precision of stimulation, which can be individualized according to clinical response or biomarkers, such as MRI diffusion tractography.[43]

Deep brain stimulation is a surgical procedure and therefore invasive. Iatrogenic adverse events can be categorized in two primary groups: those related to the surgical procedures and those related to the stimulation of brain regions. Surgical adverse events have an incidence rate of 1% to 4% and include seizures, infection, and hemorrhage.[44] Effects related to stimulation vary depending on the anatomical location of the electrodes and include worsening depression, (hypo)mania, acute anxiety, and gustatory or olfactory sensations. Unlike ablative interventions, permanent cognitive deficits have not been reported in DBS patients. Nevertheless, reversible cognitive effects (such as diminished concentration) have been described, though these are stimulation-dependent and remit with re-adjustment of DBS parameters.

The primary indication for DBS are Parkinson disease (PD) and other movement disorders, such as dystonia and essential tremor. The therapeutic approach for these conditions requires the surgical modulation of key nodes in the motor circuitry: sub-thalamic nucleus for PD, globus pallidus pars interna for PD and dystonia and ventral intermediate nucleus of the thalamus for essential tremor. As of 2019, more than 160,000 patients worldwide have been estimated to have been implanted with DBS devices.[45]

Basic and clinical research studies investigated the use of DBS for refractory OCD using various brain targets that included the anterior limb of the internal capsule, the ventral capsule/ventral striatum (VC/VS), the nucleus accumbens (NAcc), the sub-thalamic nucleus, and the inferior thalamic peduncle. It should be noted that the first three anatomical targets are very similar, if not practically the same. In 2009, the FDA approved the use of DBS to the VC/VS for the treatment of treatment-resistant OCD (under the humanitarian device exemption mechanism), thus approving the first psychiatric indication and allowing DBS to enter clinical practice in psychiatry.[46]

Several open-label clinical trials have been published using DBS for the treatment of MDD stimulating three main regions: the VC/VS (the same as for OCD), the sub-genual cingulate gyrus or Brodmann area 25 and the NAcc. Response rates (from 50%–60%) were similar for all regions.[47] Prospective randomized trials, however, have failed to demonstrate benefit of DBS in depression. A prospective randomized sham-controlled trial of DBS at the VC/VS in 29 patients failed to demonstrate superiority of active treatment compared with sham,[48] with a further study of 90 patients randomized to receive DBS to the subcallosal cingulate or sham treatment failing to demonstrate a difference between the two groups.[49] Other approaches for DBS, including changes in intra-operative targeting, are being explored, but overall, the use of DBS for depression remains experimental.

In addition to OCD and MDD, DBS is also being investigated as a treatment for other conditions that result from physiological changes in brain circuit and lead to pathological processing of affect, behavior, and cognition. A few examples under current active research include addiction, obesity, eating disorders, Tourette's syndrome, Alzheimer disease, and schizophrenia. Structures (such as the ventral tegmental area and the NAcc) are targeted for addiction and schizophrenia and the hippocampal fornix is targeted for Alzheimer disease. As we improve our understanding of the mechanism of action of DBS and its effects on key targets and we are able to develop new technologies that increase its specificity, efficacy, and safety, DBS may become a more commonly used treatment for the most treatment-refractory patients.[45]

ABLATIVE LIMBIC SYSTEM SURGERY

Concerns regarding ablative neurosurgery for psychiatric indications are understandable given the indiscriminate use of crude procedures, such as frontal lobotomy, in the middle of

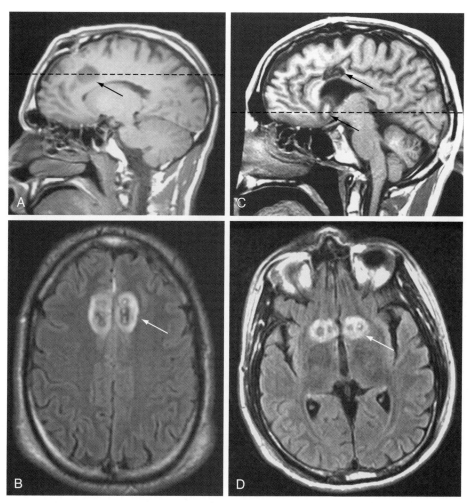

Figure 18.7 Ablative limbic system surgery. **A**, Sagittal view of anterior cingulotomy lesions *(arrow)*. **B**, Axial view (at the level of the *dotted line* in *A*) of anterior cingulotomy lesions *(arrow)*. **C**, Sagittal view of anterior cingulotomy *(upper arrow)* and sub-caudate tractotomy *(lower arrow)* lesions. **D**, Axial view (at the level of the *dotted line* in *C*) of sub-caudate tractotomy lesions *(arrow)*.

the 20th century. These procedures were associated with severe adverse events, including frontal lobe symptoms (e.g., apathy) or even death. In the latter half of the 20th century, neurosurgeons began to use much smaller lesions in well-targeted and specific brain regions. As a result, the incidence of adverse events dropped precipitously.[42] Currently used procedures include anterior cingulotomy, sub-caudate tractotomy, limbic leucotomy (which is a combination of an anterior cingulotomy and a sub-caudate tractotomy), and anterior capsulotomy (Figure 18.7). Each of these procedures uses craniotomy techniques. However, because of the small lesion volume required for an anterior capsulotomy, a gamma knife (a technique that uses focused gamma rays to create ablative lesions) can be used to perform this procedure. These procedures have been used in patients who have intractable mood and anxiety disorders; response rates range from one-third to half based on meta-analysis of uncontrolled studies.[50] Because patients eligible for these procedures have failed all other available treatments, a significant positive response to these interventions can be life-saving. Although post-operative side effects may occur, they are almost always temporary. Among the side effects are headache, nausea, and edema; more serious adverse events include infections, urinary difficulties, weight gain, seizures, cerebral hemorrhage or infarct, and cognitive deficits, all of which are uncommon.

CONCLUSION

In this chapter, we have provided an overview of neurotherapeutic interventions for psychiatric disorders that are currently available or are being studied in clinical trials. Some of these treatments have been available for many years (e.g., ECT and ablative limbic system surgery), and others (such as VNS, DBS, or TMS) have only recently been approved by the FDA for psychiatric indications. Systems neuroscience and translational neuropsychiatry research are in the path to expand our therapeutic armamentarium even further with new indications and protocols for these treatments and novel technologies.

REFERENCES

1. Fava M, Davidson KG. Definition and epidemiology of treatment-resistant depression. *Psychiatr Clin North Am.* 1996;19(2):179–200.
2. Strafella AP, Paus T, Barrett J, et al. Repetitive transcranial magnetic stimulation of the human prefrontal cortex induces dopamine release in the caudate nucleus. *J Neurosci.* 2001;21(15):RC157.
3. Trillenberg P, Bremer S, Oung S, et al. Variation of stimulation intensity in transcranial magnetic stimulation with depth. *J Neurosci Methods.* 2012;211(2):185–190.
4. Chen R, Classen J, Gerloff C, et al. Depression of motor cortex excitability by low-frequency transcranial magnetic stimulation. *Neurology.* 1997;48(5):1398–1403.

5. Pascual-Leone A, Valls-Solé J, Wassermann EM, et al. Responses to rapid-rate transcranial magnetic stimulation of the human motor cortex. *Brain J Neurol.* 1994;117(pt 4):847–858.

6. Peterchev AV, Wagner TA, Miranda PC, et al. Fundamentals of transcranial electric and magnetic stimulation dose: definition, selection, and reporting practices. *Brain Stimulat.* 2012;5(4):435–453.

7. Rossi S, Hallett M, Rossini PM, et al. Safety, ethical considerations, and application guidelines for the use of transcranial magnetic stimulation in clinical practice and research. *Clin Neurophysiol.* 2009;120(12):2008–2039.

8. Deng ZD, Lisanby SH, Peterchev AV. Transcranial magnetic stimulation in the presence of deep brain stimulation implants: induced electrode currents. *Annu Int Conf IEEE Eng Med Biol Soc.* 2010;2010:6821–6824.

9. George MS, Taylor JJ, Short EB. The expanding evidence base for rTMS treatment of depression. *Curr Opin Psychiatry.* 2013;26(1):13–18.

10. Brunoni AR, Chaimani A, Moffa AH, et al. Repetitive transcranial magnetic stimulation for the acute treatment of major depressive episodes: a systematic review with network meta-analysis. *JAMA Psychiatry.* 2017;74(2):143–152.

11. Cole EJ, Phillips AL, Bentzley BS, et al. Stanford Neuromodulation Therapy (SNT):a double-blind randomized controlled trial. *Am J Psychiatry.* 2022;179(2):132–141.

12. Fregni F, Marcolin MA, Myczkowski M, et al. Predictors of antidepressant response in clinical trials of transcranial magnetic stimulation. *Int J Neuropsychopharmacol.* 2006;9(6):641–654.

13. Fidalgo TM, Morales-Quezada JL, Muzy GSC, et al. Biological markers in noninvasive brain stimulation trials in major depressive disorder: a systematic review. *J ECT.* 2014;30(1):47–61.

14. Petrides G, Malur C, Braga RJ, et al. Electroconvulsive therapy augmentation in clozapine-resistant schizophrenia: a prospective, randomized study. *Am J Psychiatry.* 2015;172(1):52–58.

15. Espinoza RT, Kellner CH. Electroconvulsive therapy. *N Engl J Med.* 2022;386(7):667–672.

16. Hsiao JK, Messenheimer JA, Evans DL. ECT and neurological disorders. *Convuls Ther.* 1987;3(2):121–136.

17. Ward HB, Fromson JA, Cooper JJ, et al. Recommendations for the use of ECT in pregnancy: literature review and proposed clinical protocol. *Arch Womens Ment Health.* 2018;21(6):715–722.

18. Hermida AP, Mohsin M, Marques Pinheiro AP, et al. The cardiovascular side effects of electroconvulsive therapy and their management. *J ECT.* 2022;38(1):2–9.

19. Liston EH, Salk JD. Hemodynamic responses to ECT after bilateral adrenalectomy. *Convuls Ther.* 1990;6(2):160–164.

20. Drop LJ, Viguera A, Welch CA. ECT in patients with intracranial aneurysm. *J ECT.* 2000;16(1):71–72.

21. Streckenbach SC, Benedetto WJ, Fitzsimons MG. Implantable cardioverter-defibrillator shock delivered during electroconvulsive therapy despite magnet application: a case report. *AA Pract.* 2020;14(11):e01284.

22. Lunde ME, Lee EK, Rasmussen KG. Electroconvulsive therapy in patients with epilepsy. *Epilepsy Behav.* 2006;9(2):355–359.

23. Kellner CH, Knapp RG, Petrides G, et al. Continuation electroconvulsive therapy vs pharmacotherapy for relapse prevention in major depression: a multisite study from the Consortium for Research in Electroconvulsive Therapy (CORE). *Arch Gen Psychiatry.* 2006;63(12):1337–1344.

24. Semkovska M, Landau S, Dunne R, et al. Bitemporal versus high-dose unilateral twice-weekly electroconvulsive therapy for depression (EFFECT-Dep): a pragmatic, randomized, non-inferiority trial. *Am J Psychiatry.* 2016;173(4):408–417.

25. Luccarelli J, McCoy TH, Shannon AP, et al. Rate of continuing acute course treatment using right unilateral ultrabrief pulse electroconvulsive therapy at a large academic medical center. *Eur Arch Psychiatry Clin Neurosci.* 2021;271(1):191–197.

26. Bahji A, Hawken ER, Sepehry AA, et al. ECT beyond unipolar major depression: systematic review and meta-analysis of electroconvulsive therapy in bipolar depression. *Acta Psychiatr Scand.* 2019;139(3):214–226.

27. Mutz J, Vipulananthan V, Carter B, et al. Comparative efficacy and acceptability of non-surgical brain stimulation for the acute treatment of major depressive episodes in adults: systematic review and network meta-analysis. *BMJ.* 2019:364.

28. Ren J, Li H, Palaniyappan L, et al. Repetitive transcranial magnetic stimulation versus electroconvulsive therapy for major depression: a systematic review and meta-analysis. *Prog Neuropsychopharmacol Biol Psychiatry.* 2014;51:181–189.

29. Luccarelli J, McCoy Jr TH, Seiner SJ, et al. Real-world evidence of age-independent electroconvulsive therapy efficacy: a retrospective cohort study. *Acta Psychiatr Scand.* 2022;145(1):100–108.

30. Luccarelli J, McCoy TH, Uchida M, et al. The efficacy and cognitive effects of acute course electroconvulsive therapy are equal in adolescents, transitional age youth, and young adults. *J Child Adolesc Psychopharmacol.* 2021;31(8):538–544.

31. Sackeim HA, Haskett RF, Mulsant BH, et al. Continuation pharmacotherapy in the prevention of relapse following electroconvulsive therapy: a randomized controlled trial. *JAMA.* 2001; 285(10):1299–1307.

32. Nordenskjöld A, von Knorring L, Ljung T, et al. Continuation electroconvulsive therapy with pharmacotherapy versus pharmacotherapy alone for prevention of relapse of depression: a randomized controlled trial. *J ECT.* 2013;29(2):86–92.

33. Luccarelli J, McCoy TH, Seiner SJ, et al. Maintenance ECT is associated with sustained improvement in depression symptoms without adverse cognitive effects in a retrospective cohort of 100 patients each receiving 50 or more ECT treatments. *J Affect Disord.* 2020;271:109–114.

34. Tørring N, Sanghani SN, Petrides G, et al. The mortality rate of electroconvulsive therapy: a systematic review and pooled analysis. *Acta Psychiatr Scand.* 2017;135(5):388–397.

35. Semkovska M, McLoughlin DM. Objective cognitive performance associated with electroconvulsive therapy for depression: a systematic review and meta-analysis. *Biol Psychiatry.* 2010;68(6):568–577.

36. Elger G, Hoppe C, Falkai P, et al. Vagus nerve stimulation is associated with mood improvements in epilepsy patients. *Epilepsy Res.* 2000;42(2–3):203–210.

37. Nemeroff CB, Mayberg HS, Krahl SE, et al. VNS therapy in treatment-resistant depression: clinical evidence and putative neurobiological mechanisms. *Neuropsychopharmacol Off Publ Am Coll Neuropsychopharmacol.* 2006;31(7):1345–1355.

38. Kosel M, Brockmann H, Frick C, et al. Chronic vagus nerve stimulation for treatment-resistant depression increases regional cerebral blood flow in the dorsolateral prefrontal cortex. *Psychiatry Res.* 2011;191(3):153–159.

39. Rush AJ, Marangell LB, Sackeim HA, et al. Vagus nerve stimulation for treatment-resistant depression: a randomized, controlled acute phase trial. *Biol Psychiatry.* 2005;58(5):347–354.

40. Aaronson ST, Sears P, Ruvuna F, et al. A 5-year observational study of patients with treatment-resistant depression treated with vagus nerve stimulation or treatment as usual: comparison of response, remission, and suicidality. *Am J Psychiatry.* 2017;174(7):640–648.

41. Rush AJ, Sackeim HA, Marangell LB, et al. Effects of 12 months of vagus nerve stimulation in treatment-resistant depression: a naturalistic study. *Biol Psychiatry.* 2005;58(5):355–363.

42. Schwalb JM, Hamani C. The history and future of deep brain stimulation. *Neurother J Am Soc Exp Neurother.* 2008;5(1):3–13.

43. Lujan JL, Chaturvedi A, Choi KS, et al. Tractography-activation models applied to subcallosal cingulate deep brain stimulation. *Brain Stimulat.* 2013;6(5):737–739.

44. Hardesty DE, Sackeim HA. Deep brain stimulation in movement and psychiatric disorders. *Biol Psychiatry.* 2007;61(7):831–835.

45. Lozano AM, Lipsman N, Bergman H, et al. Deep brain stimulation: current challenges and future directions. *Nat Rev Neurol.* 2019;15(3):148–160.

46. Mar-Barrutia L, Real E, Segalás C, et al. Deep brain stimulation for obsessive-compulsive disorder: a systematic review of worldwide experience after 20 years. *World J Psychiatry.* 2021;11(9):659–680.

47. Kaur N, Chou T, Corse AK, et al. Deep brain stimulation for treatment-resistant depression. *Psychiatr Ann.* 2013;43(8):358–365.

48. Dougherty DD, Rezai AR, Carpenter LL, et al. A randomized sham-controlled trial of deep brain stimulation of the ventral capsule/ventral striatum for chronic treatment-resistant depression. *Biol Psychiatry.* 2015;78(4):240–248.

49. Holtzheimer PE, Husain MM, Lisanby SH, et al. Subcallosal cingulate deep brain stimulation for treatment-resistant depression: a multisite, randomised, sham-controlled trial. *Lancet Psychiatry.* 2017;4(11):839–849.

50. Volpini M, Giacobbe P, Cosgrove GR, et al. The history and future of ablative neurosurgery for major depressive disorder. *Stereotact Funct Neurosurg.* 2017;95(4):216–228.

19 Legal Considerations for Mental Health Providers

Celeste Peay, Ronald Schouten, Judith Edersheim, and Rebecca W. Brendel

KEY POINTS

- Litigation is divided into two general categories: civil and criminal. Civil matters are those involving a dispute between parties in which one party claims to have been injured by another or some other transgression has occurred that can be remedied by the payment of money (damages) or the performance or cessation of certain activities (injunctive relief). Criminal matters are those in which a party has committed an act that has been declared illegal by a governmental authority and for which the penalty may be a monetary fine, incarceration, or both.

- Anyone who has first-hand knowledge of events and facts relevant to the case can be asked to serve as a fact witness.

- To qualify as an expert, a witness must have knowledge of the subject in question beyond that of the average layperson by virtue of education, training, and experience; unlike fact witnesses, expert witnesses may offer opinion testimony, and they are generally allowed to use hearsay evidence.

- Informed consent is best described as a process in which one person, the patient, agrees to allow another person, the treater, to do something to or for him or her. The patient's signature on a consent form does not constitute informed consent itself; it is merely evidence that the informed consent process occurred. For consent to treatment to be valid in the eyes of the law, it must be based on a defined amount and quality of information, it must be given voluntarily, and it must be given by someone who has the legal capacity to consent.

- Although evaluation of a patient's decision-making capacity by a physician or mental health professional is commonly referred to as a "competency evaluation," the evaluating clinician has no authority to change the patient's legal status.

- A tort is an injury to another party that gives rise to a right on the part of the injured person to sue the party causing the injury for damages. Commonly referred to as personal injury law, tort law embodies the principle that a person injured by the acts of another should receive compensation for the harm done.

- In psychiatric malpractice claims, typical intentional torts are battery, assault, false imprisonment, abandonment, intentional infliction of emotional distress, and undue familiarity (i.e., sexual misconduct and other boundary violations).

- The four elements of a malpractice claim are often referred to as the four Ds: duty, dereliction of duty, direct causation, and damages.

- Both a failure to diagnose and erroneous diagnosis can provide a basis for unintentional tort liability if harm results.

- Of all the interactions between psychiatrists and patients that can lead to legal liability, boundary violations are among the most painful and damaging for patients, psychiatrists, and their families.

- Liability of psychiatrists is normally limited to acts of negligence and a limited number of intentional acts that occur in the course of treatment.

- Good doctor–patient communication has been shown to be an effective component of malpractice risk reduction.

OVERVIEW

The US legal system is composed of parallel systems of state and federal constitutions, statutes, and courts. The US Constitution is the controlling body of law, and any law, state or federal, that conflicts with the Constitution will be struck down if challenged. The rulings of the US Supreme Court, which interprets the Constitution, are therefore controlling on Constitutional and federal law matters. States are free to provide greater protections of Constitutional rights than the Supreme Court interprets the Constitution as requiring but they may not provide less. On purely state law matters, including most civil matters, the decisions of state courts and state statutes are controlling.

Litigation is divided into two general categories: civil and criminal. Civil matters are those involving a dispute between parties in which one party claims to have been injured by another or some other transgression has occurred that can be remedied by the payment of money (damages) or the performance or cessation of certain activities (injunctive relief). The purpose of civil litigation is to right the wrong that one party has inflicted on the other or otherwise correct the offensive behavior of the wrongdoer. Criminal matters are those in which a party has committed an act that has been declared illegal by a governmental authority and for which the penalty may be a monetary fine, incarceration, or both. Both civil and criminal trials can be held before a judge alone (bench trials)

BOX 19.1   Standards of Proof in Legal Cases

CRIMINAL
Guilt beyond a reasonable doubt
CIVIL COMMITMENT (PER THE UNITED STATES CONSTITUTION)
Clear and convincing evidence
MALPRACTICE
Preponderance of evidence

or before a judge and jury (jury trials). In a jury trial, the jury decides the issues of fact—for example, guilty or not guilty, liable or not liable—and the judge rules on the principles of law, such as the admissibility of specific evidence. In a bench trial, the judge rules on the law and is the fact-finder.

In all litigation, the party bringing the action can only prevail by supplying evidence that meets the standard of proof. That standard varies with the type of legal action involved (Box 19.1). In personal injury cases, such as malpractice claims, the plaintiff (the party claiming to have been injured) must prove his or her case by a preponderance of the evidence (i.e., the plaintiff must convince the fact-finder that his or her claims are more likely true than not). This is the lowest standard of proof. At the other end is the standard used in criminal prosecutions (i.e., the prosecution must prove the defendant's guilt beyond a reasonable doubt). In other types of cases, such as civil commitment, a standard of proof between these extremes is required (i.e., clear and convincing evidence, per the US Constitution).

There are two basic types of witnesses: fact witnesses and expert witnesses. Psychiatrists may be asked to serve in either role. Anyone who has first-hand knowledge of events and facts relevant to the case can be asked to serve as a fact witness. Fact witnesses may testify only as to first-hand knowledge; they may not introduce hearsay evidence (i.e., information they have heard from others) except under certain limited circumstances. Most important, fact witnesses may not give opinion testimony. Thus, a treating clinician testifying as a fact witness for a patient may testify about his observations obtained during treatment but may not offer an opinion regarding negligence by a previous treater.[1]

When evidence is to be introduced on a subject that is outside the realm of knowledge of the average juror or judge, testimony by an expert witness may be allowed or required to meet the burden of proof. To qualify as an expert, a witness must have knowledge of the subject in question beyond that of the average layperson by virtue of education, training, and experience. Unlike fact witnesses, expert witnesses may offer opinion testimony, and they are generally allowed to use hearsay evidence.[1]

From time to time, psychiatrists may be asked to serve as either fact witnesses or expert witnesses in litigation matters in which their patients are involved. Although a patient can generally insist that the treating clinician provide copies of records and testify as a fact witness, the psychiatrist need not, and should not, serve as an expert witness. It is generally accepted that treating clinicians should not serve as expert witnesses on behalf of their own patients because the two roles are incompatible.[2-4] For example, clinicians have a fiduciary duty to act in the best interests of their patients, whereas expert witnesses have an ethical obligation to be objective, regardless of the impact on the litigant's position. In addition, in forming an objective opinion, experts must assess the litigant's claims against information obtained from collateral sources and be prepared to reject the litigant's claims. In other words, a treating clinician serving as an expert witness must challenge his or her patient's version of events, an activity that poses great risk for the therapeutic relationship. Clinicians who agree to serve as experts but who do not follow the proper methodology for conducting forensic evaluations may find their testimony excluded under the rules of evidence.[5,6]

BASIC CONCEPTS

It is important to keep in mind that the Western notion of individual autonomy is not accepted in all other cultures and that this has important implications for patient care.[7,8]

The principle of autonomy has multiple sources in Western philosophy,[9] with the Scottish philosopher and economist John Stuart Mill quoted widely in writings about informed consent, treatment refusal, and civil commitment.[10] Among Mill's most quoted passages are the following:

The sole end for which mankind are warranted, individual or collectively, in interfering with the liberty of action of any of their number, is self-protection. That the only purpose for which power can be rightfully exercised over any member of a civilized community, against his will, is to prevent harm to others.

Each is the proper guardian of his own health, whether bodily, or mentally or spiritual. Mankind are greater gainers by suffering each other to live as seems good to themselves, than by compelling each to live as seems good to the rest.

Mill's libertarian notions had their limitations, however. He did not believe that his principles applied to people with mental illnesses,[11] nor did he believe that the goal of autonomy relieved the rest of society from an obligation to help an individual choose the course that others believe to be in his or her best interests.

The law has long protected individuals from being touched or otherwise intruded on by others, initially through the common law (case or judge-made law) and later through statutes and regulations. The early English common law, which forms the basis for the jurisprudence of many nations (including the United States and Canada), had well-established principles of trespass, which is now referred to as personal injury or tort law.[12]

Among the forms of trespass was "battery," the touching of another person without his or her consent or justification. Battery was at the heart of early malpractice cases.

Battery is just one of many legal principles designed to preserve our autonomy. That principle extends to all interactions among people, including medical treatment. US courts have long recognized the right of individuals to make their own medical decisions.[13] This right has been protected in many ways over the years, including the US Supreme Court's decision in *Cruzan v. Director, Missouri Department of Health*, in which the Court declared the right to make individual health care decisions to be a fundamental liberty interest.[14]

Autonomy is only one of the four ethical principles considered to be the foundation of clinical care; the others are beneficence, justice, and non-malfeasance.[15]

Of these ethical principles, autonomy receives the greatest attention and protection from the legal system.

INFORMED CONSENT

The development of the doctrine of informed consent extended the principle of individual autonomy to medical treatment. Both ethically and legally, the purpose of the doctrine of informed consent is to give meaning to individual patient autonomy within the doctor–patient relationship.[16]

When the patient is unable to provide informed consent, it may be obtained from an alternative decision-maker.

Informed consent is best described as a process in which one person, the patient, agrees to allow another person, the treater, to do something to or for him or her. The emphasis in this definition of informed consent is on the *process*, that is, the interactions between patient and clinician, during which there is an exchange of information and acceptance or rejection of the proposed treatment. The role of forms in the informed consent process is commonly misunderstood. The patient's signature on a consent form does not constitute informed consent itself; it is merely evidence that the informed consent process occurred.

Informed consent evolved from simple consent, which was one of the two basic defenses to a common law claim of battery. Simple consent required only that the would-be patient explicitly or implicitly agree to treatment by the physician; little or no explanation was required. The move toward requiring more substantive consent was fueled by several forces, including increased professionalization of medicine, a decline in religious fatalism, and an increased belief that health could be improved through individual effort and through science and technology.[17] Informed consent was a logical result of the civil liberties movement and the shift toward autonomy in medical ethics.

The modern era of informed consent began with a series of American court decisions in the middle of the 20th century; however, it was not an American invention. Like seminal ideas in other fields, informed consent did not arise suddenly. In fact, like many other enlightened principles, informed consent was a known concept in Ancient Greece, Byzantium, and Rome,[18] only to be lost during the Dark Ages and rediscovered centuries later. In 1767, an English court held that a surgeon and his assistant could be held liable for battery after re-breaking a patient's leg to fix a mal-union without first informing him or her of their intention to do so. The court held that "it is reasonable that a patient should be told what is about to be done to him, that he may take courage and put himself in such a situation as to enable him to undergo the operation."[19]

The following language from Judge Benjamin Cardozo's opinion in the *Schloendorff* decision in 1914 signaled the initial steps in the move from simple to informed consent later in the twentieth century: "Every human being of adult years and sound mind has a right to determine what shall be done with his body."[13] However, the next major decisions in informed consent in American courts did not come until the 1950s and 1960s. Subsequent cases held that consent to treatment is valid only if it is an intelligent consent[20] that represents an "informed exercise of choice"[21] and that failure to obtain that consent constituted professional negligence or malpractice.

For consent to treatment to be valid in the eyes of the law, it must be based on a defined amount and quality of information, it must be given voluntarily, and it must be given by someone who has the legal capacity to consent (Box 19.2).[22] The amount of information that must be provided varies by the jurisdiction in which the clinician is practicing. A small majority of states follow the "reasonable professional standard," which requires clinicians to provide the amount of information that a reasonable professional would provide under similar circumstances. A substantial minority of states use a patient-centered or "reasonable patient" standard, which requires clinicians to provide the information that would allow a reasonable or average patient to make an informed decision. Within the patient-centered school, a smaller group of states apply a standard that is more individualized (i.e., what would this patient find material in making an informed decision?).[23] Several states have hybrid standards.[24]

From both clinical and risk management perspectives, it is generally the case that the more information provided, the better. The shared decision-making model, which involves open discussion and exchange of information between doctor and patient, is

---

> **BOX 19.2** Elements of Informed Consent
>
> - Choice is based on a defined amount and quality of information
> - The amount of information that must be provided varies by the jurisdiction in which the clinician is practicing: for example, the reasonable professional standard or the reasonable patient standard
> - Consent must be given voluntarily
> - Consent must be given by someone who has the legal capacity to consent

> **BOX 19.3** Important Information to Discuss with a Patient Regarding Consent
>
> - The diagnosis and nature of the condition being treated
> - The benefits that the patient can reasonably expect from the proposed treatment
> - The nature and probability of material risks involved in the treatment
> - The inability to predict results of the treatment
> - The potential irreversibility of the procedure
> - The likely results, risks, and benefits associated with alternative treatments and no treatment
>
> Adapted from Harnish v. Children's Hospital Medical Center, 387 Mass. 152, 155 (1982).

believed by many to epitomize the ideals of informed consent.[24] Whatever the jurisdiction, clinicians who provide patients with the information listed in Box 19.3 can feel confident that sufficient information has been provided (see Box 19.3).

There are limits to the disclosure requirements, even under the materiality standard. In *Precourt v. Frederick*, the Massachusetts Supreme Judicial Court held that there must be a balancing, an accommodation, among the patient's right to know, fairness to physicians, and society's interest that medicine be practiced "without unrealistic and unnecessary burdens on practitioners."[25] In this case, the court rejected a plaintiff's argument that he should have been warned of a very remote, but real, risk of a medication when the side effect in question had never been reported when used for the treatment in question. As medical knowledge becomes more readily available through electronic media, the informed consent process will continue to evolve. There is an increasing shift toward the use of extra-clinical tools, such as pamphlets, videos, and websites, to supplement the informed consent process.[26]

Informed consent is not a universal concept, and individuals from some cultures may find application of the Western model to be inhumane.[27,28] Clinicians should be sensitive to this possibility while remembering that the process is ultimately governed by the legal and ethical requirements in the jurisdiction in which they practice.

The second essential element of informed consent is that the consent be voluntary. For the consent to be valid, it must be given voluntarily and free from direct or implied coercion.[22,29] *Coercion* is generally defined as an external force that limits the ability of an individual to make a choice.[30] Thus, an undomiciled patient who is threatened with expulsion from the hospital if he or she refuses a specific treatment has been subjected to coercion. The line between overt coercion and more subtle forces that fall within the range of everyday influences blurs rapidly, however, and draws us into philosophical discussions of free will and personhood.[31] For example, consent given by a patient who is subjected to coercion from family members (e.g., "If you don't take the medicine, we will not be able to have you live at home.") is generally deemed to meet both ethical and legal standards for valid consent.[32,33]

Individuals who are totally dependent on their caregivers, such as residents of long-term care facilities and prisoners, may be deemed unable to grant true informed consent to research or treatment due to the coercion inherent in the structural lack of autonomy in these institutional contexts.[34–36] The notion that all individuals in such situations are incapable of truly voluntary consent is open to challenge, however.[37]

The third and perhaps most critical element of informed consent is that the person giving consent must have the capacity to do so. In the absence of decision-making capacity, there is no informed consent regardless of how much detailed information was provided or the patient's assent to treatment.

It is important to distinguish between the legal concept of competency and the clinical concept of capacity, between global and task-specific competence, and between different specific types of capacity.

In the eyes of the law, all adults are considered competent, giving them status as legal persons. This means that there is a presumption that individuals have the requisite capacity to engage in activities that are necessary and common elements of everyday life, including making personal decisions regarding health care and finances, or entering into contracts (such as credit card transactions, marriage) and voting. Only a court can declare an individual to be legally incompetent.[38] Although evaluation of a patient's decision-making capacity by a physician or mental health professional is commonly referred to as a "competency evaluation," the evaluating clinician has no authority to change the patient's legal status. The clinician's assessment of the patient's decision-making capacity, which is then presented to the judge as evidence to be considered in making a judicial judgment regarding competence, is of great importance, however. In the wake of a clinical finding of incapacity and in the absence of an emergency or other exception to informed consent, clinicians are obligated to obtain informed consent from an alternative decision-maker. Although a clinician's assessment that a patient lacks decision-making capacity does not, in and of itself, change the patient's legal status, such an assessment can activate the authority of a substitute decision-maker, such as an agent appointed by a patient's health care proxy.

Courts make an important distinction between global and specific incompetence. A declaration of global incompetence strips the individual of status as a legal person, rendering them unable to make any of life's normal decisions. As a result, courts are reluctant to declare someone globally incompetent or incapacitated. Instead, whenever possible, courts note what capacities a person retains, as well as any incapacities, and limit declarations of incompetence to specific activities (e.g., making decisions about specific treatments). This is consistent with the principle that an individual may be competent to engage in some activities but not in others.

In the absence of a substitute decision-maker previously chosen by the patient or designated by statute, traditional guardianship mechanisms operate. After an individual is declared incompetent, either globally or regarding specific decision-making activities, an individual becomes a "ward," and another person is appointed as a guardian to make all decisions on their behalf. There is some variation in terminology among various jurisdictions. In some states, a "guardian" is the individual appointed to make decisions related to the person of the ward, and the "conservator" is one who is appointed to control the ward's financial affairs. In other jurisdictions, such as California, the individual appointed to make decisions is referred to as a conservator of the person or the estate (financial affairs), and the ward is referred to as the "conservatee."

In conducting a clinical assessment of a person's capacity to make treatment decisions, four elements should be examined: (1) Does the patient express a preference or choice? (2) Does the patient have a factual understanding, at the level of a layperson, of the basic relevant information concerning the medical condition and the proposed treatment, risks, and benefits? (3) Does the patient have an appreciation of the significance of the information to the situation at hand? (4) Can the patient arrive at a decision in a logical manner that considers the information provided in the context of other personal factors (i.e., is the patient rational)? It should be noted that the patient's decision may still be rational even if it is contrary to what most individuals and the caregivers might choose. Competent people are entitled to make choices that others may deem inadvisable or irrational. Such is the essential nature of individual autonomy.[38,39] These criteria are summarized in Box 19.4.

Practicing clinicians must also be aware that the legal notions of competence and clinical concept of capacity are task specific (i.e., they are assessed in relationship to the specific function or decision faced by the patient). In addition, these concepts also apply to non-medical decisions. For example, testamentary capacity (the ability to make a will) and the capacities to manage financial matters, execute an advance directive, and appoint a power of attorney all have their specific criteria for assessment. It is important to note that an individual may lack the capacity for one or more of these activities yet retain the capacity to engage in the others.[40]

Ethically and legally, we do not require the same level of decision-making capacity for all decisions.[29] Clinicians and researchers may accept as competent the consent or refusal

---

BOX 19.4 Factors to Assess in Determining Capacity to Make Medical Decisions

Does the patient express a preference or manifest a choice when asked to make a decision?
- No expression leads to a presumption of incompetency
- Is the choice stable over time?

Does the patient have a factual understanding of the information presented?
- Does he or she remember the relevant information in his or her own terms?
- Does he or she understand cause-effect relationships and probabilities in this situation?
- Does he or she understand his or her role as a decision-maker?

Does the patient have an appreciation of the situation and the consequences of various courses of action?
- Does he or she have an awareness of the seriousness of the illness?
- Does he or she appreciate the likely consequences of treatment or refusal?

Does he or she manipulate the information provided in a rational fashion? (That is, how does he or she reach a decision?)
- Does he or she weight the risks and benefits through a logical process?
- Does the conclusion flow logically and is it consistent with the starting premises?
  - Factors (psychosis, delirium, dementia, phobias, panic disorder, anxiety, depression, mania, and anger) may play a role.

- Note: Focus is on the rationality of the process, not the decision itself.

Adapted from Appelbaum PS, Grisso T. Assessing patients' capacities to consent to treatment. *N Engl J Med* 1988:319:1635–1638.

of an individual according to a sliding scale that accounts for the risk-to-benefit ratio of the proposed intervention and its possible consequences. This sliding scale approach requires less capacity for consent to low-risk, high-benefit treatments and refusal of high-risk, low-benefit treatments. Conversely, consent to high-risk, low-benefit treatments and refusal of low-risk, high-benefit treatments requires a higher level of decision-making capacity (Table 19.1).[41,42]

If a patient is deemed to lack decision-making capacity, several options are available, and these vary to some extent by jurisdiction, the nature of the treatment, and the degree and expected duration of incapacity. When a treatment is low risk and likely to be successful—for example, provision of antibiotics to a person with dementia who has a urinary tract infection—it is permissible to proceed with consent from family members or the assent of the patient if family members are not available. As proposed treatments become more aggressive, intrusive, and risky, the need to seek alternative decision-makers increases. It should be noted that whether a treatment is one that requires formal appointment of an alternative decision-maker is often determined by case law and legislation, and this view may be contrary to that of the treating clinician. In Massachusetts, for example, all antipsychotics are considered to constitute extraordinary and intrusive treatment, with no distinctions made for dosage. When incompetent individuals are to be treated with these medications, treaters are expected to obtain judicial approval.[43,44]

An alternative decision-maker may be appointed through a judicial declaration of incompetency, with the court appointing a guardian to make some or all decisions on behalf of the patient. Alternatively, although they still have the capacity to do so, a patient may execute an advance directive, such as a durable power of attorney or health care proxy, appointing an "attorney in fact" or a "health care agent," whose authority is activated after a clinical determination that the patient is no longer capable of making treatment decisions. Depending on the jurisdiction, the alternative decision-maker appointed to act on behalf of the incapacitated principal is charged with using either a "best-interests" or a "substituted judgment" approach. In the former, decisions are to be made that are believed to be in the best interests of the ward. In contrast to the best-interests analysis, substituted judgment is an approach to decision-making for incompetent individuals that seeks to honor their autonomy and preferences when they lack the ability to express them.[45–47] Substituted judgment is an important aspect of decision-making for individuals who lack the capacity to make decisions regarding treatment with antipsychotic medication.

Under certain situations, treatment can proceed without informed consent being obtained. These exceptions are generally considered to include emergencies, waiver, and therapeutic privilege.[48,49] An *emergency* is defined as a situation in which failure to treat would result in serious and potentially irreversible deterioration of the patient's condition. The purpose of treatment in an emergency is to prevent further deterioration and to reverse the clinical process. After the patient is stabilized,

however, the emergency exception no longer applies, and the treater no longer has license to continue without getting appropriate consent. This is of importance in psychiatry (e.g., when emergency treatment of an agitated psychotic patient does not give the clinician permission to initiate an ongoing course of treatment). A patient's prior expressed preference regarding treatment (e.g., refusal of certain treatments) cannot be ignored in the face of an emergency. For example, if a competent patient makes it clear that she or he never wants to have a specific treatment, that treatment refusal cannot be automatically overridden in the face of an emergency. Doing so puts the treater at risk of being sued for battery.[50]

Informed consent is not necessary when a patient competently waives consent, deferring to the judgment of the clinician or others.[22] However, clinicians are strongly advised to assess and document the patient's capacity to make such a waiver.

The therapeutic privilege exception to informed consent allows treatment to proceed, with consent obtained from an alternative decision-maker, if the consent process would contribute to worsening of a competent patient's physical or mental condition.[21,51] These situations are unusual, especially in psychiatry. It should be noted that therapeutic privilege cannot be invoked merely because the information provided might dissuade the patient from accepting the recommended treatment.

Obtaining informed consent becomes difficult when the patient can no longer speak for themselves as a result of illness. The process of identifying and appointing an alternative decision-maker can be complicated and lengthy, leading to delays in treatment. This problem can arise either because there is no spokesperson or obvious candidate or when there are several individuals who seek to control the treatment, often with conflicting views about the best treatment course. Advance directives (e.g., health care proxies and durable powers of attorney) can be of great use in these situations. These instruments allow individuals to specify treatment preferences if they lose the capacity to make their own choices. Originally developed for use in end-of-life treatment situations, advance directives have significant potential in the treatment of mental illness.[52,53] They can be used by patients to both exclude certain treatments and to ensure that treatment will be provided if the illness leads them to refuse treatment; to date, they have been under-used for a variety of reasons.[54,55] Despite the potential benefits, the use of advance directives has not been widely adopted by mental health practitioners.[56] When they are to be used, it is wise to specifically assess and document an individual's capacity to execute such a document.[57]

Advance directives are not without their problems, including the fact that the principal (the person who executes the advance directive) may include instructions that no treatment is to be provided, may insist on specific (and potentially inappropriate) treatments, and can revoke the instrument at any time. It is possible to override advance directives when the provisions conflict with civil commitment statutes or when adhering to the patient's preferences would be inconsistent with ethical practice. In such cases, standard judicial mechanisms for involuntary treatment should be followed because they provide due process protections for both patient autonomy and professional practice.[58,59]

TREATMENT REFUSAL

The doctrine of informed consent has slowly, but steadily, gained acceptance among clinicians and researchers. The idea that all competent adults have a right to make their own decisions about medical treatment is now well established, even if application of that principle continues to lead to certain ethical and legal dilemmas.[14,60,61]

TABLE 19.1 Risk/Benefit Ratio of Treatment

Patient's Decision	Favorable Ratio	Unfavorable/ Questionable Ratio
Consent	Low level of competency	High level of competency
Refusal	High level of competency	Low level of competency

Adapted from Roth LH, Meisel A, Lidz CW. Test of competency to consent to treatment. *Am J Psychiatry* 1977;134:279–284.

The advancement of notions of autonomy, informed consent, and civil rights principles, combined with growing awareness of the side effects of psychotropic medications and judicial scrutiny of conditions in publicly funded psychiatric facilities, led to significant changes in how the rights of people with mental illnesses were protected. Chief among these were recognition that (1) persons with a mental illness have the same rights to make their own treatment decisions as those with other illnesses, and (2) mentally ill individuals are entitled to have their treatment preferences honored even after loss of their capacity to express their preferences.

The introduction of these principles, which marked a shift from forced medication of a refusing patient to judicial protection of the right to refuse, was met with considerable resistance.[16] The notion of allowing an individual to refuse treatment for a mental disorder, when symptoms of the disorder render the individual unable to rationally weigh the risks and benefits of treatment or lead to involuntary hospitalization, appeared to strike at the very heart of ethical principles of beneficence, justice, and non-malfeasance.[60] Before the legal reforms in this area, patients lost all of their legal rights, including the right to make treatment decisions, upon being involuntarily civilly committed. It was only after a series of legal cases in the late 1970s, both federal and state, that states began to recognize that individuals who require involuntary hospitalization can still retain the capacity to make treatment decisions.[62,63]

The primary focus of the debate over treatment refusal by individuals with mental illnesses has been antipsychotic medication. Not coincidentally, this issue came to the attention of the courts (and eventually legislatures) in the late 1970s— approximately 25 years after the introduction of chlorpromazine. Although the widespread use of this drug and other dopamine-blocking antipsychotics allowed for the de-institutionalization of thousands of patients, the courts turned their attention to the short- and long-term side effects of the medications (such as acute dystonic reactions, tardive dyskinesia, and tardive dystonia). In many cases, even after these side effects were known, they were not discussed with patients and their families, in part because of the presumption that people with mental illnesses were not entitled to participate in the informed consent process.

Recognition that competent individuals with mental illnesses are entitled to the same informed consent process as other individuals, even if involuntarily committed, left open the issues of treatment refusal and acceptance by individuals who lacked decision-making capacity. In the United States, the approach to these issues has varied between federal and state systems and among the states. For example, Utah incorporates a judicial finding that "the patient lacks the ability to engage in a rational decision-making process regarding the acceptance of mental treatment as demonstrated by evidence of inability to weigh the possible risks of accepting or rejecting treatment" as one of the criteria for civil commitment criteria, thus tying involuntary treatment to commitment.[64] Civil commitment statutes in other states also established this issue as a component of committability.[65]

Other jurisdictions maintain a distinction between involuntary treatment and involuntary confinement. Among those other jurisdictions, there is still considerable variation in the approach to involuntary treatment. At one extreme are jurisdictions that provide administrative review of treatment refusals while ultimately preserving recourse to the courts. In federal jurisdictions, for example, antipsychotic drugs may be constitutionally administered to an involuntarily committed patient with a mental illness whenever, in the exercise of professional judgment, such treatment is deemed necessary to prevent the patient from endangering himself or herself or

others. After that determination is made, professional judgment must also be exercised in the resulting decision to administer medication.[66]

Another approach is followed in Ohio, which has a statute that prohibits hospitalized individuals with mental illnesses from being treated with surgical procedures, convulsive therapy, major aversive interventions (e.g., electroconvulsive therapy, unusually hazardous treatment procedures, sterilization, or psychosurgery) without their full informed consent. If the patient is incompetent, treaters may seek consent from "the patient's natural or court-appointed guardian, who may give an informed, intelligent, and knowing written consent." In the absence of a natural or court-appointed guardian, the treaters may seek consent from the court for these treatments.[67]

Antipsychotic medications are categorized as routine medical treatments in Ohio, and no special proceedings are required to allow forced medication. Ohio requires a guardian who is appointed to make decisions about treatment of the ward to apply a best-interests analysis with respect to the appropriateness of treatment with antipsychotic medications.[68]

Regarding involuntarily committed patients, the Ohio Supreme Court has held that the state's interest in public safety overrides the right of an individual to refuse treatment. Forced medication with antipsychotic drugs of an involuntarily committed patient with a mental illness can be ordered if a physician determines "that (1) the patient presents an imminent danger of harm to himself/herself or others, (2) there are no less intrusive means of avoiding the threatened harm, and (3) the medication to be administered is medically appropriate for the patient."[69] When the involuntarily committed patient does not present an imminent threat of harm to himself or herself or others but lacks the capacity to give informed consent, "the state's *parens patriae* power may justify treating the patient with antipsychotic medication against his/her wishes."[69] The issue of competency to give or withhold consent is a matter for judicial, not medical, determination, however, and

a court may issue an order permitting hospital employees to administer antipsychotic drugs against the wishes of an involuntarily-committed mentally-ill person if it finds, by clear and convincing evidence, that (1) the patient does not have the capacity to give or withhold informed consent regarding his/her treatment, (2) it is in the patient's best interest to take the medication, i.e., the benefits of the medication outweigh the side effects, and (3) no less intrusive treatment will be as effective in treating the mental illness.[69]

It should be noted that Ohio law specifically states that antipsychotic medications do not constitute adverse interventions.

In contrast, Massachusetts and some other states view antipsychotic medications as extraordinary and intrusive treatments, from which incompetent patients (both consenting and non-consenting) must be protected unless their rights are secured through the application of full adversarial proceedings.[43] Massachusetts requires that in the absence of an emergency, an individual who lacks the capacity to provide informed consent or refuses treatment with antipsychotic medication can receive treatment only after a two-part proceeding. These are formal, adversarial proceedings, at which the patient is represented by counsel and sworn testimony is received, regardless of dosage or purpose of the treatment. The proceedings may be conducted before the probate and family court for outpatients or hospitalized inpatients or before a judge of the district court hearing a motion for civil commitment.

The first part of the hearing is a judicial determination of competence. If the court determines the patient to be competent to make decisions, the patient may continue to refuse the treatment, absent some adequate countervailing state interest,[70] even if the patient is subject to involuntary commitment. If the court finds the patient to be incompetent, the second stage of the hearing involves a determination as to whether the patient should receive the proposed treatment. The Massachusetts Supreme Judicial Court has determined that only a judge has the requisite degree of interest and objectivity to render a substituted judgment decision that focuses on the preferences of the incompetent patient.[44] Simply stated, the substituted judgment analysis attempts to determine what the incompetent patient would have decided if he or she were able to make an informed decision, accounting for all the circumstances. These circumstances can include the likelihood that the individual will remain incompetent in the absence of treatment. The court considers, at minimum, the elements listed in Box 19.5.[43,44]

The adoption of these procedures has had a significant impact on the treatment of patients with mental illnesses in Massachusetts in terms of costs and energies devoted to the process, although most treatment petitions submitted to the court are granted. Whether this represents greater care by clinicians in choosing the patients for whom involuntary treatment will be pursued or reflects sensitivity by the judges to the appropriateness of treatment, or some other factors, is a matter of speculation.[71,72]

Patients experience involuntary commitment or administration of medications against their wishes as coercive, which in turn lowers treatment satisfaction.[73] Promoting patient autonomy and voluntary treatment early in the clinical relationship can help establish the patient's wishes in the event of later incapacitation and the need for substituted decision-making.[74]

CONSENT TO PARTICIPATE IN RESEARCH

Patients with psychiatric disorders are frequently asked to participate in psychosocial and psychopharmacological research studies designed to identify new and effective treatments for their illnesses. This poses significant legal and ethical concerns. Psychiatric disorders may compromise cognition, emotional regulation, insight, and at times the ability to reason between treatment alternatives, calling into question the validity of the consent to participate.[75] In the research context, goals such as scientific advancement may in some instances displace individualized care and may involve a greater degree of risk to the patient or an uncertain benefit. Randomized controlled trials (RCTs) with double-blinded procedures are designed to protect the integrity of the study data rather than respond to the individual needs of the patient.

Recent research has demonstrated that many patients with mental illnesses have difficulty appreciating the distinction between participation in a research study and receiving

traditional individualized care. Several investigators have attempted to identify which patient characteristics predispose patients to this therapeutic misconception and have identified low educational attainments and cognitive impairments as pertinent risk factors. It is not yet clear, however, whether severity of mental illness or the presence of psychosis correlates with a greater incidence of therapeutic misconception.[76] In addition, structured assessment instruments are being evaluated for their usefulness in determining the capacity to consent to clinical research.[77] Several leading researchers in this field have proposed a more careful and detailed consent procedure for patients considering enrollment in a research study. This discussion would highlight the nature and purpose of the research, the risks and benefits of being a participant, and whether the patient can obtain the same therapeutic interventions outside the research setting.[78] A meta-analysis of 54 RCTs examining the impact of informed consent innovations demonstrated that enhanced consent forms, extended discussion, and multi-media interventions resulted in improved knowledge on the part of those asked for consent.[79]

A significant body of research has demonstrated that people with even severe mental illnesses retain a certain amount of decision-making capacity, which can be enhanced with educational interventions,[80] including novel methods of presenting the information.[81] However, in the case of incompetent patients with mental illnesses, family members or substitute decision-makers are often called on to determine participation in a research study. In the treatment context, substitute decision-makers can focus solely on the best interests or preferences of the patient; however, consent to enroll in a research protocol has competing goals. As in the case of treatment consent, substituted consent for participation in low-risk clinical trials raises fewer ethical or legal concerns, but higher-risk studies require adherence to federal consent guidelines, state statutory guidelines, and ethical guidelines.[80] In general, incompetent patients have an absolute right to refuse participation in any study, and their refusal or expressed negative preferences are taken at face value. In the absence of such an expressed preference, substitute decision-makers can consent to research participation on the same basis as they would for treatment decisions, although these provisions vary from state to state and sometimes explicitly exclude patients who are hospitalized with mental illnesses.[4,82]

CIVIL COMMITMENT

Civil commitment is an administrative or judicial process by which the state's power is used to identify and remove an individual with mental illness from society and place them in an institutional setting. The involuntary confinement of a person because of mental illness is one of the oldest clinical interventions, if not the original clinical intervention. Throughout the ages, the purpose and justification of such confinement has cycled between protection of the rest of society and the patient's need for treatment. When the purpose is the protection of both the patient and society from the dangers associated with the illness, the state is considered to be using its *police powers*. The police powers approach focuses on the dangerousness of the patient to self or others. When the justification for commitment is the need of the patient for treatment, the state is using its *parens patriae* authority (i.e., the state is acting toward the individual citizen with the same authority and responsibility as a parent toward a child). Under this rationale, the state takes a beneficent role toward its citizens and acts in their best interests to protect them from their incapacities or disabilities.[70]

With the increased focus on civil rights and autonomy in the 1970s, the best interest or *parens patriae* need for treatment approach to civil commitment was replaced by the dangerousness or police powers approach in most jurisdictions. This approach allows an individual to be involuntarily committed to a mental institution only if the individual poses a danger to himself or herself through direct injury, if there is a direct threat of physical harm to others, or if the individual is gravely disabled and unable to care for himself or herself in the community.[83,84] The definition of danger and the level of dangerousness required for civil commitment vary among the states.[85]

The process for civil commitment is jurisdiction specific. All states provide for an initial short-term emergency confinement without the necessity of a judicial hearing. In general, such emergency certification requires examination by a mental health professional (such as a psychiatrist, psychologist, or psychiatric nurse), who documents the clinical findings required by the applicable commitment statute. After the initial emergency confinement, which varies from 2 days to 3 weeks among the states, the facility may release the patient, convert the admission to a voluntary hospitalization, or petition a court for an order of civil commitment.[4]

Commitment hearings differ in their level of their procedural safeguards. Some jurisdictions authorize administrative boards or hearing officers to conduct the proceedings, but others require a full hearing before a judge, with psychiatric examinations, witness testimony, and documentary evidence. In 1979, the US Supreme Court ruled that the standard of evidentiary proof required for a civil commitment is clear and convincing evidence that the commitment meets statutory standards. Several states, however, have chosen to require a higher standard of proof in these proceedings (namely, proof beyond a reasonable doubt) rather than offer the Constitutional minimum.

The length of these commitments also varies by jurisdiction. Most states specify a period of confinement from 6 months to 1 year, with the requirement that formal re-commitment proceedings be initiated to extend the time period. A minority of states have no explicit commitment period and provide that the commitment terminates when the patient's clinical condition no longer meets statutory standards.

Civil Commitment of Sex Offenders

During the 1980s, a series of highly publicized and horrifying sex crimes catalyzed the enactment of state statutes providing for the civil commitment of convicted sex offenders after the completion of their prison sentences. In 1990, Washington State enacted the first sexual predator law, and now 19 states have so-called sexual predator statutes that provide for indefinite confinement in specialized treatment centers after a defendant is convicted of a sex crime and is determined to be a sexually dangerous person.[86] Although each state has a different standard for such commitment, these statutes generally provide for the detention of offenders with broadly defined mental abnormalities or mental illnesses that predispose them to commit sex crimes.[87] A diverse array of interest groups have criticized these laws on various grounds, alleging that they violate civil rights, criminalize mental illness, depend on unreliable predictions of future behavior, and divert the focus away from longer or more effective prison sentences.[88] In addition, critics observe that these statutes confine patients based on a treatment rationale when it is not clear that effective treatment for sex offenders exists.[89]

The Supreme Court upheld the constitutionality of these laws in three cases. In *Kansas v. Hendricks*, the court determined that a "mental abnormality," such as pedophilia, combined with a finding of dangerousness or the likelihood of re-offense was a sufficient rationale for an indefinite civil commitment.[90] The court also upheld the validity of sexual predator laws against a claim that the treatment is so inadequate and punitive that it is the equivalent of a second prison sentence.[91] Most

recently, in *Kansas v. Crane*, the court lowered the threshold for the behavioral dyscontrol, requiring only proof that the offender has difficulty controlling his dangerous behavior rather than a "total or complete lack of control."[92] In 1999, the American Psychiatric Association task force on sexually dangerous offenders produced a report opposing the penal use of commitment statutes, concluding that they pose a threat to the integrity of psychiatric diagnosis and the therapeutic basis for other civil commitment statutes.[93] In 2006, the US Congress, however, passed the most comprehensive sex offender law in US history, the Adam Walsh Law. The law is consistent with civil commitment schemes found in the landmark sex offender cases, *Kansas v. Hendricks* and *Kansas v. Crane*, and requires the determination of a "mental abnormality" on the part of the defendant and of any volitional component to the crime.[94]

Outpatient Commitment

Although involuntary hospitalization provided a treatment setting for people at imminent risk of harming themselves or others, it did not offer a treatment scheme for a significant population of people with chronic mental illnesses who were unwilling or unable to adhere to outpatient treatment regimens. These patients were frequently re-hospitalized, only to deteriorate immediately after discharge. In response to the problem of the "revolving door" patient and a series of highly publicized violent acts by persons with mental illness, several states decided to revitalize the seldom-used outpatient commitment statutes. These statutes, previously enacted in almost every state but rarely used, allowed judges to require patients to comply with outpatient treatment regimens or face involuntary hospitalization. Outpatient commitments could be ordered on discharge from the hospital or as an alternative to civil commitment.[95]

Outpatient commitment procedures were initially heavily criticized as a violation of Constitutional guarantees of equal protection and due process of law, and an unacceptable instrument of social control. Critics also voiced concerns that despite being ordered to comply with community mental health treatment, patients were provided with inadequate treatment in under-funded programs.[96] Some of these concerns were ameliorated by two randomized trials of outpatient commitment undertaken in New York and North Carolina.[97,98] The data from these two studies, examined in light of their methodological limitations, appear to support the use of outpatient commitment to stabilize and improve the quality of life for people with chronic mental illnesses. Although the debate over the legitimacy and efficacy of outpatient commitment is still unresolved, it appears to significantly improve adherence to medication regimens and is associated with decreases in substance use, re-hospitalization, homelessness, and violent victimization among certain groups of people with severe mental illness.[99-101]

THE MEDICAL LIABILITY CLIMATE

Historically, approximately every 10 years, American medicine finds itself amid a "malpractice crisis"; the first years of the 21st century have been no exception.[102] As in the past, there is debate about the nature and cause of problems related to malpractice litigation, such as rising premiums and the cost of defensive medicine, as well as what to do about them. Are there more lawsuits and higher awards? Are insurance premiums higher and, if so, why?[103-105] Calls for tort reform routinely cite the cost of defensive medicine and the impact of malpractice on rising health care costs.[106,107]

The responses of researchers and commentators to these highly charged questions are not always consistent with the most pessimistic perceptions of the medical community. Contrary to the concern that every error leads to a lawsuit, only a small percentage of cases involving injury caused by medical errors actually become the basis for claims or litigation,[108–110] and defendants continue to prevail in most cases that result in litigation, in part because a substantial proportion of these cases appear to lack merit.[111] From 1956 to 1990, the number of malpractice claims for all specialties rose 10-fold: from 1.5 per 100 to 15 per 100 covered physicians.[112] Overall, it appears that the median malpractice award (both jury awards and settlements) doubled in real dollars between 1990 and 2001, but it has remained essentially flat since then, albeit with variation among the states.

Kilgore and colleagues[113] studied the impact of various proposed tort reforms on malpractice premiums and determined that imposition of caps on malpractice damage awards resulted in significantly lower malpractice premiums. They estimated that a nation-wide cap of $250,000 on non-economic damages would result in a premium savings of $16.9 billion per year. They also found that malpractice premiums had an inverse relationship with the Dow Jones Industrial Average.[113] This observation supports the hypothesis that insurers raise premiums to pay their stockholders when other investments are performing less well.

Support for the argument that malpractice reforms reduce costs is mixed. In 2003, Texas adopted malpractice reforms that capped non-economic damages at $250,000 for most cases. Stewart and colleagues[114] studied the impact of the reforms on general surgery malpractice claims in an academic medical center. They found a significant drop in claims from 40 to 8 per 100,000 procedures, as well as a significant drop in litigation costs. According to Paik and colleagues,[115] this did not result in reduced costs of medical care, which would have been expected had the reforms resulted in a decrease in defensive medicine.

It is certainly the case that malpractice premiums have increased over the years and that multiple causes are to blame.[116] It is not at all clear, however, that malpractice premiums have increased significantly relative to other expenses. In an in-depth analysis of data from nine regions from 1970 to 2000, Rodwin and associates[117] examined actual premiums paid (as opposed to advertised rates) relative to overall physician income and expenses. They found that premiums for self-employed physicians rose from 1970 to 1986, declined from 1986 to 1996, and rose thereafter. Premiums were lower in 2000 than they were in 1986, however, and other practice expenses continued to increase, but spending on malpractice premiums fell from 1986 (11% of total expenses) to 2000 (7% of total expenses).[117]

There is no end in sight to arguments over the causes of medical malpractice litigation,[108,118] the need for tort reform, and the assignment of blame for dissatisfaction with medical practice.[119,120] Whether there is an actual crisis or whether premiums are a relatively smaller or a larger portion of practice expenses, there is no contesting the fact that the prospect or actuality of a lawsuit can have a major impact on the personal and professional lives of defendant physicians and the relationships these physicians have with their patients.[121–124] The threat of malpractice litigation is unlikely to diminish significantly, given the Institute of Medicine's 1999 estimate that 44,000 to 98,000 deaths per year are caused by preventable medical errors. Although the personal injury system is not without its problems, hopes for a significant decrease in medical malpractice claims appear to lie with changes in how medical care is delivered rather than with doing away with personal injury law.[125]

MALPRACTICE LIABILITY

A tort is an injury to another party that gives rise to a right on the part of the injured person to sue the party causing the injury for damages.[29] Commonly referred to as personal injury law, tort law embodies the principle that a person injured by the acts of another should receive compensation for the harm done. This concept dates back more than 2000 years.[126] Medical malpractice is a subset of tort law that is concerned with injury to patients by alleged negligence of their medical professional. Medical malpractice as a concept represents the application of tort principles to the actions of professionals, and like tort law itself, is an ancient phenomenon.[17,126,127]

There are two types of torts, intentional and unintentional.[29] Both may be the subject of malpractice claims in psychiatry. Intentional torts are injuries that result from some intentional action on the part of the actor, also referred to as the *tortfeasor*, who will ultimately be the defendant if a lawsuit is pursued. In psychiatric malpractice claims, typical intentional torts are battery, assault, false imprisonment, abandonment, intentional infliction of emotional distress, and undue familiarity (i.e., sexual misconduct and other boundary violations). Each of these intentional torts is discussed later in this chapter. Unintentional torts arise out of negligent acts or omissions (e.g., misdiagnosis or failure to diagnose, failure to protect the patient from self-harm or harm to others) and are discussed later in this chapter.

Tort law serves two purposes. First, it fulfills the long-established concept that individuals who are injured by the negligent actions of others should receive compensation from the person who caused the harm for the damage they have suffered. Second, some believe that the threat of potential liability serves as a deterrent to negligent behavior.[128,129] Mello and Brennan[130] cast doubt on the deterrence idea in personal injury matters generally, and medical malpractice specifically.

Malpractice insurance also serves two purposes. First, it ensures that injured patients can receive compensation when they are harmed; second, it protects the defendant physician from having to pay damages personally, thus risking potential financial ruin.[131] Malpractice insurance is designed to insure physicians in the event that harm results from negligence (i.e., the allegedly wrongful act was inadvertent rather than intentional).

Medical treatment necessarily involves intentional actions, and liability may therefore arise from both intentional and unintentional acts and omissions that are part of the treatment. As a result, certain intentional acts are also covered by malpractice insurance. For example, a patient injured during a restraint or hospitalized against his or her will may sue for battery or false imprisonment, respectively, and the malpractice insurer will both defend the claim and pay any damage award. The same is not true if the psychiatrist punches the patient during a fit of anger as this action is outside the scope of psychiatric treatment and therefore has nothing to do with acts performed in the course of caring for the patient.[131] Allegations of personal boundary violations give rise to questions about whether such conduct is within the scope of any treatment or outside of such treatment and therefore not covered by malpractice insurance.

To establish a claim of malpractice, whether the defendant's action was intentional or unintentional, a plaintiff (who may be the injured party himself or herself or a representative of the injured party, e.g., the parent of an injured child or the executor of the estate of the deceased in a wrongful death action) must prove four things.[29,132] First, the plaintiff must prove that the defendant owed a duty to the injured party. All individuals owe a general duty of reasonable care, such that their ordinary behavior does not result in harm to others (e.g., drivers have a general obligation not to drive recklessly). The duty to behave in a non-negligent fashion toward a specific individual or group arises when there is a special relationship.[29] Thus, although a physician does not have a specific duty to a person until a doctor–patient relationship is established, after that relationship begins, the physician has a duty to perform in accordance with the standard of care of the average physician practicing in that specialty.[29]

To prove the existence of a duty, the plaintiff must establish that a doctor–patient relationship existed. Simply put, a doctor–patient relationship is established when the physician accepts responsibility for the patient's care by becoming involved with the treatment.[133] Curbside or informal consultations and even more formal consultations do not establish the existence of a relationship as long as the consultant does not assume a treatment role.[134-136]

States differ as to whether clinicians owe a duty of care to individuals other than patients with whom they have entered a doctor–patient relationship. Specifically, one may wonder what happens when a non-patient is injured by the actions of the clinician's patients.[137,138]

The second element of a malpractice claim is dereliction of duty, or negligence. It can be characterized as a departure from the standard of care that results from failure to exercise the level of diligence or care exercised by other physicians of that specialty. An error or injury does not constitute malpractice if it occurs in the course of treatment when the physician has exercised due diligence.[139,140]

To establish this element, the plaintiff must introduce evidence of the applicable standard of care. This is perhaps the most critical element in malpractice claims because the applicable standard varies according to the situation, the type of practitioner, and the jurisdiction. Specialists, or those who claim to have special expertise, are held to a higher standard of practice than general practitioners.[29] Under the "school rule," practitioners who belong to a defined, recognized school of practice or belief may be judged according to the standard of practice of that school,[141] although minimum standards of practice are expected of anyone who holds himself or herself out as being capable of diagnosing and treating illness.[29] In the past, the applicable standard was dependent on the community in which the physician was practicing. This rule, known as the "locality rule," has gradually faded with the wide availability of journals, on-line medical resources, and educational conferences, resulting in a more uniform national standard of care.[142] Although there has been a move toward a more national standard of practice, jurisdictions continue to differ as to whether residents and other trainees should be held to a standard of practice defined by others at that level of training, of general practitioners, or of specialists.[143]

The third element, causation, and the fourth element, damages, are closely tied to the first two: the plaintiff must show that the negligent behavior is the direct cause or proximate cause of actual damages.[144,145] Causation in personal injury law is assessed in two ways. First, the "but-for" test is applied: "But-for the alleged negligence, would the injury have occurred?" Second, was there proximate or legal cause (i.e., was the injury foreseeable)? The test for foreseeability is whether the claimed harm was "a natural, probable, and foreseeable consequence" of negligence on the part of the actor.[29]

Under the doctrine of "loss of chance," causation may also be established when the act or omission by the defendant-physician resulted in a lost opportunity for treatment and therefore subsequent harm.[146-148] This scenario might occur, for example, when there is a missed diagnosis, delayed referral, or delayed treatment.[149] The loss of chance rule has been rejected in professional negligence cases in some jurisdictions[150] and retained in others.[151]

Damages can be of several types. They may be economic (such as lost value of future earnings and medical expenses arising from injuries) or physical (such as the loss of a bodily function). They may also be emotional (e.g., development of psychiatric disorders or pain and suffering).[152-154] Punitive

damages may also be awarded when the defendant's behavior was so reckless as to justify imposition of added damages as punishment for egregious behavior and to serve as a means of deterring that defendant and other potential defendants who might act similarly in the future.[155]

These four elements of a malpractice claim are often referred to as the four Ds: duty, dereliction of duty, direct causation, and damages.[156] If the defendant convinces the jury (or the judge in a bench trial) that all four elements have been proved by a preponderance of the evidence (i.e., that it is more likely than not to have occurred), the defendant will be required to compensate the victim for the harm suffered.[29,156] Expert witnesses who offer their opinions on any of the four elements must testify to a "reasonable degree of medical certainty"—that is, they are confident that their opinions are more likely true than not.[157]

LIABILITY AND MANAGED CARE

Managed care has had a dramatic impact on the practice of psychiatry and the delivery of mental health services. Early on, psychiatrists recognized the potential liability associated with treatment decisions being influenced, and in some cases controlled, by insurers. One might ask, "Is the psychiatrist or inpatient unit liable if a suicidal patient is refused further insurance coverage for inpatient hospitalization, is discharged, and then dies by suicide?" In a word, yes. A psychiatrist's duty to his or her patient continues, regardless of whether the patient's insurer will continue to pay for services.[158,159]

The financial liability of employer-sponsored health plans for damages resulting from denial of health care benefits is significantly limited by the Employee Retirement Income Security Act (ERISA).[160] ERISA contains a pre-emption clause that limits the possible damages from denial of care to the value of the actual benefit or service denied, thus shielding managed care plans from liability for negligence or harm resulting from denial of care. The Supreme Court made clear in *Aetna v. Davila* that ERISA applies to all covered plans, despite state statutes that attempt to provide state law remedies for denial of care and resultant harm.[161] However, ERISA does not pre-empt state statutes that require independent third-party reviews of denials of service, according to the Supreme Court.[162]

The result of this federal statutory scheme is that physicians and health care institutions remain liable for harm that results from withholding care or from early termination of treatment even if the managed care organization has withdrawn funding. Injured patients have no recourse against the managed care plan other than a civil action for the value of the lost benefits.[163] They are free, however, to pursue traditional malpractice claims against providers. For the physician to avoid liability, he or she must protest the denial of care, appeal it to the highest level that the insurer provides, and take other reasonable steps to ensure the patient's safety. Providers themselves may pursue administrative and civil remedies to recover the value of the care provided. However, physicians' entitlements to do so are likely to be limited by their own contracts and agreements with managed care providers.

SELECTED AREAS OF LIABILITY RISK IN PSYCHIATRY

Assault, Battery, and False Imprisonment

A *battery* is the touching of another person without consent or justification.[29] An *assault* is an action that causes fear in the victim because of the reasonable apprehension that an unpermitted touching will occur.[29] Battery and assault are intentional torts. In the setting of medical malpractice, battery claims typically arise when the clinician departs from the standard of care by providing treatment without obtaining informed consent in the absence of an emergency or other exception to informed consent.[164] That is, in the absence of informed consent or an exception, treatment is an unauthorized touching, which legally constitutes battery.

False imprisonment, another intentional tort, results when the tortfeasor causes the victim to have a reasonable belief that his or her movement and freedom are constrained.[29,165] This can occur with confinement to a locked ward, room seclusion, or restraints. False imprisonment does not require actual physical restraint or physical confinement. A patient who reasonably believes that the door to his or her room is locked may claim false imprisonment, even if the door is not actually secured. False imprisonment can lead to liability for violation of constitutional rights, as well as personal injury liability.[166] Conversely, failure to restrain or confine a patient who is at risk of self-harm or elopement may also give rise to liability.

In addition to claims of false imprisonment, the restraint process also may give rise to claims of assault and battery because it necessarily involves (1) apprehension of touching, (2) the actual touching of the patient (generally without the patient's consent), and (3) restriction of movement. The legal aspects of restraint of patients on a medical or surgical ward vary among jurisdictions and are beyond the scope of this chapter and have been explored elsewhere.[167]

Malpractice claims based on battery or false imprisonment, whether they arise in the general hospital or in psychiatric facilities, are rarely successful. Successful defense of these claims lies in demonstrating that the restraint and seclusion were clinically reasonable, that no less restrictive alternative existed, that they were carried out and documented in a careful manner, that the techniques used complied with hospital policies and procedures, and that the restraint process occurred as required by applicable laws and regulations of the jurisdiction where it occurred.[168-170]

Misdiagnosis

Both a failure to diagnose and erroneous diagnosis can provide a basis for unintentional tort liability if harm results.[171] As noted earlier, a medical error that results in injury does not establish negligence if it occurred despite practice in accordance with the standard of care or the adverse outcome was an unavoidable result that might have occurred regardless of the treatment.

Failure to Treat

This broad category of liability risk includes the failure to treat an identified condition or providing treatment that is unproven, not generally accepted, or disproven. In the simplest cases, a patient who sustains injury because the physician failed to treat the condition can generally recover for harm sustained as a result. Harm allegedly resulting from administering treatments that are either unproven or not yet widely accepted can also be the basis for a claim.[172-174] The quest for effective treatments for mental illnesses has included exploration of complementary and alternative treatments.[175] Psychiatrists should be aware that the same malpractice issues involved in other areas of psychiatry apply here. Although treatment with complementary and alternative methods is a field that has not yet attracted substantial numbers of malpractice claims, significant areas of potential risk include lack of informed consent, loss of chance, failure to treat, and fraud and misrepresentation.[173-176] Psychiatry is a field in evolution, with a history of adopting apparently effective treatments that eventually declare themselves to be either unhelpful or harmful.

As a result, caution must be exercised regarding declaring certain treatments to be state-of-the-art and the failure to provide them as constituting *prima facie* evidence of malpractice.[177,178]

Abandonment

Abandonment, as a cause of action for malpractice, is the unilateral termination of the doctor–patient relationship without justification, leading to harm to the patient.[29] In non-emergent situations, physicians are not legally obligated to treat every patient who requests care. Refusal to treat a patient on the basis of his or her race, religion, ethnic origin, or disease type (e.g., acquired immunodeficiency syndrome [AIDS]) raises ethical issues and sets the stage for liability under the Americans with Disabilities Act and state anti-discrimination statutes.[179] The obligation is ethical, as well as legal.[180] Even after the doctor–patient relationship has begun, the physician may choose to terminate the relationship and may legally do so if the method used is reasonable and does not unjustifiably put the patient at risk.[29,156] Justifiable bases for terminating the relationship can include failure to pay, threatening behavior, repeated failure to keep appointments, non-compliance with treatment, and abuse of prescribed medication.[156] After the decision to terminate treatment has been made, the physician should notify the patient and inform him or her of available emergency services and alternative treatment options. Ideally, a specific referral can be provided. The treatment course, reasons and indications for the transfer or termination, the steps taken, and referrals provided should be documented in the record.[181]

Liability for the Acts of Others

Under the law of agency, as exemplified by the legal doctrine of *respondeat superior* ("let the master answer"), an employer is liable for the acts of his or her employees if they are performed within the scope of the employment. Liability arising from the supervisor–supervisee or employer–employee relationship is also known as *vicarious liability*. In psychiatry, this can become an issue in several settings (e.g., supervision of students and residents, supervision of non-physicians, and providing medication back-up).[182,183]

In all cases of vicarious liability, there are several key issues. The first is whether the allegedly negligent and harmful action of the supervisee was within or outside the scope of his or her employment. For example, vicarious liability could arise if the supervisee injures a patient in the course of a restraint but not if the supervisee and the patient were to get into a fight at a hockey game. The second issue is whether the supervisor's status was that of employer or a mere advisor or consultant. For vicarious liability to be imposed, the alleged superior must have sufficient control over the allegedly negligent actor to justify imposition of liability. Criteria include veto authority over treatment decisions, control of the amount and type of work, and hire-and-fire authority.[156,182-184] When there is vicarious liability, both the supervisor and the supervisee may be held liable.[29,185] Supervisors may also be directly liable for harm that results from the action of their supervisees. For example, an attending physician may be held directly liable for harm to a patient when he or she failed to countermand the negligent orders of a resident.[186,187]

Confidentiality and Privilege

Psychiatrists have an ongoing ethical[188,189] and legal[190,191] duty to maintain the confidentiality of information disclosed by patients in the course of treatment and may be held liable for unauthorized disclosure. Numerous ethical and legal exceptions exist to the requirement of confidentiality; these exceptions represent a balancing of the relative harms that result from maintaining or breaching confidentiality in given situations. Ethical exceptions to confidentiality tend to be permissive (e.g., "A psychiatrist may breach confidentiality. …"). These exceptions tend to be commonsense, leaving discretion to the practitioner without imposing obligations.[192] The legal exceptions, found in case law, statutes, and regulations, tend to fall into two broad categories: immunity from liability for disclosure in good faith and required disclosures.

Whether a given exception falls into the immunity for disclosure or mandatory disclosure category depends on the nature of the exception and the jurisdiction. For example, all 50 states and the District of Columbia have statutes that designate a range of professionals as mandated reporters who are obligated to report suspected child abuse or neglect to state social service agencies. Many jurisdictions also require reporting of known or suspected abuse or neglect of older adults or people with disabilities. In recent years, several states have also begun requiring physicians and others to report known or suspected cases of domestic violence to law enforcement or designated agencies.[193]

Of all the exceptions to confidentiality, perhaps the best known involves the duty to protect third parties from the violent acts of patients. This duty exists in some, but not all, jurisdictions.[139,140,194] The rationale for the duty to act to protect third parties was set forth in the California Supreme Court's decision in *Tarasoff v. Board of Regents*,[195] in which the court held that psychotherapists have a duty to act to protect third parties when the therapist knows or should know that the patient poses a threat of serious risk of harm to the third party. The court addressed the balancing issue and noted, "The Court recognizes the public interest in supporting effective treatment of mental illness and in protecting the rights of patients to privacy. But this interest must be weighed against the public interest in safety from violent assault."[195]

Liability for failure to breach confidentiality resulting in harm to third parties did not originate with the *Tarasoff* decision; preceding and subsequent cases have imposed liability on physicians for failing to disclose an individual's infectious disease status where others were subsequently infected.[196–198] Human immunodeficiency virus (HIV)/AIDS poses special problems in this regard because some states have common law or statutory obligations to breach confidentiality to protect third parties but also have prohibitions against disclosing HIV-positive status without written permission.[199] As with many other legal issues, the jurisdictions vary with regard to the duty to disclose HIV-positive status to a spouse.[200,201]

A substantial number of states have enacted statutes that address the duty to protect third parties.[138,202,203] Some states have eliminated the duty altogether; others limit its scope. States that have statutes generally limit the situations under which the duty may arise (e.g., a specific threat to an identifiable third party or a known history of violence on the part of the patient and a reasonable basis to anticipate violence). They also provide that the duty is fulfilled by taking certain steps (such as hospitalizing the patient, warning the potential victim, or notifying law enforcement). Finally, the statutes relieve the clinician of liability to the patient for good faith breaches of confidentiality, and some immunize the clinician from liability for failing to take steps to protect.

The variations among jurisdictions in the law regarding the duty to protect can lead to much confusion. Clinicians are advised, as a basic matter, to become familiar with the standards in the jurisdictions where they practice. It is important to remember that the duty represents an exception to confidentiality, which is recognized in all jurisdictions as being of paramount importance in clinical care, and that any breach of confidentiality must be justified and reasonable. It should be limited to disclosure of the minimum amount of information

necessary to serve the purpose in question. Thus, even in jurisdictions where there is a duty to protect third parties or efforts to protect are made permissible by statute, the clinician should first take steps that will protect the third party without disclosing confidential information (e.g., arranging for hospitalization). Only when necessary to prevent harm should the patient's clinical information be disclosed to the intended victim or police. The effort to prevent harm to the third party, including the decision to share information, should be regarded as a clinical intervention, with every effort made to engage the patient in the effort to avoid harm to others and the adverse consequences to himself or herself.[204]

Other exceptions to confidentiality include statutory provisions that allow disclosure of clinical information in pursuit of the civil commitment process, bill collection, and defense of malpractice claims. It is also accepted that a reasonable amount of information may be disclosed when applying to admit or transfer a patient to a hospital. For example, the Massachusetts psychotherapist patient privilege statute is typical in its exceptions to the obligation to maintain confidentiality.[205]

Passage of the Health Insurance Portability and Accountability Act (HIPAA) of 1996[206] and its implementation in 2003 have caused considerable concern for psychiatrists. HIPAA was originally designed to ensure that individuals with pre-existing illnesses would continue to be eligible for health insurance coverage if they changed employers and to increase the ease of transmission of medical information among authorized users.[207] However, in this law, Congress went far beyond this initial purpose, enacting legislation that led to the promulgation of new rules for how health information must be managed.

HIPAA imposes several requirements on practitioners, health plans, and institutions, and there have been numerous misconceptions about these requirements and their impact on patient care.[208] Many psychiatrists and other mental health professionals were initially concerned that HIPAA would prohibit disclosure of information that is required under state statutes of confidentiality that were required by state law, thus raising the specter of having to choose between a violation of HIPAA and liability under state law. In fact, there are more similarities with pre-existing confidentiality rules than differences, and HIPAA actually expands situations in which protected health information (PHI) may be released without specific consent by the patient. As with traditional rules, HIPAA calls for disclosure of the minimum amount of information necessary to fulfill a specific need when confidentiality is to be breached, even with consent.

Regarding concerns about *Tarasoff* and related dangerousness situations, the HIPAA Privacy Rule[209] allows for disclosure of PHI without the specific consent of patients in 16 different situations related broadly to public health and safety. Among them, 13 are disclosures required by law or public health authorities, reporting of abuse and neglect, reports to law enforcement, infectious disease reporting, and disclosures to avert serious and imminent harm to individuals. Thus, the rules regarding breaches of confidentiality for safety purposes are largely unaffected by HIPAA.[210]

Before HIPAA, for a physician or health care entity to release information, a patient's specific informed consent was generally obtained. In the interest of promoting efficiency in the health care system, HIPAA expressly changed this practice for covered health care providers who release information for treatment, payment, and health care operations purposes. Under HIPAA, covered entities (including physicians) may disclose a patient's PHI for these three purposes without specific consent for the release of information provided that the patient has been notified of the new HIPAA rules through a Privacy Notice. It is important for individual providers to determine whether they are covered by HIPAA to bring their practices into compliance with HIPAA. In general, physicians performing "certain electronic transactions" are subject to HIPAA; the main triggering transaction is electronic billing.[208-212]

It should be noted that HIPAA sets a minimum standard for privacy protection; where state statutes and regulations provide greater protections for privacy, they override HIPAA. Finally, physicians are not subject to direct civil actions by patients under HIPAA. Enforcement of HIPAA is strictly a function of the Office of Civil Rights of the Department of Health and Human Services. An aggrieved patient cannot file an action under HIPAA individually. However, patients are left to their long-standing civil remedies for breach of confidentiality under state statutes and common law. Violations of HIPAA can result in escalating civil and criminal penalties, depending on the nature of the violation and the frequency. In most cases, enforcement of the Privacy Rule is likely to be for corrective rather than punitive action where violations have occurred in good faith.

Among the most relevant provisions of HIPAA for psychiatrists is the distinction between general psychiatric records and psychotherapy notes. Under HIPAA, psychiatric records are generally treated in the same manner as general medical records.[209] This approach is a departure from pre-HIPAA practices in many states. The practical implication of this change is that patients are entitled to copies of their medical and psychiatric records. Patients are also granted the explicit right to request changes to the record. Whether or not the applicable staff member amends the contested information, the involved correspondence becomes part of the record.

HIPAA does recognize that some psychiatric records, defined as "psychotherapy notes," deserve special protection; however, the provision for these notes is narrow. Psychiatrists, under HIPAA, are given discretion regarding release of psychotherapy notes to patients. However, certain specific requirements must be followed for information in the medical record to qualify for the protection of psychotherapy notes. Specifically, the notes must be kept separate from the patient's medical record. Even if kept in a separate psychotherapy record, specific types of information are not subject to the psychotherapy notes exclusion; these include medications prescribed, test results, treatment plans, diagnoses, prognosis, and progress to date.[209] However, psychotherapy notes are considered as part of the medical record in the event that a subpoena is received for medical records in the course of litigation.

Psychotherapist–Patient Privilege

A concept related to confidentiality is that of testimonial privilege. The distinctions between confidentiality and privilege are as follows: whereas *confidentiality* is an ongoing obligation on the part of the clinician to maintain the privacy of information shared during treatment, *privilege* is the patient's right to prohibit the treater from answering requests to share clinical information about the patient in administrative or judicial proceedings. Under English common law, an important origin of law in most jurisdictions in the United States, the court was believed to be entitled to "everyman's evidence," and there were no restrictions on who could be called to testify. Over time, it came to be recognized that important societal purposes were served by preserving the confidentiality of relationships, such as attorney and client, married person and spouse, priest and penitent, and doctor and patient.[213-215]

The existence of the psychotherapist–patient privilege does not serve as an absolute bar to testimony or disclosure of records by the treater. First, the patient must raise the privilege and bar the disclosure of information. Although clinicians may choose to raise the privilege on behalf of the patient,[216] in most cases, failure on the part of the patient to raise the privilege, and certainly the patient's request that the records and

testimony be provided, leaves the clinician with no recourse. Second, there are several exceptions to the privilege, established by statute in most jurisdictions. The statutes in New York and Massachusetts are typical.[205,217] Chief among these is that the patient waives the privilege by putting his or her mental status at issue (e.g., by claiming emotional distress damages in a civil case or raising an insanity defense in a criminal matter). In some, but not all, jurisdictions, there is a "dangerous patient" exception. Under this exception, physicians may breach confidentiality and ultimately testify at criminal proceedings if the patient's statements indicate that there is a serious and imminent threat of harm that can only be avoided if the therapist discloses the information.[218] The existence of this privilege has raised concerns about continued erosion of confidentiality in the treatment of individuals with mental illnesses.[219]

Privilege issues can arise when patients are involved in either civil or criminal litigation. They generally begin with a subpoena that instructs a clinician to appear for a deposition, supply records, or both. It is important to note that a subpoena is not a court order, with which the clinician must comply, but rather a request. The clinician must respond to the subpoena, and this is best done by passing it on to his or her attorney for analysis and appropriate response (e.g., records are confidential and require a release from the patient). In general, clinicians should not reply to subpoenas without first seeking legal guidance. Even after legal consultation, no records should be sent in response to the request without first notifying the patient and giving him or her the opportunity to invoke the privilege.[220]

Suicide

Although suicide is not a common occurrence, psychiatrists and other mental health clinicians are frequently and appropriately concerned about their potential liability if a patient takes their own life. Although suicide is an unfortunate event, it is not grounds, per se, for a psychiatrist to be held liable for malpractice. As with other negative outcomes, a treater is only liable for malpractice if the bad outcome occurred because of the treater's negligence. Clinicians should familiarize themselves with principles of risk assessment for suicidal patients and the prevailing legal requirements for managing suicidal patients in the jurisdictions where they practice.

BOUNDARY VIOLATIONS

Of all the interactions between psychiatrists and patients that can lead to legal liability, boundary violations are among the most painful and damaging for patients, psychiatrists, and their families. Boundary violations are behaviors that involve an inappropriate departure from the accepted doctor and patient roles, as defined by societal and professional standards. They are the end point of a continuum of behavior that begins with the fiduciary duty of physicians to act only in the interests of the patient,[221] rather than in their own interests, and can end with the ultimate transgression, sexual involvement with a patient. Several studies involving disciplinary actions before state medical boards have demonstrated that psychiatrists are significantly more likely than other physicians to be disciplined for sexual relationships with patients.[222]

A large body of literature attempts to categorize the types of boundary violations and their precipitants. In general, boundary violations are conceptualized as a progression of departures from expected roles, some of which are benign and appropriate when viewed in the treatment context and some of which lead caregivers down a "slippery slope" toward patient exploitation and abuse of trust.[223-226] On the benign end of the spectrum are so-called "boundary crossings," which are deviations from traditional psychiatric practice that do not harm the patient and are at times used to advance therapeutic purposes.[227] Examples of such deviations include offering emergency assistance to a stranded or disabled patient or attending a wedding or other ceremony when clinically appropriate for the patient. The availability of personal information via social media and the ease of electronic communication between doctor and patient raise new issues regarding boundary crossings. In contrast to boundary crossings, "boundary violations" are deviations from a professional role that take advantage of the inherent power asymmetry in the physician–patient relationship for the gratification of the caregiver's needs.[228-230]

Whether a given action or event represents normative, acceptable behavior; a boundary crossing; or a boundary violation depends on its nature and its context. Certain boundary violations are egregious and clear. The American Psychiatric Association's (APA's) Annotated Principles of Medical Ethics simply and specifically states, "Sexual activity with a current or former patient is unethical."[192] Arguments for time limitations on the prohibition of physician–patient sexual relations, such that a doctor and patient could enter a relationship after a waiting period after termination of any treatment relationship, have been rejected by the APA. As of 2002, multiple states and the District of Columbia had criminalized psychotherapist–patient sexual involvement.[231] Many non-sexual boundary transgressions are also clearly inappropriate, such as taking financial advantage of patients, employing patients in addition to treating them, or using patients to gratify narcissistic or dependency needs.[230-232]

There are, however, some situations that require flexibility regarding the physician's role and an appreciation of the therapeutic context. For example, although business and social interactions with a patient are to be avoided in most contexts, a psychiatrist practicing in a rural area may have little choice but to encounter a patient at community functions or frequent a patient's retail store.[228] Similarly, although gift giving and receiving[229] are relatively common phenomena in other medical specialties, this practice has greater potential impact and meaning in psychiatry. Whether it constitutes "grist for the therapeutic mill" or a boundary crossing depends on how it is handled. The danger implicit in unaddressed boundary crossings is that they may lead to a more significant boundary violation.[233]

Breaching boundaries in psychiatric treatment can result in multiple sanctions and sources of liability. Patients may bring civil actions for malpractice based on the caregiver's delivery of negligent care. In this vein, medical malpractice insurers have resisted indemnification of alleged sexual misconduct, arguing that such conduct is both intentional and unrelated to the treatment. Interpreting the language of the insurance contracts strictly and seeking to ensure that injured patients were not left without compensation, several courts have held that such misconduct represents negligent handling of the transference and countertransference and is therefore within the scope of malpractice policies.[234,235] Under current policies, coverage for the defense of such charges is generally provided, but insurers may specify that they will not be responsible if the physician is found liable. In addition to malpractice claims, boundary violations can result in the revocation of professional licensure, expulsion from professional societies for breach of ethical codes, and even criminal prosecutions in some jurisdictions.

REDUCING MALPRACTICE RISK

In the quest to reduce malpractice risk, the clearest and most impossible solution would be to avoid all errors. Setting aside the impossibility of such an occurrence, the findings of Studdert and associates[111] that up to one-third of claimed injuries were not the result of medical error exposes the reality that even error-free practice does not completely immunize the practitioner against litigation. In addition to careful practice, several measures can be taken that effectively reduce malpractice risk. In-depth coverage of these measures cannot be accomplished adequately in this space, but general principles are worth noting. First, although individual practice behaviors are a key to reducing risk, it is important to recognize the impact of organizational and systemic issues on error rates.[126] Second, there is convincing evidence that whereas physicians with poor communication skills run an increased risk of malpractice claims, those who engage in shared decision-making, follow good informed consent practices, and represent a humanistic face run less risk of lawsuits.[236-242] Third, increasing attention has been given to the role of apology and acknowledging error as a means of sustaining the doctor–patient relationship in the event of an adverse outcome.[243-248] Fourth, maintaining a good clinical record, with documentation of all clinical activities (e.g., diagnosis, clinical decision-making, informed consent, medication changes, suicide risk assessment) is critical in defending any claims that may arise subsequently. The absence of a note in the record leaves the defendant clinician in the uncomfortable position of having to convince the fact-finder that he or she did, in fact, carry out the appropriate assessments and behaved in a reasonable fashion, even though there was a bad outcome.[156] Fifth, psychiatrists should avoid the tendency to "over-legalize" the doctor–patient relationship, for example, by asking patients to sign waiver and consent forms for minor changes in treatment. Such actions convey the wrong message about the relationship by suggesting defensiveness on the part of the physician. Forms can be important as documentation but do not replace the sharing of information that is so important to the therapeutic relationship. Finally, the value of consulting with colleagues when faced with clinical dilemmas cannot be overestimated. The maxim "Never worry alone" is well worth heeding, especially in the most difficult and uncomfortable clinical dilemmas, such as potential boundary issues.[156,237,249]

CRIMINAL COMPETENCIES

The modern era of criminal law began when English common law began to distinguish between civil and criminal matters.[250,251] Then, as now, specific procedures were required to preserve the integrity, accuracy, and fairness of the criminal process. Entering a plea by the accused was essential to start the proceedings. As of 1275, measures were in place to manage the problem of how to proceed when the defendant refused, or was unable, to enter a plea. According to the famed legal commentator William Blackstone, when the defendant refused to plead, it was left to the court to

> impanel a jury, to enquire whether he stands obstinately mute, or whether he be dumb. If the latter appears to be the case, the judges of the court (who are to be of counsel for the prisoner, and to see that he hath law and justice) shall proceed to the trial, and examine all points as if he had pleaded not guilty.[252]

In other words, if the defendant was found to be mute *ex visitatione Dei* (by act of God), the court would hear the case but take measures to protect the defendant. For defendants found to be "obstinately mute," the consequences depended on the charge. If charged with high treason, the worst of crimes, muteness was considered the equivalent of confession, and the consequences were the same: judgment and execution, with forfeiture of all property to the Crown. Muteness in the face of charges of minor crimes was also held to be the equivalent of confession, and judgment was entered accordingly. As

Blackstone reported, "But upon appeals or indictments for other felonies, or petit treason, he shall not be looked upon as convicted, so as to receive judgment for the felony; but shall, for his obstinacy, receive the terrible sentence of penance, or *peine forte et dure*."[252]

The penance, or *peine forte et dure*, in 1275 involved the following:

> [The prisoner] shall be clad in a single garment and be unshod and, laying upon the bare earth, he shall have for food but a quatern loaf of barley bread every second day, not so that he shall eat daily but only every other day, nor shall he drink daily, but on the day when he does not eat, he shall drink only water.[253]

This procedure did not consistently result in prisoners entering pleas, so by the early 14th century, the process was modified to yield the desired end: the prisoner's diet was reduced to "a little rotten bread" and "cloudy and stinking water" on alternate days, and the defendant was "pressed with as great a weight of iron as his wretched body can bear."[253] The procedure evolved further, and in 1406, Lord Chief Justice Gascoigne sentenced two accused robbers found to be "mute of malice, to delay their death . . . to have put upon them as great a weight of iron as they can bear and more . . . so to lie until death." Eventually, the prescribed process became even more detailed, going so far as to specify the amount and type of water and food to be provided, the extent of any covering, and the manner of restraint, but all with the same ultimate outcome: eliciting a plea, or death. In rare instances, prisoners who survived for extraordinary periods of time were pardoned.[253]

The motivation for refusing to enter a plea and suffering this horrendous fate can be understood as follows: defendants who died without confessing their crimes or being found guilty were not subject to forfeiture of their property, thus preserving assets for their families. *Peine forte et dure* was banned by case law in England in 1772 and by statute in 1827.[253]

Similar approaches to extracting pleadings (and confessions) were used in the English colonies of North America, most notoriously during the Salem Witch Trials. In the United States, as well as the United Kingdom and the Commonwealth countries, this brutal approach gave way to more humane procedures, and recognition that justice was not served by putting on trial a person who was unable to participate in a meaningful way in his or her own defense.[254]

It is now well established in the United States that the trial of an incompetent individual is incompatible with justice and violates the constitutional guarantee of due process under law.[254] In addition to avoiding the brutality of the ancient methods, requiring that the defendant be competent to stand trial serves several purposes. These include (1) the fact-finding portion of the proceedings can only be accurate if the defendant can work with his or her attorney with an understanding of the proceedings, (2) only a competent defendant can exercise the constitutional rights to a fair trial and to confront his or her accuser in a meaningful way, (3) the integrity and dignity of the legal process are preserved by ensuring that the defendant is competent to stand trial, and (4) the purposes of retribution and individual deterrence are served only if the convicted defendant was competent to stand trial.[255]

In the United States, the standard for competency to stand trial (CST) was established in *Dusky v. U.S.*[256] Under the *Dusky* standard, the relevant inquiry is whether the defendant "has sufficient present ability to consult with his lawyer with a reasonable degree of rational understanding, and whether he has a rational as well as a factual understanding of the proceedings against him."[256]

When the issue of competency to stand trial is raised, the trial judge must conclude that the defendant is competent by a preponderance of the evidence (i.e., that it is more likely than not that he or she meets the *Dusky* criteria).[257]

The defense of criminal charges requires numerous complex decisions. As the Supreme Court noted in *Godinez v. Moran:*

> A defendant who stands trial is likely to be presented with choices that entail relinquishment of the same rights that are relinquished by a defendant who pleads guilty: He will ordinarily have to decide whether to waive his "privilege against compulsory self-incrimination," by taking the witness stand; if the option is available, he may have to decide whether to waive his "right to trial by jury," and, in consultation with counsel, he may have to decide whether to waive his "right to confront [his] accusers," by declining to cross-examine witnesses for the prosecution. … In sum, all criminal defendants—not merely those who plead guilty—may be required to make important decisions once criminal proceedings have been initiated.[258]

Interestingly, although the *Godinez* court delineated the important rights and decisions that defendants going to trial and pleading guilty must contemplate, the court ruled against a heightened standard for competency to plead guilty.

Numerous efforts have been made to define the characteristics that distinguish defendants who are competent to stand trial from those who are not. A federal district court specified the following components of CST as meeting the *Dusky* criteria and indicating that a defendant is competent to stand trial:

> (1) That he has mental capacity to appreciate his presence in relation to time, place and things; (2) that his elementary mental processes are such that he apprehends (i.e. seizes and grasps with what mind he has) that he is in a Court of Justice, charged with a criminal offense; (3) that there is a Judge on the Bench; (4) a Prosecutor present who will try to convict him of a criminal charge; (5) that he has a lawyer (self-employed or Court-appointed) who will undertake to defend him against that charge; (6) that he will be expected to tell his lawyer the circumstances, to the best of his mental ability, (whether colored or not by mental aberration) the facts surrounding him at the time and place where the law violation is alleged to have been committed; (7) that there is, or will be, a jury present to pass upon evidence adduced as to his guilt or innocence of such charge; and (8) he has memory sufficient to relate those things in his own personal manner.[259]

There have been attempts to quantify these criteria, so that the evaluation becomes a more objective, structured clinical assessment rather than an impressionistic evaluation.[260–262]

Regardless of the assessment technique used, the threshold for finding a defendant competent to stand trial is very low, and defendants with serious symptoms of mental illness or cognitive impairment have been held competent to stand trial.[257] The Supreme Court has made clear that the standard is minimal and straightforward:

> Requiring that a criminal defendant be competent has a modest aim: It seeks to ensure that he has the capacity to understand the proceedings and to assist counsel. While psychiatrists and scholars may find it useful to classify the various kinds and degrees of competence, and while States are free to adopt competency standards that are more elaborate than the Dusky formulation, the Due Process Clause does not impose these additional requirements.[258]

As noted earlier, judges have a constitutional obligation to address the issue of CST, at any point in the proceedings, when the evidence raises "a *bona fide* doubt" as to competency.[263] As a necessary condition for the criminal process to proceed, this evaluation can be carried out without the defendant's consent.[264]

If a defendant is found incompetent to stand trial (IST), the proceedings are suspended for the defendant to be "restored to competency" as determined on subsequent assessment. The restoration process may involve both treatment of the incapacitating illness and educational efforts aimed specifically at participation in the trial process. Programs aimed at "restoring" the competency of defendants with mental illnesses or intellectual disabilities have been instituted.[265,266] Depending on the severity of the crime and the nature of the underlying illness, the charges may be dropped at this point. For example, in practice, charges of misdemeanor or non-violent offenses may be dropped when the individual has a mental illness and is committed for further treatment.

In cases involving more serious crimes, the defendant might be committed to an inpatient psychiatric facility for treatment and restoration of competency if the defendant has a treatable mental illness that impairs his or her CST. The defendant will be reassessed for CST periodically, as required according to the statute in that jurisdiction. In *Jackson v. Indiana*, the Supreme Court held that defendants who have no hope of restoration of competency cannot be committed indefinitely to state psychiatric facilities unless they meet the usual civil commitment criteria and standard procedures are followed.[267]

All competent adults, including those involved in the criminal justice system, have a right to make their own decisions regarding medical treatment, and specific processes are used to protect the autonomy and legal rights of individuals even after they become incapacitated. Individual states may choose to provide a higher level of protection than the federal standards. The US Supreme Court has handed down several decisions that set the minimum protections for individual autonomy under the US Constitution for individuals found to be IST or to lack criminal responsibility.

In *United States v. Charters*, a US Court of Appeals in 1988 addressed the issue of what procedures were necessary to protect the rights of a defendant who had been found IST and was refusing treatment with antipsychotic medication.[268] The court held that even though involuntary treatment would constitute a deprivation of certain liberty interests, the defendant's rights could be adequately protected through a process that left the decision about whether medication should be administered involuntarily "to appropriate professionals exercising their specialized professional judgments rather than to traditional judicial or administrative-type adjudicative processes."[268]

Four years later, in 1992, the Supreme Court addressed the circumstances under which an IST defendant could be involuntarily medicated to restore his competency to stand trial in *Riggins v. Nevada*.[269] The Court held that for a state to impose antipsychotic medication on an objecting defendant for the purpose of rendering the defendant competent to stand trial, the state must show that the treatment is both medically necessary and appropriate. In deciding the case, the Court looked to its earlier opinion in *Washington v. Harper*, in which it held that a state may treat an inmate with antipsychotic medication against his will if the inmate has a serious mental illness, "is dangerous to himself or others and the treatment is in his medical interest."[270]

The Supreme Court in 2003 refined its holding regarding involuntary medication of IST defendants in *Sell v. United States*.[271] Dr. Sell, a dentist accused of insurance fraud and attempting to have witnesses murdered, was found to be IST.

The government sought to treat him with antipsychotic medication, which he refused, claiming that he had an absolute right to refuse treatment. The Court held that when a defendant is charged with non-violent crimes, the Constitution permits the government to administer antipsychotic drugs against the defendant's will to render the defendant competent to stand trial only under limited circumstances.[271] The Court made clear that involuntary administration of psychotropic medication to a non-violent IST defendant can occur only when a court determines that (1) important governmental interests are at stake; (2) the forced medication will significantly further those interests (i.e., the medication is "substantially likely to render the defendant competent to stand trial and substantially unlikely to have side effects that will interfere significantly with the defendant's ability to assist counsel in conducting a defense"); (3) the involuntary treatment with medication is "necessary to further those interests and find that alternative, less intrusive treatments are unlikely to achieve substantially the same results"; and (4) administering the drugs is medically appropriate.[271]

In none of these cases did the Supreme Court hold that the US Constitution requires more than administrative proceedings before a patient can be involuntarily medicated, although appeal to the courts from the administrative decisions is not barred. This issue was recently revisited by the US Court of Appeals for the 9th Circuit in *U.S. v. Loughner*.[272] Mr. Loughner, who had shot and wounded Congresswoman Gabrielle Giffords and 11 others and killed 6, including Federal District Court Judge John Roll, was found to be a danger to himself and others and was IST. The Court upheld a lower court's order that he be medicated involuntarily, and his commitment extended to allow him to be restored to competency.

The federal approach differs from that taken by several states, which require full adversarial proceedings before involuntary medication of IST defendants and insanity acquittees.[43,273] Overall, states differ in how they address the issue of involuntary medication of both civilly committed and IST individuals.

COMPETENCY TO PLEAD, DECLINE COUNSEL, AND REPRESENT ONESELF

The reality of the criminal process is that many defendants do not reach trial. Instead, they plead guilty, usually in exchange for a reduced sentence through the plea-bargaining process. When a criminal defendant pleads guilty, he or she waives many important constitutionally protected rights, including the protection against self-incrimination, the right to a trial by jury, the right to confront witnesses against him or her, and the right to appeal the conviction. Against this backdrop, several landmark cases have addressed the issue of whether a separate standard for competency to plead guilty should be established.[259,274] In addition, acknowledging that the decision to waive counsel also entails the relinquishment of a constitutionally protected right, the question of whether a standard other than the CST standard applies in determining competency to waive counsel has been addressed.[275] Notwithstanding these inquiries, in *Godinez v. Moran*, the Supreme Court made clear that it recognizes a unitary competency standard, the *Dusky* CST standard[258]; however, the Court also commented that the states were free to adopt higher standards. In a subsequent case, *Edwards v. Indiana*, the US Supreme Court explicitly recognized that representing oneself (known as proceeding *pro se*) requires greater ability than entering a plea or even waiving the right to counsel and definitively held that states may deny the right to self-representation unless the defendant meets a higher competency standard.[276]

COMPETENCY TO BE EXECUTED

Competency is also required before a person convicted of a capital crime and sentenced to death can be executed. The standard for competency to be executed is whether the condemned person has an understanding of the nature of the proceedings and can participate in the process.[277] Requiring competency to be executed serves several purposes: (1) it preserves the integrity of the sentencing and punishment process, (2) it ensures that the convicted individual will have the ability to contest the decision through all stages of appeal before imposition of punishment, and (3) it ensures that the deterrent function of punishment is served by punishing only those who have the requisite mental capacity.[277]

The importance of the mental status of death row inmates and competency to be executed is reflected in several key US Supreme Court cases. In the 1986 case of *Ford v. Wainwright*,[277] the court held that execution of the insane is a violation of the Eighth Amendment prohibition against cruel and unusual punishment and that death row inmates are entitled to a full and fair hearing on the issue of competency to be executed.

The Supreme Court did not find a blanket bar to capital punishment for the intellectually disabled until nearly 2 decades later.[278] In 2002, the court reversed its prior rulings on this issue and held that execution of intellectually disabled individuals violates the Eighth Amendment.[279] Two years later, in *Roper v. Simmons*,[280] the court further narrowed the parameters for constitutionally permissible executions when it held that imposition of the death penalty for crimes committed when offenders were younger than 18 years of age also violated the Eighth Amendment.

The involvement of psychiatrists and other physicians in executions is controversial. The American Medical Association has taken the position that physicians should not participate in legally authorized executions.[188] Similarly, the APA took the position in a 1990 Ethics Committee Opinion that it is unethical for a psychiatrist to participate in executions. Debate remains regarding the morality of psychiatrists conducting competency evaluations for execution.[281] At a bare minimum, the prisoner must be informed of the purpose of the evaluation and the limitations on confidentiality.[282] Similarly, if psychiatrists become involved in the treatment of death row inmates, they must inform prisoners of their professional roles and the limits on confidentiality.

One of the more controversial roles played by psychiatrists in this area has been testimony on the issue of future dangerousness, a key element used in determining whether a convicted murderer will be sentenced to death. This issue has been the subject of a series of landmark Supreme Court cases. In *Estelle v. Smith*, the court held that a condemned inmate's Fifth Amendment right to freedom from self-incrimination and his Sixth Amendment right to assistance of counsel had been denied when a psychiatrist who had examined him for CST was allowed to testify to his dangerousness at the penalty phase and the defendant had not been informed of the purpose of the evaluation or his right to have an attorney present.[283]

In *Barefoot v. Estelle*,[284] the Supreme Court held that although a state cannot compel a defendant to submit to a psychiatric evaluation, there is no constitutional barrier to a psychiatric expert using hypothetical questions as a basis for testimony about a defendant's dangerousness. The court specifically rejected the APA's position that dangerousness predictions are inherently unreliable and that such testimony should be excluded entirely.

Another area of controversy has been refusal of treatment by condemned prisoners who have been found incompetent to be executed. The logical outcome of successful treatment, of course, would be death. These cases present the ethical issues for treating physicians, and the legal issue of whether a condemned prisoner may be treated against his will for the purpose of restoring him to competency, thus allowing the death sentence to be carried out. In *Perry v. Louisiana*,[285] the US Supreme Court overturned the decision of the Louisiana Supreme Court, which had held that the state's interest in rendering a death row inmate competent to be executed by involuntary administration of antipsychotic medication outweighed the inmate's right to refuse medical treatment. Noting that in *Washington v. Harper*[270] it had included "best interests of the prisoner" among the criteria for involuntary treatment of prisoners with antipsychotic medication, the Court vacated the sentence and remanded the case back to the state court for reconsideration in light of *Harper*. On remand, the Supreme Court of Louisiana held that forced administration of antipsychotic drugs to restore a prisoner's competency to be executed violates the state constitutional right to privacy and constitutes cruel, excessive, and unusual punishment.[286]

At this point in time, with the approval of the US Supreme Court, jurisdictions that use the death penalty look to psychiatrists and other mental health professionals to assess the competency of prisoners to be executed, to treat their illnesses to restore them to competency, and to assess dangerousness.

CRIMINAL RESPONSIBILITY

A fundamental principle of criminal justice is that individuals with severe mental illness or developmental disabilities are not to be held responsible for their otherwise criminal acts.[287] The concept itself and the derivative question of what to do with individuals who are found not guilty by reason of insanity (NGRI) have been the subject of much debate and have generated fluctuating standards. Few activities of mental health professionals receive as much media and public attention and spark as much controversy as testimony on these matters.

A detailed history of the evolution of the insanity defense is beyond the scope of this chapter; however, interested readers may wish to consult the classic texts on the subject,[251,288,289] as well as some of the more modern and readily available treatises on the insanity defense.[290-292]

The history of the insanity defense is a chronicle of society's struggles over moral responsibility, ecclesiastical influences, historical events, the nature and level of scientific understanding of mental illness, and public attitudes about people with mental illnesses.[290,293] For example, the episodic mental illness of King George III is believed to have had a major influence on the attitudes of the public and therefore the jurors of the time[251,290] and may have benefited some criminal defendants of the period.[290] There are numerous examples of the criminal responsibility standard being tightened after the perpetrator of a notorious crime is found NGRI (e.g., James Hadfield,[251] Daniel M'Naghten,[251,294] and John Hinckley[295]). The modifications tend to be such that the infamous defendant would have been found criminally responsible under the newly modified standard.

Before turning to the insanity defense, an overview of the basics of criminal law and related defenses is useful. For an individual to be convicted of a crime, there must be a guilty act (*actus reus*) and guilty intent (*mens rea*). *Mens rea* is considered in both a general and specific form. In its general form, it refers to the overall capacity of an individual to form the intent to commit the crime in question and thus his or her blameworthiness or legal liability. For example, an individual who takes someone else's automobile for his own use when directed to do so by auditory hallucinations or who is not even aware that he is stealing a vehicle is unlikely to be found to have had the necessary intent to be found blameworthy. In its specific or narrow form, *mens rea* is an element of a group of crimes referred to as specific intent crimes. A specific intent crime requires that the prosecution prove that the defendant acted with a particular state of mind when performing the illegal act.[296] (Under Massachusetts law, *murder* is defined as follows: "Murder committed with deliberately premeditated malice aforethought, or with extreme atrocity or cruelty, or in the commission or attempted commission of a crime punishable with death or imprisonment for life, is murder in the first degree. Murder which does not appear to be in the first degree is murder in the second degree. Petit treason shall be prosecuted and punished as murder. The degree of murder shall be found by the jury." From MGL Ch. 265 §1.)

Beyond the obvious defenses of denying that he or she committed the act or that no crime occurred, a criminal defendant has two broad categories of defenses available: justification and excuse.[287,297]

Justification Defenses

Justification defenses are those in which a normally wrongful act is committed but under circumstances that make it acceptable rather than wrongful. The justification defenses include self-defense, defense of others, defense of property, and choice of evils (i.e., a choice is made to commit a criminal act that is less harmful than the available alternative act).[287,296,297]

Excuse Defenses

Whereas the availability of a justification defense turns on the act itself and the circumstances under which it occurred, excuse defenses look to the internal mental state of the actor.[296,297] There are several related excuse defenses, including ignorance, compulsion, duress, and insanity.

Ignorance

Lack of knowledge of the crime, mistaken belief about the act, and inadvertence can all serve as complete or partial defenses under the general category of "ignorance."[296,297] There are limited roles for psychiatric testimony in such defenses because the focus is on the knowledge of the defendant, rather than on his or her mental functioning. When such testimony occurs, it is likely to be restricted to the cognitive abilities of the defendant.

Compulsion

Compulsion is a category of excuse defenses that focuses on the ability of a defendant to think and act rationally under the influence of external circumstances. Compulsions serve as a defense because the external force (not an internal influence, such as an impulse-control disorder, e.g., pedophilia) deprives the defendant of the ability to make choices that he or she would normally make.[297] The compulsion defenses represent the notion that it would be unfair to convict a defendant of a criminal act if the jurors, as representatives of the rest of society, would have behaved similarly under the same circumstances.[296,298] Compulsion defenses include duress, extreme emotional disturbance, and compulsion due to addiction or insanity.[297]

Duress. This defense is available where an individual (the actor) commits an act because another person has unlawfully threatened him or her with equal or more serious injury, such that the only way to avoid imminent death or serious injury is to comply with the unlawful instruction.[296,298] Although duress has been held not to excuse murder, it has been found to be a valid defense to robbery, kidnapping, prison escape, possession of a weapon, and treason.[287]

Extreme Passion. Extreme emotional disturbance can also serve as a partial or complete defense. Examples include situations when an individual learns of spousal infidelity or death of a loved one at the hands of another. The defense requires that the defendant prove that he or she was under extreme emotional distress at the time of the act and that his or her action was reasonable in light of that distress.[287] For example, New York penal law provides an affirmative defense of extreme emotional distress for assault charges, including first-degree murder if "[t]he defendant acted under the influence of extreme emotional disturbance for which there was a reasonable explanation or excuse, the reasonableness of which is to be determined from the viewpoint of a person in the defendant's situation under the circumstances as the defendant believed them to be."[299,300] Psychiatrists may be asked to opine about the presence and level of emotional distress on the part of the defendant, but the issue of reasonableness is an issue for the jury.

Compulsion Due to Addiction or Insanity. The compulsion defense may be raised where a defendant's addiction or insanity leads him or her to criminal conduct if the actor reasonably believed he or she would suffer death or great bodily harm if he or she did not perform the criminal act. Thus, a person suffering command hallucinations may raise a compulsion defense, just as a person addicted to drugs or alcohol may raise a compulsion defense to charges of illegal use. The Supreme Court has held that it is unconstitutional to convict substance addicted individuals of the crime of having an addiction[301] or using drugs.[302]

Lack of Criminal Responsibility

A defendant may be found to lack criminal responsibility when the defendant was impaired in his or her ability to think or to act rationally because of a mental disease or defect. The essence of this defense is that the defendant, as a result of the condition in question, has a certain status such that it would be improper to hold him or her morally blameworthy.[289,297,303] Infants and very young children, for example, are not held criminally responsible for their acts because they are not regarded as having the capacity for rational thought that would designate them as blameworthy persons in the eyes of the law.[289] Individuals who commit acts of violence due to automatisms occurring during altered states of consciousness (e.g., somnambulism, complex partial seizures, and delirium tremens) may also be excused from responsibility.[303–305]

The insanity defense is the best known of the excuse defenses. As noted earlier, the essence of the insanity defense is the centuries-old recognition that certain individuals should not be held morally blameworthy and therefore are not criminally responsible for their acts.[289] Societies have drawn a line between conditions that may relieve one of moral blameworthiness and those that do not. Like many moral issues, the line is not always clear. For example, whereas automatisms may be the basis for an excuse defense, dissociative identity disorder (multiple personality disorder) has had far less success, perhaps because of skepticism about the diagnosis.[306] Voluntary intoxication, as a state brought on by the willful act of the defendant, is not allowed as the basis for an insanity defense.[296] However, mental conditions exacerbated by intoxication or resulting from long-term substance abuse may be used as the basis for an insanity defense.[307] In many states, voluntary intoxication can be used to argue for diminished capacity, an altered mental state that does not fulfill criteria for a full insanity defense but may be used to lessen the severity of the crime of which the defendant is convicted (e.g., from first- to second-degree murder).[308,309]

Several landmark cases have marked the development of the insanity defense in Anglo-American law. The changes in the standards mark alterations between those that are purely volitional (having the ability to control one's behavior), purely cognitive (having knowledge of wrongfulness), combined volitional–cognitive standards, and pure *mens rea* standards. One state uses yet another approach, known as the "product" test.[290]

An early example of a volitional standard is the "wild beast" test, described in *Rex v. Arnold* (1723).[310] In this case, the court held that "Mad Ned" Arnold, on trial for shooting Lord Onslow, could be found NGRI only if he were completely devoid of control. The judge wrote, in part:

> It is not every kind of frantic humour, or something unac-countable in a man's actions, that points him out to be such a madman as is to be exempted from punishment: it must be a man that is totally deprived of his understanding and memory, and doth not know what he is doing, no more than an infant, than a brute or a wild beast, such a one is never the object of punishment.[310]

At the turn of that century, the insanity acquittal of James Hadfield,[311] charged with high treason after his failed attempt to assassinate King George III, turned on the court's acceptance of defense counsel's argument that those with mental disturbances short of "wild beast" status were also eligible for an insanity acquittal. Lord Erskine successfully argued on Hadfield's behalf that:

> if a total deprivation of memory was intended by these great lawyers to be taken in the literal sense of the words: if it was meant, that, to protect a man from punishment, he must be in such a state of prostrated intellect, as not to know his name, nor his condition, nor his relation towards others—that if a husband, he should not know he was married; or if a father, could not remember that he had children; nor know the road to his house, nor his property in it—then no such madness ever existed in the world.[251,290]

Hadfield was found not criminally responsible because of his illness (a delusional state that appeared to result from a sabre wound to the skull while fighting the French at the Battle of Freymar). Under the terms of the Insane Offenders' Act passed by Parliament during his trial, Hadfield was remanded to Bethlem Hospital, to be held there "until his Majesty's pleasure be known."[251]

The next major development in the insanity defense, the M'Naghten standard,[312] has remained a major component of modern criminal responsibility standards. In 1843, M'Naghten, a Scottish wood turner, shot and killed Edward Drummond, private secretary to Prime Minister Robert Peel, after mistaking him for the prime minister. He was found NGRI, thanks to his skillful counsel's success in convincing the court that M'Naghten's "partial insanity" provided an adequate basis for excusing him from responsibility.[251,294]

The public was outraged by M'Naghten's acquittal, as was Queen Victoria. In response, the House of Lords posed five questions to the judges of the court and convened them to explain the rules by which criminal responsibility would be determined.[251] The Lords first wanted to know what the law was with respect to crimes:

> committed by persons afflicted with insane delusion . . . : as, for instance, where at the time of the commission of the alleged crime, the accused knew he was acting contrary to law, but did the act complained of with a view, under the

> influence of insane delusion, of redressing or revenging some supposed grievance or injury, or of producing some supposed public benefit?[313]

In response to this first inquiry, Lord Chief Justice Tyndal explained:

> We are of the opinion that, notwithstanding the party accused did the act complained of with a view, under the influence of insane delusion, of redressing or revenging some supposed grievance or injury, or of producing some public benefit, he is nevertheless punishable according to the nature of the crime committed, if he knew at the time of committing such crime that he was acting contrary to law.[313]

Thus, if a person with a paranoid delusion killed another whom he believed was about to kill him, he could be acquitted based on self-defense. However, if the delusional belief was that the victim had libeled him, he would be convicted because libel does not justify murder.[313]

In responding to the inquiries about the proper instructions to the jury and what facts were to be considered, Lord Chief Justice Tyndal described what has come to be known as the M'Naghten rule:

> To establish a defence on the ground of insanity, it must be clearly proved that, at the time of the committing of the act, the party accused was labouring under such a defect of reason, from disease of the mind, as not to know the nature and quality of the act he was doing; or, if he did know it, that that he did not know he was doing what was wrong.[313]

Under this rule, for a defendant to be found not responsible, he had to be (1) mentally ill or suffering a mental defect, such as dementia or significant developmental disability, and either be (2) unaware of what he was doing, for example, believed he was pointing his finger when in fact he was pointing a pistol, or (3) unaware that he was committing an unlawful act, for example, believed he was defending himself against deadly attack. Notably, M'Naghten would have been convicted had this standard been applied to him.

Subsequent developments in the insanity defense, both in England and the United States, tended to expand the criteria, as knowledge and attitudes regarding mental illness changed. The "irresistible impulse test," which looked to whether a defendant had the ability to conform his or her behavior to the requirements of the law, even while knowing that the act was wrongful, made its way into English and American jurisprudence by the late 1800s.[251,290] The New Hampshire Rule, which is still the standard in that state, asks the jury to find the defendant NGRI if the alleged criminal's act was the product of a mental disease or defect.[290]

In 1962, the American Law Institute's Model Penal Code introduced criteria for an insanity defense that offered alternative bases for an NGRI verdict: either the cognitive component of M'Naghten or the volitional component of the irresistible impulse test.[296] The standard is as follows:

> A person is not responsible for criminal conduct if at the time of such conduct as a result of mental disease or defect he lacks substantial capacity either to appreciate the wrongfulness of his conduct or to conform his conduct to the requirements of the law.

> As used in this Article, the terms "mental disease or defect" do not include an abnormality manifested only by repeated criminal or otherwise antisocial conduct.[296]

By the early 1980s, 25 states were using the American Law Institute's Model Penal Code standard, as were the federal courts. John Hinckley's attempted assassination of President Ronald Reagan and his subsequent acquittal based on lack of criminal responsibility changed that, however. Hinckley's acquittal, like M'Naghten's, resulted in demands to restrict, and in some cases eliminate, the insanity defense.[314] With support from the APA and American Bar Association, Congress enacted a new standard for criminal responsibility in the federal courts:

> It is an affirmative defense to any prosecution under any Federal statute that, at the time of the commission of the acts constituting the offense, the defendant, as a result of a severe mental disease or defect, was unable to appreciate the nature and quality or wrongfulness of his acts.[315]

This standard essentially adopted the M'Naghten standard, eliminating the volitional component contained in the American Law Institute's Model Penal Code standard. It also made clear that the defendant must be unable to appreciate the wrongfulness of his or her conduct rather than merely lacking "substantial capacity" to appreciate wrongfulness. In addition, Congress specified that the underlying disorder related to the crime must be "severe" and shifted the burden of proof to the defendant. Just as with M'Naghten, the subsequent modification of the federal standard would have likely resulted in Hinckley's conviction, had it been in place at the time of trial.

The impact of the Hinckley acquittal spread beyond the federal system to the states.[294] According to Melton and colleagues,[316] by 1995, 5 of the 25 states that had been using the Model Penal Code test in its pure form had given it up, with about half the states using a form of the M'Naghten rule. Twelve states expanded the verdicts available in cases involving mental illness by introducing "guilty but mentally ill" verdicts. In these states, a defendant may be found guilty, guilty but mentally ill, not guilty, and NGRI.[294] Three states abolished the insanity defense completely and established procedures to commit guilty but mentally ill defendants, with mixed results.[295,317,318] Changes in other jurisdictions included shifting the burden of proof from the prosecution to the defendant and tightening the definition of mental illness.[295]

The insanity defense is an expression of society's view that it is inappropriate to impose criminal responsibility on individuals who are not morally blameworthy. The various criminal responsibility standards are efforts by individual jurisdictions to operationalize this universal notion in a manner consistent with public attitudes. Studies of the impact of different criminal responsibility standards indicate that mock jurors using the different insanity defense standards arrive at similar verdicts in similar cases, regardless of the standard used.[319] Mock jurors given no standards, merely instructions to use their best judgment, arrived at the same verdicts as those asked to apply specific standards.[320] From these and other studies, it appears that factors other than the technical criminal responsibility standard determine whether a jury will find a defendant NGRI. These factors include the nature of the crime, the nature of the illness, the nature of the act, and the consequences the jury sees attached to a guilty versus NGRI verdict.[290]

The question of disposition for insanity acquittees is an enduring one. In most jurisdictions, insanity acquittees are automatically committed to a state psychiatric facility for a defined initial period for evaluation and treatment. At the end of the initial period, a recommitment hearing is held; states are free to use lower standards of proof for commitment of insanity acquittees (preponderance of the evidence) than for non-criminal candidates for commitment (clear and convincing evidence). The Supreme Court has held that the government may automatically confine insanity acquittees, regardless of their crime, and hold them until such time as the acquittee can prove that he or she is no longer mentally ill or dangerous.[321]

Insanity acquittees who refuse treatment with antipsychotic medication may be treated against their will under the same rules that apply to other civilly committed patients in that jurisdiction. Civil standards apply because these individuals have not been convicted of any crime and therefore can only be held in a hospital if they meet statutory civil commitment standards.

EVALUATIONS OF CRIMINAL RESPONSIBILITY

Evaluations of criminal responsibility are, by necessity, retrospective determinations of the defendant's mental status at the time of the offense. The focus of criminal responsibility evaluations is assessment of the individual's mental state at that time using the current examination, a review of medical and criminal records, information from collateral sources, and a conclusion regarding that status relative to the jurisdictional standards for criminal responsibility. Under ideal conditions, the accused is evaluated by mental health professionals as close to the occurrence of the offense as possible. In many cases, however, the forensic evaluator may not see the defendant until months or years after the crime. An excellent discussion of these evaluations is provided by Melton and associates.[316]

Several clinical conditions can affect criminal responsibility, including delirium, depression, psychosis, delusions, panic and other anxiety disorders, sleep disorders, obsessive-compulsive disorder, seizures, and other neurological disorders. Considering this, the clinical evaluation should be detailed and extensive, with a full review of systems. Medical records should be examined and laboratory studies ordered to assess for the presence of other illnesses and conditions, including intoxication.

Criminal responsibility evaluations are complicated by the retrospective nature of the analysis, often over time, and by the fact that the sources of information are often incomplete or biased. Police reports, statements from family members, victim statements, and the defendant's self-report are also essential parts of the evaluation. And each of them is affected, to greater or lesser degree, by their own inherent bias, which is often difficult to detect. The Model Penal Code, Section 4.05, provides an outline of what the report on a criminal defendant should contain.[296]

CONCLUSION

The topics covered in this chapter represent interactions with the legal system that are part of the day-to-day professional lives of psychiatrists, especially when working with vulnerable populations whose treatment is more likely to involve the legal issues we have discussed. Over the years, many clinicians have expressed dismay over what they perceive to be intrusions by the legal system into the care of patients, as represented by the topics covered here. In fact, some of these requirements have proven burdensome and, in some situations, have resulted in outcomes that have been unhelpful, if not overtly harmful, to specific patients. Such adverse outcomes, as well as the increased non-clinical burden on psychiatrists, are frustrating. In managing these situations and our frustration, it may be helpful to keep in mind that these perceived intrusions are the result of our living in a system that protects the civil liberties and autonomy interests of all people, even when the ability to speak on one's own behalf has been lost. Ours is a system that balances individual rights to self-determination and autonomy of individuals against the rights of individuals to be safe and of states to protect their citizens. As with all human endeavors, there is imperfection, and the system does not always get it right. It is a system that is open to change and input, however, and psychiatrists have an important role to play in this regard. Basic knowledge about patients' rights and the legal system and working across disciplines are essential for providing effective care in this climate and facilitating changes that will benefit our patients.

REFERENCES

1. Cleary EW. *McCormick on Evidence*. 3rd ed. West Publishing Co; 1984.
2. Schouten R. Pitfalls of clinical practice: the treating clinician as expert witness. *Harv Rev Psychiatry*. 1993;1:64–65.
3. Strasburger LH, Gutheil TG, Brodsky A. On wearing two hats: role conflict in serving as both psychotherapist and expert witness. *Am J Psychiatry*. 1997;154:448–456.
4. Appelbaum PS, Gutheil TG. *Clinical Handbook of Psychiatry and the Law*. 4th ed. Lippincott Williams & Wilkins; 2006.
5. Zonana H, Daubert v. Merrell Dow Pharmaceuticals: a new standard for scientific evidence in the courts? *Bull Am Acad Psychiatry Law*. 1994;22:309–325.
6. Gutheil TG, Bursztajn H. Avoiding ipse dixit mislabeling: post-Daubert approaches to expert clinical opinions. *J Am Acad Psychiatry Law*. 2003;31:205–210.
7. Taboada P, Bruera E. Ethical decision-making on communication in palliative cancer care: a personalist approach. *Support Care Cancer*. 2001;9:335–343.
8. Annas GJ. Nancy Cruzan in China. *Hastings Cent Rep*. 1990;20:39–41.
9. Schneewind JB. *The Invention of Autonomy*. Cambridge University Press; 1998.
10. Mill JS. *On Liberty*. Norton; 1859.
11. Monahan J. John Stuart Mill on the liberty of the mentally ill: a historical note. *Am J Psychiatry*. 1977;134:1428–1429.
12. Arnold MS. Accident, mistake, and rule of liability in the fourteenth century law of torts. *Univ PA Law Rev*. 1979;128:361–378.
13. *Schloendorff v. Society of New York Hospital*, 105 N.E. 92 (N.Y. Ct. App. 1914).
14. *Cruzan v. Director, Missouri Department of Health*, 497 U.S. 261 (1990).
15. Beauchamp TL, Childress JF. *The Principles of Bioethics*. 5th ed. Oxford University Press; 2001.
16. Schouten R. Informed consent: resistance and reappraisal. *Crit Care Med*. 1989;7:1359–1361.
17. Mohr JC. American medical malpractice litigation in historical perspective. *JAMA*. 2000;283:1731–1737.
18. Dalla-Vorgia P, Skiadas P, Garanis-Papadatos T. Is consent in medicine a concept of only modern times? *J Med Ethics*. 2001;27:59–61.
19. *Slater v. Baker and Stapleton*, 95 Eng. 860 (King's Bench 1767).
20. *Natanson v. Kline*, 350 P.2d 1093 (Kansas 1960).
21. *Canterbury v. Spence*, 464 F.2d 772 (D.C. Cir. 1972), cert. denied, 409 U.S. 1064.
22. Appelbaum PS, Lidz CW, Meisel A. *Informed Consent: Legal Theory and Clinical Practice*. Oxford University Press; 1987.
23. Iheukwumere EO. Doctor: are you experienced? The relevance of disclosure of physician experience to a valid informed consent. *J Contemp Health Law Policy*. 2002;18:373–419.
24. King JS, Moulton BW. Rethinking informed consent: the case for shared medical decision-making. *Am J Law Med*. 2006;32:429–493.
25. *Precourt v. Frederick*, 481 N.E.2d 1144 (Mass. 1985).
26. Sawicki NN. Informed consent beyond the physician-patient encounter: tort law implications of extra-clinical decision support tools. *Ann Health Law*. 2012;21:1–10.
27. Ip M, Gilligan T, Koenig B, et al. Ethical decision-making in critical care in Hong Kong. *Crit Care Med*. 1998;26:447–451.
28. Kiesler DJ, Auerbach SM. Optimal matches of patient preferences for information, decision-making and interpersonal behavior: evidence, models and interventions. *Patient Educ Couns*. 2006;61:319–341.
29. Keeton WP. *Prosser and Keeton on the Law of Torts, 1061. Prosser and Keeton on Torts*. 5th ed. West Publishing; 1984:480–498.

30. Faden RR, Beauchamp TL. *A History and Theory of Informed Consent*. Oxford University Press; 1986.
31. Roberts LW. Informed consent and the capacity for voluntarism. *Am J Psychiatry*. 2002;159:705–712.
32. Mallary SD, Gert B, Culver CM. Family coercion and valid consent. *Theor Med*. 1986;7:123–126.
33. Grisso T, Appelbaum PS. *Assessing Competence to Consent to Treatment: A Guide for Physicians and Other Health Professionals*. Oxford University Press; 1998.
34. Gold JA. *Kaimowitz v. Department of Mental Health*: involuntary mental patient cannot give informed consent to experimental psychosurgery. *Rev Law Soc Change*. 1974;4:207–227.
35. National Commission for the Protection of Human Subjects of Biomedical and Behavioral Research. *Report and Recommendations: Research Involving Prisoners*. US Government Printing Office; 1976.
36. National Commission for the Protection of Human Subjects of Biomedical and Behavioral Research. *Research Involving Those Institutionalized as Mentally Infirm: Report and Recommendations*. US Government Printing Office; 1978.
37. Moser DJ, Arndt S, Kanz JE, et al. Coercion and informed consent in research involving prisoners. *Compr Psychiatry*. 2004;45:1–9.
38. Bisbing SB. Competency and capacity: a primer. In: Sanbar SS, ed. *Legal Medicine*. Mosby; 2004.
39. Appelbaum PS. Assessment of patients' competence to consent to treatment. *N Engl J Med*. 2007;357:1834–1840.
40. Leo RJ. Competency and the capacity to make treatment decisions: a primer for primary care physicians. *Prim Care Companion J Clin Psychiatry*. 1999;1:131–141.
41. President's Commission for the Study of Ethical Problems in Medicine and Biomedical and Behavioral Research. *Making Health Care Decisions: A Report on the Ethical and Legal Implications of Informed Consent in the Patient-Practitioner Relationship*. US Government Printing Office; 1982.
42. Roth LH, Meisel A, Lidz CW. Tests of competency to consent to treatment. *Am J Psychiatry*. 1977;134:279–284.
43. *Rogers v. Commissioner of Department of Mental Health*, 390 N.E.2d 489 (Mass. 1983).
44. *In the Matter of Richard Roe III*, 421 N.E.2d 40 (Mass. 1981).
45. Baron C. On taking substituted judgment seriously. *Hastings Cent Rep*. 1990;20:7–8.
46. Gutheil TG, Appelbaum PS. The substituted judgment approach: its difficulties and paradoxes in mental health settings. *Law Med Health Care*. 1988;13:61–64.
47. Lowy C. The doctrine of substituted judgment in medical decision making. *Bioethics*. 1998;2:15–21.
48. Meisel A. The "exceptions" to the informed consent doctrine: striking a balance between competing values in medical decision making. *Wis L Rev*. 1979;2:413–488.
49. Sprung CL, Winick BJ. Informed consent in theory and practice: legal and medical perspectives on the informed consent doctrine and a proposed reconceptualization. *Crit Care Med*. 1989;17:1346–1354.
50. *Shine v. Vega*, 709 N.E.2d 58 (Mass. 1999).
51. Dickerson DA. A doctor's duty to disclose life expectancy information to terminally ill patients. *Cleve State Law Rev*. 1995;43:319–350.
52. Srebnik DS, Rutherford LT, Peto T, et al. The content and clinical utility of psychiatric advance directives. *Psychiatr Serv*. 2005;56:592–598.
53. Appelbaum PS. Psychiatric advance directives and the treatment of committed patients. *Psychiatr Serv*. 2004;55:751.
54. Swanson J, Swartz M, Ferron J, et al. Psychiatric advance directives among public mental health consumers in five US cities: prevalence, demand, and correlates. *J Am Acad Psychiatry Law*. 2006;34:43–57.
55. Schouten R. Commentary: psychiatric advance directives as tools for enhancing treatment of the mentally ill. *J Am Acad Psychiatry Law*. 2006;34:58–60.
56. Nicaise P, Lorant V, DuBois V. Psychiatric advance directives as a complex and multistage intervention: a realist systematic review. *Health Soc Care Community*. 2013;21(1):1–14.
57. Srebnik D, Appelbaum PS, Russo J. Assessing competence to complete psychiatric advance directives with the competence assessment tool for psychiatric advance directives. *Compr Psychiatry*. 2004;45:239–245.
58. Swanson JW, Van McCrary S, Swartz MS, et al. Superseding psychiatric advance directives: ethical and legal considerations. *J Am Acad Psychiatry Law*. 2006;34:385–394.

59. Appelbaum PS. Commentary: psychiatric advance directives at a crossroads—when can PADs be overridden? *J Am Acad Psychiatry Law*. 2006;34:395–397.

60. Halliday S, Witteck L. Decision-making at the end-of-life and the incompetent patient: a comparative approach. *Med Law*. 2003;22:533–542.

61. Lo B, Dornbrand L. The case of Claire Conroy: will administrative review safeguard incompetent patients? *Ann Intern Med*. 1986;104:869–873.

62. Gutheil TG. Search of true freedom—drug refusal, involuntary medication, and rotting with your rights on. *Am J Psychiatry*. 1980;137:327–328.

63. Miller RD. The continuum of coercion: constitutional and clinical considerations in the treatment of mentally disordered persons. *Denver University Law Rev*. 1997;74:1169–1214.

64. Chapter 15. Substance Abuse and Mental Health Act part 6. Utah State Hospital and other mental health facilities. Utah Code Ann., § 62A-15-631. 2006. Title 62A. Utah Human Services Code.

65. Erickson SK, Vitacco MJ, Van Rybroek GJ. Beyond overt violence: Wisconsin's progressive civil commitment statute as a marker of a new era in mental health law. *Marquette Law Rev*. 2005;89:359.

66. *Rennie v. Klein*, 720 F.2d 266 (3rd Cir. 1983).

67. Chapter 5122. Hospitalization of mentally ill § 5122.271. Voluntary consent to treatment to be obtained; information to be provided. Title 51. Public Welfare. 2006. Ohio Revised Code Ann.

68. *In re Guardianship of Willis*, 599 N.E.2d. 745 (Ohio 1991).

69. *Steele v. Hamilton County Community Mental Health Board*, 736 N.E.2d 10 (Ohio 2000).

70. Winick BJ. *The Right to Refuse Mental Health Treatment*. American Psychological Association; 1997.

71. Appelbaum PS. *Almost a Revolution: Mental Health Law and the Limits of Change*. Oxford University Press; 1994.

72. Schouten R, Gutheil TG. Aftermath of the Rogers decision: assessing the costs. *Am J Psychiatry*. 1990;147:1348–1352.

73. Strauss JL, Zervakis JB, Stechuchak KM, et al. Adverse impact of coercive treatments on inpatients' satisfaction with care. *Community Mental Health J*. 2013;49:457–465.

74. Roberts LW. Informed consent and the capacity for voluntarism. *Am J Psychiatry*. 2002;159:705–712.

75. Appelbaum PS. Missing the boat: competence and consent in psychiatric research. *Am J Psychiatry*. 1998;155:1486–1488.

76. Dunn LB, Palmer BW, Keehan M, et al. Assessment of therapeutic misconception in older schizophrenia patients with a brief instrument. *Am J Psychiatry*. 2006;163:500–506.

77. Dunn LB, Nowrangi MA, Palmer BW, et al. Assessing decisional capacity for clinical research or treatment: a review of instruments. *Am J Psychiatry*. 2006;163:1323–1334.

78. Lidz CW, Appelbaum PS. The therapeutic misconception: problems and solutions. *Med Care*. 2002;40:V55–V63.

79. Nishimura A, Crey J, Erwin PJ, et al. Improving understanding in the research informed consent process: a systematic review of 54 interventions tested in randomized control trials. *BMC Med Ethics*. 2013;14(28):1–15.

80. Lieberman JA, Roberts LW, Butterfield MI, et al. Ethical principles and practices for research involving human participants with mental illness. *Psychiatr Serv*. 2006;57:552–557.

81. Jeste DV, Palmer BW, Golshan S, et al. Multimedia consent for people with schizophrenia and normal subjects: a randomized controlled trial. *Schizophrenia Bull*. 2009;35(4):719–729.

82. Appelbaum PS. Involving decisionally impaired subjects in research: the need for legislation. *Am J Geriatr Psychiatry*. 2002;10:120–124.

83. Bloom JD. Thirty-five years of working with civil commitment statutes. *J Am Acad Psychiatry Law*. 2004;32:430–439.

84. Slovenko R. Civil commitment laws: an analysis and critique. *Cooley Law Rev*. 2000;17:25–51.

85. Pfeffer A. Note: "Imminent danger" and inconsistency: the need for national reform of the "imminent danger" standard for involuntary civil commitment in the wake of the Virginia Tech tragedy. *Cardozo Law Rev*. 2008;30:277–315.

86. Zonana H. The civil commitment of sex offenders. *Science*. 1997;278:1248–1249.

87. Alexander Jr. R. Civil commitment of sex offenders to mental institutions: should the standard be based on serious mental illness or mental disorder? *J Health Soc Policy*. 2000;11:67–78.

88. Connor JM. Note: Selig v. Young: constitutionally protected but unjust civil commitment for sexually violent predators. *J Contemp Health Law Policy*. 2002;18:511.

89. Grossman LS, Martis B, Fichtner CG. Are sex offenders treatable? A research overview. *Psychiatr Serv*. 1999;50:349–361.

90. *Kansas v. Hendricks*, 521 U.S. 346 (1997).

91. *Selig v. Young*, 531 U.S. 250 (2001).

92. *Kansas v. Crane*, 534 U.S. 407 (2002).

93. American Psychiatric Association. *Dangerous Offenders: A Task Force Report of the American Psychiatric Association*. American Psychiatric Association; 1999.

94. Fabian J. The Adam Walsh Child Protection and Safety Act: legal and psychological aspects of the new civil commitment law for federal sex offenders. *Cleve State Law Rev*. 2012;60(?):307–364.

95. Appelbaum PS. Thinking carefully about outpatient commitment. *Psychiatr Serv*. 2001;52:347–350.

96. Hoge MA, Grottole E. The case against outpatient commitment. *J Am Acad Psychiatry Law*. 2000;28:165–170.

97. Steadman HJ, Gounis K, Dennis D, et al. Assessing the New York City involuntary outpatient commitment pilot program. *Psychiatr Serv*. 2001;52:330–336.

98. Swartz MS, Swanson JW, Hiday VA, et al. A randomized controlled trial of outpatient commitment in North Carolina. *Psychiatr Serv*. 2001;52:325–329.

99. Hiday VA. Outpatient commitment: the state of empirical research on its outcomes. *Psychol Public Policy Law*. 2003;9:8–32.

100. Swartz MS, Swanson JW, Wagner HR, et al. Can involuntary outpatient commitment reduce hospital recidivism? Findings from a randomized trial with severely mentally ill individuals. *Am J Psychiatry*. 1999;56:1968–1975.

101. Swartz MS, Swanson JW. Economic grand rounds: can states implement involuntary outpatient commitment within existing state budgets? *Psychiatr Serv*. 2013;64(1):7–9.

102. Studdert DM, Mello MM, Brennan TA. Medical malpractice. *N Engl J Med*. 2004;350:283–292.

103. Darr K. The "new" medical malpractice crisis—part 1. *Hosp Top*. 2004;82:33–35.

104. Hoffman AC. Governmental studies on medical malpractice: the implications of rising premiums for healthcare and the allocation of health resources. *Med Law*. 2005;24:297–308.

105. Shah P, Shuren AW. The current medical malpractice environment: an analysis of causes and solutions. *J Pediatr Health Care*. 2005;19:112–116.

106. Hellinger FJ, Encinosa WE. The impact of state laws limiting malpractice damage awards on health expenditures. *Am J Public Health*. 2006;96:1375–1381.

107. Mello MM, Studdert DM, DesRoches CM, et al. Effects of a malpractice crisis on specialist supply and patient access to care. *Ann Surg*. 2005;242:621–628.

108. Localio AR, Lawthers AG, Brennan TA, et al. Relation between malpractice claims and adverse events due to negligence. Results of the Harvard Medical Practice Study III. *N Engl J Med*. 1991;325:245–251.

109. Studdert D, Thomas EJ, Burstin HR, et al. Negligent care and malpractice claiming behavior in Utah and Colorado. *Med Care*. 2000;38:250–260.

110. Harvard Medical Practice Study. *Patients, Doctors, and Lawyers: Medical Injury, Malpractice Litigation, and Patient Compensation in New York*. President and Fellows of Harvard University; 1990.

111. Studdert DM, Mello MM, Gawande AA, et al. Claims, errors, and compensation payments in medical malpractice litigation. *N Engl J Med*. 2006;354:2024–2033.

112. Thorpe KE. The medical malpractice "crisis": recent trends and the impact of state tort reforms. *Health Aff*. 2004;23:W20.

113. Kilgore ML, Morrisey MA, Nelson LJ. Tort law and medical malpractice insurance premiums. *Inquiry*. 2006;43:255–270.

114. Stewart RM, Geoghegan K, Myers JG, et al. Malpractice risk and cost are significantly reduced after tort reform. *J Am Coll Surg*. 2011;212(4):463–467, e42.

115. Paik M, Black BS, Hyman DA, et al. Will tort reform bend the cost curve? Evidence from Texas. *J Empir Leg Stud*. 2012;9(2):173–216.

116. Government Accounting Office. *Medical Malpractice Insurance: Multiple Factors Have Contributed to Increased Premium Rates*. Government Accounting Office; 2003.

117. Rodwin MA, Chang HJ, Clausen J. Marketwatch—malpractice premiums and physicians' income: perceptions of a crisis conflict with empirical evidence. *Health Aff.* 2006;25:750–758.

118. De Ville K. Medical malpractice in twentieth century United States. The interaction of technology, law and culture. *Int J Technol Assess Health Care.* 1998;14:197–211.

119. Regan J, Hamer G, Wright A, et al. Tort reform in medical malpractice. *Tenn Med.* 2004;97:322–323.

120. Gunnar WP. Is there an acceptable answer to rising medical malpractice premiums? *Ann Health Law.* 2004;13:465–500.

121. Shapiro RS, Simpson DE, Lawrence SL, et al. A survey of sued and nonsued physicians and suing patients. *Arch Intern Med.* 1989;149:2190–2196.

122. Charles SC. Coping with a medical malpractice suit. *West J Med.* 2001;174:55–58.

123. Charles SC. The psychological trauma of a medical malpractice suit: a practical guide. *Bull Am Coll Surg.* 1991;76:22–26.

124. Charles SC. Malpractice suits: their effect on doctors, patients, and families. *J Med Assoc Ga.* 1987;76:171–172.

125. Institute of Medicine. *Crossing the Quality Chasm: A New Health System for the Twenty-First Century.* National Academies Press; 2001.

126. Miller NP. An ancient law of care. *Whittier Law Rev.* 2004;26: 3–57.

127. Silver T. One hundred years of harmful error: the historical jurisprudence of medical malpractice. *Wis L Rev.* 1992;992: 1193–1241.

128. Goldberg JCP. Twentieth-century tort theory. *Georgetown Law J.* 2003;91:513–583.

129. Schwartz WB, Komesar NK. Doctors, damages, and deterrence: an economic view of medical malpractice. *N Engl J Med.* 1978;298:1282–1289.

130. Mello MM, Brennan TA. Deterrence of medical errors: theory and evidence for malpractice reform. *Tex Law Rev.* 2002;80: 1595–1637.

131. Rice WE. Insurance contracts and judicial discord over whether liability insurers must defend insureds' allegedly intentional and immoral conduct: a historical and empirical review of federal and state courts' declaratory judgments—1900–1997. *Am Univ Law Rev.* 1998;47:1131–1219.

132. Gittler GJ, Goldstein EJ. The elements of medical malpractice: an overview. *Clin Infect Dis.* 1996;23:1152–1155.

133. *Santos v. Kim,* 706 N.E.2d 658 (Mass. 1999).

134. Fox BC, Siegel ML, Weinstein RA. "Curbside" consultation and informal communication in medical practice: a medicolegal perspective. *Clin Infect Dis.* 1996;23:616–622.

135. Schouten R. Malpractice in medical-psychiatric practice. In: Stoudemire A, Fogel BS, eds. *Medical-Psychiatric Practice.* American Psychiatric Press; 1993.

136. Sederer L, Ellison J, Keyes C. Guidelines for prescribing psychiatrists in consultative, collaborative, and supervisory relationships. *Psychiatr Serv.* 1998;49:1197–1202.

137. Ginsberg B. Tarasoff at thirty: victim's knowledge shrinks the psychotherapist's duty to warn and protect. *J Contemp Health Law Policy.* 2004;21:1–35.

138. Kachigian C, Felthous AR. Court responses to Tarasoff statutes. *J Am Acad Psychiatry Law.* 2004;32:263–273.

139. Tracy TF, Crawford LS, Krizek TJ, et al. When medical error becomes medical malpractice: the victims and the circumstances. *Arch Surg.* 2003;138:447–454.

140. *Dolan v. Galluzo,* 379 N.E.2d 795 (Ill. Ct. App. 1978), aff'd 396 N.E.2d 13 (Ill. 1979).

141. Waltz JR. The rise and gradual fall of the locality rule in medical malpractice litigation. *DePaul L Rev.* 1969;18:408.

142. Pruitt LR. Rural rhetoric. *Conn Law Rev.* 2006;39:159–240.

143. King JH. The standard of care for residents and other medical school graduates in training. *Am Univ Law Rev.* 2006;55:683–751.

144. *Monahan v. Weichert,* 82 A.2d 102 (NY Ct. App. 1981).

145. Young R, Faure M, Fenn P. Causality and causation in tort law. *Int Rev Law Econ.* 2004;24:507–523.

146. Short DE, Avgeropoulos P, DuMoulin FM. What are the odds? Evaluating loss of chance in medical negligence cases. *Health Law Can.* 2005;26:16–19.

147. Hayes M, Schwerin M. Recent developments in "loss of chance. *J Health Hosp Law.* 1995;28:173–177. 181.

148. Garwin MJ. Risk creation, loss of chance, and legal liability. *Hematol Oncol Clin North Am.* 2002;16:1351–1363.

149. *Dumas v. Cooney,* 235 Cal. App. 3d 1593 (Ca. Ct. App. 1991).

150. Walker VR. Restoring the individual plaintiff to tort law by rejecting "junk logic" about specific causation. *Ala Law Rev.* 2007; 56:381–481.

151. Petrilli L. Lost chance in Illinois? That may still be the case. *John Marshall Law Rev.* 2002;36:249–270.

152. Avraham R. Putting a price on pain-and-suffering damages: a critique of the current approaches and a preliminary proposal for change. *Northwest Univ Law Rev.* 2006;100:87–119.

153. Costello M. Compensating medical injury victims in the United States: there must be a better way. *Hosp Top.* 2005;83:9–12.

154. Schouten R. Compensation for victims of trauma in the United States. *Seishin Shinkeigaku Zasshi.* 2002;104:1186–1197.

155. Zipursky BC. A theory of punitive damages. *Tex Law Rev.* 2005; 84:105–171.

156. Gutheil TG, Appelbaum PS. *Clinical Handbook of Psychiatry and the Law.* 4th ed. Lippincott Williams & Wilkins; 2006.

157. Lewin JL. The genesis and evolution of legal uncertainty about "reasonable medical certainty". *Univ Md Law Rev.* 1998;57: 380–502.

158. Schouten R. Legal liability and managed care. *Harv Rev Psychiatry.* 1993;1:189–190.

159. Stone AA. Managed care, liability, and ERISA. *Psychiatr Clin North Am.* 1999;22:17–29.

160. Employee Retirement Income Security Act of 1974. 29 U.S.C.S. Sec. 1101 et seq. (1974).

161. *Aetna Health, Inc. v. Davila,* 542 U.S. 200 (2004).

162. *Rush Prudential HMO, Inc. v. Moran,* 536 U.S. 355 (2002).

163. Record KL. Wielding the wand without facing the music: allowing utilization review physicians to trump doctors' orders, but protecting them from the legal risk ordinarily attached to the medical degree. *Duke Law J.* 2010;59:955–1000.

164. *Harnish v. Children's Hosp. Medical Center,* 439 N.E.2d 240 (Mass. 1982).

165. Goldberg JCP, Zipursky BC. Unrealized torts. *Va Law Rev.* 2002; 88:1625–1719.

166. Erickson K. Constitutional law: use of force by mental health workers violated due process. *J Law Med Ethics.* 2002;30: 114–116.

167. Schouten R, Brendel RW. Legal aspects of consultation. In: Stern TA, Fricchione GL, Cassem EH, eds. *The Massachusetts General Hospital Handbook of General Hospital Psychiatry.* 5th ed. Mosby; 2004.

168. Reeves RR, Pinkofsky HB, Stevens L. Medicolegal errors in the ED related to the involuntary confinement of psychiatric patients. *Am J Emerg Med.* 1998;16:631–633.

169. Knapp S, VandeCreek L. A review of tort liability in involuntary civil commitment. *Hosp Community Psychiatry.* 1987;38: 648–651.

170. Shanaberger CJ. Escaping the charge of false imprisonment. *JEMS.* 1990;15:58–61.

171. Kachalia A, Gandhi TK, Puopolo AL, et al. Missed and delayed diagnoses in the emergency department: a study of closed malpractice claims from 4 liability insurers. *Ann Emerg Med.* 2007;49:196–205.

172. Schouten R, Cohen MH. Legal issues in integration of complementary therapies into cardiology practice. In: Frishman WH, Weintraub MI, Micozzi MS, eds. *Complementary and Integrative Therapies for Cardiovascular Disease.* Mosby; 2004.

173. Cohen MH, Schouten R. Legal, regulatory, and ethical issues. In: Lake JH, Spiegel D, eds. *Complementary and Alternative Treatments in Mental Health Care.* American Psychiatric Press; 2006.

174. Lake JH, Spiegel D, eds. *Complementary and Alternative Treatments in Mental Health Care.* American Psychiatric Press; 2006.

175. Clouser KD, Hufford DJ, O'Connor BB. Informed consent and alternative medicine. *Altern Ther Health Med.* 1996;2:76–78.

176. Cohen MH. Malpractice and vicarious liability for providers of complementary and alternative medicine. *Benders Health Care Law Mon.* 1996:3–13.

177. Klerman GL. The psychiatric patient's right to effective treatment: implications of Osheroff v. Chestnut Lodge. *Am J Psychiatry.* 1990;147:409–418.

178. Stone AA. Law, science, and psychiatric malpractice: a response to Klerman's indictment of psychoanalytic psychiatry. *Am J Psychiatry.* 1990;147:419–427.

179. *Bragdon v. Abbott,* 524 U.S. 624 (1998).

180. Emanuel EJ. Do physicians have an obligation to treat patients with AIDS? *N Engl J Med.* 1988;318:1686–1690.
181. Simon RI. *Clinical Psychiatry and the Law.* 2nd ed. American Psychiatric Association Press; 1992.
182. Regan JJ, Regan WM. Medical malpractice and respondeat superior. *South Med J.* 2002;95:545–548.
183. Kachalia A, Studdert DM. Professional liability issues in graduate medical education. *JAMA.* 2004;292:1051–1056.
184. Ingram JD. Vicarious liability of the employer of an apparent servant. *Tort Trial Insur Pract Law J.* 2005;41:1–20.
185. Jorgenson LM, Sutherlan PK, Bisbing SB. Transference of liability: employer liability for sexual misconduct by therapists. *Brooklyn Law Rev.* 1995;60:1421–1481.
186. *St. Germain v. Pfeifer, et al,* 637 N.E.2d 848 (1994)
187. Recupero PR, Rainey SE. Liability and risk management in outpatient psychotherapy supervision. *J Am Acad Psychiatry Law.* 2007; 35(3):188–195.
188. Council on Ethical and Judicial Affairs, American Medical Association. *Code of Medical Ethics.* American Medical Association; 1997.
189. American Psychiatric Association. The principles of medical ethics with annotations especially applicable to psychiatry. 2001. Accessed August 14, 2023. https://psychiatry.org
190. *Doe v. Roe & Poe,* 400 N.Y. Supp. 513 (Sup. Ct. N.Y. Co. 1977).
191. *Alberts v. Devine,* 479 N.E.2d 113 (1985).
192. American Psychiatric Association. *Position Statement on Confidentiality.* American Psychiatric Association; 1978.
193. Schouten R. Legal responsibilities with child abuse and domestic violence. In: Jacobson JL, Jacobson AM, eds. *Psychiatric Secrets.* Hanley & Belfus; 2001.
194. Almason AL. Personal liability implications of the duty to warn are hard pills to swallow: from Tarasoff to Hutchinson v. Patel and beyond. *J Contemp Health Law Policy.* 1997;13:471–496.
195. *Tarasoff v. Board of Regents of the University of California,* 17 Cal. App. 3d 425 (1976).
196. Zinn C. Wife wins case against GPs who did not disclose husband's HIV status. *BMJ.* 2003;326:1286.
197. Liang BA. Medical information, confidentiality, and privacy. *Hematol Oncol Clin North Am.* 2002;16:1433.
198. *Bradshaw v. Daniel,* 854 S.W.2d 865 (Tenn. 1993).
199. Closen ML, Isaacman SH. The duty to notify private third parties of the risks of HIV infection. *J Health Hosp Law.* 1988; 21:295–303.
200. Texas court says clinic had no duty to warn spouse about HIV. *AIDS Policy Law.* 1998;13(1):8.
201. Chenneville T. HIV, confidentiality, and duty to protect. *Prof Psychol Res Pr.* 2000;31(6):661–670.
202. Appelbaum PS, Zonana H, Bonnie R, et al. Statutory approaches to limiting psychiatrists' liability for their patients' violent acts. *Am J Psychiatry.* 1989;146:821–828.
203. Soulier MF, Maislen A, Beck JC. Status of the psychiatric duty to protect, circa 2006. *J Am Acad Psychiatry Law.* 2010;38(4):457–473.
204. Beck JC. Legal and ethical duties of the clinician treating a patient who is liable to be impulsively violent. *Behav Sci Law.* 1998;16:375–389.
205. Annotated Laws of Massachusetts. Part III. *Courts, Judicial Officers and Proceedings in Civil Cases.* Title II. Actions and proceedings therein. Chapter 233. Witnesses and evidence. § 20B. Privileged communications between patients and psychotherapists; communications to which privilege does not apply, etc. 2007.
206. Health Insurance Portability and Accountability Act of 1996. *Public Law* 1996;104-191.
207. Brendel RW, Bryan E. HIPAA for psychiatrists. *Harv Rev Psychiatry.* 2004;12:177–183.
208. Feld AD. The Health Insurance Portability and Accountability Act (HIPAA): its broad effect on practice. *Am J Gastroenterol.* 2005;100:1440–1443.
209. HIPAA Privacy Rule, 45 C.F.R. Sec. 2001;164:512.
210. Schouten R, Brendel RW. Common pitfalls in giving medical legal advice to trainees and supervisees. *Harv Rev Psychiatry.* 2009;7(4):291–294.
211. Cogan Jr JA. First-ever HIPAA conviction highlights differing views of HIPAA's civil and criminal penalties. *Med Health R I.* 2005;88:33–34.
212. Mermelstein HT, Wallack JJ. Confidentiality in the age of HIPAA: a challenge for psychosomatic medicine. *Psychosomatics.* 2008;49(2):97–103.
213. Glosoff HL, Herlihy B, Herlihy SB, et al. Privileged communication in the psychologist-client relationship. *Prof Psychol Res Pr.* 1997;28:573–581.
214. Schouten R. The psychotherapist-patient privilege. *Harv Rev Psychiatry.* 1998;6:44–48.
215. Ruebner R, Reis LA. Hippocrates to HIPAA: a foundation for a federal physician-patient privilege. *Temple Law Rev.* 2004;77: 505–575.
216. *Commonwealth v. Kobrin,* 479 N.E.2d 674 (Mass. 1985).
217. New York Civil Practice Law and Rules. Article 45. Evidence, § 4504. Physician, dentist, podiatrist, chiropractor and nurse. NY CLS CPLR, § 4504. New York Consolidated Laws Service. 2007.
218. *United States v. Chase,* 301 F.3d 1019 (9th Cir. 2002).
219. Weinstock R, Leong GB, Silva JA. Potential erosion of psychotherapist-patient privilege beyond California: dangers of "criminalizing" Tarasoff. *Behav Sci Law.* 2001;19:437–449.
220. Klinker E. It's been a privilege: advising patients of the Tarasoff duty and its legal consequences for the federal psychotherapist-patient privilege. *Fordham Law Rev.* 2009;78(2):863–891.
221. Puglise SM. "Calling Dr. Love": The physician-patient sexual relationship as grounds for medical malpractice—society pays while the doctor and patient play. *J Law Health.* 2000;14:321–350.
222. Morrison J, Morrison T. Psychiatrists disciplined by a state medical board. *Am J Psychiatry.* 2001;158:474–478.
223. Schouten R. Maintaining boundaries in the doctor-patient relationship. In: Stern TA, Herman JB, Slavin PL, eds. *The MGH Guide to Primary Care Psychiatry.* 2nd ed. McGraw-Hill; 2004.
224. Gutheil TG, Gabbard GO. The concept of boundaries in clinical practice: theoretical and risk-management dimensions. *Am J Psychiatry.* 1993;150:188–196.
225. Waldinger RJ. Boundary crossings and boundary violations: thoughts on navigating a slippery slope. *Harv Rev Psychiatry.* 1994;2:225–227.
226. Strasburger LH, Jorgenson L, Sutherland P. The prevention of psychotherapist sexual misconduct: avoiding the slippery slope. *Am J Psychother.* 1992;46:544–555.
227. Glass LL. The gray areas of boundary crossings and violations. *Am J Psychother.* 2003;57:429–444.
228. Kroll J. Boundary violations: a culture-bound syndrome. *J Am Acad Psychiatry Law.* 2001;29:274–283.
229. Hundert EM. Looking a gift horse in the mouth: the ethics of gift-giving in psychiatry. *Harv Rev Psychiatry.* 1998;6:114–117.
230. Simon RI. Therapist-patient sex: from boundary violations to sexual misconduct. *Psychiatr Clin North Am.* 1999;22:31.
231. It's the law. Psychiatr News. 2002. https://psychnews.psychiatry-online.org/doi/full/10.1176/pn.37.6.0018a.
232. Thomas CR, Pastusek A. Boundary crossings and violations: time for child and adolescent psychiatry to catch up. *J Am Acad Child Adolesc Psychiatry.* 2012;51(9):858–860.
233. Jain S, Roberts LW. Ethics in psychotherapy: a focus on professional boundaries and confidentiality practices. *Psychiatr Clin North Am.* 2009;32:299–314.
234. Rice WE. Insurance contracts and judicial discord over whether liability insurers must defend insureds' allegedly intentional and immoral conduct: a historical and empirical review of federal and state courts' declaratory judgments—1900-1997. *Am Univ Law Rev.* 1998;47:1131–1219.
235. Rokosz GJ. Princeton Insurance Co. v. Chunmuang—does the court's result signal a need for legislative reform broadening malpractice insurance coverage for the benefit of victims of physician sexual abuse? *Seton Hall Law Rev.* 1999;30:133–173.
236. Ambady N, Laplante D, Nguyen T, et al. Surgeons' tone of voice: a clue to malpractice history. *Surgery.* 2002;132:5–9.
237. Barrier PA, Li JT, Jensen NM. Two words to improve physician-patient communication: what else? *Mayo Clin Proc.* 2003;78: 211–214.
238. Hickson GB, Clayton EW, Githens PB, et al. Factors that prompted families to file medical malpractice claims following perinatal injuries. *JAMA.* 1992;267:1359–1363.
239. Levinson W. Physician-patient communication. A key to malpractice prevention. *JAMA.* 1994;272:1619–1620.

240. Levinson W, Roter DL, Mullooly JP, et al. Physician-patient communication. The relationship with malpractice claims among primary care physicians and surgeons. *JAMA*. 1997;277: 553–559.

241. Peskin T, Micklitsch C, Quirk M, et al. Malpractice, patient satisfaction, and physician-patient communication. *JAMA*. 1995; 274:22.

242. Gutheil TG, Bursztajn H, Brodsky A. Malpractice prevention through the sharing of uncertainty. Informed consent and the therapeutic alliance. *N Engl J Med*. 1984;311:49–51.

243. Wu AW, Huang IC, Stokes S, et al. Disclosing medical errors to patients: it's not what you say, it's what they hear. *J Gen Intern Med*. 2009;24(9):1012–1017.

244. Ho B, Liu E. Does sorry work? The impact of apology laws on medical malpractice. *J Risk Uncertain*. 2011;43:141–167.

245. Liang BA. A system of medical error disclosure. *Qual Saf Health Care*. 2002;11:64–68.

246. Ho B, Liu E. What's an apology worth? Decomposing the effect of apologies on medical malpractice payments using state apology laws. *J Empir Leg Stud*. 2011;8(S1):179–199.

247. Wagner P. Statements of apology—a matter of ethics. *S D Med*. 2006;59:437–438.

248. Zimmerman R. Doctors' new tool to fight lawsuits: saying "I'm sorry." Malpractice insurers find owning up to errors soothes patient anger. "The risks are extraordinary". *J Okla State Med Assoc*. 2004;97:245–247.

249. Gutheil TG. Boundary issues and personality disorders. *J Psychiatr Pract*. 2005;11:88–96.

250. Finkel NJ, Slobogin C. Insanity, justification, and culpability toward a unifying schema. *Law Hum Behav*. 1995;19:447–464.

251. Walker N. *Crime and insanity in England*. Edinburgh: University of Edinburgh Press; 1968.

252. Blackstone W. *Blackstone's commentaries on the laws of England. Book the fourth—chapter the twenty-fifth: of arraignments, and its incidents*. 1765. Accessed August 14, 2023. https://avalon.law. yale.edu/subject_menus/blackstone.asp

253. McKenzie A. "This death some strong and stout hearted man doth choose": the practice of peine forte et dure in seventeenth- and eighteenth-century England. *Law Hist Rev*. 2005;23: 279–313.

254. Note: Incompetency to stand trial. *Harvard Law Rev*. 2007;81:455.

255. *Drope v. Missouri*, 420 U.S. 162 (1975).

256. *Dusky v. United States*, 362 U.S. 402 (1960).

257. *Cooper v. Oklahoma*, 517 U.S. 348 (1996).

258. *Godinez v. Moran*, 509 U.S. 389 (1993).

259. *Wieter v. Settle*, 93 F.Supp. 318 (WD MO 1961).

260. Lipsitt PD, Lelos D, McGarry AL. Competency for trial: a screening instrument. *Am J Psychiatry*. 1977;128:105–109.

261. Grisso T. *Evaluating Competencies: Forensic Assessments and Instruments*. Plenum Press; 1986.

262. Hoge SK, Poythress NG, Bonnie RJ, et al. The MacArthur adjudicative competence study: diagnosis, psychopathology, and competence-related abilities. *Behav Sci Law*. 1997;15:329–345.

263. *Pate v. Robinson*, 383 U.S. 375 (1966).

264. *U.S. v. Huguenin*, 950 F.2d 23 (1st Cir.1991).

265. Wall BW, Krupp BH, Guilmette T. Restoration of competency to stand trial: a training program for persons with mental retardation. *J Am Acad Psychiatry Law*. 2003;31:189–201.

266. Schouten R. Commentary: training for competence—form or substance? *J Am Acad Psychiatry Law*. 2003;31:202–204.

267. *Jackson v. Indiana*, 406 U.S. 715 (1972).

268. *United States v. Charters*, 863 F.2d 302 (4th Cir. 1988).

269. *Riggins v. Nevada*, 504 U.S. 127 (1992).

270. *Washington v. Harper*, 494 U.S. 210 (1990).

271. *Sell v. United States*, 539 U.S. 166 (2003).

272. *United States v. Loughner*, 672 F.3d 731 (9th. Cir. 2012).

273. *Rivers v. Katz*, 495 N.E.2d 337 (N.Y. 1986).

274. *Sieling v. Eyman*, 478 F.2d 211214 (9th Cir. 1973).

275. *Westbrook v. Arizona*, 384 U.S. 150 (1966).

276. *Edwards v. Indiana*, 554 U.S. 164 (2008).

277. *Ford v. Wainwright*, 477 U.S. 399 (1986).

278. *Penry v Lynaugh*, 492 U.S. 302 (1989).

279. *Atkins v. Virginia*, 536 U.S. 304 (2002).

280. *Roper v. Simmons*, 543 U.S. 551 (2005).

281. Gutheil TG. Ethics and forensic psychiatry. In: Bloch S, Chodoff P, Green SA, eds. *Psychiatric Ethics*. 3rd ed. Oxford University Press; 2007.

282. American Academy of Psychiatry and the Law. *Ethics Guidelines for the Practice of Forensic Psychiatry*. American Academy of Psychiatry and the Law; 2006.

283. *Estelle v. Smith*, 541 U.S. 454 (1982).

284. *Barefoot v. Estelle*, 463 U.S. 880 (1983).

285. *Perry v. Louisiana*, 498 U.S. 38 (1990).

286. *State v. Perry*, 610 So.2d 746 (La. 1992).

287. LaFave WR, Scott AW. Responsibility. In: *Criminal Law*. 2nd ed. West Publishing Co; 1986.

288. Glueck SS. *Mental Disorder and the Criminal Law*. Little, Brown; 1925.

289. Moore MS. *Law and Psychiatry: Rethinking the Relationship*. Cambridge University Press; 1984.

290. Finkel NJ. *Insanity on Trial*. Plenum Press; 1988.

291. Finkel NJ, Parrott WG. *Emotions and Culpability*. American Psychological Association; 2006.

292. Robinson DN. Wild beasts and idle humours: the insanity defense from antiquity to the present. *J Forensic Psychiatry*. 1997;8:465–467.

293. Robinson DN. *Wild Beasts and Idle Humours*. Harvard University Press; 1996.

294. Moran R. *Knowing Right from Wrong: The Insanity Defense of Daniel McNaughtan*. Free Press; 1981.

295. Low PW, Jeffries JC, Bonnie RJ. *The Trial of John W. Hinckley, Jr*. Foundation Press; 1986.

296. American Law Institute. *Model Penal Code*. American Law Institute; 1962.

297. Buchanan A. *Psychiatric Aspects of Justification, Excuse and Mitigation in Anglo-American Criminal Law*. Jessica Kingsley Publishers; 2000.

298. Huigens K. Commentary: duress is not a justification. *Ohio State Criminal Law J*. 2004;2:303–314.

299. New York Penal Law. Title H Offenses against the person involving physical injury, sexual conduct, restraint and intimidation, 120.00. 2005. Chapter 40 of the *Consolidated Law*, part 3—specific offenses.

300. Kirschner SM, Galperin GJ. The defense of extreme emotional disturbance in New York County: pleas and outcomes. *Behav Sci Law*. 2002;20:47–50.

301. *Robinson v. California*, 370 U.S. 660 (1962).

302. *Powell v. Texas*, 392 U.S. 514 (1968).

303. Moran R. The modern foundation for the insanity defense—the cases of Hadfield, James (1800) and McNaughtan, Daniel (1843) *Ann Am Acad Pol Soc Sci*. 477198531–42.

304. Eigen JP. *Unconscious Crime: Mental Absence and Criminal Responsibility in Victorian London*. Johns Hopkins University Press; 2003.

305. Horn M. Note: a rude awakening: what to do with the sleepwalking defense? *Boston College Law Rev*. 2004;46:149–182.

306. Smythe J. Uninvited guests crash a party of one: multiple personality disorder and the criminal law's derision toward multiples. *J Law Society*. 2005;6:179–207.

307. Marlowe DB, Lambert JB, Thompson RG. Voluntary intoxication and criminal responsibility. *Behav Sci Law*. 1999;17: 195–217.

308. Perr IN. Alleged brain-damage, diminished capacity, mens-rea, and misuse of medical concepts. *J Forensic Sci*. 1991;36: 722–727.

309. Weinstock R, Leong GB, Silva JA. California's diminished capacity defense: evolution and transformation. *Bull Am Acad Psychiatry Law*. 1996;24:347–366.

310. *Rex v. Arnold*, 16 State Trials 695 (1724).

311. *Rex v. Hadfield*, 27 State Trials 1281 (1800).

312. *Regina v. M'Naghten*, 4 State Trials 847 (1843).

313. *M'Naghten's case*, 8 Eng. Reports 718 (1843).

314. Steadman HJ, McGreevy MA, Morrissey JP, et al. *Before and After Hinckley: Evaluating Insanity Defense Reform*. Guilford Press; 1993.

315. *Insanity Defense Reform Act of 1984*, 18 U.S.C. 402 (1984).

316. Melton GB, Petrila J, Poythress NG, et al. *Mental state at the time of the offense. Psychological Evaluations for the Courts*. Guilford Press; 2007.

317. Callahan LA, Robbins PC, Steadman HJ, et al. The hidden effects of Montana abolition of the insanity defense. *Psychiatr Q.* 1995;66:103–117.

318. Steadman HJ, Callahan LA, Robbins PC, et al. Maintenance of an insanity defense under Montana abolition of the insanity defense. *Am J Psychiatry.* 1989;146:357–360.

319. Finkel NJ, Shaw R, Bercaw S, et al. Insanity defenses: from the jurors' perspective. *Law Psychol Rev.* 1985;9:77–92.

320. Finkel NJ, Handel SF. Jurors and insanity: do test instructions instruct? *Forensic Rep.* 1988;1:65–79.

321. *Jones v. United States,* 463 U.S. 77 (1983).

Index

Page numbers followed by *f* indicate figures; *t*, tables, *b*, boxes.

A

Abandonment, 229
ABCB1 gene, 35
Ablative limbic system surgery, 216–217, 217*f*
Abnormal movements, patients with, 100–108
  drug-induced movement disorders, 104–106
   acute dystonic reactions, 104–105
   akathisia, 105
   antipsychotic-induced extrapyramidal symptoms, 104, 104*f*
   drug-induced tremors, 104
   parkinsonism, 105
   tardive dyskinesia, 105–106, 106*f*
  functional movement disorders, 106–107
  idiopathic movement disorders, 101–103
   Huntington disease, 102–103, 102*t*
   Parkinson disease, 101–102
   Restless legs syndrome, 103
   Tourette syndrome, 103
   Wilson disease, 103
  overview, 100–101
  patient history and physical examination for, 100–101
  tremors, 103–104
Abstraction, for patients with dementia, 163*t*
Acamprosate
  for alcohol use disorders, 185, 185*t*
  side effects of, 142
Acetylcholine (ACh), 15–17, 17*f*
  and Alzheimer disease, 167
Acetylcholinesterase inhibitors, for Alzheimer disease, 167*t*
ACh. *See* Acetylcholine (ACh)
Acute alcohol intoxication, 186
Acute bipolar disorder, lithium for, 44–45
Acute dystonia, 137*b*
Acute dystonic reactions, 104–105
Acute mania
  divalproex sodium for, 52
  lithium in, 44
Acute pain, 111
AD. *See* Alzheimer disease (AD)
Addiction, compulsion due to, 236
Adequate antidepressant treatment, 38–39
ADHD. *See* Attention-deficit/hyperactivity disorder (ADHD)
Adjustment disorders, with depressed mood, 114
Aducanumab (Aduhelm), for Alzheimer disease, 167
AEDs. *See* Antiepileptic drugs (AEDs)
Aggression and violence, attention-deficit/hyperactivity disorder pharmacotherapy, 72–73
Agoraphobia, pharmacotherapy for, 60–62
Agranulocytosis
  clozapine-induced, 93, 93*b*

Agranulocytosis *(Continued)*
  monitoring for, 93*b*
  risk of, 151
Akathisia, 90, 105, 137*b*
Alcohol
  and benzodiazepines, 62, 64
  and selective norepinephrine reuptake inhibitors (SNRIs), 64
  and selective serotonin reuptake inhibitors (SSRIs), 64
  sexual dysfunctions and, 202*t*
Alcohol abuse and dependence, lithium for, 47
Alcohol intoxication, 180, 186
Alcohol use disorders (AUDs), 179–189, 179*f*
  classifications of, 181–182
  and co-occurring psychiatric illness, 181
  epidemiology of, 180–181
  etiology of, 180–181
  overview of, 179–180
  pathophysiology of, 180
  screening and assessment for, 182–183, 182*f*, 183*t*
  treatment for, 183–189
   acute alcohol intoxication, 186, 187*f*
   alcohol withdrawal syndrome, 186–187
   brief counseling interventions for, 183–184
   fetal alcohol spectrum disorder, 189, 189*f*
   intensive interventions for, 184–185
   long-term supports for, 185, 186*f*
   motivational interviewing, 184, 184*t*
   pharmacological interventions for, 185, 185*t*
   Wernicke-Korsakoff syndrome, 188–189, 188*f*
  typologies of, 181–182
Alcohol withdrawal delirium, 187–188
  incidence of, 187
  treatment of, 187
Alcohol withdrawal syndrome, 186–187
  symptoms of, 186–187
  treatment of, 187
Alpha$_2$-adrenergic receptor antagonist, 31*t*, 34–35
Alprazolam, 62
  sexual dysfunctions and, 202*t*
Alzheimer's Association, 166
Alzheimer disease (AD), 164–169
  anti-amyloid monoclonal antibodies, 167
   safety of, 167
  clinical features of, 165–166
  description of, 164
  diagnosis of, 165–166, 166*f*
  differential diagnosis of, 166
  early-onset, 165
  epidemiology of, 164
  familial heritability of, 165
  genetics of, 165
  late-onset, 165

Alzheimer disease (AD) *(Continued)*
  long-term care for, 168
  medications for, 71–72
  pathophysiology of, 164–165, 165*f*
  prognosis of, 169
  supportive care for, 168
  treatments for, 166–168, 167*t*
   conventional, 167
   neuropsychiatric symptoms, 168
Amiloride, 48
Amphetamines
  for attention-deficit/hyperactivity disorder, 68
  use disorder, 191
   treatment of, intoxication and withdrawal, 191
Amyloid-related imaging abnormalities (ARIAs), 167
Analgesia
  independent, 113
  multi-modal, general principles of, 115–119
Analgesic pain pathway, 110
Anglo-American law, insanity defense in, 237
Animal experiments, psychiatric neuroscience and, 4
Antacids, drug interactions, 151*t*
Anti-amyloid monoclonal antibodies, 167
  for Alzheimer disease, 167*t*
  safety of, 167
Anti-anxiety agents, side effects of, 140–141
Anticholinergics
  drug interactions, 151*t*
  side effects of, 142
Anticonvulsants, 61*t*, 62
  for bipolar disorder, 52, 57*t*
  for generalized anxiety disorder, 62
  for panic disorders, 61
  sexual dysfunctions and, 202*t*
Antidepressants, 130–132
  alpha$_2$-adrenergic receptor antagonist, 34–35
  anxiety, 115
  atypical, sedative effects of, 151
  available preparations for, 30*t*, 31*t*
  bupropion, 33
  buspirone, 34
  choice of, 28–38
  clinical uses of, 28
  continuation treatment, 28
  desvenlafaxine, 32
  drug-drug interactions, 154–158, 155*t*
  duloxetine, 32–33
  electroconvulsive therapy, 213
  for generalized anxiety disorder, 62
  indications for, 28*b*
  levomilnacipran and milnacipran, 33
  maintenance of, 28
  for MDD, 114
  mechanisms of action, 27
  mirtazapine, 34

Hamilton Depression Rating Scale (HDRS)
  scores, 53
Hammond, William, 43
Headaches, 118
Health Insurance Portability and
  Accountability Act of 1996 (HIPAA),
  230
Heavy metal screening, for Wilson disease/
  autoimmune disease, 164t
Hepatic metabolism
  and antipsychotic drugs, 97–98
  drugs used, 148t
Hepatic microsomal enzymes, synthesis or
  activity of, 148–149
Histamine, 17
HIV testing, for dementia, 164t
Human genetics, 4
Huntington disease (HD), 102–103, 102t
Hydration status, and lithium, 44
Hydromorphone, potencies and special
  features of, 117t
9-Hydroxyrisperidone, 94
Hyperadrenergic crises, 133
Hyperprolactinemia, and risperidone, 94
Hypoactive sexual desire disorder, 203
Hypoglycemia, 157
Hypothalamus, 6, 7f
Hypothyroidism, from lithium, 48

I

Iatrogenic adverse events, 216
Iatrogenic movement disorders, 104
Ibuprofen, properties of, 115t
Idiopathic movement disorders, 101–103
  Huntington disease, 102–103, 102t
  Parkinson disease, 101–102
  Restless legs syndrome, 103
  Tourette syndrome, 103
  Wilson disease, 103
Idiopathic pain, 111
Ignorance of crime, 236
Iloperidone, 96, 136t
  side effects, 138
Imipramine, 31t, 86
  for generalized anxiety disorder, 62
  for panic disorder, 60
  sexual dysfunctions and, 202t
Incompetent to stand trial (IST), 234
Increased intracranial pressure (ICP), 212–213
Independent analgesia, 113
Indomethacin, properties of, 115t
Informed consent
  decision-making capacity in, 222b
  elements of, 221b
  information about, 221b
  legal cases and psychiatry, 220–223
Inositol, 80
  recycling of, and lithium, 43
Insanity acquittees, question of disposition
  for, 238
Insanity defense, 236
  in Anglo-American law, 237
Insanity defense, history of, 235
Insomnia, natural medications for, 80–82,
  81t
Insulin, resistance to, and atypical
  antipsychotics, 95
Intentional tort, 227
Intention tremor, 103
Inter-individual variability, factors
  contributing to, in drug response,
  146f
International Working Group, 166
Interpersonal psychotherapy (IPT), for
  depression during pregnancy, 122

Involuntary treatment vs. involuntary
  confinement, in law and psychiatry,
  224
Isocarboxazid, 31t

J

Jackson v. Indiana, 234
Janssen, Paul, 86
Justification defenses, 236

K

Kansas v. Crane, 226
Kansas v. Hendricks, 226
Kava, 81–82
  for generalized anxiety disorder, 63
Ketamine, 40, 159
  as dissociative anesthetic, 191
  side effects of, 143
Ketoprofen, properties of, 115t
Ketorolac, properties of, 115–116, 115t
Kinesiophobia, 114–115
Knowledge, treatment adherence, 22
Korsakoff's psychosis, 188–189

L

Lamotrigine
  for bipolar disorder, 53–54
  dosing of, 123
  drug interactions, 154
  exposure in nursing infant, 128
  for pregnant women with BPD, 123
  side effects of, 135
Language test, for patients with dementia,
  163t
Late-onset AD, 165
Lavender, 81
Law and psychiatry, 219–244
  basic concepts, 220
  boundary violations, 231–232
  civil commitment, 225–226
    of sex offenders, 226
  competency
    to be executed, 235
    to plead, decline counsel, and represent
      oneself, 234
  consent to participate in research, 225
  criminal competencies in, 232–234
  criminal responsibility, 235–238
    evaluations of, 238
    lack of, 236–238
  description of, 219–220
  excuse defenses, 236
  HIPAA for, 230
  informed consent, 220–223
  involuntary treatment vs. involuntary
    confinement, 224
  justification defenses, 236
  liability
    for the acts of others, 229
    and managed care, 228
  liability risk in, 228–231
    abandonment, 229
    assault, 228–229
    battery, 228–229
    confidentiality and privilege, 229–231
    failure to treat, 229
    false imprisonment, 228–229
    HIPAA and, 230
    misdiagnosis, 229
    psychotherapist–patient privilege,
      231
    suicide and, 231
  malpractice liability, 227–228

Law and psychiatry (Continued)
  managed care and liability, 228
  medical liability climate, 226–227
  outpatient commitment, 226
  reducing malpractice risk, 232
  standards of proof, 220b
  treatment
    refusal, 223–225
    risk/benefit ratio of, 223t
Lean body mass, and lithium, 43
Lecanemab (Leqembi), for Alzheimer
  disease, 167
Lesion studies, 2
Lethal catatonia, 91–92
Levetiracetam, 56
  for social anxiety disorder, 64
Levomilnacipran, 33
  side effects of, 132
Levorphanol, potencies and special features
  of, 117t
Lewy body dementia, 169–170, 169f, 170f
Liability and managed care, 228
Liability for the acts of others, 229
Liability risk in psychiatry, 228–231
Lieberman, Jeffrey, 86
Lipophilic drug interactions, 151t
Lithium, 39, 159
  for bipolar disorder
    acute, 44–45
    for maintenance treatment and relapse
      prevention, 45
    pediatric, 46–47
    rapid-cycling, 45
  in children and adolescents, 46–47
  discontinuation, 46
  drug interactions, 150, 151t, 152–153,
    152t
  evidence for efficacy of, 44–47
  historical context, 43
  mechanism of action, 43
  pharmacokinetics and
    pharmacodynamics, 43–44
  in psychiatry, 43–51
    for acute mania, 44
    adverse effects of, 49
    for alcohol dependence, 47
    and antipsychotics, 44
    augmentation of antidepressants, in
      treatment-refractory major depressive
      disorder, 47
    BALANCE trial in, 45
    for conduct disorder, 47
    current controversies and future
      directions, 49–50
    dosing of, 48
    drug interactions with, 48, 48t
    laboratory monitoring, 48
    for major depressive disorder, relapse
      prevention in, 47
    as monotherapy, 47
    other uses of, 47
    in pregnancy and breast-feeding, 49
    for psychotic disorder, 47
    response predictors, 47–48
    toxicity
      management of, 49b
      signs of, 49b
    treatment principles, 47–49
  sexual dysfunctions and, 202t
  side effects of, 134–135, 135b
  in suicide prevention, 46
Lithium chloride, 43
L-methylfolate, 40
Local genital disease, sexual dysfunctions
  and, 201t
Loss of chance, 228